Diary to my Daughter

daring to live purposefully with cystic fibrosis

by

Mave Salter

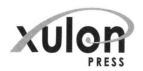

Table of Contents

Dedication

By the very nature of its title, this book is dedicated to my daughter, Claire – the love of my life, who died of Cystic Fibrosis, aged 36 years – and whom I love more than any other. At the same time however, this book is dedicated to all parents who have endured the soul-rending pain of losing a child. Thus you can transpose Claire's name with that of your own child, and know that she or he is just as precious. Each of our children is so very valuable and dear to God, so my prayer as you read this is you will see God's love for your child, just as I see His for mine.

Acknowledgements

I wish to thank my immediate family: Pat, Keith and Shirley for not only their love to Claire, but for standing by me in this great loss. Our thanks extend to all other family members and our friends who have shared this grief.

My gratitude to the three spiritual fathers who have written a foreword, as well as Claire's many other family members, friends and work colleagues who have supported her. You have all impacted her life in wonderful ways and your love and kindness in this life meant more to her than you can imagine.

I extend my heartfelt appreciation to both Claire's previous and current pastors, the Revs. Brian Edwards and Paul Pease, together with the members of Claire's church, Hook Evangelical. My special thanks to Debby Stevens for her endless expressions of support to Claire and myself, and to three older couples who prayed for Claire regularly over many years: David and Betty Simm, Ivan and Dorothy Wicker and Jim and Audrey Wilson. To my church, Chessington Evangelical, especially to previous pastors and their wives – Trevor and Val Archer, John and Pauline Tindall and Bobby and Julie Warrenburg – who through their faithful ministry helped me to trust God in the huge loss of Claire. Finally to Peter Hayden (Pastor of Discipleship) and his wife Gwyneth, my home group leaders Peter and Gita Crook, together with those from each church who have particularly cared for both Claire and me; you know who you are and only eternity will reveal how much you have meant to both of us.

Forewords

"I first met Claire in 1997. I will never forget her smile and the way she was so welcoming. Nor will I forget the way she looked at you when talking with you – her wide eyes, her open face, her leaning forward to listen to what you had to say, her genuine interest in you and pertinent questions to carry the conversation along. I was meant to have been Claire's pastor, but I can honestly say that I learned more from Claire than she did from me during the years I had the pleasure of knowing her. What did I learn from her? Perseverance under pressure. Commitment to her work. Faithfulness in friendships. Reliability in duty. How to suffer without making yourself the centrepiece. Love for the Lord Jesus. Concern for young people not to wreck their lives, but to develop them into something beautiful. Fun. Adventure. Style – lots of style. A love of life and a determination to use it well and for God's glory. As you read this *Diary to My Daughter,* you will see all these things bubbling to the surface again and again."

Paul Pease (Claire's Pastor)

"The first time I met Claire was over Sunday lunch, when she said grace for us from her high chair. We had no inkling then of the terrible battle she would later face with CF and the courage and selfless attitude she would show. When asked how she was,

Claire would immediately say, 'I'm fine' and turn the subject to you and yours. She was genuinely interested in others, even when struggling with her condition and in hospital.

"I had the privilege of visiting her in the hospital many times, the last time just days before she finally lost her battle with CF. When she said, 'It'll soon be over,' I held her hand and we prayed. I tried to lighten the situation by asking her what she thought the nurses would say if they saw this 'slightly older gentleman' holding her hand. In keeping with her wicked sense of humour she replied, 'I'll just tell them you're my bit of rough!' We laughed for ages, still laughing when her mother arrived.

This was Claire; refusing to give in to the incredible frustrations caused by her condition, and rarely letting down her guard completely other than to her close family. It was a joy to know her and witness her dignity, her deep faith and her love for her Lord Jesus. I look forward to spending more time with her in a better place where there are no more tears."

Dave McKee, member, Hook Evangelical Church

"Claire and her life were an inspiration to us all. We remember Claire's lovely smile, her non-complaining spirit, even though she had suffered with a debilitating condition, which she fought as a child and throughout her adult life. We know how she loved life in so many ways. She loved her dear family, her friends, and the church family at Hook, not forgetting her career in social services working with children. Whenever we visited Claire in the hospital, even in deep pain, her first question was always, 'How are you?' But her real love was for her Saviour Jesus Christ, whom she loved to talk about and the hope and trust she had in Him. We thank you, dear Father, for these wonderful promises in your word that gives us and has given Claire the assurance of eternal life, and where there is joy in your presence for evermore. Amen."

Steve Wigginton (Claire's group elder)

Prologue

Are parents permitted to write a love story for their child? If in the book (and subsequent film) *A River Runs Through It*[1] Reverend Maclean can say of his son that he was beautiful, I too can express my endless love for Claire in writing. Even in the face of losing a child, I believe we can find a place of shelter; as the psalmist says, "He shall cover you with His feathers and under his wings you shall take refuge," (Psalm 91:4).

If we can draw strength from our Creator, I trust we can even find growth in the face of our tremendous loss, for the death of a loved one changes everything. Rabbi Harold Kushner wrote (when recounting the effect his son's death had on him): "I am a more sensitive person, a more effective pastor, a more sympathetic counsellor because of Aaron's death than I would ever have been without it. And I would give up all of those gains in a second if I could have my son back. . .If I could choose. But I can't choose[2]." What he could choose, however, was what he was going to do with it; how he was going to make his son's death meaningful. As such, reflecting on Sheila Cassidy's words, I have written Claire's story, ". . .not in a spirit . . .of bitterness, but of love and hope." [3]

This diary is part biography, part autobiography (the latter drawing on Claire's journals written during her senior school and university years). Included also are

---

[1]   Norman Maclean, A River Runs Through It (University of Chicago Press, 1976; reprint, 2001)

[2]   Harold S. Kushner, When Bad Things Happen to Good People, (Penguin Random House 2002)

[3]   Sheila Cassidy, Audacity to Believe, (Darton, Longman and Todd, 1977)

letters written to her, email exchanges with a variety of people, as well as text messages and Facebook posts, depicting Claire's journey with cystic fibrosis (CF) and the different ways she impacted the lives of others. The book traces her life, including her career as a social worker, as well as charting the decline as her health worsened. Sadly, she never got a lung transplant.

By no means perfect, despite the looming death sentence of CF, I can truly say she lived life to the fullest, and ultimately loved God in the same way. In many respects Claire never finished her life; she left behind family, many, many friendships, a lovely new home, a job, a church and so much living to do. In other ways, though, Claire did complete her race, because I confidently believe God ordained her life and, even in death, she lives on in eternity. Had she not been, by God's grace, the lovely person she is, this book could never have been written; but I did not want her life to be an untold narrative.

So as William E. Sangster in his book *Let Me Commend*[4] extols his Saviour to his readers in the title of his work, please read any commendations of Claire as really honouring the God we serve.

In a sense, this book is a written as a memorial for children who have died or are missing from their families' lives in far more traumatic circumstances; whether that be through illness, suicide, accident, famine, adoption or as a result of war, trafficking or other atrocities. As the poet, Margaret Fishback Powers writes,[5] "My precious child, I never left you during your time of trial. Where you see only one set of footprints, it was then that I carried you." Whilst, in our grief, we stand in our own shoes, be comforted that we all stand in similar ones.

When J.G. Paton, missionary to the New Hebrides in the 1800s, buried his wife and baby son he wrote: "But for Jesus, and the fellowship He vouchsafed for me

---

[4]   W. E Sangster, Let Me Commend, Paperback (Wyvern Books, 1961)

[5]   Margaret Fishback Powers *Footprints : The True Story Behind the Poem That Inspired Millions* ©by Margaret Fishback Powers. The poem "Footprints" copyright © 1964 by Margaret Fishback Powers. Published by Harper Collins Publishers Ltd. All rights reserved.

there, I must have gone mad and died beside that lonely grave!"[6] Additionally I find so fitting what Beth Moore suggests in her study book, *The Patriarchs* (and Rabbi Kushner wrote because his son, Aaron, wanted people to remember him): "In the big scheme of things, we want someone to remember our name; God knows all our names; He knows us intimately. If we leave this earth, we want our name to continue. The bible contains the greatest story ever told and our life in Christ is meant to be a great story, becoming history-His story. Easy lives don't make great stories,[7]"

Claire, I like to think that your life was one that really counted. Oh, not in the way the spiritual giants of this world have made their mark, but in the day to day living out of your seemingly insignificant life. You never sought recognition (as Beth Moore again writes, "In the rebellion in Shinar, Genesis chapter 11 the people wanted to make a name for themselves, but God thwarted their plans because of their selfish intentions.[8]"). Humanly speaking you are the best thing that happened to me, and losing you is the worst. I pray you may be a blessing to all who read this.

---

[6] http://www.wholesomewords.org/missions/biopaton7.html (also see:) John G. Paton, D.D. Missionary to the New Hebrides, An Autobiography, edited by the Rev James Paton, B.A. (Elibron Classics © 2005, Adamant Media Corporation)

[7] Beth Moore, The Patriarchs: Encountering the God of Abraham, Isaac, and Jacob (Lifeway Christian Resources, 2005)

[8] Beth Moore, The Patriarchs: Encountering the God of Abraham, Isaac, and Jacob (Lifeway Christian Resources, 2005)

Chapter One

The Last Holiday

Dear Claire,

This diary to you is no literary genius. It is simply an honest account of your life, particularly those last months and weeks in this world and is often a rebuke to me in this regard, which I struggle with daily. This diary is, however, also an account of how life goes on, despite you – Claire, the love of my life – being now in your eternal, heavenly home, where I know I will one day join you.

"Tears in Heaven,"[9] written by Eric Clapton, is about the pain and loss he felt following the tragic death of his four-year-old son, Conor. The song was composed as a way of paying his respects to his son and telling everyone what he thought of him. I echo these words, Claire, because this diary is about demonstrating my admiration for you; telling all who read just how very much I think of you. I use the present tense because in the kingdom of your Saviour, you are more alive than ever.

In this way I hope to "record each treasured moment, capture every thought. . .make these hungry, empty pages come alive,"[10] Yet how will I find the

---

[9] Tears In Heaven, Written by Eric Clapton and Will Jennings, from the album Rush, Warner Bros. Records, January 1992

[10] Source unknown

words to tribute you as you fully deserve? What "language shall I borrow?"[11] You never liked to make a fuss of your health problems and that is why you would not discuss them openly, nor try to command an audience every time you were ill. But now you are gone I feel a deep need to tell people that, although you did not allow your illness to define you, it actually made you the person you were; caring, empathic, determined. As I begin my diary (which shows the fascinating and all too real life you lived) to give readers a little background into the time preceding your final hospital stay, I'll start with your thirty-fifth birthday in 2010. Incidentally, this was ten years after you wrote your chapter for *Horizons of Hope*. We had visited Gunwharf Quays in Portsmouth to buy you a dress for a wedding you were attending and we had lunch in one of your favourite restaurants, Giraffe. I'll never forget you crying that you hadn't achieved much in life, and I'll never forget thinking how very wrong you were! You had said that nothing in your life counted; that you were invisible to others. Truth be told, Claire, you were so visible, so valued.

You had a veggie burger with French fries, together with a smoothie, while I had a traditional beef burger, followed by that proverbial cup of coffee. We chatted happily about the holiday you and your friend Emma T. were planning to take to New Zealand and Australia, breaking the journey in Singapore. Looking back, the fact that you went on that trip was a miracle in itself, as you were still recovering from swine flu only a year prior. During your travels you were far from well, and at one point you thought you may need to return home early. You managed to keep going, however, and that was so typical of your strength and a real answer to prayer.

Of course, I was naturally very concerned that you were thousands of miles away and feeling so ill at times; but I knew you would never dream of coming home early if you were feeling okay. Emma was such a star to travel with you. You had said how vulnerable you felt so far from home, but you persevered. You

---

[11] O Sacred Head Now Wounded, composed by Hans L. Hassler 1601

certainly loved every minute. Of course, you had no idea this would prove to be your last long haul holiday.

I had written in your Christmas card for that year:

As I write this you have just left New Zealand; I so admire your courage and your, "Life is an Adventure – Dare It," philosophy. As I have said before, you have had a profound effect on my life with your courage and your down to earth attitude of just getting on with things, despite very often feeling really unwell and when most of us would take to our beds. Life may not have been the party I hoped for you, but I so admire your Christian approach: "While I am here, I might as well dance!" I know you have had more health problems the latter part of this year and I wish I could make things better for you. Time waits for no one; treasure every minute you have and be assured that many, many look at you and admire your sheer grit to do as much as you can while you can.

"He will cover you with His feathers, and under His wings you will find refuge," Psalm 91:4.

As I write now, in 2015, the inclusion of this verse was quite remarkable, Claire, because it was the verse that was to be God's encouragement throughout your hospital stay on that last admission.

On your return you shared your tales of adventure and we laughed together, trying to avoid until absolutely necessary the underlying topic at hand; it was evident a lung transplant was much needed and imminent. We discussed it eventually and both agreed you would have to upsize your home to provide enough room for your increasing medical equipment. I would also need a room in order to stay with you for an extended period of time.

Soon after Christmas in early 2011, you displayed my birthday presents so beautifully on your kitchen worktop, and even took a photo. Looking back now, Claire, I see these were so many touches of God's goodness. He knew in those moments that in years to come just how deeply I would treasure those presents and the little note you left that read: "Please read the poem entitled 'Your love' in the little present wrapped up for you." I did, Claire, and it read: *"Your Love. Mothers endure every illness, every grief, every anxiety suffered by their children-often powerless to help. Only able to wait, to love. Thank you, for that love is what I hold on to."* It came from the little book: *Thank You Mum for Everything,*[12] by Helen Exley.

In response I wrote:

Dear Claire,

I wanted to say a very big thank you for all the lovely cards and presents I received for Christmas and my 65th birthday from you. Words can't express your kindness and care of me in the many gifts so lovingly chosen. And, if all that isn't enough, the trip to look forward to on Mother's day on the Orient Express! The tea at Richmond Hotel was fantastic, as was our take-away. Claire, you put so much thought into what you do and give me that I am lost for words at all your love and care. Thank you so much. Only eternity will reveal what a very special and precious daughter you are to me. As I have said so often, you are my reason for living and I've had the time of my life being your Mum.

You seek so often to walk in another's shoes and attempt to understand what life is like for them and I am so very proud of you. You are such a caring, compassionate and sensitive person. So many people have commented on your sense of fun and humour, together with your inner strength and determination. When the going gets tough, as it does frequently, God

---

[12]   Thank You Mum For Everything, Helen Exley (Helen Exley Giftbooks, 2007)

is still there, worthy of trust. Please know that you have never, ever been a disappointment.

In closing, if I may just offer one word of advice: You slowed me down, Claire, and that was so necessary, for I fear you have learned your busyness from me and it is a lesson that pays a high premium-high in the sense of never having the time to sit and reflect. I hope you manage to do it in your new home.With all my love and prayers for 2011 and beyond, Mum.

Reader, little did I know then that the beyond was going to be heaven.

You would be hospitalised in February that year with your first bout of pancreatitis, a side effect of CF. It was a family birthday and people were coming to me; however, as happened so often through your life, when you became ill plans had to be cancelled. Instead we spent a gloomy twelve hours in the Accident & Emergency room at the hospital before you were transferred to a ward. It was one of many painful experiences, and hospital visits, but you endured and we still managed to smile.

True to past experience, illness is no respecter of person or plans and the following month on the day before we were due to go to New York, you had a further flare up of pancreatitis. We went to bed that night not knowing if you would make the trip. Being the strong woman you are, you wouldn't hear of cancelling, although the flights were a story in themselves. You seemed to love every minute of our travels, and I am so very pleased we went as it would become a very special last holiday Auntie Pat and I shared with you.

What a wonderful trip we had. We arrived around lunch time on Sunday and, not deterred from the long flight, you wanted to go straight to the Rockefeller Centre and up the observatory tower. After that, we had coffee in one of the department stores and then an evening meal before returning to crawl into bed at the famous Waldorf Hotel (chosen by you, of course, and so very special). Breakfast was had at the local Starbucks on the street until we discovered the hotel's own Starbucks. My daily duty then became getting our breakfasts and bringing them back to the room.

On the Monday it was a little dreary, so we decided to hit the shops. You bought a gorgeous necklace at Tiffany's, then we shopped at the illustrious New York Macy's and various other fine stores. By afternoon, we were ready to see *The Phantom of the Opera.* Quite the charmed lives we were leading.

On returning to the Waldorf, we ordered hot chocolates for a nightcap and laughed that it cost us twenty-eight dollars for the three of us to have a cup! Our tour of New York the next day was extra special. I had been twice before and you once, but I believe you had never gotten a grasp of the city before this visit. The tour took us down to the culturally rich Chelsea neighbourhood, and once we had fed our civilized sensibilities we decided to have an evening meal in Little Italy to feed the rest. The following day, we continued the tour and you so enjoyed visiting some of the places you had seen on TV, going into famous bars and various pubs. Our last day found us hitting the shops again and you bought a DKNY watch (now owned by Sophie H.G.), as well as a pair of shoes. Then it was time to ascend the Empire State Building just before visiting our final destination before flying home – Ground Zero. It was sombre and reflective, to say the least.

We arrived home late because the plane had to be de-iced prior to leaving, but nothing could dampen our spirits after such a joyous trip. On our return from New York, you continued to look at various houses, and in this time your breathlessness became increasingly apparent. I remember the sales person waiting empathically for you as you tried to catch up with us. You bought Plot 45 on the estate we looked at previously, because it not only had a south facing garden, but it had "The Green" outside the front door, giving a great feeling of space. Throughout the summer of 2011, I cherish the memories we spent so fondly, viewing the progress of your new home to be and looking around the show house. You spent hours meticulously choosing your colour schemes in preparation for the big move. It was you who came up with the brilliant think-outside-the-box idea of me downsizing and moving into your current home in Chessington. It was a genius thought, and we now had our plan!

Little did we know, during that Easter of 2011 when I had cleared the loft at my home, that a year later you'd have only a few weeks to live. Little did I know too, that when you were telling me I would need to learn how to blow-dry your hair and style it with your hair straighteners while I was thinking about lung transplant, you already knew that your days were numbered.

We reminisced over some toys and baby clothes I had kept, and you remarked they were very '70s! I laughed and agreed that, yes, you were born in that era, after all! I remember over the Easter period, amid the excitement and mirth of packing and getting ready to move you into your new home, you had been on seven Intravenous Antibiotics (IVABs) a day for three weeks and it proved exhausting for both of us.

So yes, it's true, you had some very hard knocks in your brief sojourn here, Claire (despite your middle-class lifestyle for which some would give their right arms). Yet throughout your physical and spiritual struggles, the Lord was ever faithful to keep you. Oh, to be sure, it became rocky. During some of these severe trials, I was not always conscious of you opening your Bible or praying, but who am I to judge? Especially when the very same has been a failure of mine so often, and yet you clearly surpassed me in holiness. As is want of us all as Christ's followers, we return to the God from whom we cannot escape, and retrace those tentative steps back to Him. As the scripture says: "After this many of his disciples turned back and no longer walked with him. So Jesus said to the Twelve, 'Do you want to go away as well?' Simon Peter answered him 'Lord, to whom shall we go, you have the words of Eternal life,'" John 6:66-68.

Having professed Christ, we cannot disown Him; in our brokenness He is all we have to which to cling. We are answerable to Him alone, and He draws us back. Often He uses our Christian friends, and often just the sheer knowledge that we cannot live life without Him, however much we may want to try.

I remember buying you a small devotional book at a particularly dark time in your life. I found it seemingly untouched in your bookcase when going through your precious belongings once you'd passed. I remember realizing that God had drawn you back without that devotional, Claire; my efforts to manipulate and control were not required. God was all you needed and in this I am reminded again that He watched over you and cared for you far more than I ever could have hoped to do. As we come sobbing, sorrowful, repentant back to Him, He promises to always wipe the slate clean. As the Psalmist says: "As far as the east is from the west, so far has He removed our sin from us," Psalm 103:12.

How do I know this personally? Oh, because I have had to do it, so very many times; vehemently telling God I didn't want Him in my life anymore; that it was about time you and I got a break. I would scream and shout in defiance and yet, as with all His wayward children, He gently cradled me in His arms, quietened my rebellious spirit and simply told me He loves me. I guess that to a lesser or greater degree we have all experienced this.

In the words of Sheila Cassidy, she too had

Run from the Hound of Heaven until she wearied but now was deeply happy and fulfilled. . . .Values which had loomed larger than life scuttled back into line like naughty children. There they stood, health, success, fame, achieve-ment, in a silent row, reduced to their proper place among all the other things on the face of the earth, to be used or discarded in the measure in which they assisted or impeded the pursuit of the will of God.[13]

---

[13]   Sheila Cassidy, Audacity to Believe (Darton, Longman, Todd, 1977)

Similarly as she expresses later in her book: "So I sat there and somehow stretched out my hand to the God who seemed so far away."

This is part of your legacy also, Claire, as it is true for each one of us as Christ's followers; the knowledge that we are helping others who will one day wake in the huge company of the redeemed. These are the great cloud of witnesses (Hebrews 12) when our testimony will join in unison with the Patriarchs of old, giving others the strength to fight the fight, to endure the faith, to finish the race.

The fact that you were in relationship with Him whilst on earth and, despite going through the proverbial valleys, continued to seek and honour Him is what brings your heavenly Father joy. Claire, you have loved so many others and have been Christ to them and, in your struggles and subsequent bravery, you have shown us what it means to truly be alive in God. As David Rhodes reflects regarding his writings in *Faith in Dark Places*: "This book is a book about failure and hope. People . . .physically so ill who can yet show us things of immense value; people who live close to death but who reveal to us what it means to be alive."[14] Indeed, Claire, no one could ever accuse you of being so concerned about dying that you never lived.

As said above, I am not saying, Claire, that you were always trusting of and always submissive to God's will, always doing the right thing. At times, you admittedly went your own way, did your own thing and inwardly questioned His plan for your life. Nevertheless, what mattered was that when God pursued you, you were ultimately willing to allow Him to bring you back. Yes, He does so for each one of us, in our questioning, our disobedience. As Rhodes continues: ". . .What sort of real and loving relationship forbids any expression of anger, frustration or pain? What sort of friendship is it where one person does not genuinely want to hear how the other person feels? If God cannot take occasional rage and frustration,

---

[14]   David Rhodes Faith in Dark Places, (Triangle, SPCK 1996)

then he is not the God of the Christ who questioned in his pain and dying: 'My God, why have you forsaken me?'"[15]

By the time May 2012 arrived, although you were weakening physically, you were strong in the Lord. You bravely and proudly represented Him with joy and hope, albeit tempered with the maturity of spiritual discernment. This is evidenced in an email you sent to your friend Paul before a prayer meeting on May 2:

Hi, Paul. Thanks so much to all for praying tonight, I'm so grateful to everyone. Please pray for the following: Tomorrow will be a month in the hospital with a week's break at home at the beginning. It's been a tough admission in many ways due to intensity and persistence of chest infection, pancreatitis over the weekend, and side effects to drugs have also had an impact on me physically and emotionally. Please pray I remain focused on returning to my health baseline and hopeful and strong in mind and body. There are a huge amount of chemicals going into my body, please pray my body remains strong and manages changes in chemicals. Dare we pray for a full recovery?

Please pray for Mum and Auntie for strength and comfort for them, pray for wisdom for the doctors and medics who have care of me, pray my fast heart rate settles, pray I remain strong and positive re: the future. Thanks, Paul, so much and thanks for being a wonderful and fun pastor and a substitute dad to me. I value you a lot. I'm so blessed to have a church like Hook. Please tell them that if you can that I love them a lot, too. Thank you, Paul, xxxx.

You were only three when Myra Bluebond-Langner wrote in her book, *The Private Worlds of Dying Children* (predominantly those with leukaemia and cystic

---

15   David Rhodes Faith in Dark Places, (Triangle, SPCK, 1996)

fibrosis), *"I will become an anthropologist, get a Ph.D from this study. These children will not become. There is never enough time. Life is a terminal illness for all of us. It is just that some know the end before others. I have failed unless this study contributes to the memory of these children, to those who cared for them and to children who still must suffer."*[16]

Thankfully, people with cystic fibrosis no longer die in childhood; indeed their lifespan can reach into their forties and beyond. Even so, like this author, Claire, I want to contribute to your memory; to those thirty-six years that were uniquely yours, but which you shared so lavishly with many of us. In this way they also became ours. Bruce B. Wilmer has written many poems, but my favourite was one printed on a scroll that I bought on our first trip to America, and that you would have seen in a prominent place in my home often, titled "To My Daughter." I do not have permission to print it within the pages of this diary, but it poignantly describes daughters being precious treasures and our days being complete because of you. Wilmer,[17] in writing these words of his own daughter, reflected what you mean to me.

Yet as I start to write, I am ever-mindful of the countless numbers who have lost loved ones, particularly children, who mourn as I do and yet learn to move on with their lives. May the following pages bring comfort and hope to them, too.

---

[16] Myra Bluebond-Langner, The Private Worlds of Dying Children (Princeton University Press; First Edition 1978)

[17] Bruce B. Wilmer, Feelings, 1987 Wilmer Graphics

Chapter Two

Your Early Years

Dear Claire,

When you were only eighteen months old, I began writing letters to you. In January 1977 I wrote:

My darling little Claire, the day you were born was the happiest day of my life. You came into the world a precious little 5 lb. bundle and I walked on air for months after. As you grew you were my pride and joy, so friendly and adaptable, very beautiful and everyone loved you (nothing has changed)! I'm sorry that sometimes, even as young as you are, I got cross with you, but you were a busy, active little girl and because I was ill, there just wasn't enough time in the day to get everything done. We had some great times together, particularly holidays and Christmas, but also just playing at home, in the garden in the summer, lots of walks in the winter. God provided a lovely house for us to move into, but then I became more unwell and had to go into the hospital. You wondered why Mummy had disappeared, but you used to come in and see me every day. You were cared for by the family and also Tracey and Jane's Mum, Pat W. [kind neighbours who lived a couple of doors away]. Then Mummy had to have a big operation and just in case I didn't come through it, I wrote you this letter to tell you how much I love you and what happiness you gave us all. My one prayer for you, above all others, is that you will come to love God and trust Him as your Saviour. With all my love.

On thirty July, 1975, shortly after midnight, you were born. Oh Claire, how your beautiful face lit up my heart. Due to your low birth rate the hospital classified you as "premature," but in my eyes you were absolutely perfect.

During my pregnancy I was, however, thoroughly convinced you were going to be a boy. You gave me so much anxiety! Instead, looking at your tiny, though perfect body in the Special Care Baby Unit, no one in the family would have exchanged you for a football team of boys! When I held you in my arms for the first time, there was a joy so indescribable it changed my life. I suppose only the universal language of music could make some sort of attempt at capturing my love for you and, as such, the first time I looked into your face I was reminded of the timeless song sung by Roberta Flack (written by Ewan MacColl), who certainly captured my (and I guess every lover's) sentiments: "The First Time Ever I Saw Your Face."[18]

You were dedicated to God on nineteen October of the same year; this simple act was to thank Him for your life and to commit you to His keeping. Little did I know how important that was going to be. Before I knew it, you were growing and growing and growing! I have some of the loveliest photos of your first year, particularly down by the river in Surbiton, as well as in Richmond Park. Despite a bout of pneumonia as a baby, you were always relatively happy and radiant, it seemed. I had no idea the implications of you having pneumonia at the time, and just thought it was a rare occurrence. Thankfully, those summers of 1975 and 1976

---

[18]   Roberta Flack, The First Time Ever I Saw Your Face, From the album First Take (Atlantic 2864, March 7, 1972, Written by Ewan MacColl)

were particularly hot and inviting, and you were healthy otherwise. As Chas E. Cowman's beautiful poem says,

> *The soft sweet summer was warm and glowing,*
> *bright were the blossoms on every bough.*
> *I trusted Him when the roses were blooming,*
> *I trust Him now.*[19]

I trusted God then, Claire, but as your life panned out, the question refused to remain buried: "Can I still trust Him?" When I was discharged from hospital after my surgery, Claire Malc's mum cared for us both and I will never forget that family's kindness. Claire would become one of your very best friends, and although you would also come to long for a brother or sister, it was sadly never to be. I was eager for you to have lots of friends, though, with whom you could play in your younger years and I think this was one of the reasons our house was often the place all of you congregated. In the summer months the garden swing and large paddling pool were attractions for the neighbourhood children, and this made me very happy.

I think back to how adorable you were; such a happy, vivacious child. One day, early in your life, I came face to face with a parent's worst fears. After moving house, you decided you would climb over the garden wall and, with your doll's pram in tow, you confidently made off down the road. Needless to say, many desperately anxious moments were had until I found you, thankfully safe and sound. This was yet more evidence of God's hand upon you, and that would come to be our ebb and flow, Claire, our loving dynamic; your fearless zest for life and my prayerful (fretful) reminders from our Heavenly Father to allow you to live life to the fullest.

When you were two and a half, you started Sunday school with your friends: Alison, Hannah, Jo, Nicola and Rachel. You absolutely loved it, though mainly

---

[19]   Chas E. Cowman, Bird In A Winter Storm (Cowman Publishing Company Inc., 1962)

because Auntie Pat and Auntie Peggy were Sunday school teachers. You also started in the church playgroup at the same time, but weren't so keen on my leaving you for that time. It was one of those heart-rending yet heart-warming moments, where I felt so very valued by my child, yet didn't want you to feel any sadness or fear. To my surprise and more mixed emotions, as soon as I left the hall you stopped crying!

You were always a very family-oriented child, and we were blessed to be surrounded by so many loving, caring family members. When I returned to work for just one morning a week, Uncle Keith would look after you (aided somewhat by his lady neighbour). Auntie Pat and Uncle Pete also took you out most Saturdays and you would excitedly visit playgrounds and farms with them.

As you know, we always celebrated birthdays and Christmases in style, and you so enjoyed the many toys you received from all the family. Of special note over your childhood years were countless dolls, a pram, a crib, a doll's house (made by our resident family carpenter, Uncle Keith), Home Pride cooking utensils and mixing bowls, as well as plenty of puzzles and books.

Grampsie also used to have you for an hour while I did the shopping, since you screamed inconsolably every time I put you in the supermarket trolley. (Of course, as soon as you hit your teen years, we could never get you and your friends out of the clothing and shoe shops!) When you were two, Grampsie made a scrapbook for you to mark the Queen's Silver Jubilee, so that you would have it as a keepsake when you were older. I found it when going through your boxes in the loft, and smiled to myself at how you managed to keep it safe and treasured through all those years.

I still have the sweetest article clipping, complete with a photograph from the *Surrey Comet* newspaper, dated seventh July 1979. You were only three years old, but performed like a star in front of five hundred people, along with your little group of ballet pupils! You and your dance mates wore the cutest nightwear, while the caption beneath the photo read: "Rehearsing for a matinee performance of 'Dances and Dreams' at the dancing show in Surbiton." That was your first public photo, and I'll never forget how proud all of us mums were of our little girls!

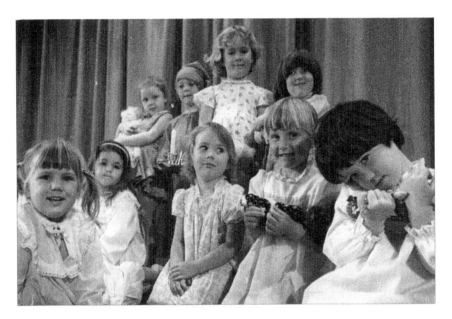

Performing 'Dances and Dreams' (Claire is second from right, front row)

I also have two other newspaper cuttings from your early years, showing you clearly in the picture at Surbiton Hill Nursery School's Harvest Festival and then Long Ditton County First School. Even now, I recognise familiar faces from the first friendships you formed, some of which lasted well into your adult years.

When you were about four, I bought you your first hat for a wedding. True to form in those days, you hated wearing anything that wasn't comfortable, and the following morning in church (much to the amusement of the congregation), you pulled the hat off and promptly threw it at me! You have always been your own person, Claire. As your childhood years progressed, you came to love Cindy and Barbie dolls like the authentic little girl you were. Much to your delight, I would often knit custom clothes for them. Jo R.'s mum passed the patterns on to me, so it was an easy way to see your beautiful eyes light up in that way I love so much.

Holidays were spent at the family caravan, where you loved playing on Highcliffe Beach in Dorset with new friends you met each summer. Those were such magical times, and you especially loved crabbing on Mudeford Quay and visiting relatives on the Isle of Wight, and in Somerset. You never wanted to leave but eventually we had to make our way home, and after the tears and pleading, before long you were happily playing with your friends on the estate where we lived. The residual joy of the holiday always carried you well into the following months.

It felt like mere days before you turned five and were ready to join your friends at primary school. Sadly, Claire Malc's family soon left to return to New Zealand. Another New Zealander family came in, however, and then a Danish family too, next door to them (who still remain friends). Mums and kids would walk down the steep hill to school all together, but it was not nearly such fun coming back up when you were all tired and hungry after your long school day. Sports days were always great fun and I am sure all parents have photos of doing the proverbial egg and spoon race after you had all completed your races.

During that year you became very unwell with pneumonia again and were admitted to hospital, the first time of many when you were administered intravenous antibiotics. I was concerned, of course, but still felt reasonably sure your condition was a rarity, and would soon be taken care of by the antibiotics. After several weeks you were diagnosed with Cystic Fibrosis. Despite my nursing background, I was admittedly terrified and confused. Words can't explain a mother's anguish on delivery of such news. All I could really do was cry and pray. I wasn't permitted to stay overnight, but spent all day, every day at the hospital with you. It would be the first of many such dark times.

At the time, I hadn't realized how traumatic the experience was for you. Years later, when going through your social work folder on "Group Sharing," I found an entry that broke my heart all over again. You had all been asked to recount, in an exercise together, your earliest, painful memories (I guess to mirror the experiences that children in your care may feel). You had said that you hated me leaving you in the hospital when you were ill. I realise this is why you wanted me to stay in those last, dark, fearful nights as you approached the end of your life.

Thankfully, I was permitted to stay with you when you were an in-patient at the hospital in London. You also wrote in your chapter for *Horizons of Hope* the importance of a doctor's bedside manner and of the great relationship you had with the paediatrician. We were indeed very fortunate to have Dr. S. care for you. Because your sinuses were also affected, you would come to have regular bi-lateral antrum washouts. These were so painful, yet you were extremely brave, as you have always been with the myriad of agonising or downright uncomfortable treatments and investigations you and all those with CF have had to endure. After that first hospital stay, and the delivery of that terrible news, I knew I would need to always be one step ahead, and ensure I had plans in place in case you had to go into the hospital on short notice. As Jodi Picoult suggests in *My Sister's Keeper*: "It takes only 30 seconds to realise that you will be cancelling all your plans."[20]

Reader, when we become parents – and dare I venture to say, especially mothers – the thought of losing our children, unless they have a life-threatening condition, is never further from our minds. We look at that gorgeous bundle of joy in the crib and although the thought of, "What if?" may cross our minds, we quickly banish such thinking and focus on the happiness we feel. But what happens when that longed-for child is seriously ill? When we can't banish the thought because reality looms over us, dark and sinister? Claire had pneumonia as a baby on numerous occasions, but her bad chest was thought to be familial, in that my father had bronchitis and asthma. It was assumed the same trait had simply shown

---

[20]   Reprinted with the permission of Atria Books, a Division of Simon and Schuster, Inc. MY SISTER'S KEEPER by Jodi Picoult. Copyright©2004 Jodi Picoult

up in her. I was to learn, however, that she had a far more serious chest condition and that moment was terrifying. Here's the thing: life goes on and many parents experience juggling illness in the family within the daily round of living. It's just something that simply must happen. Hand-in-hand with parenting are the many other tasks that need doing and, even though I often got bogged down along the way, one has to simply carry on.

Despite the difficult news we had received, Claire, I was determined to give you some cultural experiences, and going through photos, I found one of you at age six on the steps of St. Paul's Cathedral in London. The trouble is, for the life of me, I can't remember taking you there! You also had guitar lessons in St. Mary Infants' school and started piano lessons when you progressed to junior school. When you were eight, Uncle Keith moved to Dartmouth, which gave us a completely new holiday area to explore. It was a good job you had practice walking up the hill from school each day, because Dartmouth is really hilly and your uncle lived on one of the steepest climbs.

When I think back, my heart warms knowing we had so many good memories during your early childhood years. There were too many places to list where we had such wonderful times, but they included: the local library, walking through Oxshott Woods, tadpoling in Ewell Court Farm, visiting Claremont Lake and Gardens, playing around fishponds, black-berrying, feeding the ducks on the Thames River, spending time in Richmond Park, Home Park and Bushey Park. I remember, together with Sara and Jo, we'd catch the ferry across the short expanse of the River Thames and walk through to Hampton Court. Those were the days when entrance to the beautiful grounds was free! Looking back, although I miss you so dearly, I am comforted you had many rich experiences as a child. I know they meant so much to me, and I hope those magical trips and times were a great experience for you at that impressionable age.

It was especially entertaining to watch you become so fascinated with your schoolwork and hobbies. You went through a stage of stamp collecting as well as a project on "Flowers of the Bible," where you collected and pressed flowers, reeds and more. In my collection of your achievements there is also an assignment you did on Hampton Court from a junior school visit. Your teacher wrote regarding this project, "Good, neat work. I like the personal approach to this topic." All these were carefully preserved by you Claire, and now it is my great pleasure to continue to treasure them.

In 1983 at age eight you gained a distinction in your Bible Exam and that same year your school report read: "Creative writing is fluent and imaginative. All work is extremely well presented. Claire deserves praise for her progress this year; she has worked consistently and well. She is a happy and friendly girl; a really delightful member of the class."

I can almost hear you saying, as I write: "Oh, mother, every child gets a good school report at that age; stop showing off!" However, I had forgotten all about so much information regarding your teen and childhood years and now that I have waded through papers to find it, I want to remember it. Why should I not write about it, too? Like me, Claire, Meg Woodson recognised that when Peg died, she had not only lost an adult daughter, and mourned the passing of her at every age, but reprimanded herself that she could not remember every event of Peggie's life. I feel such an affinity with this mother and thank God for that seemingly casual event (although I know now that nothing is casual, but ordained by God) when I picked up her book as I dashed off to the hospital that fateful morning of the second of May 2012[21].

Your mind was expanding and your intellect developing tremendously. I was proud that your emotional life appeared to be developing equally well, despite

---

[21]   Meg Woodson, Turn It Into Glory, (Hodder and Stoughton, 1991)

some difficult life experiences you had to endure at such a young age. At age eight, you wrote the following regarding Grampsie's death:

My grandpa died on the 30th September, 1983. This is to remember him. When I was little we went to his house and he gave me lots of sweets, but I had to make them last all week. When I was little he said that if he lived until I was six that he would be happy for the rest of his life, and he lived until I was eight years old and two months. We used to go to Ewell Court Farm with him; while I was on the swings with my friends he sat and had a cup of coffee and chatted to my mum. When he was too frail to come with us, after school my mum used to take me and my friend, Laura, to the Care Home he was in and sit in the garden with him. He never let my mum take him back to his bedroom. He would only let Laura and me take him and we felt very grown up.

I felt for you, but you handled Grampsie's passing very well. I could tell the richness of the memories you retained while coming to terms with the fact that he was no longer part of this world. Time passed so quickly when you were young, and it seemed like your birthdays came and went so rapidly. Since your birthdays were in July, the weather was normally good enough to have your parties in the garden when you were small. They were simple affairs with the usual games of pass the parcel, musical chairs, etc., plus you always had a delicious cake either made by Auntie Pat or Auntie Anita. Being entirely social, you so loved sharing these occasions with your school and church friends.

I also remember the year you went to Tiffin Senior School. Anita made you a cake with the Tiffin school badge on it. Some feat that was! Your other childhood enjoyments were the November fifth bonfire parties at Brockham Village (it had one of the largest bonfires and firework displays in the vicinity at that time).

Afterward, we would all walk back to Elisabeth and Erik's home for a delicious supper. Another annual event was a circus where you would bring some of your friends, too. The more I think back, I am truly thankful for so many memories of such good times.

In 1985 at age nine, courtesy of the Les Evans Holiday Fund, you went to Florida in the United States with a group of kids who also had CF. I got talking to other parents as we waited at the hotel to have one-to-one conversations with the doctors travelling with you, and I learned that you were one of the healthier kids. It was quite a reality check for me to find out that for some of the children, this would be their very last holiday. There is truly a camaraderie in sharing the same illness, and I have never forgotten some of those children. You didn't keep in touch with the older ones, but with those of your age you firmly became pen pals.

Similarly, as your life progressed you loved making friends with fellow hospital patients, and in the ward's kitchen we parents would also gather to share stories. We were a great help to each other, too, even with simple things such as regarding where to park and to how to obtain a disabled badge. We also naturally compared notes on how you were all doing. I know you had the same empathy. There was a special strength in unity, but also a unique grief we shared as a group when one of the patients would pass. You loved that American holiday though, and it was your first time out of England (besides visits to Belgium to see your cousins). I believe that trip gave you your great zest for travelling that would feature so significantly in your later life.

You revelled in new experiences (daunting though they seemed at first), and true to form you retained all the keepsakes from your visit: the flags from Disney World, the scrapbook you made on your return (including the "Bon voyage" cards you received), the notebook you kept during that "holiday of a lifetime," and the special relationships with the children that accompanied you. In the scrapbook (among other things) you glued brochure cuttings of Florida itself and the theme parks, your Pan Am *Flying Fun Kit*, the St. Pete Beach Chamber of Commerce gift certificate, a Peppermint Patty's flyer, your hotel room card and the programme from "An Evening of Fun, Food and Fellowship for Great Young People visiting from the UK," organised by St. Petersburg Rotary Club. As I've said before, one of your defining traits has to be your indomitable desire to live life to the fullest. One major expression of this was your love of travel, and I'm so very happy you discovered this at such a young age.

In fact, as I think back, Claire, it is only fitting this book should begin with an excerpt from the chapter, "Life is an adventure–Dare It" that you wrote for *Horizons of Hope*[22] in 2000, when you were twenty-five years old. So the reader understands the context and significance of the book, the following is quoted from the book's back cover:

Dealing frankly with the subject of disability, *Horizons of Hope* chronicles the stories of a number of Christians who have lived through the reality of personal crisis, and have a testimony of faith to share. . . .The book is moving for both its honesty, and the fact that through their difficulties all concerned can see that there is a plan in their lives. *Horizons of Hope* is an unsentimental, candid admission that Christians struggle, and can even experience despair, despite their trust in God's sovereign plan.

You wrote it at the request of Brian, the book's editor, who was also the pastor of Hook Evangelical Church during your childhood. Brian wrote by way of your chapter's introduction:

Claire has recently completed a post-graduate Master's Degree in Social Work at the University of Reading. As a child she was diagnosed as having cystic fibrosis, a progressive and life-threatening lung disease. Claire is no stranger to emergencies and hospitals, but she remains active and

---

[22]   B.H Edwards, Horizons of hope (Day One Publications, 2000)

determined to put into life all that she can. Here, she allows us into her private world of fear, frustration, faith and hope[23].

I believe Brian had excellent insight into your passion for life as an adventure, as we'll read in the following excerpt you wrote:

Life is an Adventure – Dare It

Descending the steps to Eliot dining hall at the University of Kent, I was confronted by chatting of students, the clatter of crockery and the smell of food. It wasn't exactly cordon blue cookery, but it was my university and I loved it. Eliot halls are strategically situated so that the huge dining room windows provide a panorama over the city. This particular autumn evening offered a magnificent view down the hill where Canterbury Cathedral could be seen, lit up in all its splendour in the distance. Ali and I had never met before, but we happened to sit next to each other at dinner that evening and when she coughed, it sounded so familiar that it was rather eerie. We introduced, and she told me she was Alison Browne. We chatted about irrelevancies initially but I just couldn't get her cough out of my mind. I remember feeling quite rude when eventually I asked her if she had cystic fibrosis (CF). I just had a feeling that she did, but it would have been a terrible assumption if I was wrong. That was when our friendship began and I always admired Ali. I was touched with how brave and comfortable she was about her disease; cystic fibrosis was part of her and she was not ashamed of it.

Whenever we saw each other on campus we would check to see how we both were-there is companionship in sharing the same illness. We often bumped into each other in sick bay or in the medical centre, and Ali and I

---

[23]   B.H Edwards, Horizons of hope (Day One Publications, 2000)

were also treated by the same hospital. It was there that I saw her before she died-just before the end of her course. We hugged and said goodbye, little knowing that was the last time we would see each other. I found Ali's funeral extremely difficult personally, and cried very much. The church was absolutely packed and it has left a lasting impression on me. So let me tell you a little bit about the illness Ali and I shared.

All I can remember about my diagnosis was that the boy being tested before me was crying so much he was almost hysterical, although the test was quite harmless. Although I was put off by the little boy screaming, I also remember having lots of attention. Of course at the age of five I didn't know the seriousness of the issue, but to me it was brilliant because my family were so attentive to all my needs, especially my love of chocolate!

I had been ill on and off during my infant years and had pneumonia a couple of times as a baby (not that I remember any of this). Prior to the diagnosis being made, my Mum was certain that there was something wrong with me, but the doctors thought she was being over protective. She took me to the local hospital (Mum is a nurse) and I was then transferred to a London hospital that specialises in heart and lung conditions and was a regional centre for cystic fibrosis. However, at Epsom hospital, the paediatrician was a great support and someone who was to oversee my care locally throughout my childhood. I got to know the consultant very well and she always spent time explaining to me what was happening and why she was prescribing various treatments. She had a fantastic bedside manner, something I think is very important in any doctor, and I constantly badger friends who are training to be doctors just how crucial this is for patients.

There is an abnormality of salt transfer within the cells of people with CF, which results in the production of sticky mucous in the affected organs. The lungs are the main organs that are affected as the thick mucous is difficult to clear and is an ideal breeding ground for bacteria, leading to lung damage. Cystic fibrosis shows itself by lots of chest infections so antibiotic treatment plays a major part in trying to combat infection. Chest physio-therapy goes hand in hand with this and although the mode of delivery has changed over the years, it continues to play a major part in treatment of the disease. Altogether the physiotherapy takes about fifteen minutes, three times a day-well it's supposed to if done properly. I'm afraid physio is not one of my priority activities!

My younger years

My Mum was told she could either wrap me up in cotton wool or let me lead a normal life –she chose the latter; had she not, I would probably have chosen that route anyway. She was good in allowing me to do such things as sleeping under canvas, even though the damp conditions were not the best environment for me to be in. However, certain boundaries were set when I was a young teenager, that I was not so keen on, such as ensuring I was in by certain times so I wouldn't get overtired. The reason given was that there was physio and other health needs to attend to when I got home in the evening, but leaving church or other social events dead on time often made me resentful as I felt I had lost face with my friends.

When I was younger, I had a lot more energy than I have now! One of my first memories was that in primary school I could take time off if I felt unwell. Because the teachers knew I had cystic fibrosis, if I said I was ill they were very concerned about what would happen if they made me stay at school and I became seriously ill. I'm afraid that I used to play on that a bit, especially when I was keen to go home and watch television-which was much more preferable to lessons!

I have vivid memories of being in hospital when I was younger: memories of falling out of bed and giving myself a nose bleed, riding on the rocking horse in the children's play room, which I did constantly, and having my first intravenous antibiotics (IVABs). This was quite traumatic for me, especially as the doctor kept swearing because he couldn't find a vein to put the needle in. I remember thinking that because I had been in hospital for so long and was now on a 'drip' I was very ill, because when I used to see other children with drips I thought they were seriously ill. However, I also remember thinking it was quite funny because I didn't really feel too bad. I can't say that I ever wanted to be in hospital, but there were times when I enjoyed it because I made lots of friends. When I meet up with some of the other CF patients I got to know in hospital, it's interesting to compare ourselves with one another. We chat about the hospital staff who looked after us so well, and generally catch up on news.

But there were other things to be getting on with. Part of living a normal life for me was camping under canvas with the youth group at Hook Evangelical Church in Surbiton. It was at one of these camps that I became a Christian. Church activities had been a part of my life since I was a baby, and as I became older, I learned that God, in his love, had sent his Son to die for my sin and I needed to repent. It didn't matter whether my sins were great or small, none of us live up to God's standard and I needed to say sorry to God. By doing this and asking him to come and help me and share my life, I became a Christian.

Youth camp was an annual event and I have definitely benefited by such positive experiences of being able to do all the things my friends did. I even enjoyed camp food, except the dessert we called 'slop' that was served from a bucket! My auntie, who was one of the youth leaders, made sure I was OK. However, she did have an annoying habit of doing some of my physio in the breakfast queue. This involved 'clapping' my back in front of all my friends and I found that very embarrassing! I didn't want to be any different from the other children, but this was like advertising it to the world. My CF wasn't that much of an issue when I was a child, at least not to me. I just had all my treatment and went into hospital when unwell, had two weeks off school watching TV and I didn't think too much of it. I knew I had cystic fibrosis and that meant I had a bad cough most of the time, but I didn't grasp the impact and consequences of it until my teenage years.

When I was nine years old, I was given a great opportunity. I went to Florida by courtesy of a charity that sponsored 'holidays of a lifetime' for children with life-threatening diseases. It was a really fantastic experience. In Florida the main aim of the trip was to go to Disney World and Sea World; this was brilliant for a nine-year-old who had never dared to dream of such experiences. We went to other theme parks in Orlando and it really did prove to be a holiday of a life time. However, that was the first time I came into contact with a lot of other CF people and it was quite a shock to me, because at that stage I was very well compared with some of the others. This was the first time I remember feeling guilty about my better health compared with theirs. I shared a room with a little girl called Rachel and she seemed very ill to me. Lots of the children were thin, and when we had our physiotherapy they coughed up a lot of mucous, yet when I had physio I hardly coughed at all. Some were wheelchair bound because of their breathlessness. It was very sad to see them and I found it hard to understand how ill some of them were. It dawned on me that there were other people who had CF far worse than me. I wondered why I was so well and why they seemed so ill.

Despite all this, it was a wonderful holiday; I never thought I'd ever have the privilege of visiting America. Sadly Rachel died a couple of years after we returned from Florida and that was my first experience of death. I was upset, but at ten I didn't really grasp the full implications of someone dying from CF. I wondered why Rachel had died and not myself. I was upset that I had not had the opportunity to say goodbye and I felt sad for her family too. I was also aware that this had implications for my own life and death; however at that age I couldn't fully understand. I remember fooling myself into thinking that maybe she had died from a car crash and not CF and that made me feel better about it.

Ah Claire, your passion for living was so evident for everyone to see. After you died, I found a photo on your Facebook page from May 2011 with you and your book group girls, attending the reunion of Tiffin Girls' School. I asked your friend, Ndullee, where it originated from and she replied:"It was taken in the quad in the old Tiffin building at the Tiffin Old Girls' Association reunion. The other photo was taken afterwards in Browns, in Kingston where we went for dinner and cocktails, which is a bit of a tradition! Happy memories! Love, Ndullee, xx."

I didn't know half the things you did, because obviously you were an adult and had your own life, so finding these little gems has been so meaningful.

You also had so many friends, not only because you were social, but because you cared deeply for people. That included anyone, no matter their age or station in life. A special example of this was, with the lighter evenings in May, you were keen to continue to keep in touch with our neighbour you used to clean for when you were at school. Over the prior few summers we regularly met him for a meal and also to see the Harry Potter films that he loved so much. In 2011, his mobility had become very limited and he tended not to go out on winter evenings, but you so much wanted to meet with him. Dennis had been a part of our lives for so long and is still a great friend, despite the age difference. Then again, that is you all over; age did not matter when it came to the people with whom you kept in touch.

Your big heart was always so visible to everyone. That May, together with your close colleagues at work – Helen, Jo and Marianne – you organised a large cake sale at your office in aid of the Cystic Fibrosis Trust (of which you were on the fund-raising committee for the local group) and you were positively thrilled with the result. Sue C., who worked in the Early Years department, encouraged her colleagues to support the sale and the two of you had a lovely email exchange following:

Hello, my lovely. Well done, Chuck, on a successful cake sale. I hope all the hive of activity paid off for you in terms of cakes this morning. The Victoria sandwich cake that your colleague Jo S. made was simply delicious. Jo's given me the recipe and I'm going to try it out for Andrew this weekend for his birthday. It's lovely seeing you at work, always your bright and cheerful self. I do admire you; you are such an example to us all. I rallied the troops and Early Years were out in force today. Do let me know how much you raise. Definitely worth repeating again next year! Lots of love, Sue.

To which you responded:

Hi, Sue. Thank you so much to you and your team for such a great turnout today. We raised £175.00 and counting, so I'm over the moon. I had hoped for £50.00 at the beginning of the day. Please, would you thank your team so much? Especially Julie, very kind of her to donate her cake. I really value your support and the lovely things you said. I will, of course, let Mum know too what a trooper you are!

Your church friends – as well as Pat and Kelly – made cakes, but who would have known that a year later you would be in the hospital, never to leave? Similarly,

June of that same year found you enjoying Wimbledon tennis from seats on Centre Court. We had applied for tickets through the lottery, and how good God was to give you seats (and thus not to have to queue for hours, plus stand when you got into the grounds). That, of course, was the last time you enjoyed watching one of your favourite sports. As your health grew worse, and the business of your house move began to engulf us, I wrote you the following in a card for your birthday. I had no idea it would be your last.

Dear Claire, how quickly your birthday has come round this year. I do pray that all goes well for the rest of this significant year, both house and health wise. I know a little of how disappointed and concerned you are re: your increased health problems following your emergency admission to the hospital earlier this year, but despite it all our paths are set for us by God's hand. We may not have what the world or even other Christians have, but the happiest people have the ability to make the best out of a bad job (your "While I'm here, I might as well dance" philosophy), and you certainly have that, Claire, in your "Life is an Adventure – Dare It" approach.

Charles Schulz (1922-2000) said something along the lines that the people who make a difference in this sad world are not those with the most qualifications, the most money or the most accolades; they are simply the ones who care the most about others, and that is you. Your role, Claire – as with all of us who are the Lord's people – is to bring Him glory and you certainly do that. With my love and prayers for a happy birthday and the rest of 2011, Mum.

Following this birthday, your last on Earth which was full of anticipation for your pending move, you wrote a card that said:

Dear Mum, I just wanted to say a very, very big thank you for giving me such a lovely birthday last weekend. I love all of my presents, from my Links necklace (my favourite) to my kettle and toaster for my new kitchen. . . With lots of love, Claire. Xx.

You are such a grateful woman, Claire. I suppose that is one of the blessings in disguise people speak of when a child is critically ill. These phrases often sound so cliché, yet clichés are born out of enduring truths; your suffering may have made you extra-appreciative of even the little things in life.

In September you attended a charity ball at Epsom Race course with Jo, Leah, Kate and Zoe and wore a beautiful dress that, true to form, you had bought in a sale. In October you went to your friend and colleague Marianne's retirement evening. You and Jo R. had a few days in Tenerife prior to the move to set you up for all the hard work of packing up your previous home and moving into the new. You had more episodes of pancreatitis that month and ended up being ill in the Canary Islands on your short holiday with Jo. Things were beginning to career downhill. When you returned from that time away, you texted Auntie Pat after your hospital appointment: "Feeling rough, but going home on intravenous antibiotics again as they don't have a bed, otherwise I'd be in."

Sadly, the builders reneged on their plan to move you in for July/August, then pushed back even September/October, so we had to settle for November. I emailed a couple of my friends:

October 2011. Still no moving date yet, but hopefully beginning of November. Claire has been very unwell with both chest and pancreas and is back on IVABs at home yet again, as no beds to admit her. I realise even more these past few weeks that I need to simplify my life as Claire's health gets more complicated. She is very low at present and thus irritable (who wouldn't be?). She has said some quite significant things to me re: the future and what she feels about it: e.g. Resigning from her job (that's a real biggie as far as Claire is concerned); her health and how it is impacting on her life, the fact that she doesn't know how "normal health" feels. It doesn't get any easier the older I get, but I also count my blessings.

Then a couple of weeks' later:

Claire had hospital appointment today to see two different consultants. She needs to think about the future and the treatment they think will be necessary, and she became very emotional and tearful yesterday evening. One of the consultants talked more about the future than the immediate and I was disappointed they didn't do what their last letter said, but we will get the move over and then talk to them again.

Claire, to coin yet another cliché, we know hindsight is always twenty-twenty. As your health began to deteriorate, I'm not sure if it was my mind subconsciously trying to distract me from the impending reality, or if I believed I would be more useful busying myself with getting your moving arrangements in order.

Sadly, this would be the beginning of a pattern for me. Like the dad in the classic song below, I grew to wish I had spent more time *with* you, instead of spending time *for* you. I kept this in my work diary for years, always exchanging "Dad" for "Mum." I only brought it home Claire, (where it remains) when I retired, but I suppose that is a story for a future chapter.

Cat's in the Cradle

My child arrived just the other day

He came to the world in the usual way

But there were planes to catch and bills to pay

He learned to walk while I was away

And he was talkin' 'fore I knew it, and as he grew

He'd say, "'I'm gonna be like you, Dad

You know I'm gonna be like you."

And the cat's in the cradle and the silver spoon

Little boy blue and the man on the moon

"When you comin' home, Dad?"

"I don't know when, but we'll get together then, son.

You know we'll have a good time then."

My son turned ten just the other day

He said, "Thanks for the ball, Dad, come on let's play

Can you teach me to throw?" I said, "Not today,

I got a lot to do." he said, "That's okay."

And he walked away but his smile never dimmed

And said, "I'm gonna be like him, yeah.

You know I'm gonna be like him."

Well, he came home from college just the other day

So much like a man I just had to say

"Son, I'm proud of you, can you sit for a while?"

He shook his head and said with a smile,

"What I'd really like, Dad, is to borrow the car keys

See you later, can I have them please?"

I've long since retired, my son's moved away

I called him up just the other day

I said, "I'd like to see you, if you don't mind."

He said, "I'd love to, Dad, if I can find the time

You see my new job's a hassle and kids have the flu

But it's sure nice talking to you, Dad,

It's been sure nice talking to you."

And as I hung up the phone it occurred to me

He'd grown up just like me

My boy was just like me. . .[24]'

Chapter Three

Your Senior School Years – 1987 & 1988

C laire, I am intentionally beginning this chapter with a section from your *Life is an Adventure – Dare It* chapter in *Horizons of Hope*. As this chapter in *Diary to My Daughter* reveals, long before you ever wrote your chapter for *Horizons of Hope*, you embodied everything you would one day write about. You simply preached what you practiced, Claire. Even at the tender age of eleven, when you started senior education at Tiffin Girls' School. It took you a while to settle in to secondary school, as your early school reports show, but once you had put down roots, you appeared to love it (as your chapter in the above book gives testimony). Your journals would seem to say otherwise, of course. One thing you always did particularly enjoy was participating in poetry competitions and school plays. I will never forget your role in 'The Rebels of Old Bridge Street."

When I look back on your teen diaries it appears that you were, to a degree, Wednesday's child, full of woe. However, I am so glad to know you were, without a doubt, God's child and with your love of the TV series "Fame," on your promotion to Heaven, you did indeed "learn how to fly." If truth be told, Claire, I lived in denial by hoping, praying that a cure for this awful disease would be found soon. You never let much dampen your spirits, as Section Two of *Life is an adventure-dare it* attests:

Life is an Adventure – Dare It

My adolescent yearsAs I grew older I had more of an inkling that I was a bit different from others. Of course I knew I had CF but I don't think it really affected me at the time. Every year I would go into hospital and have intravenous treatment and try my best not to miss too much school but then, when you are ill, you're ill. However, I hated being away and missing out, and I was absent for only about two or three weeks a year. I enjoyed my time at secondary school, despite all the hard work and the pressure to do well. I met a lot of very caring friends with whom I still keep in touch. They continue to maintain an interest in me and I appreciate as well as value their love and support.

I tried to be as active as possible, though sometimes I felt I was losing the battle. I was never very good at sports, as my lung function didn't allow me to be. Even if it had, I don't think I'm a particularly "sporty" person. But I used to try and run the 1500 metres because I was the only person who volunteered! What a mug I was, as I was always lapped, but at least my classmates cheered me on and thanked me! All the teachers knew that I had CF and looked out for me. It was that sort of school and I did appreciate it. I may not have done brilliantly academically but the ethos of the school was great.

I was involved in school plays and I enjoyed English, particularly poetry. I wrote an article for a Christian magazine about living with CF. My Mum had written the previous article and I wrote the second one. I really enjoyed this and for a while after that I wanted to be a journalist! I felt I was giving back to society in a way by letting people know about CF. The article also helped me to be able to talk about my illness, which I had not done so publicly until then. Along with another pupil in the school, who also had

CF, we spoke about it in a school assembly to promote CF week. I hated standing up in front of the whole school but at least I was known after that.

Cystic fibrosis is the most common genetically inherited disease in Britain, and I had friends at both school and university suffering from it. Approximately one person in twenty-five carries the defective gene for CF. Carriers are completely healthy and can be tested to see if they carry the gene. If both parents are carriers, there is a one in four chance that a child will be born with the disease, a one in two chance that a child will be a carrier and just a one in four chance of being completely clear.

During my secondary school years I started helping with the seven to elevens in the church youth group. I loved this work and tried as much as possible to take an interest in looking out for others and I do try and empathise with people. For the past few years I have worked with older teenagers and find this a great privilege as well as challenging at times. I was also a prefect in my sixth form and enjoyed the social side of things at school. During the sixth form in my spare time I worked for an older neighbour. He needed his cleaning done so I was earning some money and that made me feel quite independent. My Mum used to get infuriated with me at what she called "burning the candle at both ends." I guess I am a firm believer in living life to the full, even though I do get so tired. I knew I had cystic fibrosis, but that was that; everyone knew so I didn't have to tell anyone. It was accepted and no explanation was needed. I felt very safe and secure.

1986 Form 1B

For someone who did not like Math at senior school level, you came second, with 90% in your last year of junior school. I sincerely believe that when you went to Tiffin, you were so overwhelmed by it all that your confidence just took a dive. Within a couple of weeks or so of your arrival at Tiffin, everyone in class had to write a project, the title of which would be "All About Me." I chuckled to myself when I found your project among your souvenirs. One of the first things that became clear in this project was your forthright and vocal disapproval of your new school at first, categorizing it as one of your *dislikes!*

Interestingly, Claire, even then you wrote a poem that included the line, "I hate sad goodbyes." This sentiment would last throughout your life and I have commented elsewhere that you were well aware your years were numbered. In your list of likes, you fondly made mention of your friends from junior school and I remember your years there with happiness, as I do all the friendships you made throughout your life.

In this project you also listed church friends, in addition to those you had already made at Tiffin. You had to include topics such as: vital statistics, how you spent your time, your favourite food, likes and dislikes, family tree, an ideal day (including ideal clothes), a poem about pets and, lastly, a survey. I was most impressed that you put one of your hobbies as playing the piano!

Concerning your rabbits you wrote:

> I have two albino rabbits,
> They are both nearly two.
> They are very lovely
> But also very mucky!

> Fluffy is a female and Snowflake male.
> Fluffy has had three lots of babies (by mistake!)
> I clean them out once a week without fail.
> I line their cages with straw and feed them carrots and cabbage,
> always ensuring they have enough water in their bottle to drink.

My uncle made a run for them and we try to let them use it as often as we can. It is well protected from foxes.

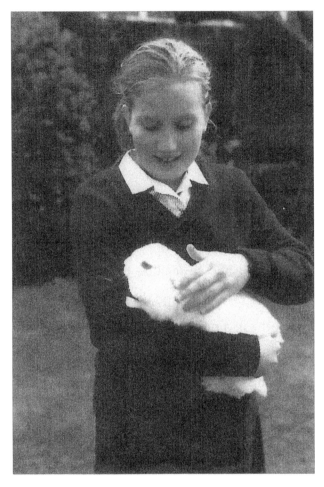

With 'Fluffy', Claire's rabbit

You also list your top ten favourite songs and also included a family tree. Of yourself you wrote:

My name is Claire

I am very fair

I have blonde hair.

I like to play

The piano everyday

I try not to let it slip away

I have blue eyes

And hate sad goodbyes

I have dreadful sighs

I like to say

that everything is ok

except on school days!

And of your friends you wrote:

They're the ones

Who I really trust

They keep all my

Secrets safe as houses

They're the ones

Who I really like

For they stop me crying

When I feel like sighing

They're the ones

Who I can call my own

They always ring me

On the phone.'

For each letter of your Christian name you wrote something of what defined you:

C=Clever *[on reading this, it made me smile, Claire, that you, who were the epitome of modesty, should say this of yourself!]*

L=Loveable

A=Ambitious

I= Interesting

R=Reasonable

E=Exciting

Your teacher commented that the following poem was cleverly written: "I Hate That Subject"

Steps are always included in it

Poems and rhymes are always a part of it

Many people have to take part in it

Dance

I hate that subject

Moving is a strong part of it

Hitting is the hurtful part of it

Balls are a special part of it

Hockey

I hate that subject

Decimals and fractions take part in it

Adding and subtraction are all of it

Multiplying and dividing are in it

Maths

I hate that subject

"I Like That Subject"

Liquids are always part of it

Bunsen and Tripods take part in it

Skeletons and Fossils are part of it

Science

I like that subject

Saxon invaders are part of it

Tudors and Stewarts lived in it

We will be part of it

History

I like that subject

I did happen to notice you did not comment on another disliked subject – Latin. Latin was part of the school curriculum for the first two years; you did not find it easy and I had never studied it, so could not help you when you struggled. I suppose this would be in the category of some of the more difficult memories.

Each pupil had two annual reports; in January and July each year. Your first term report at Tiffin showed the only "C" grade you received was in Math. Apart from that your marks were virtually average – sometimes a little under, but also sometimes above. The tutor comment from Mr. C. read: "Claire did not find it easy to settle in to Tiffin at first, but she seems happier now and I am sure that her work will continue to benefit from this next term." Lacking confidence in your own ability did not mean that your marks were low; it just meant that your tutor felt that increased self-confidence would lead to improved results. Indeed, many others in the first year had plenty of friends from their junior school who also went to Tiffin, while you, having attended an out of Borough school, knew no one.

In Art, Mrs. L wrote: "Claire puts a great deal of effort into her work. She draws well and has some interesting ideas." In Music, your exam result was spot on the average again and Mrs. T commented: "Claire has made good progress this year. I hope she retains her motivation and determination in order to continue improving her standard."

In Science, your exam result was below average for the class, but this improved in your second year, as you settled more into school and felt happier. Even in Physical Education, that was not easy with your breathlessness, your report read: "Claire has worked hard, made a good start to both Athletics and Tennis and achieved promising results in sprinting events."

You write so passionately in your teen diaries, Claire, that you needed to concentrate more at school and work harder. However, as your school reports show, not only were you industrious but you were popular among teachers and pupils alike and gave your all to your studies, despite struggling with some subjects. Of note, your teachers reference your hospitalisations and ill health, which meant you fell behind at times, but this was no fault of your own and they said you always made up your work.

As you well knew, life was not all about working hard; hence you played hard too, to which your diaries bear testimony. One summer for your birthday we went to Thorpe Park with a few of your senior school friends (in fact, as many as we could comfortably and legally get in the car!). You absolutely loved it, Claire, and so did your friends. It makes a parent so full of joy to see her child happy. For another birthday you all went ice-skating when the rink was still open at Richmond, and just about every weekend saw you hanging out with both church and school friends.

1987

In 1987, you and Beth paired up to write an anthology of poems on feelings, composed for an English Literature project. Looking at your poetry, Claire, knowing how deeply your poems reflected your beautiful soul, I find myself holding the pages to my heart. I want to touch and handle everything that you touched, created, and of which you were a part. Yet I know this is only until we are reunited in heaven.

One poem read:

Feelings of hope

Feelings of scorn

Feelings of joy

Of the right to be born

Feelings of fear

Deep down inside

it's so unfair

Why me every time?

Feelings of peace

Less of the pity

Inside you feel warmth

A new day has dawned.

Love, emotion

Full of devotion

But then crying, sadness

No one who cares

Pain and suffering

Little discussing

Depression, sighing

Fed up of trying

Laughing, singing

Till all ears are ringing

Day after day

A new me I display.

Your end of year report for 1987 read: "Claire has found a place for herself within the form now and this has seemingly enabled her to feel happier, which in turn has led to an improvement in her academic standard. I hope that things will continue to get easier next year."

Mr. N. also wrote that you seemed to have settled into the school and the class and were producing better work. In French, the year average was 84% and you had improved to 82% in your exam. Mrs. H. wrote: "Claire has made every effort to improve her French and thoroughly deserves her pleasing examination result."

In Classical Civilisation, the average was 75% and you achieved 77% in the exam. In History, you were spot on the average and your tutor wrote that you treat your work seriously and had tried very hard to raise your standard.

You had significantly more absences in your second year, due to three hospital admissions. In the autumn term of 1987, Mr. C. wrote: "Claire is working hard in a subject which she finds difficult and is to be commended for this. She still adopts rather a low profile within the form and I am sure that her progress will improve further with greater self-confidence."

At the age of twelve, you were kindly invited to Switzerland to spend a week with Margaret (a friend with whom I went to senior school), her husband Balz, and their daughter, Sara. I found this precious note that said: "Things to ask Mum when she phones on Monday night: How are the family and everyone at church? How's the extension to the house?" You also wrote this lovely postcard to your family: "I am having a nice time and the weather is good. Went on bikes this morning and took photos. We are going into town tomorrow to have a meal out. We shall go near the river. See you on Sunday. Love from Claire."

You also kept a sweet little notebook of your holiday there, with the Swiss flag and picture of the Alps entitled: "Visit to Switzerland 17th-26th July, 1987 by Claire Salter." You wrote regarding family life (visiting Sara's grandparents,) cycle rides, and playing board games as well as cultural visits and general outings. You especially loved the Alps (including the Alpine flowers) and your visit to Oberdorf and the lakes. You took plenty of stunning photos whilst site-seeing, which I am thankful for as it makes me think of how happy you were during that trip. You were so blessed to experience several different holidays, but I remember you spoke about this particular one often.

1988

By the time 1988 arrived, you had settled in and although you still had moments of struggle, I was glad to see you becoming far more focused and confident. Your July school report read: "Claire is still reticent in form time, but takes her work very seriously, indeed. She is conscientious and reliable and always polite."

The general consensus was that you were working competently, to a good standard, and making progress.

In History, Mrs. B. said your research topic was thoroughly prepared. Equally, in Geography your exam result was above average and Mrs. F. said: "Claire works hard and with interest. I am pleased with the progress she has made this year."

In Religious Studies, your exam mark was again above average and your tutor wrote: "Claire has worked well throughout the year and produced a very pleasing examination result."

Even in Maths, Mrs. A. wrote: "Claire's efforts during the year have been most pleasing and she has made progress. The algebraic content of the course causes her problems and it is this area to which she needs to give special attention."

In Music, you were well above average and your tutor commented that you had made excellent progress, particularly in composition and performance (so your piano lessons out of school were paying off!).

Chapter Four

Your Senior School Years – 1989's Journals

From your diaries, I found this was the first year you began writing a daily journal; you were thirteen (and a half) and in your third year at secondary school. I have only selected parts of them; not that I do not want to disclose all of your entries, but rather I would not want to disrespect your privacy entirely. For interest's sake however, it was very important for me to include these excerpts so the reader may gain an idea of the authenticity of your love and charm, while also seeing very real struggles and immense durability. As such, here are your diaries from 1989:

January 1989

Sunday, January 1, 1989: Our youth group church House Party has ended; going home is quite sad and most people want to stay.

Wednesday, January 4, 1989: Back to school and Drama rehearsals for the school play are going to be quite frequent. Had chats to my friends about all our problems, i.e. boys!

Monday, January 9, 1989: After school I had an appointment at the hospital. I got off the bus and Mum was waiting in the car. We made it just in time to see the consultant (my mum hates being late and I hold my breath sometimes as we dash through the traffic.)

Tuesday, January 10, 1989: Our Religious Studies teacher told us today she was a Christian; interesting. Drama rehearsals are not only at lunchtime, but also after school (Mum comes to collect me sometimes; otherwise I am so late home if the buses are full).

Wednesday, January 11, 1989: We have to choose our GCSE options by 27/2, but I feel it is too early to decide what subjects I want to take; that's obviously necessary when deciding on a career. Along with this, all the decisions to make about boys and who to go out with are too much for me. I'm worn out already by Drama rehearsals and they've only just started! We couldn't play hockey because the field was flooded. Mum came to collect me from Drama, but I was nearly an hour late (Miss F. kept us until we learned the dance steps perfectly), and she was mad, shouting at me, as she had to be out again by 7:00pm. However, when she came home she apologised to me for her behaviour, and so she should!

Thursday, January 12, 1989: My cauliflower cheese in Home Economics turned out quite well, but then, what can go wrong with such a simple dish! Got off bus in Surbiton to look at shoes, but they didn't have my size so I went into McDonalds, but was a penny short – how embarrassing!

Saturday, January 14, 1989: Had a lay in and just messed about in my room until 12:00, but Mum was very cross as we were meant to go to the Kings

Road in London to buy new jeans for me. Still not dressed by 1:30, so I was told off again and Mum not happy in car as we were running so late.

Tuesday, January 17, 1989: Catherine did a brilliant drawing of a rabbit today. At lunchtime I went to get some tickets for the School Drama Production; six altogether, two for each night for family to come. I looked at the programme and it had everyone's name on it apart from mine! I felt so awful I almost cried. I told Ms. F. and she apologised, saying she would have my name put up on a projector at the end of each evening. When I told Mum about my name being left off, she was furious; I should think so, too!

Wednesday, January 18, 1989: Apparently other people had had their name missed off the programme, so it wasn't just me. We had to sign a list of all those who weren't included. I came out of Drama early as I had a hospital appointment. My mum was 15 minutes late and I shouted at her, but got my head bitten off because the traffic was so bad. We were late getting to the hospital, but the consultant's clinic was running late, so no panic.

Thursday, January 19, 1989: It was hockey today and I could have got out of it because of the chest infection the consultant said I had yesterday, but I wanted to play, although it was freezing. I even scored! I was so cold when we came in that Kate rubbed my chest really hard in an attempt to get me warm. In the school play there is going to be a slide up and a piece of paper on each seat with the names not in the programme.

Friday, January 20, 1989: Kate was upset today because she had had a row with her mum. I tried to comfort her after her good turn to me yesterday. My tapes that I'd taken in didn't get played.

Sunday, January 22, 1989: At Bible class today I had a really bad cough and Maria, one of our leaders, prayed for me. I was very touched because this chest infection is taking its toll on me. We had people back from church for lunch; roast dinner as usual. Mum thinks I'm going vegetarian and she could be right!

Monday, January 23, 1989: I was thinking what stupid things I do and say at times. Sometimes I hate myself so much. This is what Mondays do to me generally; low self-esteem takes an even deeper dive.

Wednesday, January 25, 1989: A month since Christmas; lots of people are asking me to do things, but I have no time! I have all my homework to catch up on, acting in the school play and I feel I need at least a week off school to recuperate from this chest infection. I never seem to be happy anymore, though I know with just a month to choose our options has a big impact on how I feel. "Why do I bother?" as my Mum would say, and my rhetorical response: "I won't bother." Mum was in a bad mood and I had to creep around her to get a lift to Craftsmen at church.

Saturday, January 28, 1989: Had a lie in today and then Mum took me to get the video, then to Alice's to meet Zoe. We arrived at Richmond station 20 minutes late and walked to Kate's from there. Then back to mine, to meet up with Catherine, Rebecca, Beth and Emma for yet another video. Zoe joined us afterwards.

Sunday, January 29, 1989: Our pastor spoke on the subject of illness and suffering and I felt God was speaking directly to me. Mum is determined that we don't spend many more holidays at the caravan and she is definitely going to pep things up for me, so Auntie Pat and I are going to join her in America in July (after she goes out on a Nursing scholarship). New clothes for me are a must!

Monday, January 30, 1989: We had a good laugh on the bus this morning and once at school rehearsed the whole play from 9-5pm. As "The Rebels of Old Bridge Street" is set earlier this century, my costume is one of my Mum's dresses, cut down to size. Well, that must be a first! By the end of the day everyone was tired and we hadn't rehearsed to the best of our abilities. Roll on our first formal performance this evening. (Mum is coming this evening and Auntie Pat tomorrow.) S. told me he liked me.

Tuesday, January 31, 1989: Thalia and I were the only ones in our form that made it to school by 8:30. Everyone else came at 9:00. Feedback from Ms. F. today re: the school play was that we were: B*** brilliant and b*** marvellous. Boy, that made us feel as if we were walking on air! However, I feel my academic school work is slacking and I must try harder. I know I'm not as brilliant as some of my peers, but come on, Claire, you can do better. Is it just that self-fulfilling prophecy, bound to fail? Another hospital appointment today to see if my lung function has improved, so Mum came to collect me from school and we drove directly there. I had to almost shout at Mum to get me home so I could do homework. Mum gave me a lift back to school this evening for another performance of the play and it went well. Ms. F. gave us all a carnation.

February 1989

Wednesday, February 1, 1989: School again today for the Award Ceremony and a feast following all our hard work in the production. I was the only living thing wearing a skirt. No, that's not entirely true; there were a couple of others.

Tuesday, February 7, 1989: Bang goes my diet. It's lunch time and I nearly fainted. Mental note to self: Must eat something mid-day. Breakfast at 7:00 and dinner at 6:00 is not enough to support a growing gal! What with Maths and French tests too, it's all so unfair. I am so appreciative of supportive friends. Where would we all be without each other? My mum often says she is sad I'm an only child.

Sunday, February 12, 1989: it was Catherine F.'s last day at Tiffin today and we bought her loads of presents. It's sad to see one of our peers leave when we are such a close bunch. Okay, we fall out with each other at times, but on the whole "support" is our key word.

Wednesday, February 15, 1989: Hooray, half-term and we went ice-skating. Mum gave us a lift in and we caught the bus back. This week has been taken up with both hospital and dental appointments, doing all the homework we were set, practising for my piano exam and when time, seeing friends/watching videos.

Monday, February 20, 1989: Back to school and up again at an unearthly hour. This is the problem of catching two buses to school. I wrote another poem for English on "Feelings." Yep, just about right, I have so many mixed up feelings. Not great marks for Biology and Chemistry, but this is what life is all about – a challenge!

Wednesday, February 22, 1989: I felt bad today. Why can't I be pretty and witty all the time? And would you believe it, another chemistry test tomorrow; why don't they give us more notice? I'm going to be on the video today, doing "Bread" in our English lesson. Not sure what it entails, but we are using two ideas, one of which is mine, so am looking forward to it.

Thursday, February 23, 1989: Parents' evening tonight went well. It seems that most of the teachers are quite pleased with me (not of course, I dare say, as those that are far more academic than me, but it has chuffed me anyway). Miss S. Said, "I love teaching Claire," and Mr. G. said "Claire, yes a very clever girl – she'll do very well in Information Technology." (I'm the only Claire in the form, but were they really talking about me?!)

Friday, February 24, 1989: I'm not entirely sure what options I'm going to take; ah well, *c'est la vie.* I talked to Mr. H. today about it; he said to meditate or pray before I go to bed, like he does.

Saturday, February 25, 1989: I had a bit of a lie in today, but only a bit. . .Mum made sure of that. I needed to do my homework before meeting Hannah in Surbiton, where I bought Zoe's present. I get so mixed up when blokes say they like me; what do I do about it all, and why do the blokes I like not like me?

Monday, February 27, 1989: I gave my option choices in: I'm going to do Biology, Information Technology, Geography, History and Drama (I don't need to take Religious Studies at GCSE level just because I want to do it at A level, so that's good). Of course the non-optional subjects are Maths, English Language, English Literature and French. So that's my nine.

Tuesday, February 28, 1989: Although I woke up in a good mood, the day gradually went downhill. I feel so confused about so many things but don't want to discuss them with anyone.

March 1989

Wednesday, March 1, 1989: A great start to a new month – I was late for school because I felt so ill. I feel I am lapsing in my school work and I don't know why; maybe I am just not applying myself, but I do know feeling so unwell often doesn't help my concentration levels. Dr. S. at my last hospital appointment said to take time off when I am ill, but if I do that, I will fall further behind. In English, we watched the video of our work and it was interesting.

Friday, March 3, 1989: I felt so ill this morning and caught the bus late. Mum didn't overly sympathise with me and I slammed the door. Coming home I had to walk up the hill with my heavy bags and I thought I was going to collapse; why is life so hard?

Sunday, March 5, 1989: It was great to relax with school friends today; there were 8 of us altogether. This evening it was youth club at the church, with Alison, Hannah, Jo, Rachel and the boys. I'll swear I'll be grey before I'm 30 because I worry so much. I'm just like Mum – I make work for myself. I don't check things enough and then I have to catch up later with it all. I guess as teens we all feel like this from time to time. Maybe it's because I'm an only child; I don't talk about it enough to others. I really don't know what the answer is.

Tuesday, March 7, 1989: It was Comic Relief Day today when the wealthy and illustrious wear objects on their noses to raise money for those not so well off. Our school was raising money, too. Drama was good, and joy of joys, I found my hockey stick! We played other forms in our year and although we didn't win, we did well and it was fun.

Saturday, March 11, 1989: Had a sleepover with school friends at my house last night. I was really tired but went to collect for Cystic Fibrosis with my Auntie Pat outside the local shops. People were so generous and we raised £65.00 in one and half hours! My friends came to see me and also donated. It was S.'s birthday today and I thought people could have made more of an effort for her, so it was a good job some of us did.

Thursday, March 16, 1989: Miss E. was quite nasty today, but I stood up for myself and showed initiative. The name Salter is probably dirt in the staff room, but so be it. I haven't even packed for Belgium yet and Samantha asked me to the cinema this evening, but I said no. I told Mum about it and she agreed it wouldn't be worth it either, as time was at a premium. There was no hockey at lunch time today and we stayed in at recess because it was raining. When I saw Miss E. later she was quite nice. So, my taking the initiative was good; I must stand out more and be ultra-confident. Two of our teachers left today and it was sad to see them go. It felt as if we were losing a big asset to the school. We were all absolutely worn out this term and most of my friends are going away. K. is going to Florida, A. is going to Switzerland and two or three of them are going to Scotland. C. is going to France, and me to Belgium so we can compare notes on our return. It was raining still when we left school and we had to walk down the Richmond Road because the buses were full. My hair was drenched and it seemed like I saw every single boy I knew.

Friday, March 17, 1989: The end of term and we are all heaving a sigh of relief. It has been such a busy time and I have felt so ill most of it. I hate the winter as I have more colds and chest infections. I have started having intra-venous antibiotics at home and it is hard work and so time consuming what with hospital appointments, physio and everything else. Going to Belgium to stay with my Belgian family means I will really miss my school and church friends. My piano lesson didn't go well today, but I know I don't practice enough. Huh, what time do I have to practice?

Saturday, March 18, 1989: I got up quite early this morning, as the light woke me. I made some flap jacks before going to Auntie's. Everyone was popping in to see her new bungalow. Uncle Keith said he would take me to Wimbledon tennis in the summer. I will really look forward to that. I cycled home really quickly as I had to leave to meet Beth. However, Mum had a phone call to say Beth was ill, so that put paid to that. We decided to go and see Mum's cousin, who was very ill with cancer and in hospital. I was a bit upset before we actually saw her, but after we said hello, she asked "Why?" How can one word be so powerful and yet so sad? I think it just summed up everything. That one word just hit me so hard. Yes, you see it on television but to experience it in real life is something else. Edna started to cry and so did I. The mystical essence of a human life.

Sunday, March 19, 1989: In Bible class today we acted out 4 play-lets from the gospels. I was nearly in tears as everyone apart from me is going to the Fellowship of Independent Evangelical Churches' (FIEC) conference. After class, we swarmed around the honey as usual; it seems we are drawn to them. Hannah was so sweet as she didn't seem to mind that Jo was coming with me to Dartmouth in the summer after we get back from America. It will be her turn the next year.

Monday, March 20, 1989: March is soon over, then we will be in April, June and July. Yippee, off to the States! I hope I fit everything in. I went into Kingston with Hannah today and bought this bronze nail varnish. Not quite the colour I expected when I put it on. I then had a hospital appointment this afternoon. Hooray, the consultant says my chest is clear. This evening I realised that it was all systems go from now on. Help, I need somebody!

Tuesday, March 21, 1989: Today was a complete disaster; everything went totally wrong. I, or rather my mother, sorted out my wardrobe. Then we went shopping in Kingston for clothes to take to Belgium, but there was nothing that I liked so that was a waste of time. We stopped for lunch and then shopped again. Still nothing I liked. Mum got cross. "Surely," she said, "out of all these shops there is something." She then said she was going home and I could come in the car or get the bus, but I bumped in to Kate H. so I decided to stay. We went to the dentist later and he said my teeth were looking nice. Edna died today and that made me so sad.

Wednesday, March 22, 1989: My auntie gave me some money for clothes to buy for our American holiday and also to join Surbiton Lawn Tennis Club. I am so lucky. I must remember how fortunate I am always, always!

Saturday, March 25, 1989: It is 12:04 and I go to Belgium today, but I'm not even asleep yet. In church Trevor A. spoke on, "I'm not afraid of dying, I just don't want to be around when it happens." I thought this statement was very true. I still feel sad at leaving my Christian friends behind, but I keep telling myself it's only for a week and what's a week when we will spend eternity together? Today I am flying alone as a "young flyer" to visit family in Brussels! We phoned the airport to ask what time we were to arrive. Having said goodbye, I got safely on the plane when they suddenly said I would be going to Ostend instead of Brussels because there was a strike on! Mad panic! All the children travelling unaccompanied were given a drink, some grapes, sandwiches and arrived in Ostend within half an hour. We could see the ground most of the way there. We were hurried on to a coach, then completed our journey in a hired car. Anne and Ben, the younger two travelling with me, fell asleep. It was 113 km from Ostend to Brussels and along the motorway. No one from British Airways was with me. At least we travelled in style; a Mercedes, I think it was. When we finally arrived in Brussels airport, there was no one to meet me, but a quick phone call to my aunt and they were on their way. After dinner (I don't think anyone knew I was vegetarian) we washed up, went for a walk and went to bed. *Bon-nuit!*

Sunday, March 26, 1989: Easter Sunday. I had a restless night, then choked on my breakfast due to a coughing fit. I'm a bit nervous about the language, etc. *Dans le matin, je suis allee aux Bruxelles avec mes cousins, ma tante et mon oncle. C'est bon.* During our sight-seeing tour we saw the Grand Place. I thought it was one of the most beautiful architectural places in the world. We came back, ate, washed up and I had my first French lesson that Auntie Lesley is giving me while I am here.

Monday, March 27, 1989: Easter Monday. Today we went to the baker's to buy our rolls for breakfast. In the afternoon, we went for a walk in the forest; it was pretty with the sun glistening through the trees. During my week in Belgium, I went swimming, chilled with my cousins and their friends and experienced Belgian shops as well as the Metro (it was really clean and fast). The Cede Park is like a tropical paradise containing so many water sports and I just loved the choice of swimming pools, Jacuzzis and slides/tubes and wave machines. Then we dried off on the sunbeds. It was brilliant. I cried when I left Belgium because I don't like saying good-byes.

April 1989

Sunday, April 2, 1989: I miss everyone in Belgium, especially my cousins. I felt like crying today. I really want to go back and hope I can soon. Normally when I return from holiday, I develop a bad mood and that's so today. I didn't really know my cousins before I went; they were just cousins, but now they are people. I showed my friends the photos and they thought the girls were pretty. M. said we had the same eyes! I just miss Belgium like crazy.

Monday April 3, 1989: A new term began today at Tiffin Girls' school and what a day. Firstly, I became deputy form captain (so not everyone must hate me!). But we were all thoroughly fed up with being back. I was pleased, though, as a few people said I looked tanned. I said it was from lying on sun beds in Belgium.

Tuesday, April 4, 1989: My bus didn't come on time this morning, so I was cross. I must remember to collect the form register each morning, part of my job as form deputy. I'm sure I'll forget! Now it's summer term, we will be doing athletics and will start with high jump next week. I'm really looking forward to that. Tennis also features, so I'm excited. It was a horrible, wet day and sleet fell after school. Still missing Belgium and worrying about loads of things, though I tell myself not to, but there's so many things on my mind.

Wednesday, April 5, 1989: So much for it being the summer term; it was an extremely wet day today and it even snowed; more snow than in December and January. We all wondered if we would get sent home early, but of course we were not. Education comes first and all that! In Chemistry today we made a nylon thread and it is one of the best lessons I have been to. We managed to bus-hop today, so got home at a reasonable time. I'm going to really try and get my work up to a better standard this term so that I can prove I am a hard worker.

Thursday, April 6, 1989: I had a really bad day today as everything went wrong. The weather was miserable and was just like how I felt. I woke up late; my Latin test was a mess, but surprisingly I passed. I didn't understand our physics lesson and my ruler fell out of the window. I didn't bring my tennis racquet as I thought Miss E. didn't teach tennis, and I forgot to bring socks to change into. Even K. commented on the things that were going wrong. I wanted to start a new term and get good results, but did I? No! I got a B in French, however I did get an A for my homework, so was really pleased. We had a table tennis lesson with a new teacher and he was so sweet. My yoghurt I made in Home Economics tasted great and Mum agreed.

Friday, April 7, 1989: I don't think I will travel home on the bus any more with S. and S. I have come to the conclusion that they only have one thing on their minds, and it is not doing me any good. I have better friends in my form and at church and can travel home on the bus with others.

Sunday, April 9, 1989: Bible class was ok today and Mum took us all home afterwards. We had a nice lunch in the garden, the first time this year. Mum and I went to look at Surbiton Tennis Club grounds. It was exciting, the thought of me joining.

Monday, April 10, 1989: Up early for school again and it was great sharing our weekend happenings together: Who was going out with who, etc. In athletics we did a track relay, but on finishing we were all told we were unfit. Huh!

Tuesday, April 11, 1989: I was supposed to go jogging with Mum at 6:30 this morning. I heard her getting ready, but dived under the covers and pretended to be asleep. I made up for it later at school, though. We had 15 minutes of jogging round the track. After school at my piano lesson, I learned I am to take the written paper in June and the practical in July.

Wednesday, April 12, 1989: I was going to Rebecca's today. I left the house at 3:30 but didn't get to her until 4:30 as the traffic through Kingston was diabolical, but others were late arriving, too. We watched *Oxford Blues*, showing the great American spirit. T. phoned when I got home as she was really upset and was crying. I tried to comfort her and give good advice. Why is life so hard at times and why can't be people be happy and fulfilled instead of sad? Life sucks for so many.

Thursday, April 13, 1989: I went to school depressed today and it got more depressing. I only got a C for my homework, but at least I handed it in on time, which is more than can be said for some people. Less than 2 weeks ago I was in Belgium. It seems far away now; too far. I want to be successful, imaginative, show initiative, to have fame, good looks, long legs, long hair, but it goes so wrong at times.

Friday, April 14, 1989: Normal routine today. My cooking (pizza) in Home Economics turned out well. It was our first day of extra Maths. Sometimes I feel unintellectual and unsure of myself, but I guess lots of teenagers do. Mum came in earlier than usual; I went to our church youth group looking my worst, but we all enjoyed ourselves. Had a good chat to the boys. My last page of my first ever diary – the end of an era. (I have written so much in it since the New Year that I have run out of space!) Well, it's the end. Farewell, *au-revoir,* but not *adieu.* (I say *au-revoir* because I expect to see you again. I don't say *adieu* because that would mean I wouldn't expect to see you again.) You've been great fun! The End. Read it and weep!

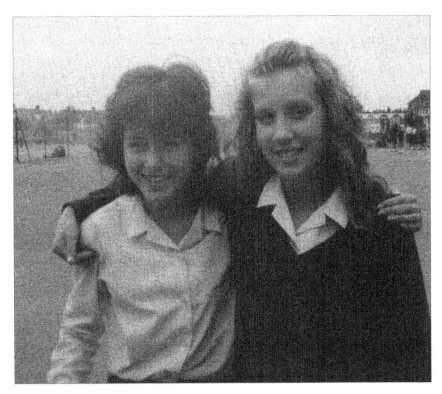

#3 Close friends from Tiffin Girls' school, Ndullee and Claire

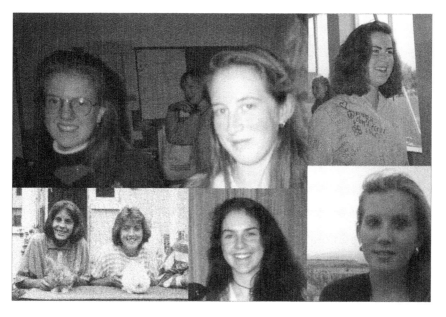

#4 More friends from Tiffin Girls' School:

Top:L-R Melanie, Claire E, Zoe

Bottom:L-R Beth, Catherine, Faye, Claire

On reading this I weep, too, Claire. Like most parents I do not know where your childhood and early teen years went to, let alone the rest of your life. My heart wonders how the time slipped away like a vapour. I am reminded of the Abba song "Slipping Through My Fingers:"

Schoolbag in hand, she leaves home in the early morning

Waving goodbye with an absent-minded smile

I watch her go with a surge of that well-known sadness

And I have to sit down for a while

The feeling that I'm losing her forever

And without really entering her world

I'm glad whenever I can share her laughter

That funny little girl

Slipping through my fingers all the time

I try to capture every minute

The feeling in it

Slipping through my fingers all the time

Do I really see what's in her mind

Each time I think I'm close to knowing

She keeps on growing

Slipping through my fingers all the time

Sleep in our eyes, her and me at the breakfast table

Barely awake, I let precious time go by

Then when she's gone, there's that odd melancholy feeling

And a sense of guilt I can't deny

What happened to the wonderful adventures

The places I had planned for us to go

(Slipping through my fingers all the time)

Well, some of that we did but most we didn't

And why, I just don't know

Slipping through my fingers all the time

I try to capture every minute

The feeling in it

Slipping through my fingers all the time

Do I really see what's in her mind

Each time I think I'm close to knowing

She keeps on growing

Slipping through my fingers all the time

Sometimes I wish that I could freeze the picture

And save it from the funny tricks of time

Slipping through my fingers

Slipping through my fingers all the time

Schoolbag in hand she leaves home in the early morning

Waving goodbye with an absent-minded smile.[25]

Although that small notebook could not contain more than half way through April, you continued in another book:

Saturday, April 15, 1989: Today I had a lie in and went to Kingston. E. is still depressed about Dave. We all had a good laugh trying on clothes. We saw L. in Miss Selfridge and dashed out again; she didn't see us, luckily. Saturday club at church was okay. I got beaten at almost anything and everything. It was an utterly brilliant day, hm-hm!

Sunday, April 16, 1989: I felt lousy when I woke up this morning; everything was against me. Grandma and Granddad came for the day and Jo came in the afternoon. I felt so low that I cried in church.

Monday, April 17, 1989: I was so depressed today. Mum had a go at me for not eating breakfast. School was okay apart from high jump. Miss S. helped me a lot, so I am grateful to her. I phoned Mark – I expect too much from him.

Tuesday, April 18, 1989: Nothing interesting happened today except that the bus home was really late and crowded. I felt ill – everything seemed against me. I can't cope anymore. I'm so depressed and fed up. I think I'll emigrate to Australia, then I can leave my unhappy memories in England.

---

[25] Slipping Through My Fingers, SONGWRITERS: ANDERSSON, BENNY/ULVAEUS, BJORN by permission of Bocu Music Ltd. Photocopying is illegal without the consent of the Publisher.

Wednesday, April 19, 1989: School was long today. I got 75% in my French test. I had a brilliant Drama lesson. After school I visited Auntie Pat's new home–the Jacuzzi was lovely. Uncle Keith was there, too.

Thursday April 20, 1989: I didn't feel brilliant today, considering I was on the bus for nearly an hour, but I had a good tennis lesson and Miss E. made positive comments on my back hand!

Friday, April 21, 1989: I felt really awful today. I was so hot. My Home Economics turned out well. When I got home I didn't feel at all well, so Mum rang the doctor, who said we should go over. The GP gave me a new antibiotic and said that if we were worried we should see the hospital consultant next week. Overnight I was quite ill. Shock, horror!

Saturday, April 22, 1989: Mum rang the hospital this morning and they said to bring me over. My chest was congested, but there was no sign of pneumonia. I had an x-ray and it was decided to put me on intravenous antibiotics again. Mum left me at 12:00 and I did nothing until 5:00, when family came to visit. My friends were concerned about me and phoned. I had another bad night.

Sunday, April 23, 1989: I woke at 6:30, now that's what I call a Sunday lie in! I had my drip inserted this morning. After a lot of messing about, the doctor managed to find a vein. Jo, Hannah, Rachel and Mum came, bringing loads of goodies. Mark gave me a letter! Zoe and Kate came later with Mum. After supper, Julius phoned. I had loads of fluids with my intravenous antibiotics overnight.

Monday, April 24, 1989: I had another bad night, not at all enjoyable. They took my drip down at 11:00 as the needle had tissued (when the medication is by-passing the vein), causing my arm to be very swollen. I then had a bath, what luxury! The drip was then changed to my right hand, so my writing is now impaired. It hurt and I made a fuss.

Tuesday, April 25, 1989: I had so many visitors today – 16 in fact – made up of family, neighbours, school friends, church friends and was totally shattered by the evening. The doctor said I was unfit, but I don't know how he can come to that conclusion when I play so many sports: tennis, hockey, athletics, basketball, swimming! I got a present and card from my school form. I've got so many good friends and I am very fortunate.

Wednesday, April 26, 1989: Loads of visitors again today. I went for a walk in the hospital grounds and it was good to get out. We had a good laugh with the medical student. My drip played up again today. *C'est la vie.* Amy, the young girl in the bed next to me, doesn't know she has CF as her parents haven't told her. I find that very weird.

Thursday, April 27, 1989: I actually enjoyed myself today as the nurses and I really laughed. Again, I had loads of family and school friends who visited. I went to the physio gym this afternoon but it wore me out as my chest is still bad and I'm very breathless. More blood tests as the pathology lab messed the previous ones up, yet again! And again my drip needed re-siting; the doctor found another vein quite easily. I'm getting so many really nice presents from my friends and family. I'm really lucky.

Friday, April 28, 1989: Today was quite depressing. I came off my drip and may be able to go home on Sunday, as my x-ray was much better. Again loads of family and friends visited. Rick Astley definitely looks like my doctor. I'll have to sleep with a pin-up of him under my pillow!

Saturday, April 29, 1989: It felt a sad day today. I am most probably going home tomorrow. I don't really want to go as I've had so many visitors, but all good things must come to an end. Again, loads of family and friends today. It's 4 weeks since I returned from Belgium; hopefully I can go back soon. The airline has sent me a ticket. It's not long till Mum goes to America. Time goes too quickly. My last hospital night (I think). Rick Astley, the latest heart-throb!

Sunday, April 30, 1989: The last day before May and I'm still in hospital. Yes, can you believe it; I've got to stay until Friday! Another 5 days, but what can I do? I only hope my favourite doctor is on duty. I even started packing my bag until the doctor came to tell me; I just couldn't believe it. My school friends and family came up trumps in visiting again today. Some of my school friends are finding life hard. We worry about each other, but I feel out of it whilst in hospital. All my summer term ambitions have flown out the door because of my health status.

May 1989

Monday, May 1, 1989: The first day of May. A new beginning. I was allowed out of hospital for this afternoon and Auntie took me to Kingston. I saw a few girls and a teacher from school. I missed some visitors while I was out, and they kindly left some flowers. I feel so guilty with them making an effort and me not being there. Geoffrey and Mark cycled and were not too pleased to wait 2 hours. But it was so nice of them. Mum has a cold so did not come; we have been warned that what a cold virus is to some, can become a bacteria for those with CF. My drip again tissued and had to be re-sited.

Tuesday, May 2, 1989: Today was not the best of days, but then it wasn't the worst. Again, loads of visitors as my school and church friends come so often and it is a heck of a way to travel for them. We went into Epsom Town Centre and had a milkshake in McDonald's. I didn't feel much like socialising with the ward staff today. I just want the drip to stay in, continue to get my intravenous antibiotics and get back to school, etc. I feel I am missing so much and will have to work so hard to catch up on all my lessons.

Wednesday, May 3, 1989: I had a mixture of feelings today: loneliness, happiness, depression, ugliness, selfishness; it was quite good in one sense but horrible in another. All my visitors came at once today. I made a cushion this morning via the occupational therapist. She came to give some structure to my day and I enjoyed this project. I've really enjoyed being in hospital, especially talking to the doctors and nurses. The weather was good today and I had a walk outside the hospital. I have no good points anymore, but did I ever? I am selfish and ungrateful.

Thursday, May 4, 1989: I was visited by one of the Bucks Fiz band! Shock, horror and great! I have continued to do some homework.

Friday, May 5, 1989: Very mixed feelings today as I came out of hospital; part of me really pleased to be able to continue with normal life, but at the same time really missing everyone, both staff and patients.

Saturday, May 6, 1989: We went to Kingston this morning although I still feel very unwell, but I want to get back to school on Monday, so this was a dummy run to see how I manage. I bought a nice dress. The party I went to was okay, but I am feeling very unwell still. I missed both the doctors and nurses today. I went to bed early, as I had little sleep in hospital.

Sunday, May 7, 1989: I'm glad I made it to church as it gave me a sense of belonging. School tomorrow and I feel so out of touch, despite loads of friends visiting me in the last couple of weeks and keeping me in the loop.

Monday, May 8, 1989: My first day back at school. Sheer bliss! What fun! (Actually, it was better than I expected.) I didn't take part in the 200 metres as I wasn't allowed to. Loads of people are going to audition for the school play. It was so hot today, but we still have to wear our blazers. The 6th form no longer has to wear skirts when they wear mufti; they can wear trousers. Tiffin Girls' is definitely going downhill; trousers indeed, in this day and age! The new rule went down so well, as all the 6th form turned up in trousers! Miss them like crazy.

Tuesday, May 9, 1989: It was a struggle at school today and I didn't feel like doing anything. I did games, but I realise I should not have done 'cause my breathlessness was so bad and I felt ill.

Wednesday, May 10, 1989: Life is becoming one hard slog and I doubt anyone makes sense of it. Work, rest and play. Boy, do I like the weekends!

Thursday, May 11, 1989: I know I am still convalescing as I don't feel my usual self. I get so tired; I am concerned that I am not catching up with all the work I have missed.

Friday, May 12, 1989: It was weird today, as Ben would say. First I was sad, then I was happy; now I am fed up. I refuse to let all the work I need to do drag me down. With others of the form, I came second place in the Young Poets' competition that the Royal of Borough of Kingston ran for school pupils. We have to go and read them out at an awards ceremony in the Guildhall. It was great to be back at church this evening.

Saturday, May 13, 1989: We went shopping today, my mum and me. I got quite a few things that are quite nice, but I'm not entirely sure about them. I got a pair of sandals. Mum seems to have started packing my case already for July, just typical! She says she wants to make sure I take what I should and not bung things in at the last minute when she isn't here. She tells me she has so much to do before she goes next month, so she needs to get organised! I beat the boys at skipping at church this evening, although I didn't beat them in running.

Monday, May 15, 1989: I am told to stand up for myself; well that's what I did. I got in an argument with Mr. H. as he said I had to do the work I had missed. I explained that I was doing my best to catch up, but that wasn't good enough for him, hm! Walking up Herne Road from the bus after school is really hard, I find, since being ill.

Tuesday, May 16, 1989: I was so tired today and my piano lesson was the last straw. I got an A/B for my self-portrait in art. Athletics was really hard, but I beat some of my form at hurdles, getting a time of 7.94, so I was well chuffed. I could excuse myself from games if I wanted to, but I just don't want to. I want to carry on as normally as possible.

Wednesday, May 17, 1989: One day nearer the exams and I am dreading them. Here I am, still trying to catch up with my homework, let alone do any revision. I know I want to do as well as I can. Not long to go until church camp either. My school friends still tell me I'm preaching too much. I wish people would tell me these things before I make a fool out of myself; but no, they just let me carry on.

Thursday, May 18, 1989: My hospital appointment went okay, but the doctor said I am still getting over the severe chest infection I had and needed to be "kind" to myself. Our Drama lesson was really good. Uncle Keith was up from Devon and he says we should have a good time when we visit him in the summer.

Friday, May 19, 1989: The last day of the school week and everyone at school seems really down at the moment. I don't know what I've done, but I keep offending people. Shame on me. It was sweltering today, very uncomfortable. Church youth group was fine as we saw some old camp photos. It's amazing how people have grown up over two years, as we all have. Soon we're going to be OAPs. Just thinking about it makes me worry, and worry I do!

Saturday, May 20, 1989: I knew my trip to London would end in disaster and I was certainly right. I got so annoyed with Mum and she got annoyed with me. Hannah was great. We walked from Oxford St. to Waterloo and Hannah came back for tea. I just don't know how I got to Claire's party on time but I managed it eventually, although I was worn out in the end.

Monday, May 22, 1989: The day started off well and then gradually deteriorated. The bus didn't come and when it did, it was packed. We managed to get on one at 8:20 and got to school at 9:00. The day went quickly downhill. My Biology exercise book (together with others in my class) was taken in to be seen by an Inspector, picked at random. Aren't we privileged!

Tuesday, May 23, 1989: Today was hot, muggy and sticky; at least it was a change from rain. It was a long day today. Next time I go to the hospital for physio, I'll need to take my walkman to pass the time away. As usual it was all touch and go everywhere. I managed to have a shower before I went to read my poem at the Guildhall. I wasn't as scared as I was last year. We all did our best and got free T-shirts!

Wednesday, May 24, 1989: Buses – who invented them? I walked for 50 minutes, got on a bus but it was packed. I felt so worn out when I finally arrived at school. It was so humid today and then relieved by a thunderstorm. When I got home I finished packing for camp. I hope the weather is good.

Thursday, May 25, 1989: I know I am still struggling after my hospital stay. I didn't think I'd last the day today. I felt like collapsing. But things were okay after a while, though. I don't think I could cope with very much more! I felt very uplifted on the bus this morning as I remembered Mr. H. got 40 tickets to go to a popular roadshow. I can't go because of camp. I hope all my problems disappear by tomorrow. Fat chance!

*Friday May 26, 1989-Tuesday May 30, 1989-*Church Camp!

Wednesday, May 31, 1989: I didn't write a diary for camp. It was really good in some ways, but it was a love-hate sort of feeling. We all got on well together, especially on the last day when there were hugs all round; a day to remember for many years to come. I went to Jo's today and it was quite relaxing. I have fond memories of camp which made my heart thump passionately. Other times I felt different. Let's just say I'll never forget the summer camp of '89.

June 1989

Thursday, June 1, 1989: A fun-filled day. I had another lie in. The phone didn't stop ringing all day and only one of the calls was for me! I did my revision today; well, I tried anyway. We watched a video that we had seen before. It hadn't lost its loving feeling.

Friday, June 2, 1989: Another fun-filled day, I don't think! Revision and eating filled the day, although I did make lunch and had my hair done. Why should I bother anymore? Mum goes soon; she'll be away for more than a month. I hope I'll manage with the arrangements in place.

Saturday, June 3, 1989: I tried to do some revision today, but it didn't last very long. I doodled about all day and achieved nothing. Saturday Club was okay. Info re: the guys, etc.

Sunday, June 4, 1989: It was a perplexing day today on many fronts. Mum's last day today before she goes to the USA tomorrow ahead of us. Our pastor interviewed her this evening.

Monday, June 5, 1989: I left for school, but then doubled back to say good-bye to Mum again. She got on the plane safely and should be arriving in America soon. I hope she'll be okay. The music exam was not particularly brilliant, but there we go. We did the 800 metres today and I came 6th in the class. I was very annoyed as my time was poor and I should have done much better. However, Miss E. said that, considering I was still in hospital this time last month, I had done pretty well. Hm! The only excuse for me is my cold I now have. Auntie Pat helped a lot this evening. A good few weeks before we join Mum. Will it ever arrive?

Tuesday, June 6, 1989: I don't feel like working now. Mum rang this evening. She sounds very distant; not surprising really. Apparently she has been to the Whitehouse and Capitol Hill. It is very hot out there. Mrs. White wasn't too overjoyed with my theory work today. It's all systems go in preparation for the exams and everyone is bogged down with revision. At present I go from high to low in a matter of minutes.

Wednesday, June 7, 1989: There is not a lot to say, really. The usual routine. The weather was pretty bad for June again today. All go for the exams. Not that I'm going to do well. I wish I would surprise everyone I know by getting some good results. Wednesdays seem long, but in reality they go quite fast. Drama was good today. Things are going okay at home, although I forgot to put the potatoes on. Typical!

Thursday, June 8, 1989: I can't think of anything positive apart than Mum just rang. She is fine but didn't like the YMCA in Washington, so she has moved to a hotel for the duration of the conference she is attending. It is now very late and I am writing my diary by torch-light.

Monday, June 12, 1989: The first day of the wonderful exams. Biology and History. I don't think I did very well and they're subjects, among others, that I'm taking for my GCSEs. I can't afford to allow my mind to wander. I got a letter from Mum today, which was very hard to translate and typical of her writing; that's why she normally types everything! Mum has been gone a week now but it seems much longer. Exams are on the brain.

Tuesday, June 13, 1989: Panic! This was the main essence of the day. We waited for the bus as usual and it didn't come. At 8:25 we managed to get on a bus after waiting 40 minutes! By 9:00 I was in school, thankfully. The Chemistry exam was quite enjoyable and English was okay, but I didn't have time to check through my Maths and I couldn't remember how to work out some of the formulae, so much so that I was quite upset this evening.

Wednesday, June 14, 1989: The exams were okay today, although I knew I didn't do fantastically in them. It was humid, hot and sticky and I was sat right in the sun for the whole of the day which didn't do me any favours with my cough and cold. Not only that, but I was told off for coughing and told in future I must sit exams in a small room by myself – the injustice of it all. Mum just rang – she was worried about me when I told her what the teacher said. I don't blame her at all. God knows the results of my exams; I don't know that I want to!

Friday, June 16, 1989: Another day in the life of C.R. Salter, *le premier.* Maths was easier than I thought, but by no means fantastic. Latin worse, as I didn't revise for it. Exams finished until next week, hoorah!

Saturday, June 17, 1989: What a day and a rush this morning. I went shopping with Auntie. The netball tournament was embarrassing. We lost 3 games and drew one, not our brightest and best hour. 3 weeks ago we were on camp; it doesn't seem at all possible.

Monday, June 19, 1989: A very hot day. Piano results and I got 81% overall. The doctor didn't say much about my health; rather a waste of time going.

Tuesday, June 20, 1989: No exam results today. I'm not going to worry myself about my marks this year. I'm not going to Wimbledon tennis tomorrow as it's going to be too hard to get over there. Sleep tight!

Wednesday, June 21, 1989: Some exam results today; some good, some not! Mum rang and seems quite chirpy; I told her some of my marks. Although I am cross with myself, I refuse to slag myself off. Forget the past, relax; be nice and don't worry about anything. If only!

Saturday, June 4, 1989: It was an okay day today. I woke up early and now it's catching up with me. Hannah and myself wandered around Kingston and then to Richmond. We walked everywhere for lunch but didn't find anything apart from M&S, so we bought sandwiches and ate them on the Green. It was really good. We popped to see the local fair on the way home and that was my Saturday gone. Sometimes I really want to spend a lot of time with my friends at school, but other things get in the way so often. Until *le matin*.

Sunday, June 25, 1989: I'm discovering different things about me that I didn't know. I hate my voice. I'm totally fed up; I'm not happy anymore. I should be fun to be with. I should bring sparks into other people's eyes. I want to keep this relationship, but I know this relationship doesn't want to keep me!

Monday, June 26, 1989: I had a really good time today, 81% in English, 3rd in 1500 metre, which was okay. Uncle Keith came to get me from school and we went to Wimbledon tennis. It was great, in fact *magnifique.* I saw so many famous tennis players in the grounds and well as seeing play on Centre Court! We met Uncle Keith's friend, Wendy, who let me use her ticket. The tennis was great; 5 hours and I didn't get bored once. There is some nice talent around there. Go to Wimbledon if you want to meet real people!

Tuesday, June 27, 1989: I woke up half an hour late at 7:00am and what a rush to get to school on time. My hospital appointment was good as I saw my bubbly nurse. Zoe was after me in piano lessons, so we had a great time chatting. I'm fed up with being depressed, but it comes so naturally nowadays. I'm hardly ever happy. I'm running out of depressing things, but not finding any happy ones.

Thursday, June 29, 1989: Ndullee is coming back to school tomorrow which will be great, as she, Beth and myself can hang out again. I had a good chat to Daniel on the way home about the old times. I enjoy his company a lot. Until we meet again!

Friday, June 30, 1989: Ndullee's first day back at school. She hasn't changed at all after her year spent back in Greece. It was great to see her. I met someone from my old school who said: "Last time I saw you, you had a disease and were going to die in the next 2 years." That really cheered me up.

July 1989

Saturday, July 1, 1989: There was a great lack of sleep last night, past 1:00am before anyone nodded off. It was okay, but I just wanted to come home. I felt so guilty coming home, but I was so tired. Mum flew to Dallas and phoned today. She sent me some stuff through the post about American music, etc. Not long now 'til we join her.

Sunday, July 2, 1989: The majority of today was good. I've worked out who I think will be in the women's finals, but the men's is rather more of a tough decision. Church was good both morning and evening. However, we heard that it was a very sad day for our sister-church a mile or so from us; a family has been killed in a car accident. It doesn't bear thinking about, as the car caught fire. I am so grateful that we will have life eternal.

Monday, July 3, 1989: Wimbledon will be over on Saturday for another year. It's my birthday this month, almost 14 years old and growing stronger; well, almost! Nothing to report on the home front. Is there ever? Oh, well, another close to yet another typical day.

Tuesday, July 4, 1989: American Independence Day and in 16 days I'll be there, although what I'll be doing, I am unsure. It hasn't really sunk in that I will be going in just over 2 weeks. My Art result wasn't very good today and I'm in a slight dilemma about my party, as I don't really know what to do. Should I invite both my school and church friends or not? Would they get on together? I am both wondering and worrying. My discus throwing was pathetic today and I wonder if life will ever improve. My oral antibiotics are making me feel sick all the time.

Thursday, July 6, 1989: The weather today was horrible; humid, hot, sticky. Even Ndullee wasn't used to it. Help; there are so many things to arrange before I go on holiday. I can't keep up with them all. In our tennis lesson we won a game, which was pretty good fun and that's the highlight of the day. I lost my cheque for Drama, which wasn't too fantastic; however it was okay as a man rang the school and I got it back. Ah, well, must close after another typical day. Until tomorrow, I can share all my problems with you, dear Diary.

Friday, July 7, 1989: There was a thunderstorm last night; quite a bad one. I even woke up, along with the rest of the south east of the country, as it rattled through. The rain continued, but still it was hot and humid. The Read-a-thon went okay, apart from not sitting on proper seats. It's all go for the holiday; I really hope we get it all done in time. I personally don't think we will. Mum rang; she seems a little tired and I don't blame her, travelling in so many different states and trying to observe in hospitals, as well as write up her project as she goes. Sight-seeing at weekends, though, is light relief, she says. This week at home has been diabolical. Hockey at church was hot stuff this evening.

Saturday, July 8, 1989: I'm writing my diary today almost a week late, oh well. I can't remember what I did today. Oh yes, Auntie came to visit me. I was 30 minutes late for meeting Catherine in Kingston. Saturday Club was a disaster. Oh well, not to worry, maybe next time or sometime I'll have a brilliant day and everyone will be happy, me included. Some dream of a perfect day!

Saturday, July 9, 1989: Quite a reasonable day today. Everyone is so tired, though. I'm dreading saying farewell; in fact I haven't thought about it very much. Ah, well, I'll love you and leave you *mes amies.*

Monday, July 10, 1989: I arose at 6:15 this morning; I'm catching up now, though, with this interminable diary. I was told that my poem was expressed very emotionally and with feeling. A few sniggers could be heard, but apart from that I survived the insults. Self-assessment pretty naff today; I couldn't think of anything to write, so I asked Mr. H. what he thought of me; he said serious, sincere, warm, friendly. "Codswallop," I thought. My party plans are becoming rather *tres* boring but *c'est la vie.*

Tuesday, July 11, 1989: Why do normal people suffer from tiredness? I wouldn't know; I'm not normal. I felt unsociable today and I must get in trim for the big event tomorrow. Mum rang this morning; she sounded well. D. rang – it was quite funny. Anyhow, better close now. See you in the morning, love. Don't wait up. Life is too short to be sad or depressed!

Wednesday, July 12, 1989: Sports day! A fantastic time – our class certainly was pants for team spirit! I ran the 1500 metres and came 14th out of 16. (the other two dropped out!) Miss E. said: "Why do they put you in for it,

Claire? You are wheezing like there's no tomorrow and your lung capacity won't take it." Well, I'm glad she realised it. Rebecca broke the record for shot, which was really good. It's my party tomorrow and in the words of Lesley Gore (1963), "and I'll cry if I want to. You would cry too if it happened to you."

Thursday, July 13, 1989: Today was quite good. This afternoon I went to Kingston with Auntie. It was quite funny, trying on clothes and especially shorts. Auntie bought loads of stuff for me – silly nightshirts and all. I felt so guilty not paying for things. Well, the party went okay, so all that worrying for nothing! Ndullee stayed an extra hour, which was great. I opened some of my pressies –was very spoilt.

Friday, July 14, 1989: I was alone all day today, ahh. Quite sad, really. To earn some extra pocket money for America, I did a work plan for cleaning Dennis, our neighbour's home and very thorough it was. The highlight of the day was going to Craftsmen. Everyone was so kind to me. Not long to America. I just wish I could take all my friends with me.

I got my end of year report today and it commented on my hospital admissions this year, especially when I was in for 3 weeks, just before the exams. Mr. H., my form teacher, wrote: *Claire is a helpful and friendly member of the form. She performed valuable services in her role of mission monitress last term, arranging for financial support for the causes the girls support. She is a generally active member of the form. Claire is a very friendly, polite and supportive form member, too. She is warm and sensitive to the feelings and needs of others. She takes an active part in form life and makes most valuable contributions to it.*

My French exam result was spot on average, but obviously our teacher doesn't expect us to rest on our laurels and she wrote: *Claire has worked conscientiously throughout the term; however she must make an effort to participate in class as she lacks confidence.* For History, my exam mark was spot on the average and Mrs. B. wrote: *Claire's work has matured in the third year and her project was well researched.* In Religious Studies Mrs. G. wrote: *Claire's class work has been thoughtful and thorough. She is learning to argue her point of view well.* In Biology Miss C. wrote: *Claire has worked with application and interest. She has made good progress and should be pleased with her examination performance.* In Chemistry, Mr. H. wrote: *Claire needs to make more effort, in her written work; however her examination mark was pleasing.* Similarly in Physics, Mr G. wrote: *Claire has found Physics difficult but has worked hard to overcome her difficulties but needs to continue her hard work.*

Even in Maths Mrs B. was pleased with my progress and hard work and my Drama exam result of 76%, was above average, which prompted Miss F. to write: *Claire obviously enjoys drama and has shown commitment to the subject both in lessons and outside the curriculum. Claire's assessment performance was sensitive, thoughtful and promising.* She continued: *Claire has shown unfailing commitment to the Drama course and, as a result, has made marked progress. Her level of confidence appears to have risen, particularly with regard to showing her work to others. I was most impressed with Claire's monologue work.* In Technology I got an A and Mrs. S. said: *Claire has learned and mastered many new skills this term and always works with dedication. Her mole was mechanically excellent.* *Sunday, July 16, 1989:* If I had actually written this on the 16th, I would probably have been devastated. The day was good up until the evening, then it went down-hill fast. The evening service was very distressing. I said goodbye to all of my friends and managed to hold back the tears, but got big hugs from most of them.

Monday, July 17, 1989: Today felt quite enjoyable. The lessons were brilliant; I can just see myself as a lawyer! D. came round; I had a feeling he would. He cheered me up; he knew I was upset yesterday and just listened to me. Everyone needs a shoulder to cry on, etc.

Tuesday, July 18, 1989: What a day today; I can't really remember school as I was probably half asleep, but never mind. I hope I awake for the 4th year!

Wednesday, July 19, 1989: My last day in England. How will I ever miss it. *Je ne sais pas.* I quite enjoyed school today; we had the junior presentations of awards during the afternoon. I said bye to all my friends. I felt upset and guilty. I know I'm a spoilt brat and don't deserve this holiday, but then a lot of my friends go abroad more than once a year. Ah well, a woman's got to do what a woman's got to do! So it's to the US of A tomorrow. *Bon voyage,* Claire; we'll meet again.

Thursday, July 20, 1989: America! L.A. airport, then to University Hilton. Mum was so excited to see me after so long. We start our brill coach tour of California, Arizona, Nevada and Hawaii tomorrow.

Friday, July 21, 1989: Los Angeles

Saturday, July 22, 1989: Disneyland-Orange County, Palm Springs, Radisson.

Claire, at this time you also enjoyed writing plenty of postcards to both family and friends:

We have been travelling around quite a lot. We spent a day at Universal Studios and saw a new ride at the Studios which looked fantastic – it was so real to life. We also saw *Jaws* and many other famous film sets. Yesterday we went to Disneyland, which everyone enjoyed. We shopped along Main Street and went on lots of rides. The standing in line took so long, though! This evening we will be in Phoenix and last night stayed in a beautiful hotel in L.A.

Sunday, July 23, 1989: Palm Springs-Phoenix, Arizona

Monday, July 24, 1989: Phoenix-Grand Canyon

Tuesday, July 25, 1989: Grand Canyon-by plane to Las Vegas.

Wednesday, July 26, 1989: Las Vegas

The following is a card you had sent:

Dear All, we are having a good time in the USA. So far we have been to Disneyland, Universal Studios, the Grand Canyon, Phoenix, and now we are in Las Vegas. The weather was hot – 115 degrees F in the desert in Arizona. The Grand Canyon was fabulous. We watched the sunset and then got up at 4:45am to see the sun rise – quite unbelievable. See you soon. Love, Claire.

Thursday, July 27, 1989: Las Vegas-Bishop, California (also known as the Golden State)

Friday, July 28, 1989: Bishop-Senora

Saturday, July 29, 1989: Senora-Lake Tahoe

Sunday, July 30, 1989: My fourteenth birthday: Lake Tahoe. Sacramento then on to San Francisco. Excellent; no other word to describe it.

Monday, July 31, 1989: San Francisco (including Sausalito and Alcatraz)

August 1989

Tuesday, August 1, 1989: San Francisco, shopping and riding the cable cars.

Wednesday, August 2, 1989: Left S.F. and did the 17 mile drive. San Luis Obispo.

Thursday, August 3, 1989: San Luis Obispo –Santa Barbara. Los Angeles Airport – Hawaii! Had a brilliant week in Hawaii, we were meant to go to morning church on a boat, but no one picked us up! Enjoyed it immensely; beach, swimming, shopping, eating, island hopping.

As an aside, Claire, I had gone out six weeks ahead of you and wrote/phoned to see how you were often. I wrote on June 30, 1989:

This time next week I'll be in Tucson, so every plane journey moves me nearer to the west coast and meeting up with you. Tomorrow (1st July) I'll be able to tell myself I'll be seeing you this month, so roll on July 20th, what excitement. Claire, they naturally have a thriving CF charity out here in the States and at the Emory Children's Hospital I was at yesterday they had premature twins, approximately 2lbs in weight and they were doing physiotherapy on them with an electric toothbrush!

Our "Wonders of the Golden West Tour" of sixteen wonder-packed, west coast-based USA sites followed by seven days in Hawaii was our first holiday in the States. The main foci of our trip (but including some great stop-offs) were: Los Angeles, Palm Springs, Phoenix, Grand Canyon, Las Vegas, Bishop, Yosemite National Park, Lake Tahoe, San Francisco, Monterey, San Luis Obispo and then on to Hawaii from L.A. In Los Angeles – you have an envelope stuffed full of advertising paraphernalia and on it you wrote, "Los Angeles, the place to be" – we visited Disneyland, Universal Studios, Hollywood (including the Walk of Fame) then stopping off to do some gold-panning, Sacramento, and San Francisco. We just loved shopping at Fisherman's Wharf, where you bought your Levi jeans and you were one for keeping as many souvenirs as you could, including your Levi tags and the Hard Rock Café T-shirt. We loved riding the cable cars, visiting the Fairmont Hotel, Alcatraz Island, Sausalito and traversing the Golden Gate Bridge. We visited Santa Barbara, San Luis Obispo, Bishop, Palm Springs, Yosemite National Park, Senora and Lake Tahoe (you celebrated your 14th birthday with a dinner cruise on the lake) and the Sierra Nevada mountains, Monterey in California, Phoenix and Scottsdale, Arizona, the Grand Canyon (I think this was one of our favourite places, Claire and we loved seeing the Colorado river deep inside the Canyon. One of my favourite photos of you is the one taken at one of the lookout points on the rim). Then on to Sedona, (another of our favourite places) and Las Vegas. We didn't go into any of the casinos, but spent our time either in the hotel pool or the air-conditioned malls! One day found us at Wet and Wild to try and keep cool in the intense heat. Next we went to Lake Mead and Hoover Dam, Nevada, then once back in L.A we flew over Monument Valley, although you did not want to take the trip. I'm sorry

I rather bamboozled you into taking it, as I thought we would never be this way again and thus my thoughts were to take it while we could. Our last flight west was on to Hawaii, where we also visited the smaller islands, watched volleyball on Waikiki beach, swam out to the float anchored out to sea, and you even attended an Elvis evening with Auntie Pat, having first visited Hanauma Bay, where one of his films was shot.

I am so pleased you enjoyed this holiday, and the photos you took bear testimony to that. You snapped photos of Chevys and stretch limos, Hollywood, Monument Valley, gold panning, Sedona, Grand Canyon, riding the cable car in San Francisco, the lights of Las Vegas and of course we crooned over the beaches in Hawaii, too. It was hard coming back to England, but nevertheless you had missed your friends and were keen to tell them of your new experiences, whilst also listening to their school vacation adventures. Your diary continued:

Friday, August 11, 1989: Back from USA. No words in the human language to describe the disappointment.

Saturday, August 12, 1989: Went home – packed. Saw Belgian cousins briefly as we are heading to the caravan to sleep for the week! Tired, thrilling. Asleep in car – Safeway to shop. 6:15pm bed!

Sunday, August 13, 1989: Wake up, brekkie, sleep. Lunch, sleep. Tea, sit outside. Church. Then to Highcliffe to say hi to Rachel.

Monday, August 14, 1989: Beach in morning, although cloudy. Saw Peter and his grand-daughter Kelly. Came up from beach. Rachel and Rebecca came for lunch. Shopping in Christchurch.

Tuesday, August 15, 1989: To Poole with Rachel and Rebecca. Looked at shops and good art gallery. Lunch by harbour, but it was windy.

Wednesday, August 16, 1989: 12 years ago Elvis, the King of Rock n' Roll, died. I can't really explain my feelings. I don't suppose he could either. Swanage *avec* Rachel and Rebecca. Ferry to Studland Bay then on to Durlston. Walk, ice-cream. Shopping. Drive to Corfe Castle. Photostop. Really nice day.

Thursday, August 17, 1989: Rachel and Rebecca's flat, rained. No swimming, no beach, windy. Sunbathed once rain stopped. Highcliffe on bikes, beach again, then to Mudeford Quay in the evening.

Friday, August 18, 1989: Beach all day. Sun, swimming, wind breaks then lunch. Relax/farewell, *adieu*. Drive home. Panic, frenzy/angry. Sleep. Wow, what a holiday-packed summer this is. Tomorrow I am off to Dartmouth while my mum catches up with the laundry, prepares her scholarship report and goes through the mountains of post.

Saturday, August 19, 1989: to Dartmouth. Had a great time with Jo, staying with my Uncle Keith, but I'm not going to keep a diary. I need a rest from writing!

Monday, August 28, 1989: Back from Dartmouth

Tuesday, August 29, 1989: Convalescing Day as missing everyone.

Wednesday, August 30, 1989: One month ago, in San Francisco. I can't say I miss Dylan, though he probably doesn't know my name and has forgotten about me. I like his style. He's different; I like that in a man.

Thursday, Tuesday, August 31, 1989: Zoe's house, and bike ride along toe-path to Sunbury for lunch.

Notes for August. Dylan. It doesn't hurt to change. Hang loose. I will be right here waiting for you.

September 1989

Friday, September 1, 1989: Tennis with Jo. To Kingston with Hannah. Saw a lot of people I knew.

Sunday, September 3, 1989: A real church service with real people and a real ministry. It was so good (well, you know what I mean) to be back at my home church. I think people have an inner part to them, deep down in their soul which nobody knows about and something that will always be kept a secret. I wouldn't say that I'm an extrovert, but I do hide the part of me which I feel to be private. My opinions change frequently. I need someone to care for me. You don't need a boyfriend. You know nothing about life really; neither does anyone, I doubt.

Monday, September 4, 1989: The travelling was good today, all around London before we ended up at the hospital. Doctor said I need to stay on antibiotics continuously, which isn't too great but never mind. I had a blood test, but I didn't worry. I was actually allowed a gown this year for my x-ray, big deal. Over the past week I've never seen so many Volvos in my life (a reminder of someone who travelled in one in Dartmouth last month). It's not that I've been looking out for them, but somehow they spring up from nowhere. Rubbing salt in! The summer is over and I'll have to wait until next year for any more fun. I suppose it is an end of an era. I'm one of millions who looks forward to tomorrow with anticipation as well as excitement (I don't think!). I wish I was happy back on holiday.

Tuesday, September 5, 1989: 1st day of new term, indeed new school year. It was unpredictable today. At first everyone wanted to get warmed up; a new form room filled with different people, but not strangers. Just different. It's hard getting used to being a year older and acting it too. More mature than six weeks ago, more experienced in some ways. I think today it sunk in that we were hardly going to see each other anymore in lessons, as we have now chosen our General Certificate of Secondary Education (GCSE) Options. Although we will be further apart, maybe it will do some good. Teachers and the time-table are annoying; no free periods anymore. However, life within the class hasn't changed. Summer romances are the topic of conversation.

Wednesday, September 6, 1989: Full day of lessons and the day seems much longer than last year but maybe even better than last year? We have officially started our GCSE coursework which, in some respects, is frightening. The big exams, as it were. It suddenly hits you that you are working for the exams that will determine your future. Well, now there is only GCSE coursework to look forward to in life, but I'd much rather be thinking of something else. It's odd saying to friends, "What lesson have you got next?" Mr W., what a heart-throb and nice with it. Geography was very s l o w. English was expressionless but okay.

Sunday, September 10, 1989: Students ahoy, it was our turn to host the church student lunch today, so many of them. Mum was fortunate to have cooked enough food. Luckily, too that our brains were switched on for their academic minds!

Tuesday, September 12, 1989: A month ago today there were tears all around. I wish, well ya know how I feel. I miss it, I loved it; it's just part of me. School was nothing to write home about, but that's not unusual.

Thursday, September 14, 1989: The worst day of school so far this term as not feeling particularly happy about myself. Computing is like a foreign language. C. is good to me. I do feel neglected and maybe that's why I'm not feeling too confident in myself, but I chide myself because I have loads of friends and even now am making close connections with the girls in my option groups. L. can't come on Saturday so that was upsetting; well annoying. I hate being let down, but today was just one of those days!

Sunday, September 17, 1989: Bible class and church were okay. Lunch good. This afternoon I played tennis with Jo although we had to wait a long time for a court. Mum was in a foul mood; so was I but we had a good chat and now things look promising.

Wednesday, September 20, 1989: A month ago today I was so happy. All I could want. I just wished I'd thought more. You never know if I had I might be an even happier girl today. I look at Volvos but don't see who I want to.

"I'll be right her waiting," but I expect he didn't give me another thought after our natter.

Thursday, September 21, 1989: There are very few things I hate about my mother, but one of them is making my illness an excuse. I don't mean to get angry, but sometime it's just a reflex action with her. She infuriates me so much sometimes. It's like she's making people feel sorry for me, which I don't like. I know my family loves me, but sometimes they hardly *see me* anymore.

Friday, September 22, 1989: Tiffin was absolutely great today. I talked to Daniel on the way home. "See you around." That's so meaningful and I just can't describe how I felt.

Saturday, September 23, 1989: I blocked the world out this morning as I was so tired. I had a weird dream. I saw Steff P. today and caught up with the news about everyone, although it was a bit weird. If at St. Mary's I could see myself now, I would cry. Things change and people change. It hurts real bad when you think about it. The dinner party at ours was good, but I want to be a shoulder to cry on.

Sunday, September 24, 1989: I felt so at home today with new people and new food. We had an American family over for lunch. It sure was awesome. The dessert was great; in fact, there was nothing wrong with the food, only our accents. They were so cute and extroverted. I had a little chat with Ben. The Harvest Festival was good. I wish I had courage and faith. Maybe that is the answer!

Monday, September 25, 1989: Today things went wrong and I can't explain them. It was a day of ups and downs; more downs than ups – quite strange. The highlight of today was talking to myself!

Tuesday, September 26, 1989: Tomorrow after today. Martin Clarke is going to teach us for Basketball. Why do the actions of some of my friends make me panic? Do they really know how dangerous they are? We had Biology assessments and if that was the exam, I would have failed. That's being optimistic. "Appreciate your Mum" is a lesson to be learned. Mum was feeling better today as she was shouting and giving me advice about boys. Take opportunities when they arise!

Thursday, September 28, 1989: I remember too well. It's hard to describe the way I feel inside this term. I've been too introverted and thus not said a lot. In some aspects I've been breaking in two. This doesn't worry me unless people notice. I enjoy my own company, but I also love socialising. I suppose the change from holiday to school has cut me like a knife. I miss everyone and everything. I've just blanked most of it out of my mind, which I don't think is a wise thing to do as this just hurts people more. I want to care about people. It doesn't seem possible that I've only been back at school a month; quite unbelievable. I want to hang on to the memories and hold on to everything that goes with them. Oceans apart, still I can't stop the pain.

Saturday, September 30, 1989: Great time today. I really enjoyed seeing my cousins and Auntie. I can talk to Auntie now, though sometimes I say too much. Saturday Club was good and the Hoedown was excellent. What with Mr. Sayer and Mark, what more could a girl want? Repeat the act of human contact.

October 1989

Sunday, October 1, 1989: It's weird how people change. Well things, not people. I've changed, so have friends and people I love around me. I know I'm sentimental; it helps to overcome these changes and it's important to recognise. I remember laughing with the friends I cherish, but not any-more. I don't see them or talk to them now. I haven't got many chances left if this is all we have of the best days of our lives. I think mine are over. My days, the people I've loved, gone. Pain. I hate feeling sorry for myself and sometime I hate caring. It's harder for them than for me. Maybe the memories should be forgotten. Huh!

Monday, October 2, 1989: Monday mornings. These, a legend in their own time. School didn't seem anything marvellous; the class seems to be drifting in various corners somehow, but I guess we are less cohesive as we all have our different tutorial groups.

Tuesday, October 3, 1989: I know this may sound awful, but it is weird bitching about people. Sometimes people love it, other times – in fact, *always* – we have a guilty conscience in one way or another. It's like a sport; winning and losing. I hate people bitching about me. Every time we see the person who we have just been bitching about, it makes me inwardly smile and I think of her in a different light; sometimes this is a good idea and other times not! I don't like people who put on fronts either. It's lying to other people; it's like acting and not very nice; it's hard to be controversial and make a sentence in a word.

Thursday, October 5, 1989: We all "copped it" at Drama this evening. "The older ones should look after the younger ones. The older ones are not mature enough to go to the Workshop. There aren't any places. We've been worried about you for some time. All your teachers have noticed." One teacher has been with us for one term only. Don't they realise because we haven't got a good teacher, we don't work as well? Can't they see the comparison? I don't believe it. Jimmie said we were better than the Wednesday group. Don't they understand we can't express what we feel when the problem is surrounding us? They need to sort it out, not us! Well, that's passing the buck back to the powers that be, isn't it!

Friday, October 6, 1989: Babysitting this evening –yes, it's brought back memories of "The Way We Were"; that's one of my favourite songs in my teen years. The children were good. It was quite a good laugh, actually; very interesting. I wasn't scared either, which is a sign. But what sort of sign, I wouldn't like to say.

Monday, October 9, 1989: Good day, my foot! My nail broke at 6:45a.m, demonstrating what sort of day it was going to be. Oh yes, I know I am a teenager, so just give me licence to believe in fate (although I am a Christian!). Actually, I survived this Monday. Drama was good today. I got a lift home from school so bang goes my social life on the bus. E. had a better weekend than planned by the sound of it. Let's hope the ending is happy. I'm thinking a lot about the past, as usual. Past, present and future.

Tuesday, October 10, 1989: It wasn't a very good day at all today; in fact, I can't think of anything I enjoyed apart from Basketball with Martin C. Recently I've been making subtle but bitchy comments about people, which hasn't been very nice sometimes. I can't resist getting a word in edgeways – it seems I must always have a say in the matter.

Wednesday, October 11, 1989: Another normal day, nothing old. In fact, everything old but nothing new. There is nothing important to say unless I discuss other people's lives in depth and that won't be too interesting. Last Saturday I wanted to do something and this Saturday no one is doing anything. English was good. Jo wasn't in when I phoned her after school.

Thursday, October 12, 1989: Today was more like tomorrow, i.e. not the 12th, but Fri. 13th. One of my friends told me she didn't want to come to church anymore and she even apologised. There was nothing to apologise about, it was me who should say sorry. I haven't done my duty as I should have done. I knew it was coming and didn't do anything about it. This may mean that we grow apart. I don't feel close to anyone at school anymore or for that matter, at church. I don't even know if I am close to myself. It's like I'm two different people and I don't show the real me all the time. "Why am I afraid to tell you who I am?" The book by the author of *Why Am I Afraid to Love?* contains insights on self-awareness, personal growth and communication with others. Why do people continually hide their real selves from the people around them? Why are so many so insecure and afraid to open up? The answer, supported by John Powell, is that maturity is reached by our interactions with others. This book considers the consequences our real self faces if no one else ever finds out what we are like.

Well, that's a bit of intellectual writing, Claire; you surpass your journal jottings at times. No reader, it's not me, it's what Powell suggests.

Sunday, October 15, 1989: I had an awful dream last night. It's funny to think of my cousins when they're so far away; I miss them. I keep thinking the worst, which annoys me. I suppose I just feel sorry for myself. Me! Me! All the time. I doubt people think in the way I do. They probably don't always put themselves first! Tomorrow is a new day, whether filled with good or great things.

Monday, October 16, 1989: Another weird evening yesterday. I wonder if dreams do play a part in your sub-conscious; they must trigger something. Drama was weird today too, both sessions. I couldn't make my body want to move to get up and do anything. I know this current chest infection is wearing me down, but I can't blame it all on that.

Tuesday, October 17, 1989: Jo's 16th birthday today. She was fine and happy, which is the most important thing. Everything is excellent. Jo will never have a 16th birthday again, can you believe it?

Wednesday, October 18, 1989: San Francisco had an earthquake today; over 200 people killed. It devastated the whole city. It's strange to think that it could have happened a couple of months earlier. I can't believe how pathetic I look with my hair this colour in my school uniform. "Foul" is the only word in the human language that could possibly describe it. One only really sees these things happening in movies and not in real life-except in mine. It's strange to think what an earthquake can do to a whole city. Not long until the house party now, only a few days or so. Who's counting this year?

Friday, October 20, 1989: Church youth group house party but puncture on way so arrived at 1:00am. Fell into bed exhausted. Rain and more rain; the poor leaders.

Tuesday, October 24, 1989: Vicki became a Christian, which was a great encouragement.

Wednesday, October 25, 1989: The worst thing about going away is returning. I didn't feel like doing anything today, but I did. I miss everyone; the house, the atmosphere, the laughter, the food but most of all the people. It is sad to see people go, let feelings go and then react again. Feelings change slowly, but paradoxically quickly. I don't know how I feel or why I feel it, but I know I do feel it. In our heart to hearts together in our dorm, my friends said how they have the same kind of feelings. It was so great, and yet you only really appreciate it when it's over. . .gone away. My last one, maybe the last closeness.

Thursday, October 26, 1989: I couldn't settle down to work today as much as I would have liked. I keep having flashbacks of the house party and of how I miss it. Normally I would have been in floods of tears, but today I just feel sad. That's weird, I hate to say it but maybe I've changed a bit, from bad to worse. I enjoyed seeing *Macbeth*.

Sunday, October 29, 1989: Hannah's birthday today, 14 years old. She took care of me so well. Was willing to put herself out. I really enjoyed it. Special missionary weekend today and then visitors back for lunch. Hannah got a walkman as well as many other things. Mum is worried as she thinks we don't have a relationship anymore. Get a life, Mum, weren't you a teenager once?

Monday, October 30, 1989: I was depressed today and I couldn't hold it in and ruined things. Mum dropped me at Surbiton Station although I would have rather stayed at home. I'm fed up with my marks and with school; I know I don't try hard enough. There needs to be more motivation on my part. Went to the hospital and the doctor said I should have a long line (a long tube inserted into my arm to give intra-venous antibiotics and to save me having venflons, for which I need to stay in hospital). They feel this current chest infection has been rumbling on for too long and need to zap it. I am having the long line put in on Saturday and it seems like a scary experience. We all know why this came about, now don't we? Shh! I don't want to hear it repeated, that same old record of me not taking care of myself enough.

Tuesday, October 31, 1989: I didn't go to school today as I was feeling very unwell. It's good to know your friends do care about you when they ring up to ask why you are absent. Jo may have glandular fever, which isn't very nice. Poor love, that's all she needs at the moment. Hannah didn't sound too happy on the phone. I put it down to the poor quality of the tap water – well, we must blame something. But another explanation could be the time of the year, with winter bugs proliferant [sic]. There's always the spring to look forward to and those hot, summer, lazy days that everyone longs for when it's minus 5 degrees outside.

November 1989

Wednesday, November 1, 1989: Pinch-punch. . .the things we used to do when we were little kids. The fireworks can be heard now. It makes me look forward to ours at the weekend. I've told a few people about my life-line. I feel guilty telling people about it. It's like I'm wanting to gain as much attention as I can. There was a moody old lady on the bus today. I'm glad I didn't speak my mind, though. I was expecting to go over her knee any minute. The day seemed long today but it was survivable. Back to the dark evenings now. The sooner the better when spring and the longer days arrive again.

Thursday, November 2, 1989: In the words of the Beatles song by John Lennon and Paul McCartney, "My troubles don't just belong to yesterday. Nope, they're here and they won't go away!"

Drama was very enjoyable this evening. Marion took it again and we acted out some scenes about anorexia, rather scary. I got my photos back today from various holidays from the summer, which I really enjoyed seeing.

Saturday, November 4, 1989: I had my hair cut this morning –very nice too! I also spent the day at the hospital. After much ado, and 2 hours in the treatment room, hack-saw in hand, mask over face, the doctor managed to get the long line in on the 5th attempt. What more could I ask for. . .3 nurses, warm blankets, copious bowls of hot water to warm my veins. Success, but so painful. Mum now has the job of administering by antibiotics 3 times a day for 3 weeks. At present we have no idea how long it will take the both of us to do this. I came home with copious bags of syringes, needles and anti-biotic vials. If this is a welcome to CF taking on its next stage in my life, all I can say is, "Help!"

Sunday, November 5, 1989: Remember, remember the 5th of November. How could I forget? I felt ill this morning; the tube stung. Going to church was a mistake. People were very nice. Went to the hospital as antibiotics still stung. It was decided that the line wasn't in the vein but had tissued, so out came the line. Painful again and plasters where it was inserted. Felt an idiot and attention seeking, but hey, it wasn't exactly fun having it put in or taken out, so much for a long line meaning to last 3 weeks, less than 24 hours and loads of pain was what I got.

Monday, November 6, 1989: I didn't want to go to school today as I still felt so ill and of course I'm not getting the antibiotics through my veins that I need. The bus was cramped and awful; I hated it. I know it's wrong to be moaning, but I just couldn't stand it. Talking of not standing it, that's exactly what I had to do all the way to school, stand on the wretched bus when I was so unwell. At my piano lesson I had to explain to Mrs White all that had gone wrong over the weekend and why I couldn't play very well.

Tuesday, November 7, 1989: Basketball today and I wonder, should I have gone? Well, I did anyway. A face in the crowd? Maybe. I felt quite happy at lunchtime today but I feel as if I'm not really happy.

Wednesday, November 8, 1989: I don't know how I'm feeling today. I think wallowing in self-pity and sadness. Several reasons why; three come to mind but I'd better not say anymore. People have different moods at different times, me too. The Home of Compassion was quite good; well, I'm not sure that's the word but when one wants a part time job for the school holidays, you have to take what you can get. I was very nervous but it was okay. My mind keeps wandering to different things so I must learn to concentrate more. I wish I could be someone else for a minute and look at myself and hate it or like it.

Thursday, November 9, 1989: Great day, I wish. What sarcasm. I've got a great chance of getting in to the basketball team now. I got a B+ for my Drama essay. There are so many things worrying me at present; they seem like a long line of lead dragging behind me everywhere I go and whatever I do. L. is a bit upset. I wish I could think for myself and be a light in the darkness in a dead world.

Friday, November 10, 1989: Rainy day, but don't blame it on the rain. It was okay, I suppose. Biology was awful, but I cheered up as the day went on. Catherine is still unwell and away from school.

Saturday, November 11, 1989: I went to see *Shirley Valentine* with Ndullee, Beth and Rebecca. It was quite good, but rude. Now I know how my mother feels. We were chauffeured back and forth and saw an Elvis movie. Then we had a slap-up meal at Ndullee's, so an excellent day.

Sunday, November 12, 1989: Remembrance Sunday. It must be awful for all those people who remember poignantly the war/s that they either fought in, lost loved ones in, or read of/saw films of. I would have hated to live in those days. D. was upset today and I don't know how to help her; it's not as if I know what she's going through. S. and I aren't close anymore. I don't know how to handle that either. M. is lovely but I know she gets fed up listening to it all. In short, everything is a shambles. Oh, can't you see it, baby?

Monday, November 13, 1989: Memories. . .light the corners of my mind. "The Way We Were" is the title song to the 1973 movie (I read that in a book, too.) Sometimes it hurts to think about things that happened a long time ago. . .or even yesterday. I didn't socialise very much today. H. and J. aren't too excited about life at present. Guess who's going on the house party? It's all right for some; two house parties in three months! This news gave my warm blue eyes a green, icy glaze.

Wednesday, November 15, 1989: Tension within the form of IVB today, but I chose not to notice it until it knocked on my door. T. is fed up with L. and everyone else, including me. Apparently there are other tensions in form IVB. D. rang but I feel so nervous when we speak; my heart just pounds. It's unnerving. There are so many things I want to say, but I end up saying nothing.

Friday, November 17, 1989: Feeling ill again today, so actually stayed in this evening and watched "Children in Need" on TV, which was very sad. Among other stories it featured a lovely girl, Caroline, who risked so much for her sister. I wish I had that much strength and courage. Felt respect and proud to be living in the same country as her.

Saturday, November 18, 1989: Mum and I started to make the Christmas cake this morning, which was rather late to allow it time to mature, but never mind. Then we went up to Oxford Street, which was an experience. No, we didn't fall out. I got a skirt and a cardigan and a top. All very nice and I was quite thrilled in actual fact. And of course, a coat which is rather nice, but it drowns me. Tea at Auntie's and off to the swimming gala at

Epsom, which was okay, but so hot with the heat of the pool. We have very sore throats from shouting our encouragement.

Sunday, November 19, 1989: I didn't go out this morning – what a naughty girl but I just can't shake off this latest infection. I did go to church this evening, though, as I need to go to the hospital tomorrow and wanted a dummy run at being out.

Monday, November 20, 1989: Mum told on me to Dr S.; thanks very much, Mum. I have to go back in a couple of weeks and then the decision will be made about whether I have the long line or not and what will become of me.

Tuesday, November 21, 1989: I didn't go to school again today as I just wasn't well enough. It is easy to take life for granted; there are so many sick people in the world who will not see the beginning of the new year. I've decided that TV is boring and not worthwhile, though I did see the opening of Parliament, plus the situation in El Salvador. Yes, I have been watching the news for once. I should take life and my education more seriously. We are lucky to have this opportunity; some people do not.

Wednesday, November 22, 1989: Today was a hassle; I went to school, and tried to make it through until lunch time. My fever was causing me to get disoriented and after several failed attempts, got through to Mum who said I would be going into hospital tomorrow. I then blurted out to those around me what was happening. I don't reckon I'll have to stay in long, at least, I hope I don't have to. Piano was rushed. Then to "The Beaux Stratagem" in London, a comedy by George Farquhar. On return I had so much to do to prepare for tomorrow that I got to bed at 12:00.

Thursday, November 23, 1989: Hospital

Friday, November 24, 1989: long line in after 3rd attempt

Saturday, November 25, 1989: hospital until 30th November.

December 1989

Friday, December 1, 1989: I got a get well card from the class today, ah. I felt really ill last week but am better now, out of hospital and completely happy. I saw Hannah at the last minute and she's much better. We had a little chin-wag.

Saturday, December 2, 1989: We went Christmas shopping in Epsom. The meeting this evening was challenging and God spoke through Paul H. I've heard the Gospel message so many times now, but different speakers give their own distinctive view.

Sunday, December 3, 1989: The mission went very well again today and there were lots of people in church. Sang one of my favourite hymns: "And can it be, that I should gain, an interest in my Saviour's blood. . . . .My chains fell off, my heart was free," (Charles Wesley, 1738).

Monday, December 4, 1989: Back to school with a vengeance.

Wednesday, December 6, 1989: It was Catherine's birthday today and a very fine one at that.

Thursday, December 7, 1989: Ever since the beginning of the 4th year, the class doesn't seem to have its previous relationship bond that we had in the second and third years. We have less than 2 years of each other now, before we go our separate ways for 6th form or college to do A levels and then some of us may never see each other again. It's gone so quickly and it's hard to believe we're in the 4th year now. D. seemed depressed today, but there was little I could do to comfort her. I just don't seem to come out with the right notions or empathy anymore. I had to say goodbye to S. and K. and it was very tear-jerking and upsetting, but I pulled through. I say hello again to one friend and then in another breath, goodbye. It's scary.

Friday, December 8, 1989: Not a great evening. I had to tell someone and Mum was the only person I could tell. She gave me good advice, but I don't know whether it worked.

Saturday, December 9, 1989: I was still worried this morning but managed to survive; it's horrible when things like this happen and I worry it's my own fault, but having thought about it incessantly I know deep down it wasn't. I was on time to meet my friends in Kingston but it was heaving with the pre-Christmas rush and I still haven't got all my presents. Mum was really kind to me today, and the Panto for the Sunday school party went quite well but not brilliantly, especially as the Beanstalk fell down before the axe touched the root!

Tuesday, December 12, 1989: A free day was not spent wisely; there were fewer people in Kingston, considering how close we are to Christmas and compared with weekends. I'm finding Maths hard, but I must spare a thought for those who are worse off than me.

Wednesday, December 13, 1989: Mum really makes me feel so uneasy when she is sighing and tutting; it's very hard to remain sane. The reason was because we were late for physio and the Christmas traffic was worse than usual rush hour.

Thursday, December 14, 1989: We had another letter from Auntie Lesley today telling us of her concerns. I wish my family would give me more credit for my mature outlook on some things; yes, I can be very mature at times and feel strongly that I should be listened to. I can imagine myself as an old granny remembering my teenage years with relief that they are over. It is not nice to worry about others this much.

Saturday, December 16, 1989: Today I stayed in, apart from going into Surbiton for five minutes for a last minute gift I had forgotten. I spent the day wrapping presents and writing cards.

Sunday, December 17, 1989: The family came to lunch today and it went quite well. Mum got a bit frantic, which was understandable up to a point as there were lots of us, but we survived.

Monday, December 18, 1989: I'm getting more and more like my mother every day and I'm getting worse. I speak about the same things and it's getting boring, but I can't do much about it.

Wednesday, December 20, 1989: The final day of school for this term and it was great; we all thoroughly enjoyed ourselves. We ate, drank and were happy, but it was sad saying goodbye to everyone and it will be sad next year when we have to do the same, especially as it will be our final Christmas altogether. I just love my class so much on days like these; they are very understanding and lovely. This evening Hannah and Jo came round, but as usual we didn't do much and sat around watching a video and as soon as it ended their parents came to whisk them off home.

Thursday, December 21, 1989: The first day of the Christmas holiday! I know it sounds stupid, but I missed my class; I missed the atmosphere. We were sorely beaten at basketball – 69/25, ouch!

Friday, December 22, 1989: Why is the world so corrupt and why can't everyone live in harmony with their neighbour, whoever that may be? War divides the world, whether caused by religion, poverty or greed. No amount of money can replace love.

Saturday, December 23, 1989: The eve of Christmas Eve. I am concerned, as I anticipate the joy of Christmas, that so many around the world will go without. Why should many suffer, when others have in abundance?

Sunday, December 24, 1989: As I jot my diary entry I've got mixed feelings, mostly about boys. I feel anxious because of various things. I am excited about tomorrow; it will be a fun day. But in myself I don't feel complete; something is missing although it shouldn't be. I had a reasonably okay day. The carol service was heaving with people. Zoe came and enjoyed it very much.

Monday, December 25, 1989: I am really grateful and pleased with my pressies. The day worked out pretty well. Keyboard, toiletries, tapes, bracelets, earrings, chocolate, slippers, nightie for Christmas '89. Oh, to be a fourteen and a half years old forever! (Dear Diary, does that sound rather paradoxical as I peruse my last weeks of entries!)

Tuesday, December 26, 1989: Boxing day: We had the usual family and friends for the day today. I say the usual because they come every year. Next to Christmas day, I love Boxing day.

Wednesday, December 27, 1989: These are the last few days of 1989; I can't believe I've been alive for 14.5 years; I've got a lot to learn.

Thursday, December 28, 1989: I stayed in today; friends from church came. I went to stay at Zoe's for the night; in fact, the morning as we didn't get to sleep until around 5:00am.

Friday, December 29, 1989: There is not enough time left of 1989; the year when there were huge highs and deep lows. I can't really write anymore for this year. It has been memorable for so many different reasons. If I don't stop now I, who hate goodbyes, won't be able to bid *adieu* to this year of 1989.

Chapter Five

Your Senior School Years – 1990's Journals

Dear Claire,

With you having told me how much you had enjoyed writing a journal, in the diary I gave you for 1990 (the year you turned fifteen) I wrote these words, but have no idea where I found them, (and having searched online, I am still none the wiser.) I wrote: To Claire, "record each treasured moment, capture every thought, make these hungry, empty pages come alive."[26] I believe you accomplished this and more.

January 1990

Wednesday, January 3, 1990: Last lie in before school starts tomorrow. Went to the hospital. I will need to start seeing the cystic fibrosis team in London. My shared care between the two hospitals is coming to an end. I shall be so sad, as I really like Dr S. I need to give my all this year.

---

[26]   Record each treasured moment, (Source unknown)

Thursday, January 4, 1990: Phone call from doctors in London – I need to go up and have a consultation there. I feel boring and bland. . .back to reality. I watched too much television today – I think we should get rid of the TV. Then there would be so much more time, but I know I would miss it. I don't think I'll audition for the play this year –it takes up so much time and all rehearsals are on Sundays, and I need to put my faith first. I believe God was speaking to me today about keeping his Sabbath day holy. Our pastor and his family came for lunch today; it was good to see them.

Monday, January 8, 1990: It seemed a long day. . .must have seemed an even longer one for those who suffer. Basketball practice was good. We are improving, yeh!

Wednesday, January 10, 1990: It is the first day of the exams – geography was okay because I understood and had revised answers to the questions (isn't it good when such questions appear?) It's the 21st anniversary of Grandma Inch's death today (of course I never knew her). We know she is safe in heaven and that we will see her again.

Thursday, January 11, 1990: We had two hours to revise before our first exam of the day, but doing so in a noisy classroom is not ideal. However, I must be grateful I am in school, in a church, am taught well; so many in third world countries don't have such privileges. So many of my friends feel like I do; confused, uncertain, lacking in self-worth. . .

Friday, January 12, 1990: I'm glad I spoke with E. today – I want to help in any way I can. It feels the form is closer when we all have the worry of exams. School is satisfactory at present; I hope we will always be as close as we were in the third year. Together forever.

Sunday, January 14, 1990: It's so long since I've seen my friends from my previous school. We vowed never to lose touch, but times change, life moves on. Middle school is probably the best time in a child's life, learning and discovering life outside the furnace that awaits them in secondary school. Throughout my exams I have been more cheerful than usual, which has helped. During the summer holidays, Hannah and I are going to get up to a little monkey business but unfortunately not on the Costa Del Sol, but another thriving resort.

Tuesday, January 16, 1990: Exams over. As I trundled back from school and had my shower, I didn't feel as relieved as I thought I would. I was very tired and lonely. Mum came in at just the right time to drop me at the bus stop to meet my mates. My cousin is unwell; embedded fears and hidden worries. Communications about feelings are so important in every aspect of life. Why do we always feel we have to be as good as, or even better than the next person? People do need others to look up to in life – it needs a purpose. I guess God is that purpose, but so few recognise Him as the answer.

Friday, January 19, 1990: The school birthday proved a success. Gemma proposed a lovely thought of dedication and I so appreciated it. I will treasure it. London. here I come. After an enjoyable ride on the tube, blood tests, talking to the hospital staff, the doctor told me I may need to have an open lung operation – part of my lung removed. The news panicked my Mum a little. It's strange to be told such things. After the hospital visit,

Mum and I went on a shopping spree to Oxford Street and arrived home with many nice sale purchases. Visits to hospitals have their plus side. But looking around London today reminded me that the world is so large; "corrupt" was the word that stood out in my mind. The sullen buildings and murky sidewalks were depressing. The dogs smelling the litter and other creatures enveloping the alleyways. Over the years, everything has changed and developed, most of which is for the worst. "Before it hatches, don't count them."

Saturday, January 20, 1990: Today I have experienced new knowledge, some of which would have been best unknown and forgotten about completely. Family matters are very important to me; I want to know what concerns my family and I don't like secrets being held from me; I am 14 and old enough to be in the know. Similarly at my age I am old enough to tell people how I am health wise and for them not to keep asking my mum. I wasn't feeling great tonight at church, and maybe people could see I was unwell.

Monday, January 22, 1990: There is always a sluggishness on a Monday morning, but my concern is that the form is not as close as it used to be; there seems to be some fraying at the edges. Maybe we are just growing up more, but surely we still need each other just as much, if not more. I can hear the wind crack against the gables outside; the howling of the atmosphere surrounding the house. Each person is complex and incomprehensible, unless we are that person.

Tuesday, January 23, 1990: The day started off grim, although it improved by the end of it. As I walked aimlessly to the biology lab at lunch time the sky grew a shade darker, but my exam mark was acceptable – I gave a long sigh of relief. My exam results as a whole have not been totally nerve-wracking, but it will be this time next year when I take my GCSEs that will be the real test.

Friday, January 26, 1990: As I have not auditioned for the school play this year, I decided to volunteer to be in the costume department. It was hectic today in readiness for next week when there will be full dress rehearsal, but I got by on a wing and a prayer. After school Mum was a little cross with me and my behaviour, but I have to take responsibility for myself now. I'm 14 years old. She understands about my exam results, however, which helps a great deal. She recognises that illness has played a large part this last year or so. There were many injuries yesterday and lives lost due to the weather. It seems that we will have to expect more of this in the future as this is part of the greenhouse effect and will continue. Insignificant is how I feel.

Monday, January 29, 1990: The sun shone so brightly today and it lifted my spirits. I could've been walking down a Spanish dirt track, but it wouldn't have mattered. We received two more exam results today, after teeth-chattering and nail-biting. They weren't as bad as I thought, so thank you, God. My piano lesson wasn't great, but I know I worry too much and am such a self-doubter. Think vertical.

Tuesday, January 30, 1990: I didn't make the basketball team; sometimes I feel so worthless and stupid, but Ms. E. said that obviously my lungs are not great and that has an effect on my energy levels, which begs the question: Why does CF have to get in the way of sport? But I'm not the only one to feel upset. D. was so depressed and it seems nothing will cheer her up. She said she hated herself, no one liked her and life was awful. I told her that just wasn't true that we all go through these kinds of feelings but that we all adored her. The need to sustain sanity. The car got bashed by another mother outside school today. Mum was none too happy, but very polite. It was embarrassing as I know the other girl. I haven't watched hardly any of the Commonwealth Games this year.

Wednesday, January 31, 1990: The form seems happily satisfied with each other at the moment, which is a good place to be.

February 1990

Sunday, February 4, 1990: After Bible class it was my turn to do church crèche – the little ones are so sweet; there is a baby boom coming up again soon, so we will be overcrowded and may need to change rooms. This evening's sermon was on Revival – we are so consumed with our lives, careers, families that we give such little time to God and what He wants us to do. My key word for today is, "priorities."

Monday, February 5, 1990: It was a manic Monday today. We were all slightly aghast, but too polite to really say so at D.'s comments. Hopefully she will return to her normal self soon. Mum and I went into Kingston for an hour as she collected me from school.

Wednesday, February 7, 1990: It seems as if it should be the end of the week, not just the middle as I am always so tired. The consultant said this is natural when you have a lot of chest infections and on antibiotics; she suggested I try to equate it to how people feel when they have flu or just getting over it, i.e. lethargic, difficulty concentrating, etc. I guess that makes sense. When I am old I expect I will look back on this diary and the pages will scream at me: "Hello, I was fourteen and half years old when I wrote this; here are my views on abortion, nuclear waste, the environment and yes, us humans are complex beings, too complex for man to fully understand." I sincerely hope I will get wiser as I get older. I guess even the successful get worried at some point. I want to be my true self with God's help, instead of thinking of myself as an outsider to my own life. It was good to chat to Hannah, Jo and Rachel after church. Key word for today: "chameleon."

Sunday, February 11, 1990: Nelson Mandela is to be freed today. It is now 13:45 and he should have been freed at 13:00. All the world is watching; the crowds have gathered in huge anticipation – this is a real watershed in history. Post script; he was released at 14:12; at least that is when we saw him among the cheering masses. I am so pleased to have witnessed this great event. Today was quite relaxing for me, although Mum works so hard. Church was good, but I need to concentrate more. I find at times that my mind wanders all over the place. If I call myself a Christian, I must behave like one.

Monday, February 12, 1990: Hospital appointment after school to collect the new nebuliser. I hope it will be as effective as the last. I saw the physiotherapist and need to do lots more physio each day and she said she is going to keep on at me! Hospital appointments are so tiring after school because I get home late, we eat late and I start my homework late, ugh. Apparently the hospital has signed me up for a medical trial. They asked for my permission and I said yes, but only if I didn't have to go more often, because I told the doctor how difficult it is to get over to Epsom from Kingston at the end of a school day and in the rush hour.

Tuesday, February 13, 1990: Basketball at lunchtime in the Hall was a treat, especially as we couldn't get out at recess because the rain was so heavy again today. Mum was waiting for me at the bottom of the hill as I got off the bus, so it was good not to have to walk home as sometimes it's the last straw at the end of a long and busy day. Christian Union meetings have now changed to Thursday lunchtimes, and I must give these priority.

Monday, February 26, 1990: It was good to be back among all my school friends today, my travelling companions on the bus were all pleased to see each other (my Mum drops me off on her way to work, so it saves the walk from our house down the hill, but coming up the hill on the way home is, of course, a battle). I had my interview for Bourne House Care Home today. I have applied to work as a kitchen assistant one evening a week straight after school. I have no idea if I gave the correct answers or not, but I got the job. (Big deal!)

Wednesday, February 28, 1990: I doubt everyone is happy; in fact I know they are not. Many of my peers are confused and intimidated despite our outward appearances.

March 1990

Thursday, March 3, 1990: I started my new job at Bourne House this evening. I have had to persuade Mum to let me take it, arguing that it is only one evening a week for 3 hours, and so close to home. She is not keen that

I am going straight from school, but she knows how much I want it so we have decided to give it a go.

Friday, March 2, 1990: I must admit I don't like Bourne House; it is very old and gives me the creeps. The residents, however, are lovely, although many are deaf and I hate shouting; it seems rude. My job is to lay the tables for tea, heat the soup, take the sandwiches and cakes from the cook and put them on the table once the residents are seated. I then make their cups of tea, and when they have all finished (being careful not to rush them), I then have to clear up, wash and dry up (no dishwasher) and then prepare the cups for their evening drink prior to them going to bed. I then lay the tables for breakfast. It is a full on 3 hours and I felt good to have learned what to do so quickly. The owner of the Home, a doctor, seemed quite pleased with me, but boy the washing up takes ages. Mum was waiting for me on the doorstep when I got home, anxious to know how it went. I feel so privileged living in the west, I know I should think of myself less especially as I am a Christian, but it is so hard when I feel inferior so often.

Saturday, March 3, 1990: Help! I do take after my mother although I would never admit publicly to it, but I guess you pick up family traits and are like the people you live with, to a certain degree.

Sunday, March 4, 1990: We stayed in this afternoon and relaxed as Mum is working herself far too hard. I need lessons on relying on God more. D. was upset/confused at church this evening but weren't/aren't we all, with so many things to contend with? I'm worried about the future, and not just my future. What will this generation be like as adults? What are we going to do? How can we make the world better? Can we all work together for peace? (It's not been achieved yet.) Life is lived on tenterhooks. A step towards tomorrow could be what we are dreading most. Are people really so bitter that they can't forgive? Why am I such a hypocrite? What am I doing towards world peace? Days/time is short and we have the solution, God, but we have to tell the world.

Church was a real challenge this evening. (I love Youth After-Church at our Pastor's house, but if it goes on too late I hate having to leave early as I have to fit my physio and medication in before going to bed.) I am shallow and unconcerned for the salvation of my friends and family members that don't know God. But how do I not feel superior when talking with them about Christianity and how do I tell them of the need for Him when they say I am preaching? I have so much to learn. D. is worried about J., and vice versa, and none of us know what to do to help.

Monday, March 5, 1990: It wasn't a bad Monday morning today, but it was Monday without doubt. The light coming through the window early this morning is good; the days of getting up in the dark have gone for the summer. The class felt whole today and not bitty as it did last week. It takes a while to get used to school again, even though it has only been the weekend. We had some worthwhile lessons, which I enjoyed. I need to concentrate on schoolwork and stop doing the unnecessary, silly things I do with my time before it's too late. Take heed to what parents say; they are more educated than us.

Tuesday, March 6, 1990: We played hockey today and I've come to the conclusion that there's nothing like a good game of hockey to get the muscles moving, especially in key positions like goal. This was followed by contemporary dance. I felt a bit more of the class today, which I haven't recently.

My mind is wandering again and I feel we should have a long retirement in our teens instead of being worked so hard. They say the teens/being young are the best years of your life, so why not have time to enjoy?

Retirement in your sixties sounds like one is just waiting for death. Waiting must be awful, especially as you realise you are not getting younger and life is betraying you. Whichever way you look at it, it still spells the same verb: restless.

Wednesday, March 7, 1990: I can't believe I messed that phone call up so much. I've waited 3 weeks for it and I had to ruin it. I am so stupid. What must he think of me? The lesson on abortion went okay, although I was accused of being totally biased against it. Yes, one can debate the pros and cons of subjects, but at the end of the day, if you are not true to yourself and your Christian convictions, what can you be loyal about? I think our side of the debate deserved a better response, but I don't feel embarrassed about making my stand. I was shaking, but managed to control myself. 37 for abortion with 25 against – not as bad a result as I thought. I continue to not understand myself and until I can, how do I go about sorting my feelings out? Key word: "Mouth zip."

Thursday, March 8, 1990: I felt so worthless today and miserable, but what can I expect from a loser like me? I don't understand why people always put themselves first, why they so often change their opinions of people; why people don't understand themselves or those around them; why people fantasize, hide their true feelings and put up a front. "Nicholas Nickleby" is a very good play and I really enjoyed it.

Friday, March 9, 1990: Today seemed more like a Monday than a Friday. I should enjoy school more, but then does anyone really do so? Considering I wasn't going to go in today after Mum's outburst last night, it wasn't a bad day. Maybe she knows something about growing up, too. Think before you speak next time, Claire. I learned that I should try hard to understand people more before I criticise.

Christian Union was good today, over 50 of us, very encouraging. We got our school reports today and I wasn't as psyched up about it as I thought I would be.

Saturday, March 10, 1990: The adults in my family seemed a little confused today and I can't blame them; life even as an adult must seem a little scary at times too. My cousins do understand about their parents' break up to a degree, but are much too young to fully comprehend it. It was "shake a tin" day for cystic fibrosis again today, although the Lifeboat Brigade seemed to overpower us. I guess it is all charity anyway. Going by train to Guildford to shop with Hannah was good. I got my school bag; it was okay, but not fantastic. It was a different shopping experience than Kingston and had lots of interesting precincts. We must go again in the holidays.

Sunday, March 11, 1990: I was furious about the situation this evening. I needed more self-control, but didn't have any. Here's where I ended up: worse than before. My mind is too tired to question; my head too full. Why do people behave so weirdly? Why are we in such foul moods at times? South Africa looked quite beautiful and it was good to see what was going on there. The language of love pulls us together, never apart. Key words: "A cry in the dark," "mixed emotions," "self-control." My piano lesson was okay, but I left my music bag there which was such a pain as we had to go back for it. Key word: "Dull."

Tuesday, March 13, 1990: I had a day off school today – my fever was really high from tonsillitis and I felt better for sleeping.

Wednesday, March 14, 1990: Another day off school. I always felt girls off sick with tonsillitis were weak, but boy, now I know differently. I feel I should be at school, or at least up and doing things; I must have a problem with guilt. 2 weeks today and my piano exam will be over. Friends phoned, so that was nice.

Thursday, March 15, 1990: I went back to school today – it takes a while to get into the swing of things and to feel welcome. I still don't feel myself, as my mother would say; my throat still really sore, but one can't laze about forever. I had Christian witness opportunities today but unsure if I handled them well. I received my first two wage packets today, which was nice. After all, that's why I'm doing the job, to get some extra pocket money. It wasn't too hard an evening and good job, considering how I felt.

Friday, March 16, 1990: I felt in a positive mood this morning (note past tense). I was annoyed with Mum again at dinner time. I just wish the world was just one big, happy family. There must be something that can be done about this world of friction and sadness; something that can draw us together again; to break the chains of sin.

Saturday, March 17, 1990: It's funny how I always seem to argue with my mum these days; it never used to be as bad as this. I don't think she has any patience at all and she makes work for herself. She is annoying to the limit. What I say in private is very different to what I say in public. It was a lovely sunny day and we had lunch in the garden again, I love eating *al fresco*. Do you know where you are going to? Do you like the things that life is showing you? If at first you don't succeed, try, and fail again. I need strength and support and confidence. It's a cruel world.

Sunday, March 18, 1990: I was interviewed for an article that came out today, in *the Independent on Sunday*, by Sharon Kingman: "Cruel Genes Make Hard Choices." She said I had clear views on abortion when I argued that: "If I had been terminated, it would have been a waste of a life." Some of my friends and people from church said I was testament to that. I like to think I have made a difference in some small way to this little corner of the world.

Tuesday, March 20, 1990: Was late up this morning that didn't prove too popular with Mum. She gets into a fluster, insisting on doing things her way and will not listen. We travelled up to London for my hospital appointment. She did pick holes in the receptionist, which I thought was a little unfair. Apparently I'm doing okay health-wise. I'm quite a weepy person and have no self-control. I bite back at everyone systematically and don't care about their feelings or concerns at all. My friends seem to be in an equal state of disrepair as I am; I want to help them. I miss D., we all do.

Wednesday, March 21, 1990: I was even later up this morning and Mum was even less ecstatic than yesterday, but cooled down quickly. Everyone was being nice to me today but I doubt it will last long, not because of them but because of me. It was all drama this evening at home; Mum had four phone calls back to back. I had two, one that didn't go too bad until I reflected on what I had said. He didn't have a good impact on me; I didn't get excited at all. I think I will have to make up my mind before it is made up for me. Coughing, nose running, full blown infection again. Sticks and stones will break your bones, but words will never hurt me. How false that is. We are all hurt by people's unkind words. Work wasn't so bad today. People there are talking to me more and help a bit as I think they realise how hard it is to do all that work in 3 hours. I don't want to hurt him, but I really don't know what to do or say. Key words: "Mission impossible."

Friday, March 23, 1990: The sun was shining this morning, despite the feeling of gloom and despair all around. Other people have so many problems. I just want to get all my coursework out of the way forever, but of course that is not possible. I know so little about myself and that is worrying, to say the least. I bought some new Converse boots today!

Saturday, March 24, 1990: Mum and me went to Guildford today and it was rather good, although I can't remember exactly all that we did. The shops are much better in Guildford, as we found out. It was quite a struggle climbing the hill, though. Finding where to park was also a bother, but we managed to do quite a few things in the 2 hours we were there. I continue to be worried about various matters. I wish my nose would stop running with this cold. I wish also that I could stop coughing.

Tuesday, March 27, 1990: My piano exam didn't go as badly as I thought it would, PTL! I need to ask God to help me decide on my future as I'm not sure what I want to do. Someone, somewhere, is worse off than you.

April 1990

Tuesday, April 3, 1990: Today is so hot, we don't even need our blazers; something to chalk up for the beginning of April. I can't believe I'm going to Belgium in a couple of days. I handed my computer coursework in, which was quite a relief, especially as I was up until nearly mid-night doing it (only 3 of us handed it in on time). No wonder I am so tired today. My chest infection is still not better and that's why I feel *tres* fatigue.

Wednesday, April 4, 1990: It is now 2:50 in the morning, and Mum, if you ever read this, please don't go mad. I have a perfectly reasonable explanation (even though I cannot think of it at this present moment!).

Thursday, April 5, 1990: This afternoon at school was brilliant. I really felt wanted and people were so kind to me. I could hardly believe it. To what do I owe this pleasure? As the last day of term, quite a few people are off on their travels and it seems we'll have circled the world between us soon.

Wednesday, April 18, 1990: Being back in England is not such a great shock to me. Sometimes I feel just too tired to feel anything else. I can't believe I lived through yesterday, to touch and feel it with my emotions. I loved being with my cousins and being with all their friends. I left a part of me there, which I believe will always be in Brussels. Now I look to the future but don't forget anything that has happened in the past. I feel better to know that maybe I will see the people I met again, that we'll be back together again someday. I'm sorry that things were bad for one person in the group, but I am sure situations happen for us to learn from. Paradoxically, I was pleased to be home for various reasons; yes, it was good to be home again.

I wanted to spend time with the family; to sleep in my own bed; to feel wanted at home.

Friday, April 20, 1990: Having spent time with my grandparents, they brought me home and then I went to work. I was looking forward to Mum coming to help and I think that's what kept me going. If she hadn't been there, I don't honestly think I could have managed it by myself at all and I probably would have been quite upset. A quick transformation in the car and all was in order, a Wonder Woman-type job. The basketball gig was quite enjoyable. A ray of light down a dark tunnel.

Sunday, April 22, 1990: We watched Uncle Keith complete the marathon this afternoon; his time was 4 hours, 45minutes and 5 seconds. So many people running – they all looked like spare ribs wrapped in their tin foil. The atmosphere was great; we were scanning the whole area for him and eventually found him. So proud of him; he deserves his long bath.

Monday, April 23, 1990: I suppose it was good to be back at school and among friends again today. It felt like a normal school day, with all the usual hustle and bustle of getting to lessons on time, etc. I passed my piano exam, great news.

Tuesday, April 24, 1990: Another game of basketball this evening and loved it.

Wednesday, April 25, 1990: This time next year we will be in the 5th form and it will be some people's last term at Tiffin. Not everyone wants to stay on in school into the 6th form, so they are opting to go to 6th form colleges instead. Some people influence us more than we realise.

Friday, April 27, 1990: It was a lovely morning today and my mind was in the summer term mode again. I think of all the faces who I so very often see and talk to everyday, but only a few are mentioned by me at home.

There must be so much going on in a school which we never hear about and will never do so, and this is quite worrying because it baffles me as to the real ins and outs to a school. Who will tuck my conscience to sleep now?

May 1990

Saturday, May 1, 1990: All this teenage strife is silly and wrong, especially as it was another lovely, hot day today and we've had so many lately. I can't believe we are into the 5th month of 1990; a day of sport and nice things. But despite all this, I didn't really enjoy school today; however, who really does? We enjoy being with our friends and also some lessons, but not exactly school in its bare sense at all. I am pleased he rang again today.

Thursday, May 3, 1990: Apparently we are in the middle of an official heatwave, but it is hard to say exactly how long it will last. I'm so glad my friends came to Christian Union with me today; I hope they continue to come. Working in a steamy kitchen was really difficult in the heat, especially as this current chest infection seems to go on and on. I am off intravenous antibiotics, but the oral ones still make me feel less that great. But one thing I do know – the summer climate suits me much better than the winter. I doubt I'm the only one who likes to be busy, because then we don't have to think about things so much. A cycle ride this evening with friends was fun. One thing becomes more apparent every day (and here I go again) – we all battle with feelings of low self-esteem, wondering who we really are, and what others think of us. I think Mum knows there is something wrong but she is unsure (as I am) as to what it is. The situation does worry me as I suppose she feels the same away, although I'm unsure of that but that is just one of those things. I'm not content about anything, just worried too much.

Tuesday, May 8, 1990: School was basically fine today and I guess in many respects it always is; I just make it more of a problem. So many of my friends need help and I hope my efforts are sustaining them enough until they feel they can ask others, too.

Friday, May 11, 1990: The last day of school with the 5th and 6th formers today as then they all have exam leave. Odd to think it will be us in the 5th year next year. We all need to believe in ourselves more.

Tuesday, May 15, 1990: I have to be so careful of some of the company I keep. Some parents are not as discerning regarding what their children watch and I need to be able to extradite myself from situations that I should not be in. How does one do this without causing offence? But as a Christian I must.

Sunday, May 20, 1990: Mum insisted we go to the hospital today (why does she feature so much in my journal? I guess, Dear Diary, we could answer that either positively or negatively, though methinks the latter is the correct response) and I wasn't really in a dominant position to argue. We went and did I have a nice doctor? Yes, a very nice doctor indeed, which made me very happy, despite feeling so ill. The poor little boy who wouldn't eat anything was just skin and bones; I felt sad and upset to look at him. I was so sad to see his grandma (in a wheelchair) unable to comfort him or have him on her lap. She must have felt such frustration and heartache. How do people in those situations cope? I don't understand life.

Friday, May 25, 1990: It was quite a good day at school today, without too many hurdles to cross, and thus relaxing. I always feel a bit nervy and upset when I am at school, but today was very teary, though maybe it's all the antibiotics kicking in. However I feel, I do know that I am a sociable person and love being in contact with people, strange as that seems! Exams looming and I hardly see any school friends outside of school, but we are all in the same boat. Poor loves, they (and I) are in the middle of such a worrying time. Church Camp this weekend!

Wednesday, May 30, 1990: I looked to see what I had put in my diary this time last year. My feelings now are more subdued and not so strong, so maybe that is a good thing. I certainly felt camp withdrawal symptoms today and was extremely tired, sad and fed up but I suppose the feelings were and should be natural in many respects. I felt quite ill, depressed and tearful with my thoughts, "Misty water coloured memories at the way we were," (I have the words to it now.) Mmm. Mmm.

"The Way We Were"

Mem'ries

Light the corners of my mind

Misty water-colored memories

Of the way we were

Scattered pictures,

Of the smiles we left behind

Smiles we give to one another

For the way we were.

Can it be that it was all so simple then?

Or has time rewritten every line?

If we had the chance to do it all again

Tell me would we? Could we?

Mem'ries, may be beautiful and yet

What's too painful to remember

We simply choose to forget

So it's the laughter we will remember

Whenever we remember

The way we were. . .

The way we were. . . .[27]

Auntie Pat collected me today and it was nice to see her. Auntie Shirley, also. I love my family so much and I don't know what I would do without their support – all the times they have encouraged me and stood firmly beside me. I love them.

June 1990

Monday, June 4, 1990: I didn't want to see him today, but surprise, surprise he came to collect me. Sometimes there is no one I can talk to about this, apart from God. I feel I let down my church friends, but going back to school today it was good to see everyone again. I don't want to portray Christianity as a life of negatives, but at times, one has to take a stand. I

---

[27] The Way We Were Words and Music by Alan Bergman, Marilyn Bergman & MJarvin Hamlisch © 18th May 2015, Reproduced by permission of EMI MUSIC PUBLISHING LIMITED, London W1F 9LD

love being a Christian and am so thankful for such a supportive church, which is behind me all the way. We don't have to see the consultant until September, which is great as I take that to read that I am very well. Mum gets frantic about me, but there is no need to worry. I am fine and always will be. A poor child lost his life in Chessington today and I must stop worrying about my feelings (my dairy, whilst writing about friends too, is mostly about myself; how selfish can I get?) when a whole family has been torn apart. Christian Union today was great; our pastor came to speak and loads of my friends came. I needn't have worried all morning. It certainly had that panic feeling, although totally unnecessary. How relieved I was that all went well. I am trying to be really supportive to those who have problems and I want to say the right words; do the right thing. How much I need God's help. Altogether it was a good day, feeling close to people; feeling happy.

Sunday, June 10, 1990: June should be a happy, warm, glowing month, full of airs and graces, a good summer fun time which everyone enjoys. But I need to stop fantasizing, sort my confusion out on so many things and concentrate on the important aspects of life. Maybe I could scrape my face up from the floor and smile again. I love the sound of the ten o'clock news on ITV (Independent Television). It makes me feel quite happy and it has a certain peace connected to it. Together with loads of classmates I gained a bronze award (some got gold, others silver) in the British Association for the Advancement of Science.

July 1990

Sunday, July 1, 1990: I have given up my job in the Care Home because it was really interfering with my homework on Thursday evenings too much. I wrote: "I am writing to inform you that, due to increasing homework, it will be necessary to cease employment with you. However I do hope that in the future I may have the opportunity of working here again." I am so pleased I did it for three months, but I pride myself on the vibes I feel about certain places and I got bad vibes from there; not from the staff or the residents, but from the old building. Normally I love old building, but no that one! I earned £10.50 each evening and that went a long way to buy clothes over the summer.

I had a nice reference from them today. It read: "1st March-19th July 1990: Kitchen Assistant, Bourne House Residential Care Home: We found Claire hard-working, pleasant, trustworthy, reliable and eager to learn." And to me: "Please let me know if you want to work for us in your school holidays."

Friday, July 6, 1990: This weekend Mum took us (a group of my school friends and me) down to the family caravan in the New Forest in Dorset. We soon unpacked, decided where we were all going to sleep and then drove down the road to get fish and chips for supper. Then we sat in the car and let Mum chauffer us to where we wanted to go.

Saturday, July 7, 1990: New Milton supermarket was our first stop this morning to buy food for today, then back to the caravan for lunch and then to the beach, which brought back happy memories for us all and which we could all relate to. Then on to Bournemouth via the garden route, which I personally thought was brilliant. I love Bournemouth because it is so welcoming and happy and joyful. It was fun. The beach was lovely; the steps down and the garden area leading to the beach were, too. Burger King for tea (which we all enjoyed), sharing a window seat, and then to the beach again. Later in the evening we watched Wimbledon tennis, then a film. We talked (at least they did while I fell asleep and missed all the fun) into the early hours.

Sunday, July 8, 1990: I woke in a mad panic thinking that Mum was not up, but all was okay. We messed about, talked and had breakfast. We went to the beach again and enjoyed ourselves; felt quite refreshed and windswept. But the result was definitely worth it and we felt the better for it. Then to Christchurch, which, again I love. Between us we bought out the cake shop. We ventured into novelty shops and into the Quay. My mind is full of happy memories of the weekend and I just can't believe what a good time we had; it was so enjoyable. We then returned to the caravan and packed up all our stuff, walked to the lake and around the holiday home site and then hopped in the car to leave. I was hungry although the others weren't, so we waited until we reached Guildford to picnic before driving on home.

Saturday, July 21, 1990: Dear Diary, I just haven't found the time to write daily, but you will know that I am away on holiday with my church friend, Hannah and her family on the Isle of Wight for my fifteenth birthday.

A very early start today, I meant to be awake at 4:00 but it was 4:30a.m until I came into the land of the living. I was collected at 5:00 and we were in Portsmouth to catch the ferry by 6:30. We made an early visit to the beach at Ryde, then for lunch and onward to the caravan site at Whitecliffe Bay. The bay is lovely and very much reminds me of Blackpool sands in Devon.

Sunday, of course, found us in church. A United Beach mission team was in the service, too. I have applied to serve on a team next year (when I'll be old enough), so it was good to see them.

I, of course, brought the "must have" reading with me: *I Know My First Name is Steven* (Mike Echols, Pinnacle Publishers, 1989). This is an extremely worrying book. The poor child, as no one would have ever understood the pain, trial and torment he went through for seven whole years. We can never begin to understand all of his anxieties, how emotionally mixed up he must have felt and totally scared about how he was mistreated. What a disgusting and mixed up world we live in, to say the least. How can we educate our children to live happy, normal lives when there are monsters of evil all around? It makes me feel sick. No one could understand Steven at all; no one really wanted to try. He didn't have a social worker or someone he could speak to properly about his guilt, which never should have been lain on his shoulders. If only there could have been someone he could really confide in, young as he was.

Sunday, July 29, 1990: We enjoyed visiting so many places on the Island but today it clouded over, so we spent the time to the best of our resources, hunting for rock pools. The last hours of my fourteenth year approach, I feel remorse, not happiness. Today was thoughtful, reminiscing on my first years as a teenager. I have looked back with a mixture of good and bad memories, but none of which I can forget. I know that I don't want to grow older. Fifteen. I dreamt of being fifteen, but that was so long ago and so hard to remember, but there is no turning back now. I need to work much harder, be a better friend, get good GCSE results and most of all to serve God in all that I do.

August 1990

Wednesday, August 1, 1990: My first new month as a fifteen year old. A new beginning. We spent most of the day sunbathing and relaxing on the beach. The sea was cool, but deliciously inviting after the hot sand – the swim very refreshing. This evening we enjoyed a volleyball session on Sandown beach with the United Beach Mission team. I was surprised to see so many teenagers there. I'll never see that team again; maybe I will work with teenagers. Key words: "Heart yearning."

Thursday, August 2, 1990: I'm going to miss Hannah and her parents and Whitcliffe Bay. I love holidays and am often spoilt for choice. The Isle of Wight looks quite a distance from us now. I love the South Coast of England. I dread the time when there will be no caravan, no Hampshire, Dorset, Devon, Somerset – indeed all the old haunts.

Monday, August 13, 1990: It feels strange being back home again, but sort of good and enjoyable. Home! I sorted my room out today and then spent hours on the phone catching up with friends. Joni Eareckson-Tada spoke at a local church this evening. She had a great sense of humour and was just so caring toward us, her audience. Even though she was in a wheelchair, she obviously is so used of God, and there is no sense of any bitterness toward her accident that paralysed her from the neck down. I'd love to work with the marginalised in our society. Show me the way Lord, please.

Wednesday, August 15, 1990: I cycled to the "mentally handicapped" club today. I don't like that name, but that's what the Local Authority refers to it as on the forms we have to complete if we want to help. Terry wasn't there;

he wasn't well, poor love. I felt so sorry for him. They had the bouncy castle today; it was lovely to see them so happy and contented. Helen was very upset today, demonstrated by lots of head banging and there was nothing we could do to stop her or take her mind off it. I hate to see children so disturbed when they have enough to cope with in life. I feel a great deal of empathy for their parents, too.

Thursday, August 16, 1990: It didn't sink in today that my Belgian cousins will be arriving this evening. Lunch with Catherine from school was nice. We are going up in the world, dining at the Next Café and it was good to speak of our friendships together. I came back home, but only Laurent was there; my twin girl cousins were out. We decided to go to Chessington World of Adventures tomorrow. We are so fortunate to have it on our doorstep. Then the day after we will all go shopping in Kingston.

Sunday, August 19, 1990: A traditional family lunch, followed by my cousins and Auntie Lesley coming to church and I was so pleased they came with me (Auntie Lesley, when she was growing up in Chessington, used to come with her friends in their day). We took up a whole middle row; fantastic.

Monday, August 20, 1990: Our big day out today. London, here we come, but before that was my boring physiotherapy, then my cousins and I met "the Clan" at Surbiton station. The sightseeing tour of the Capital was great; Big Ben, Houses of Parliament, the Tower of London, St. Paul's Cathedral, Westminster Abbey and Buckingham Palace. I don't know if my cousins enjoyed the sight-seeing tour but I thought it was marvellous; extremely enjoyable and fun! We had lunch by the river, then on to Oxford, Carnaby and Regent Streets before heading home in the rush hour crush for a meal and a relaxing evening.

Tuesday, August 21, 1990: An early rise this morning. They have left, gone just after 7:00a.m. It was good to share a goodbye hug because touch is so important in most relationships, but especially with family and friends. I didn't want them to go and it is hard to say goodbye to a little part of you because you feel you have lost something. All I really wanted to do was pretend they were still here when I got home from Kingston seeing friends, and then I just wanted to be by myself in my own mind and thoughts.

Wednesday, August 22, 1990: Today was set aside for working, but as usual I did not get down to the nitty-gritty as I was supposed to do. I lazed about all day feeling quite neglected and in a state of remorse. I don't really know how I feel; maybe a bit sad but on the other hand, incredibly okay. Baby-sitting this evening was fine. Claire (my name-sake) put on her ballet shoes and danced around; Karen is such a darling; all three of them are like porcelain dolls. I was ever so pleased to help; it was so enjoyable. For my younger English cousins it is a time of confusion, following the break-up of their parents. Good job. Auntie Shirl is such a constant in their lives. Why is life so rewarding and yet also difficult at times? Why does it hurt so much? Solemnly, we are the next generation, as the adverts say, but what are we going to do about it? An argument with my mum was sad. I sobbed because I don't know what's wrong with me.

Saturday, August 25, 1990: It seemed strange to be in Dartmouth again as we descended the steep hill past the Naval College, looking at all the places with their great memories when Hannah and I had come down last year to stay with my Uncle Keith. I loved the town this evening –the vibrant lights. If I ever fell head over heels in love with a place, it would definitely be Dartmouth.

Sunday, August 26, 1990: When I turned around and saw his face, my tummy kept giving me butterflies. I glanced around again, but he was gone. It was so strange to see the people we were so friendly with last year, and yet 12 months on we are different people. I loved him maybe? It was a relief and yet it broke my heart to see him. Key words: "I'll get over you. I know I will."

This afternoon we went for a superb walk right out to Sugary Cove (I love that name!). It was beautiful – deserted, despite it being an August Bank Holiday weekend, when everyone wants to catch the last of the summer before returning to another academic year at school, etc. I just can't describe the setting; it is truly out of this world. I love it.

Then this evening, after watching my uncle play in a tennis doubles match (great that he and his tennis partner won), we walked by the boat float. It was so good to just walk; feel free and safe. I need this place! Dartmouth Regatta is definitely the week to be down in the West Country. Following our walk, my uncle had his tennis friends back for drinks. I love serving them all and chatting while I do the rounds, glancing occasionally out the window to the view from my uncle's house. You need to see it to believe it. The Red Arrows (the Royal Air Force Aerobatic team) gave a superb display over the river and the fireworks were definitely better than last year.

September 1990

Sunday, September 2, 1990: Up early this morning to see the last of the tennis and also for us to play a game on the Naval College courts before heading home. So sad because this is also the end of our summer before returning to Surrey and thence to school for our 5th year. Not a little sad to say goodbye to this beautiful part of South Devon.

Monday, September 3, 1990: Back home in Oaks Way. I'm glad I spoke to Hannah at length today. I just can't abide coming home from holiday; it is one of the worst things in the world, whatever anyone says to disprove that fact. I stayed in today because on days like this it is not a wise decision to venture out. It was a relaxing day, which I think I needed. It's strange being back home and I miss the views in Dartmouth. I miss the people and I miss most other things about it, too. How anyone would want to live in a city compared to Dartmouth, I really don't know.

Tuesday, September 4, 1990: It was good that I was busy this morning. I didn't feel like doing an awful lot, but I was quite content with the manner in which all things turned out. The hospital appointment was okay. I really feel as though I wouldn't mind going in there for a while to rest, but then that's hard to imagine, despite the lovely but energetic and tiring summer and now being back to school tomorrow. Mum's job is worrying her a little so I do feel sorry for her, but it looks as if things are on the up again after so long, although I don't know what I could do apart from giving her advice, which I may not be fantastic at. Life has to be hard to make me push myself. Life is too short to fail.

Wednesday, September 5, 1990: The fifth year and only one year left before some of my form leave to go to 6th form college, while those of us that want to stay for the 6th form at school will remain together. I couldn't wait to get to school, there were many stories to tell by us all. However, sometimes I can't act as if I condone all that my friends do. I also have to be true to my Christian faith.

Thursday, September 6, 1990: I didn't enjoy school today. (Are you meant to in the fifth year?) None of us seem mature enough to be worthy of our standing and thus it is worrying. Maybe we just need a few more days to get used to it. I'm worried about the coming year; we have our mocks in two months' time. I felt very nervous going into the new youth group – Cornerstone – this evening, but it was fine. I certainly need to stand up to my Christian convictions more, both inside of and outside of church.

Thursday, September 13, 1990: Despite my feelings concerning myself at times, school was good today and I enjoyed talking to people. I spent ages on my Geography coursework, but at least it is done. Mum met me and we went into Kingston for a while. Sometimes I think I tell her too much of what's going on in my life. However at the same time I know some of my friends (school and church) are not very happy and I must try and help them more.

Sunday, September 16, 1990: Church this morning was lovely; little Bethany dedicated to God. I had an argument with Mum. I do feel that I need to let out some steam at times. I feel so nervous and worried sometimes, as if life is just a shambles, but don't we all? I get so nervous being around the boys I've grown up with in church, although why should I?

Monday, September 17, 1990: Monday morning again. One day I will wish my whole life away and that will make me cry.

I'm glad I spoke to the doctor about my medication. It was a good piano lesson this evening.

Tuesday, September 18, 1990: Mind over matter; surely I was fine today although knowing me it was quite difficult to tell when I feel so vulnerable. Quite a few people were away today, which was quite strange. Whether they were "bunking off" or not, who knows? Each day is precious, as we only have a year together before we split up. Additionally, we are only on earth for such a short time and then we spend eternity somewhere we don't know and don't particularly understand or, at our age, want to. We English are such a weird race; we are so reserved, but surely emotions are always welling up inside of us all. Why are we so pompous and insecure?

Wednesday, September 19, 1990: My moods seem to change quite frequently. Often I'm on a high and quite enthusiastic about lots of things, but in the space of an hour I can feel quite down in the dumps, which sounds a little better than depressed. Puberty is such a difficult time. I like school, but at the same time can't wait to get home; and then home is much worse than school, but then school worse than home. Oh, gosh I am so mixed up. No one in the class appears to have serious boyfriends at present.

Thursday, September 20, 1990: Thirteen months ago and thirteen months too young; I'm so pathetic. I need to mature and become stronger in my faith, as God would want me to. Saw *Empire of the Sun* today (story of a privileged English boy living in Shanghai when the Japanese invaded and all foreigners forced into prison camps). How anyone could have survived the war and still live with all the hurt and sorrow that goes with it is truly heartbreaking to hear. The unimaginable torture of those who never saw their families again. This film helped me glimpse and understand a little of their suffering.

Friday, September 21, 1990: Church was good today, but I wish people wouldn't give me sympathetic looks every time I cough. I'm not an invalid, but maybe that is me being too harsh on people who genuinely care about me. I feel bad that Gwen was sitting by herself, but I just couldn't change seats without making it obvious. There is a lot of sense and empathy in me and I need to tap those resources more. I do believe I am consistent in my witness. I don't want to be a bore, but if I believe that God wants us to live for Him, then it makes sense I will be unpopular at times. Life offers so much and we take, take, take from it, but do we give anything back? There is more to it than school, college, uni, career, marriage, kids, retirement, death. Well, I certainly need more of a pattern than that. It was nice to see K. today – I was surprised with how depressed she was, but later she seemed to deal with it better. I hope I am not dull, but I will not be pushed into things I don't want to do. I have my principles and that is important.

Saturday, September 29, 1990: The weather matched the mood of today because no one appeared happy by any means. We (Auntie Pat, Mum and me) talked about the upcoming holiday next year. I would prefer to delay it until 1992, but the consensus is to go in '91.

October 1990

Monday, October 1, 1990: I can't believe we are into October already. It's good to know that you can always have friends. I've felt much better for that, both content and happy. I enjoyed reading a part in *Macbeth* today, although my speech therapy lessons when I was three years old do creep into mind. I remember back then I had a lisp, but so did loads of my little friends back then too. It was good to go as a group and talk to our youth leaders this evening – I think we all felt very nervous and worried going, but it was a good session. I do hope it didn't influence others to share my views.

Tuesday, October 2, 1990: Off school ill today, and lots of phone calls this evening enquiring how I am. So sweet of everyone, but I don't want people to pity me or for me to feel self-pity either. I managed youth group this evening. When I was young I didn't know boys existed! Oh, take me back to those carefree days. I have a dream of us all, in future years, sitting around a fire with our spouses and reminiscing of these years as teenagers; happy to be together. I want to experience so much, I want adventure, but I also want to follow God's will.

Saturday, October 6, 1990: I seem to be drawn between two worlds: the Christian and, somewhat up until now, a protected world, but then another full of materialism, jealousy and greed. Walking along the Kings Road in London today the tug of war was definitely noticeable because I was walking among the cream of the crop, but on the other hand, maybe I am doing these people an injustice. Life can be so corrupt; it worries and unnerves me. Too many people and not enough time; that must be the essence of this world. Life is what you make it and I want mine to matter, though I don't want to show off and appear to outshine others.

Monday, October 8, 1990: Our Geography project was fine today. Maybe I am being lured into a false sense of security, but so far the coursework is less challenging than I expected; however I am still very worried about the coming year. I think we all are in one way or another, but I have so much to be thankful for. God has kept me well these past few weeks which has meant school attendance has been good, although life is so strange, and scary and worrying at times. I know all the homework we are getting (so much coursework to do) means my journal entries will be shorter, but hey ho, that's life.

Tuesday, October 9, 1990: I was ill in the night and my temperature is still up so Mum won't let me go to school. Maybe I spoke too soon yesterday! I was worried and feeling sorry for myself because my chest felt so tight and breathing a problem. "Up the antibiotics," is what the doctor said.

Wednesday, October 10, 1990: It's good to be back at school today and among friends. Visit to orthodontist means I need to keep my brace on for another 18 months, but my teeth are straightening out and loads of us are wearing braces. As the saying goes: No pain means no gain.

I don't know what my friends in youth group feel about me playing the organ. I am not too impressed myself but if I don't, who will?

Wednesday, October 24, 1990: Half term and after 14 years of living next door, oh, why do people have to leave? The removal vans came today so I'm glad I said goodbye to Graham and Janet. Every day in the car when I was little, waiting to see if their garage door was open, and whether their car was there or not – could we play together, or were they out? Since Daniel and I have been going to different senior schools, I haven't seen a great deal of him nor his brothers and sister, but nevertheless we spent our infant and junior years together, and being young and carefree was very special to me. It will be very sad without them. I wish I had told the family over the years how important it was to me to have them next door. Memories, that's what's important in life; playing in each other's gardens, houses, making camps, jumping in and out of the paddling pool. So they left – a new start, a new life. To me, my next door neighbours will always be the Thorpe's. To end a nostalgic day, I came last in bowling in youth group! My mum said that someone has to, and it's not the end of the world.

Friday, October 26, 1990: Christmas cake made today. Mum did her Christmas shopping yesterday, my goodness, whatever next! Her excuse is that she never knows when I will next need to be in hospital and come out on IVs, so her motto is, "Forewarned is forearmed."

Saturday, October 27, 1990: Canoeing with Cornerstone today. Why did Louise and I have to fall in? I knew it would be me. Scary.

Sunday, October 28, 1990: My Belgian cousins arrived today and we had a great time in London again – Oxford, Regent and Carnaby Streets. Tomorrow Catherine is coming to school with me.

November 1990

Thursday, November 1, 1990: Piano theory exam today and I knew quite a few of the pupils taking it.

Sunday, November 4, 1990: Laurent and Catherine returned home today. The journey isn't too long over the channel and they must be safely in bed by now. Lots of childhood memories flooded my mind this evening: trips to Margate, people coming to see me at different times in hospital.

Thursday, November 8, 1990: D. is very insecure and it worries me.

Friday, November 9, 1990: I quite enjoyed school today as there was a sense of wholeness within the form. First night of me being a helper in Spectrum Youth Group at church. Sixteen were there, then off to baby-sitting, which helps supplement my allowance now that I am no longer working at the care home.

Wednesday, November 14, 1990: I want to help people who are going through tough times. I want to say the right things and do what is supportive. How grateful I am not go to a school where bullying is part of the culture.

Friday, November 16, 1990: Emma and Sarah's birthdays today and it was really quite good fun. Went into hospital after school today.

Saturday, November 17, 1990: I had quite a few visitors today. Nice nurses, but my intravenous drip played up.

Sunday, November 18, 1990: Not feeling great. Really nice doctor today, but loads of church and school friends came and we chatted about euthanasia.

Tuesday, November 20, 1990: Drip still playing up and needed re-siting in different veins, not once but twice.

Wednesday, November 21, 1990: Can't remember if Margaret Thatcher resigned today or yesterday. John Major, Michael Heseltine or Douglas Hurd to replace her. People on the ward are so nice and friendly with lots of nice doctors and nurses, too. Drip fine today.

Friday, November 23, 1990: Small baby next door (the baby unit of the ward) with CF. No visitors today apart from Mum, but no worries as had so many mates visit this past week.

Sunday, November 25, 1990: I felt very sad to be going home today as everyone's been so nice. I feel selfish and angry, but then teenagers have very confusing thoughts. I needed to cry; I still need to cry.

Monday, November 26, 1990: Straight back to school and I found it so hard to concentrate in mock exams. We have them all week, so I must get used to it. English and Computing weren't bad at all. I am so stupid, because when I get good marks I worry that they have made a mistake and will come back and tell me I have failed!

Friday, November 30, 1990: Spectrum was good this evening and it was great to be back among the youngsters.

December 1990

Sunday, December 2, 1990: It felt good to be back in church today. I thought the sermon was good; it was certainly powerful and quite challenging. Are we really Christians, all of us, or is it simply a pretence? I wish I could turn back the clock. Create in me a clean heart, oh God (Psalm 51). Longing for Christmas to come.

Saturday, December 8, 1990: Last exam yesterday. It snowed today; the fields looked very beautiful. Auntie Lesley has had a lump removed and we all hope she will be okay. I feel so sad that I can't do a thing to help. Hopefully, we will be able to go to Belgium to see them all soon. Prayer is the only thing that we can offer until we can see her. My exam results are not as good as I hoped, but they are not all bad either. My mum tried to reassure me that being in hospital immediately before them couldn't have helped.

Thursday, December 13, 1990: I really enjoyed travelling to Heathrow today on our school trip. It was fun answering the telephones; the people were so friendly and kind. The weather is bitterly cold.

Saturday, December 15, 1990: I fulfilled my dream today by going up to Oxford and Regent Streets in London for my Christmas shopping. Seeing so many friends was also great. I want to mature much more and show my faith in words and actions.

Sunday, December 16, 1990: Great today with the family visiting. The nativity went well in church, too. I need to demonstrate Christian values in my life more, but things have a strange way of "becoming," as my mother would say; but she is not as wise as she sounds and certainly not as patient! Long suffering is not her forte, and the times she needs to apologise to me for going off into one of her rants bears testimony to that. There is so much suffering in the world.

Monday, December 17, 1990: The school carol service with those that sang in the choir doing Tiffin proud. It was a nice atmosphere and good to be together.

Tuesday, December 18, 1990: The Museum of Jewish life was very worthwhile for our school cultural visit today. The events that happened in the Second World War were truly awful. Our guide, Solomon, told us how he survived a concentration camp. Hearing him recount his experiences was so sad and unbelievable. I would have liked much more time there, but we spent more time on the coach than at the museum. I definitely want to go into one of the helping professions. There is so much need in the world and people need love, support, dignity.

The countdown to Christmas shopping days is very rapidly decreasing and can be very worrying if not all presents are bought.

Friday, December 21, 1990: As form 5B, we will never, ever share Christmas together again. It's really sad. It's weird thinking that, this time next year, those people who we were close to, we may have lost contact with. Together forever is fast running out. A day like today will never be experienced again.

Saturday, December 22, 1990: Why does everyone seem to feel so vulnerable? I have come to the conclusion that it just isn't me alone.

Monday, December 24, 1990: I am really pleased some of my school friends came to church yesterday. It was good going round to Auntie's today. I enjoyed both being with the family and also seeing friends. I must feel guilty this Christmas because I am so lucky. I have a home, friends, relatives that care for me deeply, food, presents and so many more daily things that are so often taken for granted. I need to think of those people at Christmas who lack so much, and most importantly as we celebrate Christ's birth, the one who gave up everything for me.

Tuesday, December 25, 1990: It was a lovely day today; the family was together and there was so much happening. We left church having seen so many friends. I was spoilt rotten and had far too many presents, but I enjoyed every minute of them and of the day. I love both giving and receiving. Yet it is not just about our family when so many people globally lack so much. Christ's birthday, but once church is over, do we think of Him as the centre of our day? I can no longer curl up in my own, snug little world and remain cosy when others lack so much.

Friday, December 28, 1990: I quite enjoyed the mentally handicapped club today, but we need to always remember we are there to help the children and not carry on our own conversations. We (Hannah and me) had to do a couple of sentences "report back" that could be used to encourage other helpers. We wrote: "Throughout our time at the Centre we both enjoyed the relationships we developed with the children, the sense of achieve-ment it brought, and the signs of affection they showed us. It was both a real learning, but also humbling experience."

It was nice to spend the evening with Mum; we don't achieve this often, in the busyness of church, school and work.

Saturday, December 29, 1990: This morning's sermon was quite a telling off; it had to be because we face a new year and cannot just take Christianity as something on the side; it must affect our whole lives. I know I am so selfish and stubborn (the list could go on) and need to change.

Monday, December 31, 1990: On the eve of a new year, there are so many feelings to express. So many things have changed, and yet so many things have paradoxically stayed the same. I need God more than ever this next year. 1991 is so important in terms of qualifications.

Chapter Six

Your Senior School Years – 1991's Journals

January 1991

*T*uesday, January 1, 1991: There are so many people in the world that others are oblivious to people who suffer each day; people no one will ever acknowledge. These include the ill, the old, handicapped, young and also those who have mental health problems, to name but a few. Life is sacred, but so short, too short to do many things that are so important to try and do, to say; to enjoy and worship the God of creation. The years go fast now; there is not much time. It's also important to cherish those people/things that are central to our lives. A new year should resonate change, wholeheartedly embracing the future.

Wednesday, January 2, 1991: Mentally handicapped club (I prefer to call it a club for the educationally challenged, and yet that does not do these lovely people justice; they may not have the same intellectual capacity as some other people, but they have a great capacity for love and enjoyment of life) was great today as everyone had a superb time. The look on the faces was that of absolute delight; it was nice to see them so joyful and happy. However, I know there were times when they demonstrated concerning behaviour, like head-banging and rocking; what goes on in their minds to cause this I don't comprehend.

Saturday, January 5, 1991: It's weird to think that this is the year I'll do my GCSEs, get my results in August and then go on to A levels.

Wednesday, January 9, 1991: It seemed odd walking into the form room today and meeting everyone once more, some people not too happy about their romances. Teenagers, particularly, need truthful comments from their friends as so often we get fake compliments and words spoken just because they appear nice things to say. I am concerned with the amount of friends I have, in and out of school, who don't feel the need to save sex for marriage. I know that sounds humbug, but as a Christian I need to say it, despite people calling me old fashioned and judgemental. If people didn't bring the subject up, I wouldn't need to speak out, so it cuts both ways.

Monday, January 14, 1991: It felt almost spring-like today as the sun was shining brightly, but I know we have a few months to go before it actually arrives. I like winter and I like spring too, with all of its new life and dazzling but simple and ornate beauty, the crocuses like a carpet of colour, with the appearance of one large art canvas.

Tuesday, January 15, 1991: Our society is so conservative and toffee-nosed. That poor man on the bus, who obviously did choose to look as he did, but it was disturbing that no one took the seat next to him when so many were standing. People under no circumstances should be judged simply by their outward appearance; the inside qualities are so very often disregarded and not examined. He was the first one to reach out and steady the old lady as she stumbled. Well, I hope those that saw the incident were challenged by his kindness. Today is the deadline before the possible outbreak of war; 5:00a.m tomorrow morning will determine whether we will start killing each other again. Human lives are sacred; whether a soldier, dustman or whoever – they all play a role in society. It is, after all, just another word for murder.

Wednesday, January 16, 1991: The deadline has passed; the Americans and Allied Forces are lining up on the border of Kuwait to fight Iraq. There are tanks surrounding London Heathrow Airport. Blood will be shed, as if it is worthless. Mothers may never speak to or see their sons again (or their daughters, for that matter). So many can be widowed; children left parentless; parents left childless – we need to see the conflict from both sides. We call ourselves a superior race; intelligent and knowledgeable. I call us barbaric.

Thursday, January 17, 1991: The troops have attacked Iraq in order to rescue Kuwait. The whole of the Middle East is threatened. There is no longer a chance for peace, because the war that everyone was dreading and hoping would be averted has now begun. The threat regarding chemical weapons, so we hear, is real. The bombardment of Iraq is frightening. Despite the campaigning for peace, war is a reality. We must pray and not be selfish about ourselves, but think of others.

Saturday, January 19, 1991: This war is at the forefront of my and so many others' minds. Whether the problem central to all this is oil, or dictatorship, or foreign relations is not up for grabs in my mind; the real problem is us all, the human race. My prayers for peace have never been so real and earnest. My support for Amnesty International is equally earnest, because this is as much about the abuse of human rights as any other cause – there is no sanctity of human life.

Thursday, January 24, 1991: It appears that many people are beginning to accept the war as *fait accompli* and, like all atrocities, after a while we get used to it; like the Northern Ireland violence. Propaganda is rife and the distant nightmare edges towards reality on our TV screens night after night. Saddam Hussein has now set oil fields alight in Kuwait. Despite the many peace protests around the world, it seems this war will not be over quickly.

Monday, January 28, 1991: Day 12 of the Gulf War; day 12 of mass murder and infinite ignorance. Day 12 of hatred, disobedience, starvation, sickness, injury. Day 12 of madness, mental stress and worry beyond measure. Day 12 of wondering whether your relative will be alive one hour from now. Day 12 of wondering if your children will ever see their father again. Day 12 of ignoring the plea to save lives. Day 12 of incomprehension. I will continue to write about the Gulf War until it ends, so outraged am I.

February 1991

Friday, February 1, 1991: It seems impossible that a month of the New Year has disappeared already. What happened to January? A month, it seems, has been erased from memory but as time passes so too will years be erased, blotted out and diminished, no more to return. This is why keeping a diary, if I can, is so important to me. Childhood is a sacred part of a precious life and is wiped out so quickly – there is no turning back. Life is cruel and hard once teenage years are thrust upon one. Innocence seems to be forsaken and life no longer appears pure and clean. There is nothing to cling on to that one can save from a corrupt, deceitful and out of perspective world that teases and chides and can corrupt such a pure and young mind. Faces of troops killed in their early 20s. No words.

Saturday, February 2, 1991: It was nice to spend time with Auntie today as I enjoy her company. I also needed to spend time at home; to relax and enjoy the surroundings of my room. It felt nice to be home, but this house does not always feel like home; it is very strange and weird. I like my house but I'm not sure whether I'd always call it my security blanket, but then maybe that's why God has put Eternity in our hearts. I'm not sure what home is or what it means. Home is somewhere you can go to relax and feel free from any bounds. It is somewhere you can look forward to going to and feeling free and happy. Home is where you find rest. Home is happy and comforting. Home should console you when you are sad. Sometimes I really want to go home; maybe many of the troops yearn for their homes, too. Eternal freedom.

Wednesday, February 6, 1991: 'Twas the school play today and the music was vibrant. I always feel music brings out the best in people. The characterisation was good and I felt I could relate to the lead role, Kathy. The choreography was great; there had been so much work put into it. There was joy in the air and the whole audience seemed to capture the excitement and energy.

Thursday, February 7, 1991: Pessimism seems to have resulted from optimism! I was surprised to see the amount of snow that had fallen as it was absolutely astounding. Everyone seemed happy to venture in; we expected to be told to go home again, but unfortunately this did not happen. It was worth going in, even for the morning because everyone was enjoying themselves at lunchtime. We had a really massive snowball fight and also built a snowman that we wrote on: "5B rules OK," that led all the way round the hockey pitch. We'll never have a snowball fight again in the class as a whole.

Sometimes I think the class is already drifting apart; there seem to be a few strings tying some bonds together, but eventually the knot will snap. Things will be said, promises made, but I doubt that everyone will keep in touch. A flake of snow, slowly dissolving and then it disappears for good. Maybe a description of form 5B.

Friday, February 8, 1991: It seemed like a holiday today, not going into school. There was quite a lot of snow and now the big freeze has affected most of the country. The pure, un-driven snow is absolutely beautiful; it's innocent. There's certainly enough snow for tobogganing. I miss my childhood years when we all used to play together in the street where I live, those years when a convoy of us walked to the little school down the hill, when my gloves were threaded through my coat sleeves with elastic to prevent me losing them. When, even younger, I wore a red jumpsuit and ear muffs to keep my head warm, when my wellies were the right size. Those were the days. I was more secure then than I am now; I was happier and contented in my own little world, where nothing could harm me. A child can cling to their childhood, as I do because it is sacredly pure.

Saturday, February 9, 1991: it was good to go tobogganing in Oxshott Woods today. It snowed again overnight, and there were even some people on skis, so great fun for us all. God knows more about me than I do; one minute I'm confused, the next everything is perfectly fine. Maybe I'm just the stereotypical teenager.

Tuesday, February 12, 1991: Sometimes I feel so lethargic and I am sure my CF is making me feel this way, but I need to be tough and not give in. The Gulf War seems to be almost forgotten; overtaken by something as menial as the weather. . .as if they can compare.

Wednesday, February 13, 1991: Our first actual GCSE exam today; although it seemed much more relaxed than I had imagined it to be, but results will tell. Quite a few of the girls in the form have boyfriends now; I guess it is the coming of age when this is rife in teen relationships. This is the time I suppose that my mother warned me about; to stand up and be proud of my identity as a Christian, and to choose opposite sex relationships wisely. Well, I don't feel at all proud; I just feel left lying in the gutter, tossed aside (although there are plenty in the class who *don't* have boyfriends). There has been quite a lot of build up for Valentine's Day tomorrow, not just on the media, but all over the place; peer pressure, etc; "If you have any worries, you can contact. . ."

Thursday, February 14, 1991: I felt out of it today. "And I will always love you" (Dolly Parton, 1973). How many couples will vow their love for each other today, but more importantly, how many of us will be able to say, "We love Him, because He first loved us"? (1 John chapter 4, verse 19.) Yes, I did get a Valentine card. . .from Chris, yeah!

Friday, February 15, 1991: Thankfully school went quickly today as I was longing to come home again. (So much for my previous journal entry on what home really means!) Everyone has problems in life, thus everyone is in the same boat. Things may seem difficult for me, but they really are just a few minor hitches compared to most other problems in the world. We got our exam timetable today, which was rather scary. However, a good swim certainly brushed the cobwebs away!

Thursday, February 24, 1991: Life appears so shallow at times; what would I do, where would I be without a faith in God? Although I must admit my mind was wandering all over the place in the sermon this morning. I need to be an encouragement and a role model to others; not have a mind that is so unfocused. Sometimes I hinder more than I help. I need to repent of my selfish ways.

Tuesday, February 26, 1991: For my Information Technology coursework I designed an improved drip stand. (It's very frustrating, being in hospital and having to exercise in the corridors with the physios, when the wheels from the wide base of the stand get in your way; even the physios get cross.) Hopefully the design means that patients can walk without the risk of tripping over it. I had to undertake a patient survey before the design, but thankfully passed the project.

Thursday, February 28, 1991: The good news is that Kuwait City is free; Hussein's troops surrendered and there has been a ceasefire (as long as Hussein doesn't renege about the United Nation's resolution). How much of this was accomplished by the prayers of believers? The prayer of a righteous person has great power as it is working (James 5:16b).

March 1991

Sunday, March 3, 1991: Arguments, arguments; our family is very good at them, despite our faith. Mum is very difficult sometimes, but she is not the only one. I really enjoyed the sermons today because I was able to understand all or most of what was being said. I must watch my tongue, though; I am far too opinionated in many respects and moody into the bargain! I seldom portray the image that I know I should and also yearn to.

Monday, March 4, 1991: Class felt rather empty today as so many were away. There is so much to do that some just need time off to work through it all. At some point of the day I felt like flinging myself on the bed sobbing, and that's the truth. It's not an exaggeration to say that I'm not the only one that feels this way as all of the form feel fed up and over-worked. But A levels will be worse, so we keep being told, and once we get to them it will be "roll back the GCSEs."

Wednesday, March 6, 1991: It was lovely to see on the news the prisoners of war being freed from Iraq and the camaraderie they had with each other; however one must not forget all those who gave up their lives in yet another war. There are so many things that I don't know how to answer concerning my Christian faith, but I do know when Joe Public holds views contrary to the Gospel. I don't want to argue with people; I just long for them to know that God loves them, and respond to their questions or statements in a loving way. And how do I explain words like "predestination" in simple, everyday terms? I have so much to learn.

There are a few in the class who are worried about D.; we have decided that while she has to take responsibility for herself, she may get very hurt in the process. It has been a joint (group) decision to respond if she asks us for help, although not to interfere in case she gets defensive. I hope this isn't showing our weakness, but how can we judge others; barge in with telling her how to live her life when we know it's not what she wants to hear? I feel sorry for her and if only she kept private things to herself, others would show more respect, rather than stir things up.

Saturday, March 9, 1991: Auntie Lesley is coming over in 2 weeks to stay again. I feel very sorry that she is so unwell and I hope the rest does her good. Mum is always working more in a day than I'll ever work and is so faithful and just with all the work. I'm not appreciative enough and yet Mother's Day should be when we show them how much we truly love them. I must learn not to complain; to hold my tongue and to be happier (if only the latter came more easily), as self-centred is my second name. Oh, if only I could show more positive attributes. I feel so lost at times, but if I gave more of my time to others I am sure I would feel better about myself.

Our Drama GCSE tomorrow and I'm so nervous, but I know from talking to people that all of us are in the same boat. I'm worried that there aren't enough props or creative ideas for the set, but a little late in the day to concern myself with that. While everyone is saying, "Fingers crossed," it's Louise and me who know that we need to pray about it.

Wednesday, March 20, 1991: The blossom on the trees seems to have appeared out of nowhere, and yet it is so beautiful and intricate; how good God is to provide such detail in creation. Daffodils line the grass verges as we gaze out of the bus window. We performed our Drama again today for the rest of the school and interested parents. I was astounded at how many turned up to watch.

Thursday, March 21, 1991: The grey sky was reflected in the puddles, but in contrast to the cherry blossom and spring flowers that were expressive of colour and fine detail. I know why spring is one of my favourite seasons.

Friday, March 22, 1991: People hurt and scar deeply. When you stare at a person at the bus stop or simply glance at them as they walk down the street, it's impossible to know any pain they are suffering. Broken homes, war, rape, murder. . .How can people live feeling so much pain? Search for happiness, yearn for peace, live not for yourself but for others, crave unselfishness. Do not be self-seeking, humble yourself, keep watch for anyone in trouble and seek righteousness. It didn't seem like the end of term at all today. I hope those that are going have a great ski trip. In many respects I wish I could go, but another holiday to the States in the summer has ruled that out. I will still be looking forward to that when the others return.

Saturday, March 23, 1991: I watched too much TV today in an effort to unwind at the end of term. There appears to be so much pressure from the media on romance, and if that weren't enough, the subtle and not so subtle provocative situations are worrying.

Monday, March 25, 1991: Hannah and I helped at the mentally handicapped club today. I feel this is such a happy way to return some of the blessing I get out of life, by giving/spending time with those who are not as fortunate as I am. I wouldn't say it is easy, though; one has to be aware of each child's dynamics and the capacity they have of fitting in with each other, but I find it very rewarding. I learn so much from them; their vying for attention, the subtle ways they can play one leader off against another, the devious (and not so devious) ways they try and hurt each other. But who am I to judge them? I am sure this is all learned behaviour and I must be held to account for my role in society where this education takes place.

Tuesday, March 26, 1991: Fruitfulness was not the aim of my day today. In fact, I was very unfruitful. Some of my conversations with friends were not profitable and I must learn how to disagree/disapprove, but without judging them. Not that I want to disagree with them for disagreement's sake, but if I am here to be salt and light, then I have to be accountable. It is understandable that teens will not always get along with their parents, or with peers in church, but as Romans 12.18 says, "If it is possible, as far as it depends on you, live at peace with everyone."

It was good to spend the evening with Auntie Lesley; she always looks so smart and trendy. She told us how her drip was removed so callously by medical staff; there is no way a patient would be able to endure all of that trouble and pain without support. As the Beatles' song (John Lennon and Paul McCartney, 1967) reminds us that we will manage when we have "a little help from our friends."

Wednesday, March 27, 1991: I was very selfish today and very unpleasant, unkind and frustrated with many things. I think that I really wanted Mum to suffer as a result of the pain she caused me. However, she stuck up for me greatly.

Friday, March 29, 1991: Good Friday. I enjoyed this morning's service very much. The time of prayer with Cornerstone was really profitable. We all learned from each other and, I felt, grew far closer as a result.

Saturday, March 30, 1991: Easter Saturday. A trek to Kingston this morning to have a look at the Good News Bus. Evangelising scares me, but having an older person showing me the ropes certainly helped.

April 1991

Monday, April 1, 1991: Easter Monday. I can't believe we're into another new month. It has been lovely spending the weekend with Auntie as it's lovely to have an aunt who cares and does so much for me.

Saturday, April 6, 1991: My work experience at a London hospital. I received my programme; I get to spend time with the social worker, occupational therapist, on the ward (as an observer, of course) and in various other departments. It seems I will be in for a good few days of learning.

Wednesday, April 10, 1991: School again and we have only got 4.5 weeks together as a class before we all disperse, like blossom on a tree, to have exam leave. I have prepared a card for my peers: it says:

To: All of 5B, Vicki, Faye, Lynne, Gina, Helen, Catherine, Emma, Miranda, Isabel, Beth, Rebecca, Kathryn, Rebecca, Kate, Lorna, Gemma, Kate, Caroline, Sarah, Jacquetta, Sarah, Ndullee, Helen, Sam, Alice, Hannah, Thalia, Zoe and Catherine. . .Good luck with all of the exams. They'll soon be just a faint memory! With best wishes for the future. Keep in touch and take care of yourselves. School days are the best days of your life. I'll miss you all. With lots of love from Claire. Xxx

It seems strange to think you have seen someone every day for the past five years but soon Form 5B, the Class of '91, will be no more. My fellow pupils have been such an important part of my life; part of my living. My bus rides to and from school will soon be coming to an end for the summer. The world is so hostile; speaking at a bus stop seems forbidden, you mustn't make eye contact or smile either. I wonder if other people, as I do, imagine these people in their everyday lives; the men and women who get off at Surbiton station to catch the train to Waterloo and then in to the City. What kind of jobs do they do? What is their working day like, their families, their leisure time? And without being too stereotypical, the females, who get off the busy in Kingston town centre, no doubt working in offices or shops. I find it quite embarrassing not talking or speaking. I think now it's time to give up. We have no relationship, no conversation, nothing in common.

Thursday, April 11, 1991: That distinct smell of summer has almost arrived. It's quite disorientating when the weather is so good less than 2 weeks into April. It was lovely to be part of the Christian Union again. Prayer time I found to be particularly encouraging. I guess at present, my conversation with Mum regarding baptism made me feel a little pressured and I realise that it must be my own decision, seeking to do what God wants me to do. I may well feel more comfortable sharing my baptism with some of my friends, but I need to give it more thought, though at the same time knowing that this is a command from Scripture.

Friday, April 12, 1991: Well, this hot weather has certainly brought the best out in people; there is a spring to our steps, the summer wardrobe has come out early and it's interesting to see the plethora of sunglasses designs. It was good to take the Spectrum kids to the field to play rounders this evening. Cornerstone was also spent outside, despite the fading light. I don't know how I really feel about running Christian Union at school, as I feel that a C.U. leader must be totally committed to that, and also the first year of A levels may be too much. Thankfully I have a few more months to decide. I feel I must devote more attention to Kate (not the Kate in my class, but lower down the school). There's been a problem for her since our 4th year and I just didn't take much notice. I felt embarrassed for her; she wants people to tell her if there's something wrong all the time. I think she feels quite sorry for herself in a way and quite fed up. I don't know how and if I can help her. I'll feel stupid if I just end up saying the totally wrong thing.

Saturday, April 13, 1991: Today found me in Kingston hanging out with school friends, but I – like so many others – am responsible for the materialism in the world. We have so much of everything, yet at the same time, watch the TV almost detached from the images displayed. Kurds fighting for their lives with nowhere to go, no food to eat and no clean water to drink. The situation is absolutely horrendous but we just sit back, detached, in our own little world and watch these people dying whilst we have everything.

Monday, April 15, 1991: How many teenagers are really themselves? How does one class "normal"? Why do people need to put up a front and not be their real selves? Why aren't I myself? What are the social effects on our character? Are certain types of personality hereditary? Who am I? What will the future bring?

Why do we judge people by outward appearances? Didn't Jesus ask us to look at man's heart? What I am trying to say is that everyone deserves a chance; this is the message of the gospel, after all. Are qualifications the only thing that matters? Oh, we know the social situations many find themselves in at cocktail parties. "What do you do?" or, "What school did you go to?", as if in the big scheme of things any of this matters. We could be a Hitler or a saint, and in the big scheme of things, what we do for a living, etc. does not matter one jot.

Thursday, April 18, 1991: Countdown again. It seems strange that we only have 16 days left as a form; as a real class that we have been made up of for five years. Who would have thought that in the first year (1B), half would be leaving in five years' time? But to divert my mind away from the break-up of our precious class, I am drawn to reflecting how I wish I had played the game (but it is definitely not a game, it is so real) of life differently. If I were given another court to play on, I would make sure this time that the ball would go over the net. If I were given another life, what would I change? I think the answer to that is that it would have to be everything. If I were given another dream to dream, or race to run, what would it be this time? Whatever happened to pure childhood? But it is no use feeling nostalgic; we are given one life only to make of it what we will.

Monday, April 22, 1991: Should I speak to our pastor about baptism, or would this be presumptuous? Okay, I can give a short talk in the youth group and pray in a small group of peers, but I don't really live my life for God. Would I be frowned upon, seen for the imposter I am?

Friday, April 26, 1991: There are only a few days left of us as a form, a few days of the "B era"; it's hard to believe that we've been together for nigh on 5 years and it must all come to an end so quickly. What kind of a profound effect have we had on one another since we met up that first tenuous day in 1986? I knew absolutely no one then, but what a difference now. What will happen to each and every one of us in a quarter of a century's time? It was lovely to see Mrs, Smith, my junior school teacher, again today, and Caroline too. It's strange to think that it was almost five years ago since I left St. Mary's (and the friends I had) behind. Oh, if only it could be, "Yesterday Once More" (Richard Carpenter and John Bettis, from the Carpenters 1973 album). All those old memories, still so dear to me.

Saturday, April 27, 1991: The Youth Training Day was profitable and it was good to be around fellow Christians, enjoying fellowship. The talks were light-hearted, but at the same time, there was a measureable depth to them. When we visited Mr. Rhoades later, he was well-ish, but one could see deterioration since the last time we saw him.

Sunday, April 28, 1991: I am so challenged by Christians who are willing to lose their lives in God's service. How can I possibly claim to be a Christian? How dare we as a nation even call ourselves a Christian country when so many overseas risk their very lives to follow Christ? Signing the petition in church today I really was a hypocrite, writing my name and address illegibly so that if there was any come back, I would not be recognised. Oh, Claire, where is your commitment, your faith, your allegiance to your Lord?

Monday, April 29, 1991: There was a time when I couldn't wait to leave Tiffin Girls', but now half the class is leaving to go to college for their A levels, I am pleased I will remain with the others staying on for the 6th form. GCSE exams are approaching ominously, and there just seems too much to think about all at once. I do hope the school can find me a work experience placement with Social Services; if I want a career in the helping profes- sions, I need to have some insight into what I am letting myself in for. Time seems to race by so much more quickly since I reached my mid-teens and it is frightening.

So the dreaded exam leave is here, followed by the dreaded exams themselves. Well, the less said the better.

All us 5th years had to prepare a post-16 Record of Achievement (the idea being that those who were not staying on at school for A levels would have a record of their achievements at Tiffin). I must say they looked really professional and each one was signed by the Head, for her to put her stamp on it, as it were. I feel confused and low in self-esteem, unmotivated, lazy. I have a nasty mouth, I feel self-conscious, sorry for myself; hectic, busy, guilty, ugly, embarrassed, stuck in a time warp, immature, humiliated/ hated by boys. I care about what people think of me, I feel alone, don't really fit in anywhere, so much to do, such little time to do it, I get so jealous of other people. Well, that's the summing up of my feelings and my rant is over. Maybe I'm just silly; after speaking on the phone to Rachel, I feel much more at ease!

We returned for the final day of Form 5B today to say our farewells and to collect our end of year reports. Here I go with the photocopying in the library again. The headmistress wrote: Claire is a caring and unselfish young lady with a generous and loving nature. She has enjoyed excellent relations with her peers and staff alike. Her contributions to the well-being of the form have been outstanding. Despite her health difficulties, Claire has been an example to all through her positive, uncomplaining attitude. Signed: Sandra B.

And from Des H., my form tutor in the 5th year: I am delighted that Claire will continue to be a member of my form in the Lower Sixth. (I like to paste these in my journal; they will remind me in later years how teachers fabricated the truth! No, I don't mean that; they will remind me that I was thought of in a good light on occasions.) The rest of the day was spent enjoying our form party and writing in each other's hymn books; a tradition on such an occasion as this.

These are excerpts from mine:

Ndullee: Thanks for always being around and for being a really great friend. We've had a few laughs, haven't we?! Keep in touch, okay? Love you lots.

Ruth: You are one of the most wonderful, kind-hearted persons I have ever met. My experiences with you at Tiffin will be cherished forever.

Laura: Thank you for putting up with my moaning all year and for being so encouraging!'

Faye What can I say except thanks for everything? The list is too long, but you know what I mean.

Beth: How can I forget you, Claire? You're a brilliant friend and I'll miss you loads. Keep in touch. Xx

Gina: Claire, good luck; keep being nice to everyone.

Kate H.: Thank you for making Tiffin what it has been. Take care and always keep in touch. Love you lots. Xx

Zoe: I'll miss you lots and lots; you've been such a great comfort and help throughout the years. Take care of yourself, sweetheart. Lots of love. Xx

May, June, July

So came the end of our 5th Form and the next day we journeyed to Gatwick Airport for our flight to the States. For our 1991 National Parks and Cities tour we visited Los Angeles. We arrived a day earlier than the tour started and spent the day on Venice beach, cycling on cycle tracks of Santa Monica beach, swimming and generally chilling. The Tour proper started the next day and took us through the famous Californian fruit orchards in the San Joaquin Valley to Fresno. Then to Yosemite and San Francisco (where we had visited two years previously. We stayed overnight in the Park, and took the shuttle bus valley tour, stopping off at Yosemite Village for a coffee. Boarding the coach, we drove through lush redwood forests to San Francisco, where we stayed overnight, taking the opportunity the next day to visit Mum's friends Howard and William via the Bart railway to Walnut Creek. We saw the marvellous array of doll houses that William had made through the years.

The following day saw us leaving San Francisco and journeying up the coast to Eureka. I had my 16th birthday (30th July) in Eureka with a "Sweet Sixteen" banner plus cards and presents in the hotel room, before going next door to Denny's for a free breakfast –people with birthdays were allowed breakfast "on the house," and I even made a journal entry as to what I had: strawberries and cream hot-stack, cinnamon roll and milk, before travelling on to Redwood National Park while still in California (partaking of BBQ lunch in Richardson Grove, among the redwood trees), then visiting Coos Bay, Oregon Dunes National Park - we ran up and down the sand dunes and loved it – before reaching our hotel in Newport at 7"00pm, where I again celebrated my 16th birthday at Sizzler's, photos on the beach, and opened more cards and presents.

Back on the coach the following morning and on to Portland and then to Mount Rainier National Park (an ice-packed, dormant volcanic peak with glaciers reaching down the mountainsides – yes, you can tell I am reading out of the holiday brochure!) in Washington State. Had a meal in the cafeteria and walked to Myrtle Falls just below Mount Rainier – very picturesque.

The following day found us going to Seattle for lunch and shopping (interesting how we always found time for this!) before crossing into Canada and visiting Victoria and also Vancouver Island in British Columbia (BC).

Mave: On the ferry crossing there is a photo of you engrossed in a book –you read avidly, Claire and I guess this is what led you and your equally book worm friends from senior school to form a book group in your adult years. Back to your holiday journal:

Our evening in Vancouver included chancing our feet on the Capilano Suspension Bridge –took a lovely photo as we crossed, enjoying every minute of it, unlike my initial concerns.

On our way to Kamloops (BC), the coach drove past the Fraser River valley to Devil's Gate. I absolutely loved that part of the journey, for we saw some of the traditional freight trains the U.S. was famous for in the '90s. We saw a black bear way up in the mountains, just near Mount Robson National Park. The highlight of our tour took us through the scenic Rocky Mountains to see the Columbia ice fields, Jasper National Park and *en route* we saw Maligne Canyon and waterfalls. Again, in my mind's eye, I can see the photos we took. We took in Lake Louise, Banff National Park, Calgary (all in Alberta), before journeying back into America to Kalispell in Montana.

Mave: Little did we know then that the following year the film *A River Runs Through It* (directed by Robert Redford) would be made, and we would fall in love with Montana all over again. Claire, anyone reading this would think that you and I were inseparable, always sharing a love of the same things. Elsewhere in this diary I have made reference to the fact that you were so independent and whilst with similar tastes, you had a very strong identity of your own!

Back to your journal once more:

From there we journeyed to Glacier National Park where a few of us had a row boat on the lake. The following morning we were up early to sit on the balcony and take in the sites before a ride in the red bus along "Highway to the Sun" (extremely picturesque, snow-capped mountains and deep valleys). We thoroughly enjoyed experiencing white water rafting in the afternoon, before our onward journey to Flathead Lake and Deer Lodge.

The following day found us journeying down virtually the whole state of Montana, stopping at Mousslim, Butte (shopping mall) and Ennis, a lovely old town like Sedona and where I bought jewellery in a half price Indian jewellery sale. (Some habits don't die hard with me!) Our next stops were Yellowstone and Grand Tetons National Parks in Wyoming, with Jackson Hole thrown in for good measure. We took a walk from the hotel in the lazy summer evening and were thankful we were in Wyoming. I just loved the thought of visiting so many different U.S. states and this was another one we could proudly add to our list. The next day we had lunch in Jackson, an old west town – lots of shops, a real treasure – before travelling through Idaho and on to Utah.

Salt Lake City in Utah was our next stop and we weren't overly ambitious about this (sorry, Utah residents!). But I did love our next stop, Bryce Canyon National Park. (The opportunity to go down into the canyon and experience it, something we were not able to do with the Grand Canyon, was very special.) My Auntie and I went on a "chuck wagon evening." We went to Page for our flight through Monument Valley the next day.

This afternoon's drive included taking in the vast Navajo Indian Reservation and with my love of American history, this was special to me. Zion National Park and then to the Grand Canyon where, having spent all afternoon admiring the sites, we dashed back to the rim again in the evening to Sunset Point before eating supper with Edgar and his family. As if we had not had our fill of this amazing beauty, we were up at 4:45 the following morning to see the sun rise over the canyon before I walked along the rim back to the hotel for breakfast. (This was a great repeat of my previous visit to the Grand Canyon.) Left the Canyon, and on to the Hoover Dam and Lake Mead (having previously visited these in our 1989 tour) before one of our last stops to Las Vegas, where we swam, sun-bathed, had a meal and took our last opportunity of shopping for souvenirs and gifts for those at home. It was a really long day!

Our last day found us heading back to Los Angeles (today's journey included a visit to Calico Ghost Town, crossing the Mojave Desert and into the San Bernadino Mountains) to catch our flight back to the UK. Thus our second American dream holiday came to a close. A great sight-seeing holiday with many happy memories of the USA. And again, I kept a variety of different brochures and information as I traversed the west coast of America and Canada so that I could make a scrapbook when I returned home. I bought some beautiful Indian postcards to retain, rather than send to people. As I loved looking at maps, tracing the journey as we travelled, a stickler for "living the moment" and entering into the very depth of the experience was my forte.

I think this song as part of my thankfulness to God at this time sums up my feelings: "What a Wonderful World," written in the late 1950s by Same Cooke along with Lou Adler and Herb Alpert and sung by Louis Armstrong.

I wrote to Thalia W., one of my class mates, (but never posted it!) from Kamloops. It read:

Dear Thalia, I hope that you are having a great holiday in America. At the moment I guess we are not far away from you. We are having a lovely holiday over here and the weather is so hot. There seems to be a drought here and we have to preserve water as much as we can. I'm eating so much, too. Almost every day we have pancakes for breakfast and we're eating a load of French fries for dinner, very unhealthy! We have been cycling and walking lots. The horse riding looks very inviting but appears rather expensive here. Having crossed the border, we are now in Canada. Take care, hope to see you soon and enjoy the summer. With lots of love from Claire. xx

August 1991

Saturday, August 17, 1991: I certainly live life in the fast lane, because no sooner were we back in England that I was off on Beach Mission and very scary the first day was too, without even time to get over jet-lag. It seemed so hard to settle back to life in the UK but Dave and Anita, family friends, were on holiday in Broadstairs and they came to see the team and cheered me up a little bit.

Through the week we had family games on the beach, Bible story time for the kids, and of course, the proverbial *[sic]* sand castle competitions. I soon settled into the routine and loved it, but at the same time yearned to be back in Surrey. So at the end of a tiring and busy week, Saturday found me back home and into a nice soak in the bath. My Mum had placed a book in my room and wrote:

August 1991

Dear Claire, just a brief note to welcome you home. The enclosed book, P.S., I Love You, is to congratulate you on your exams and on being made a prefect.

I bought the book at Fort McCloud, Alberta, when we were on holiday; as the title and explanation behind it made me think that I don't tell you often enough how much I love you and also one day soon you will be left home forever. Will I be writing to your or will you be close enough for phone calls, I wonder?

The following are examples of "P.S.s" that Jackson's mum would write at the end of her letters to her two children:

(Although you haven't had your exam results yet, I thought that the P.S. on page 5 was timely):

-"What you are becoming is more important than what you are accomplishing,"
(and also page 9):
-"Dearest Daughter, you don't have to prove yourself. You've done your best and that's all that matters."

-*"You can make more friends in two months by becoming genuinely interested in other people than you can in two years by trying to get other people interested in you." (Dale Carnegie)*

As an aside, Claire, I feel this was so very true of you throughout your life because, as each of your spiritual fathers relates in his Foreword, one of your defining characteristics was your interest in others.

- *"I know you have an impressive wardrobe but of all the things you wear, your expression is the most important. If someone remembers your dress and not your smile, you didn't smile enough."*

- *"One of God's greatest miracles is to enable ordinary people to do extraordinary things."[28]*

So Claire, I am so very proud of you and hope you are proud of yourself. Christians are allowed to be proud of their accomplishments because it is God living in us, changing/helping us. So welcome home, congratulations on being made a prefect and I hope you enjoy the good advice in this little book. Enjoy being 16. P.S., I love you!

Sunday, August 25, 1991: It's impossible to describe all my feelings today. In many respects I feel really numb and quite pathetic. I don't really know how to feel, what to think and how to react. It was lovely to see my Belgian cousins today. England does not seem the same, nor life in general, either. As said, no words can describe how I feel.

---

[28] PS I Love You, Compiled by H. Jackson Brown, Jr. 1990 Rutledge Hill Press, Nashville

Monday, August 26, 1991: Now I feel as if I've been back in England for many days and do not feel at all different. I still haven't got over my jet lag. It was a lazy morning but really quite enjoyable, too; it was nice to do virtually nothing and basically try to relax. I watched lots of TV programmes. It was sad to see Mr. Rhoades but it was also lovely to see him, too. It was lovely to see Auntie Pat this afternoon. It doesn't seem possible that we've been all that way around America and Canada and in many respects it seems so sad we are back. One's mind can only take in a certain amount and with Beach Mission last week, I feel overwhelmed with different things from church. Jo and Rachel are so wonderful.

Tuesday, August 27, 1991: The first day of Holiday Bible Club (HBC) at our church today; so many things seem to have been taken from Beach Mission ideas. We only had about 40 children, which is our lowest number ever and quite sad; however, we shouldn't go by the amount of children. It's quality, not quantity as the saying goes, and all of them heard the gospel. The weather today was really hot, but still so much enthusiasm from the leaders as well as the children. It was lovely to see Ndullee again. It was really weird to walk past Hampton Court this afternoon. So many visitors flood there every year but because it is on our door step, we don't give it a second look. Shame on us with all its history.

Thursday, August 29, 1991: It was sad to leave HBC today. We arrived at Heathrow, which was so disorientating as we felt as if we were going on a plane. The journey down to Dartmouth on the coach was really scenic. We had a nice time getting a taxi, going across the river Dart on the ferry and then down to the tennis courts. The fireworks were amazing too; ooh, aah, better than last year.

Friday, August 30, 1991: Today we watched the tennis and helped with the teas. We walked to Dartmouth Castle and then on to the Pottery.

Saturday, August 31, 1991: Although we had big plans for today, we did not manage to fulfil them. This morning we watched the tennis. Uncle Keith won the Men's singles, then lunch, followed by the Men's doubles, where they came runners up. The Awards Ceremony was a time of celebration.

September 1991

Sunday, September 1, 1991: It felt peaceful to be in church today, followed by lunch and a good afternoon. We had a lovely meal out this evening and our last look at Dartmouth.

Monday, September 2, 1991: We arose quite early this morning as we had to get back home. We said goodbye to everyone, including Rob and Chris. We then took the ferry over to Kingswear and went into Paignton. We had a lovely view of the Torbay area. The coach trip was scenic and went very quickly. Summer holiday, gone.

Tuesday, September 3, 1991: It was very daunting going back to school. I guess this was because it's like starting all over again and beginning something new. The A level options were hard to decide and I feel as though we didn't really get a wide enough choice, or counselling after our GCSE results. I certainly felt as if I needed to talk to someone seriously about the choices I was making before I may make a mistake in choosing subjects.

It was good to see everyone again, but the school just didn't seem at all whole now that half of Form 5B had left. It seemed empty and quite depressing. So many faces were missing; people who I just expected would be there and in the end had decided to go to 6th form college rather than return here. Their faces flash across my mind now; friends of yesterday but also hopefully friends forever. I do know some of the teachers, but not all of them. I'm a bit apprehensive about starting a new course, but at the same time there is an element of excitement toward the unknown and undiscovered. The prefect role does not sound at all glamorous now; it appears as a grueling task; but in for a penny, in for a pound, I'm now committed to it. The summer holidays seem such a long way away. I don't want to examine my feelings.

Wednesday, September 4, 1991: In many ways today just seemed the normal routine, but yet very different and bewildering. It felt like a new term, but didn't have that ring of depression. The whole approach appeared more relaxed, an air of carefree attitudes. It was great to have a visit from some of our mates who popped in, as their college doesn't start until next week: Zoe, Catherine, Beth, Helen and Jo. It was such a surprise, but then again, almost normal to see them. We used room 6, a great haven, and remnants of the 4th and 5th years were still very visible, breathing and living.

The prefect duties were given out but it seemed hard to tell the new first years what to do. The whole day was stretching on the mind but exciting and worthwhile. It's going to be a lot of hard work, though.

Thursday, September 5, 1991: The 6th form still doesn't seem real to me, although all of the others seem to be relaxed. Our form is not really cohesive yet, but I suppose that's because a lot of them are spending so much time in the common room. With the 6th forms above us, they all seemed so mature, but I feel about as mature as a new pea in a pod. Poor D. is having a hard time of it at the moment; they all seemed so happy together in June, but that could all have been part of a front. The situation must be difficult for everyone.

Friday, September 6, 1991: It's hard settling back into school and I don't think it helps that it is some sort of fashion show as we all turn up in mufti each day. To my hospital appointment today and surprisingly the time went really quickly. My lung function I had to do over and over again; maybe they just couldn't believe how bad it was. My x-ray was a disaster. I hate the thought of all that radiation everywhere, despite being told the risks are small. I was excited to be returning to Spectrum this evening and the children definitely were, too.

Saturday, September 7, 1991: It was really strange today, just sleeping and sleeping but I really felt as if I needed it after the Cornerstone night-hike yesterday – not exactly wise after a whole week at school. I just felt so completely tired and exhausted.

Sunday, September 8, 1991: It doesn't seem that I have been away from Hook at all; in fact it just seems the same. People are sun-tanned, hair has been cut in readiness for the new school year; outward appearances may change, but people are just the same inside. It seems unbelievable that this time last week we were still in Dartmouth. I enjoyed having Jo round today; it would be my dream to be half as nice as she is.

Monday, September 9, 1991: Daunting is how I describe it, the trip down the middle aisle of the hall in Assembly when us prefects are paraded before the rest of the school. It seemed very strange returning to Room 6 to see a class has taken over our notice board.

Tuesday, September 10, 1991: As Louise said today, life just seems to be one big meeting. We were given all our text books for our two-year course, but the highlight of the day was General Studies with Tiffin boys. It wasn't as compartmentalised as I thought it would be.

Wednesday, September 11, 1991: We've only been back at school a week which seems virtually impossible, as it seems an age. We are expected to work by ourselves more, and I guess this is usual for A level studies. There are a lot of things we are encouraged to get involved in, such as voluntary work, but I guess it is finding the time (saying that emphasises how middle aged I sound, but I get haggard and physically exhausted) and also a balance between Christian Union at school, continued youth work at church and other extra-curricular activities. Also I will be working each week for Dennis from now, so that's another commitment. However, I did sign up for weekly visits to the care home for senior citizens (we get two free afternoons a week, so one I will spend at the care home and the other doing my neighbour's cleaning; he pays me well).

Thursday, September 12, 1991: The week tends to feel as if it gets longer and I don't feel I am back into the swing of school yet. I had another bout of *deja vu* today, so I guess that I must have dreamt of this day before.

Friday, September 13, 1991: The Spectrum youngsters were great again this evening; they are so enthusiastic and excited to come each week.

Tuesday, September 17, 1991: We've only been back at school for two weeks, but I've completely exhausted my mufti wardrobe already. Soon I'm going to give up and just wear different coloured jeans with a colourful top. School keeps us all so busy; it is tiring and if we don't share subjects together, one doesn't see much of one's friends.

Thursday, September 19, 1991: Speech Day today and we were form 5B again for the evening; it felt lovely to be back together and fantastic to see everyone again. We had time to speak to one another before the ceremony began. The evening was much more relaxed than I had imagined it. The teachers all wore their black gowns. It was nerve-racking going up on the stage to receive prizes, but very acceptable at the same time. Being the selfish type, I quite enjoyed people looking at me for the moment. We all sang the school song with pride.

Friday, September 20, 1991: I still feel worried about telling pupils off (if the need arises) during my prefect duties, so I need to increase my authoritative skills!

Monday, September 23, 1991: Swimming again today and Miss E. says I am naturally buoyant. Phew, at least something is in my favour. We are well and truly ensconced into Christian Union now, but am I as good a Christian as the others; or should I just stop any comparisons and know that I don't reach God's standards? For that matter, none of us do. Should I always check things out, or follow my intuition? I guess this is a steep learning curve for each one of us who are leaders now and only time will tell.

Thursday, September 26, 1991: Mum has been fantastic today and particularly kind and friendly towards me. We had news from Auntie Lesley today; it was very sad news and it is understandably horrific. Auntie Lesley's cancer has now spread to the pelvis.

Friday, September 27, 1991: We received our prefect badges today but if truth be told this was not such a highlight because I still miss our previous peers who have moved on to other 6th form facilities.

October 1991

Tuesday, October 1, 1991: A new month already, although it doesn't distinctively feel like autumn yet. Everything seems like a blurred vision of despair; not for me necessarily, but for others. The news is inevitably full of doom and gloom and I find myself wondering why God allows suffering to continue unabated. But as we learned on Sunday, from Ecclesiastes (ch 1, verse 2) "Meaningless! Meaningless!" says the Teacher. "Utterly meaningless! Everything is meaningless." Until, of course, we see it all under God's perspective. Christian Union was exciting today. (Well, it was when we got over the panic!) We had a good number come along. But following that panic, another set in; I haven't even started on my essays yet and I'm worried that I won't get them done in time. I guess it's all about balance and life is just that, one big balancing act.

Friday, October 4, 1991: Today a lift down the road from none other than the headmistress! It was really scary actually, but she was ever so nice and comforting and she made me feel so welcome and wanted. It was nice to feel that I was able to speak to her one on one.

Monday, October 7, 1991: Swimming was good again today, learning new strokes, and although Miss E singles me out to tell me not to exhaust myself, I think she has my best interests at heart. I must admit I get very breathless after a few lengths, but that's life with CF. However, I don't want excuses to be made for me; I just want to be one of the crowd.

Tuesday, October 8, 1991: Another day in paradise began okay today, but as is the norm, gradually deteriorated. Actually, it wasn't too bad, but my opinion of life is pretty drab at present. I don't know myself. Sometimes I wish I'd never heard the word "baptism." The lady in Superdrug was so nice to me. Sometimes I just feel so deflated. I guess I just need reassurance; for someone to tell me that everything will be fine and not to worry about anything. Sometimes I feel mad that things go so wrong, but I can't help feeling sad for myself because that's the type of person I am and life is such a pickle.

Thursday, October 10, 1991: Autumn definitely has arrived with more leaves on the ground than on the trees. Shades of yellow, red, orange and brown carpet the streets. The Tearfund lunch for Christian Union went okay. I wish Mum was as understanding as she was today always and I wish life would gradually improve and I would be ever so grateful if life was much more enjoyable and fun. Auntie Lesley being ill is not fun. Whenever I go to Dennis' I don't feel at all pressured yet I thought I would, but I just get worried beforehand and then panic. God seems quite distant at the moment but a paradox really, because at other times quite close.

Saturday, October 12, 1991: I still feel about thirteen or fourteen; a stop button must have been pressed because I'm just totally in turmoil and haven't matured at all (that's why I have to remind myself that I am valued and mature and loved). Life seems to be full of many ups and downs and the distance feels further when heading for the ground. I am so damned impatient and unrealistic, basically; I guess because I've inherited it from my mother, which is nothing to boast about.

Thursday, October 17, 1991: My Jo is 18 today! I remember when we used to play with Cindy dolls and have jumble sales. It was all good, clean fun; we will never play with Cindy dolls again and that is quite sad and sentimental. Looking back on life as it was, I guess it's because I enjoyed life then. Open Evening was good and it was really nice to see Emma again. I want to keep in touch with all of my friends; I want to write to them and hear about their husbands and get photos of their kids in school uniform in years to come. Maybe I'm asking too much of them; maybe even too much of myself. I really like it when the school feels cohesive; that's when it feels like home.

Friday, October 18, 1991: It felt really weird not going to school today, but my trip into Kingston was actually quite successful and I even managed to buy a pair of shoes. Dennis' was surprisingly okay and I actually felt pleased that I went because the work was quite rewarding. Cleaning out cupboards I think has been my favourite so far, although I don't know if I'll ever have such a good day again. I'm really scared about getting baptised. Despite feeling muddled and confused, I'm sure everything will work out okay. Maybe I take things far more seriously than I should.

Sunday, October 20, 1991: It seems impossible that a week from today I'm going to be baptised. Rachel and I tried on our baptismal dresses and they looked absolutely awful! I feel so nervous about standing up in front of all those people and giving my testimony and pretending I'm really close to God and know everything that there is to know.

Monday, October 21, 1991: Half term and it was a bit of a funny day today as there was so much of a catastrophic nature about it, although it was quite a good day too. I went to see the consultant, who was extremely kind and helpful; she was so lovely and really did support me while I was feeling pretty down in the dumps and nervous. She told me that I had a "mild" form of CF, which really helped me and made me feel a little happier about myself and about life in general. She seemed pleased to hear about my mum and everything like that; she was really encouraging and had time. She didn't rush me; she was just kind and considerate and loving. I really don't want to have another doctor because all I know is Dr S. and that is someone who is really comforting and friendly. I really hope that I can be of the same help to somebody soon.

Thursday, October 24, 1991: It was really weird to see Caroline and Michelle today from my primary and junior school days, although it was so exciting, too. We had so much to catch up on; neither one has intrinsically changed. Yes, their expressions and appearances have, but they are still my friends and people who I care about deeply. I had missed their friendship and there were so many things that I had forgotten that now sparked my memory. We had shared so many good school times together, as well as bad, yet we are still really close. There are times over the years when I've felt sad because St. Mary's was the place where I felt secure, safe and loved before the unwelcome world of senior school hit.

Friday, October 25, 1991: When we went to our baptismal class today I wasn't very happy at being encouraged to share in my testimony that I have Cystic Fibrosis. I guess I'm being silly because I am now worrying about it. There will be nothing to be afraid of although I can't help think how people will react, although of course my school friends who will be there know, as do indeed the majority of people. I just need to grit my teeth and have faith in God, who will be with me.

Sunday, October 27, 1991: Today was very fulfilling and very lovely. It was a special day and one that I will certainly remember. Before we went into the church, both Rachel and I were quite nervous, but by the time we reached the pulpit, all our fears seemed to disappear and we relaxed. It seems odd to say that it felt like my birthday. Mum made it a special day and efforts were not in vain.

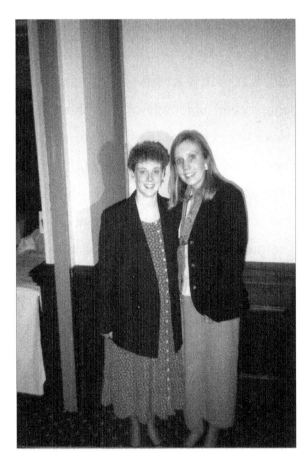

Rachel J, one of long-standing best friends, and Claire after their baptism.

I received some lovely letters (good old photocopying again!):

From Dr. Wright (on the occasion of my baptism): *"My dear Claire, just a wee note to say how glad I was to hear your testimony this morning. I was very moved. You spoke splendidly and I could hear every word; you were so relaxed and joyful."*

From Mum: *"Dear Claire, we're very proud of you. You were really great today."*

Rachel J., who I was baptised with: *"I want to tell you of the joy that I feel that we are sharing this special day together. It is a day I will never forget."*

And from Fleur: *"Your testimony was so clear this morning that even the children could understand what it means to be a Christian. . ."*

Monday, October 28, 1991: Today felt like the day after my birthday or Christmas. I suppose that it was because I was really excited about yesterday; it was really special. Looking back on yesterday I felt I had a truly marvellous day with so much to look forward to, to praise God for and also to appreciate. I felt really happy after yesterday and really pleased that so many of my friends came.

Tuesday, October 29, 1991: Back to school today and now there is a whole fresh half term ahead waiting to be discovered and also explored. Let's hope for the best. I felt really strange about accepting to speak in assembly with the focus on Christian Union.

November 1991

Friday, November 1, 1991: It was really odd looking at my school hymnbook today and realising how many of my previous peers have gone; some gone forever. Those pages, back and front, filled with messages from them to me, just as I had messaged and signed in theirs. I don't know how some of my form can have weekend jobs, but I guess my weekends are full of youth leader commitments and church, so it maybe balances things out. But let's not worry about things like that; there's so much to look forward to and enjoy, even though it's hard. I'm looking forward to having the house to myself tomorrow and just relaxing.

Thursday, November 7, 1991: Today I felt quite relaxed; maybe I have come to the point of beyond worrying and feeling sorry for myself. I've just looked back to what I wrote in January this year; those feelings have been around for quite a while and yet they are not prominent in everything; they are not ultimately the first thing on my mind all of the time. So far this year, change has been okay. Being a teenager is an experience, yet I think that the feelings we have will always be remembered and perhaps not understood. Life seems to be a bit of a problem for most people and yet they nearly always pull through. I believe, equally, that school is a bit of a problem for most people, too. Poor Auntie Lesley; why am I complaining when I've got the world and she has virtually nothing as far as health is concerned? We're definitely going to see Auntie Lesley in Belgium at the end of the month, which I'm looking forward to.

Sunday, November 10, 1991: It was quite a nice, relaxing day today. At present I like having quiet Sundays at home with not too much going on.

Monday, November 11, 1991: My friends were so kind today in supporting and encouraging me with my exam; it really meant a lot to me and I was so relieved that I could answer the questions adequately. I hope I am becoming less nervous of situations that in the past I would have found difficult; it's nice to speak to people who have the same worries as me. It was a time today to remember the fallen in the Great Wars. So many over the years; young men, merely boys, older men too, husbands, fathers, and then much older men. A time to give thanks for those that lost their lives for us. Mum performed her annual attack with the needle for my flu vaccine today and now I'm suffering the consequences!

Friday, November 15, 1991: The school day was okay today and everyone seemed to be pleased it was the end of the week. I enjoyed working at Dennis' this afternoon and did some ironing instead of polishing the wood floor. I continue to enjoy voluntary work at the care home, and that is genuine. Even if people do voluntary work only to put it on their UCCA or PECAS University forms, that's up to them, but believe it or not, it's one of the highlights of my week. I want to be popular, but also just be myself. Just totally 100% myself and no one else. But that won't happen at all. Why do I waste my time thinking about stupid things when I've so many memories to cherish, so much to look forward to? I can recall such brilliant things that otherwise I wouldn't have experienced. My friends are so supportive and kind to me. Someone has failed Sociology. Thankfully, it wasn't a person in my form. The school is not pleased with this happening; being a grammar school, a teacher's head is bound to roll.

Monday, November 18, 1991: People kept telling me how pale I looked today and yes, I was feeling grotty. Sometimes I wish that I could just fall into bed without a second thought at all and sleep. A fifth year that left to go to college has now returned. I didn't know her very well but I feel so sorry for her as it was a bit of a let-down, leaving, then having to come back because things hadn't worked out. In Sociology today we looked at a portion of *Roots* and were asked to give our reactions. I felt ashamed to be white and would not blame the whole black race if they hated all of us. Similarly, walking through Cardboard City outside Waterloo station evoked so many feelings in the group that we talked about it for ages after.

Robert gave me reassurance in myself and a definite confidence. I guess he made me feel as though I was someone who was worth something.

December 1991

Tuesday, December 3, 1991: It seems impossible that yesterday we were in Brussels and today we're back in England. Why was I born into this English family? Obviously I was meant to be, but why weren't the other two babies born too; why was I the only one out of the three of us? If truth be told, I am jealous of my twin cousins. It must be lovely to have someone to talk to and really appreciated; someone who can understand you; that you can relate to and who is always there caring for you despite tearing your hair out at them sometimes; someone who you can completely depend on and can go back to time and again. Someone you can laugh with and remember the good old days, family holidays and different relationships. Someone who is always part of your life, whom you have always shared with and always will.

In Religious Studies today we were asked for our views on euthanasia, AIDS and homosexuality. A long and sometimes heated discussion. I need, as a Christian, to form my opinions aligned to God's Word but at the same time loving those who are different.

Saturday, December 7, 1991: Spectrum was good yesterday evening and I really enjoy it when I am permitted to do the talk. The doctor and nurses were really nice and friendly to me when I had to go to the hospital today. I couldn't believe that this long line didn't hurt at all and it was no trouble, though I don't relish getting up even earlier for Mum to do all my IVs, nor having to be in at a certain time at weekends at the other end of the day for them.

Monday, December 9, 1991: School was not at all bad today and my English result was surprisingly good, I am pleased I read *Pride and Prejudice* with detail and precision. It pays off when I pay attention to things!

Thursday, December 12, 1991: It was great to see Zoe, Catherine and Beth today and pick up with them virtually where we all left off after the summer holidays. Lucky them to have come to the end of term already, while we slog on! I am so sorry that Cecilia has left church. We can only do a certain amount to make people feel welcome, because at some stage they are responsible for themselves.

Sunday, December 15, 1991: A really good day with the whole family to ourselves for the day. As Christmas approaches, I am humbled by those who give up a day with their families, the 25th December of all days, to work in soup kitchens and hostels so that those less fortunate can at least have food in their stomachs and a roof over their heads and feel wanted and cared for. How guilty I feel in a centrally heated house in the London suburbs, clothes on my back and food on the table, that I am so fortunate. As my mum reflects, what makes one person born a king when another is born a pauper?[29] Oh, for there to be more equality in this sad world. What's more, I am sickened by people who abuse children. We have looked a bit in Sociology regarding social work and the need for child protection. Not only am I sickened that we live in such a society; but how dare parents abuse their own children? I am reminded of the book *Colour Purple* (Alice Walker, 1982, Harcourt Brace) and Celie's father saying to his neighbour that his daughter, "Ain't fresh." Of course she was not fresh! He knew, because he was the abuser; he was raping her!

Friday, December 20, 1991: The last day of school this year; the last time of being friends for another year; the last of many things and only a few good-byes not accounted for. Still seems so odd not to be back in our old form 5B at this Christmas time and celebrating together. I guess that I really enjoyed today, although poor Ndullee was ill for this last day of term with flu. Thus the last day of our first 6th form term and, in general, a whole new outlook on life.

Saturday, December 21, 1991: Mr. Rhoades passed away this afternoon. At Home for Christmas, free from all his pain and able to walk and speak again with no difficulty. Mr. Rhoades was always ever so kind to me, friendly and joyful. He was always asking after my welfare and was wanting to know how I was, even though he was bed-bound during his last months on earth. He cared about others; he will never be forgotten and he will live on in memory. I hope in time I can show his kind of sensitivity.

Tuesday, December 24, 1991: I am sure the Creator did not want us to be this busy, this involved with materialism at this special time of year.

---

[29]   William Sangster, 'He is able' (Wyvern Books, Epworth Press 1962)

It is meant to be a festival for Christians, but everyone (or at least nearly everyone) has joined on the band wagon. A time for giving, not forgetting, a time to love, a time for peace. A time for hating and fighting to cease.

Wednesday, December 25, 1991: Christmas day 1991. 6:10 a.m. I get up to get ready for church and this is really exciting. It was a lovely day; the church service so special, with the children having fun up on the stage showing their presents to the congregation. Mum and I then went to the hospital where she works, which was special. We spent time specifically with James and Jean, two patients who didn't have visitors. There was so much traffic on the London roads, which I was quite surprised to see. The rest of our day was spent at Auntie Pat's, a great day in all.

Thursday, December 26, 1991: Boxing Day. It was an enjoyable day with a lazy morning; a good atmosphere, television to watch and family and friends for lunch and tea. We had a superb lunch. It was lovely to especially see Auntie again, albeit we saw her two days in a row! I did so well with my presents again this year from both friends and family. A fantastic Christmas.

Friday, December 27, 1991: "Rainy days and Mondays always get me down." (I can't remember which song these words come from, but I think The Carpenters sing it, but it sure was raining today.)

Saturday, December 30, 1991: Almost the last day of 1991 and it has gone by so fast. I hope that in 1992 I can fulfil some of my aspirations and be selfless rather than selfish and help other people as so many help me and generally be much kinder to my friends. There is so much to think about.

Chapter Seven

Preparing for University

November 14, 2011

Claire, as you began to conclude your senior years of school at the start of 1992, and prepare yourself for the bold new world of university, I think back to another time that found you nervously excited. After seemingly endless preparation, November 14, 2011 found you moving in to your beautiful new home! All the shopping in preparation for your move meant you tired very easily and your lack of energy was constant. Astoundingly, this rarely ever held you back, and in time I came to a realization, that despite your beautiful and feminine persona, you were tough as nails. Still, we wondered how you had avoided going into hospital immediately following the tremendous effort of the move, and all it entailed.

The ironic part was that likely due to our constant struggle against CF, I was less protective over you than many parents who did not face the same struggles. There are certainly many parallels that can be drawn living with CF and I remember the all too frequent times your friends and I stopped for a coffee break to give you a rest when on shopping expeditions and the like. Because we loved you, it just became part of the excursion. I do think, Claire, that you knew before any of us that you were seriously ill. True to form, however, you kept going, resilience in the face of adversity. Resilience can come at a price however, and after having moved into your new home, you became too unwell to stay by yourself.

I stayed with you, and even though you weren't feeling on top of the world, you emailed from work:

"Mum, thank you for all your love and support to me over the last few weeks. It has meant so much to come home and know that there is some-body there to care, love and support me in everything."

You always kept going Claire, never one to give in easily, and always up for some fun. You even accompanied Penny to meet Yasmine in Reading one Saturday. To my relief, this was a halfway point to Yasmine and thus a good venue.

Life at No. 10

Prior to your move we took your coffee table to the furniture shop to match up the colour for a larger dining table for which you now had room. We meticulously measured all the windows for curtains and blinds, arranged a date for the intruder alarm company to come and fix the alarm, and drove to Ikea to buy the kitchen shelf and window blinds.

We had it down to a fine art on moving day regarding tea-making facilities and to provide lunch for all the help you had. Praise God Steve W., your group elder, had arranged a tremendous removal team from church, whilst your friend Rhys P. drove the delivery van. Peter H., the Pastor of Discipleship at Chessington E.C., called in to me early on the morning of the move just to see if all was in hand. I also had help from my church home group, packing boxes into the church minibus a couple of days before in readiness for the team from Hook to deposit in your home once it was cleared of your furniture. This was a double move that certainly required a lot of planning, especially as you had been so unwell and still on treatment at home. We not only had to empty everything from my bungalow, but had to fine-tune the moving of your furniture so that my boxes and furniture could be put in yours! As you were upsizing, you had done your part in ordering the new furniture you required from Dwell and Next for delivery once you had moved in. Auntie Pat was in charge of refreshments that day, but it was your job to go round and take the orders for everyone. We laughed because you looked in vain for the man fitting the aerial, until I suggested he may be up in the loft. When you found him, he was so pleased indeed to be offered tea and cake! It was all so exciting, and well planned, I am just so sad, so very sad, that all the hopes and dreams we both had for you living there were cut acutely short.

The following day I got cross with you because you wanted to re-arrange the bed-room furniture that had been carefully placed by the men the day before. Claire, I am so sorry I made you cry; I think we were both just totally exhausted, but you especially. I did move the furniture around, however; not for my convenience, but for yours. It was oh, so worth it, because you were so very happy with your new layout. The next day saw Steve and Cliff putting some fixtures and fittings up in the shower room and family bathroom, while we took your clothes from the hanging rails and put them in the large fitted wardrobe in the en-suite bedroom. Oh, how you loved that wardrobe, Claire! On Thursday we unpacked some of the kitchen boxes, whilst on Friday of that week we headed to Kingston to shop for the incidentals you still required.

Because your previous house had all my boxes deposited in the lounge while renovations were being done, I stayed with you as you were so unwell by then, you said you could never have managed without me. Right up until you went into hospital there were still things that needed to be done in the house. Having read so many of your texts, Claire, I am now aware of how very ill you felt for so long. I pray I gave you the support you desperately needed and so deserved.

Cliff and Steve continued to come each Wednesday morning to help with D.I.Y jobs, right up until Christmas, and we were so grateful to them. Pete, our handyman, was great at coming to our rescue when the landing light broke one weekend, as he had been so many times previously. We managed to get the loft ladder and flooring put in to store some of your boxes from your earlier years for which I no longer had room. You loved your new home so much, Claire. Even if you were only able to enjoy it for a few weeks, it was worth every penny and every effort in getting it exactly how you wanted it. We went to Brian and Rosie's wedding in December, but still the builders and contractors came in to the house regularly to put right the "snagging," as they called it; the little defects and shifts the house makes after being built. We had to continually remind them of what needed correcting. This extended to outside, like the garage and the front garden that needed some work.

Do you remember all the deliveries you were expecting? No one seemed to know where this new housing development called Hinchley Park was, while the GPS system directed them to other roads in Esher. I used to go down and wait at the entrance to the estate, for fear they would give up and go away with your precious items undelivered. That even extended to pizza and Indian takeaways, which we ordered at the end of a busy day. We'd unpack and put things into their new places as we enjoyed our much anticipated dinners. I'll never forget you were so chuffed to know that a Red Rose Indian take-away was opening up in Hinchley Wood. We also went to the Prince of Wales (one of your favourite pubs) for a meal and into either Cobham or Esher to Carluccio's often, both before and after you moved. Carluccio's was also like home from home when you were in hospital in London, with a restaurant just opposite South Kensington station.

Your texts at this time to your pastor, family and friends probably best revealed your thoughts, hopes and fears:

"16th December: Been at hospital today; didn't admit me as no beds but Mum has to stay with me for a while as infection quite bad."

Although I suggested you didn't "do" Christmas 2011, I was amazed how you found time to shop for the many presents you normally buy. I was feeling probably twice as healthy, yet didn't do half as well as you. We did, however, manage to get in to Kingston to buy your lovely fur coat from the sale in Coast! Although you only got to wear it a few times, it made me so happy to see how much you loved it.

Sadly, you were not well enough to make and ice a Christmas cake as you had done in previous years. How you managed entertaining at Christmas, Claire, I have no idea, but you wanted every one of your friends to have a meal at your spacious dining table, or at least to have coffee in your roomy lounge. Nat and the children came, so did Hannah and Mark, Rich and Caroline, Rach, Saj and Asha, together with Bernie, Edwin and Timmy. Louise and Suzanne also, as well as Elisabeth and Jessica. It so blessed my heart you were always surrounded by so many wonderful friends. You also had your book group for dinner and hosted Bernie's birthday for her work colleagues. (Bernie also celebrated in style for her 40th in London.)

As you got into the swing of things, you and Jo R. attended a cupcake decorating evening and brought home the most delicious and cleverly decorated cakes. You, who said you weren't much of a cook or baker, turned out trumps on many occasions. Together with Jo R., you headed up to Westfield shopping centre, where you bought PJs in readiness for your lung transplant. Again, I am in awe of you accomplishing this trip when you were already very ill.

As I write, I have located the gift card you gave me your last Christmas morning:

"To Mum, this is a make shift ticket (authentic ones to be collected from Waterloo station box office) to "The Railway Children" on Monday 2nd January at 5:00pm. I love you so very much, Mum. Thank you for all you do for me day after day, year after year, it never goes unnoticed. Lots and lots and lots of love from Claire."

You had no idea how much those words would comfort me in years to come. In the same way, your Christmas card read:

"To Mum, wishing you a very wonderful Christmas and happy 2012. Thank you so much for all you have done towards my lovely and beautiful home."

For my last birthday, you gave me a card with an orange Gerbera which read:

"To Mum, I love you so much. Wishing you a very happy birthday. Thank you for your unending daily self-sacrifice and love and support to me."

There are so many things I wish I would have done differently, Claire, but these cards, completely undeserved by me, help so much in the moments I struggle.

As New Year's Eve rolled in, you celebrated it with Jo R. and some of her friends, while I spent the evening at No. 10. (There was nothing I enjoyed more than staying put on damp, cold, dreary evenings.) On New Year's Day, however, we enjoyed another meal at the Prince of Wales in Esher, which you loved so much. As the year kicked off and we got into January, we had a couple of visits for coffee in Carluccio's in both Esher and Cobham again. Time and again, Claire, I reflect on the last six months or so of your life realizing there was definitely a strong sense of foreboding. I knew you were very ill, but at the same time you were being seen frequently in out-patient clinics. Of course, we all fully expected you to be admitted, have a work-up for lung transplant at Harefield Hospital and give up work while you waited. One of the nurses had visited you at home to discuss transplant and I thought it was a foregone conclusion. We all assumed you would keep recovering as you always did from these bouts, enough at least to have the lung transplant. I had no idea the hospital was not as meticulous in their assessments as I expected. I certainly did not know your days were numbered.

Perhaps it was your unquenchable spirit, Claire, that threw off my deeper alarms of intuition. Looking back at your senior school years, you were ill through those too, yet you always came through. You were (despite the typical teenage angst) such a joyful person, Claire. As I've said, perhaps it's a mother's denial of the impending brutality life can sometimes dish out, but I suppose I believed things would carry on as they always had with my precious Claire enjoying her new home, socializing and working hard, just as she had done in senior school.

From 1992 and 1993 you may not have seen it, but you were developing into the beautiful adult you came to be. Thankfully, we have your journals to see this remarkable process unfold.

Chapter Eight

Preparing for University – 1992's Journals

January, 1992

Wednesday, January 1, 1992: Such was the seriousness of the eldership at Hook in commending their youth leaders for their work, that an annual Youth Workers' Covenant service was held where the church pledged to pray for us all.

Friday, January 3, 1992: Phil Rhoades funeral. I am so very sad; he was such a lovely man.

Tuesday, January 7, 1992: Back to school and a couple of us joint-leading the school C.U. meetings. The Kingston Schools' Work Trust Senior Worker, Ian Fry is coming to observe. Help!

Saturday, January 11, 1992: I enjoyed today because nothing happened and I didn't have to go out anywhere. There was nothing happening at home. As Mum would say, it's nice not to rush around. Badminton tonight was okay; the atmosphere surrounding me was good and I was relieved by that. Going to Jaquetta's was also fun.

Sunday, January 12, 1992: I'm helping with a group known as the Young Disciples; those who have come to faith and who meet regularly on Sunday mornings.

Monday, January 13, 1992: This term we have swapped from swimming to squash. There is so much to do at school, to learn and also to be thankful for. In Religious Studies we are taking a broad look at other religions and asked to form our own opinions, so no one can say we have a narrow perspective of different faiths and it is about appreciating that people have different viewpoints. Again, it was a good day to be around friends. I feel really overwhelmed at times at the state of the world; the evil of mankind versus those who work for world peace, etc. I need to get a lot more enthusiasm when working with the Spectrum children. My zeal for the work has waned rather over Christmas, and I need to get the enthusiasm back; be an example of what Christian living is about, not only with Spectrum but within my group of peers in Cornerstone. I also need to feel more relaxed talking to my Christian friends about God.

Wednesday, January 15, 1992: This evening at church it was the Youth Commissioning Service, when all of us who work with young people re-dedicate ourselves to the work and are prayed for by the church. It served as a reminder of how much we need to watch our personal walk with God so that we have the aroma of Christ as in 2 Corinthians 2.14. I wish I could begin to be a good leader and helper. Sex, lust and money are not what we should be entertaining in life.

Thursday, January 16, 1992: After my positive exam result today I was really touched by the flowers I received. I couldn't have thought of anything better to congratulate me, really.

Saturday, January 18, 1992: It was Grandma and Granddad's Golden Wedding yesterday, but the party today at our home went really well with loads of relatives and friends cramming in.

February, 1992

Monday, February 3, 1992: People are already starting to plan their summer holidays and this made me think back to last year and how exhausted I was, both physically and emotionally while I was on Beach Mission. I guess that was because I only had a day between coming back from the States and its commencement. Then afterwards, within a few days, I was back at school. I was warned I was doing too much, but hey-ho. I remember playing with the kids in the sand, sand everywhere and all I wanted was a nice shower. It was really good to speak to Kirsten on the telephone this evening. She was one of my very best friends at St. Mary's and we used to play at each other's houses.

Thursday, February 6, 1992: Part of our prefect duties include returning to school for open evenings; this time it's for 3rd years and then next week it's the 5th years. Do I live in the reality of my dreams, or the reality of life itself? I cough so very much and I am sure this puts people off.

Wednesday, February 12, 1992: Yep, I've hit the 6th form and I knew my diary entries would become less frequent. Two more days before Valentine's

Day and it will be very embarrassing to wake up and find no post, but one must always live in hope.

Friday, February 14, 1992: My fears of having no Valentine's cards have been unfounded and I have six – beat that!

Sunday, February 16, 1992: Mum has got so tired with her M.E. so that's no fun at all. I did lunch today and it was good.

Thursday, February 20, 1992: I feel mean about giving those girls a detention. I want everyone to like me; fat chance of that now. However, school rules are meant to be kept, not flouted and I did give them a second chance but to no avail.

Friday, February 21, 1992: I am relieved today is over and that I'm in bed; such a relief to be here after so long. It seems I've been awake for eighteen hours. My first problem was finding the correct road for the care home voluntary work today and I was so pleased Melanie was with me. The next hurdle was getting over the Spectrum lesson, but spring over it I did. I know I shouldn't be so concerned with such inconspicuous goings on, but they are important, especially at the end of a hectic week.

Wednesday, February 24, 1992: A good mid-week prayer meeting this evening, but I didn't pray out loud because so many of the adults were praying that I found it difficult to start a prayer before someone else jumped in. I am petrified of starting to pray at the same time as someone else does, then what would I do?

March, 1992

Friday, March 6, 1992: School was unproductive today, so it was really nice to come home. Overall at the local shops this evening we collected £78.50 for the CF Trust, a mark of everyone's kindness. The Camomile Lawn was so sensual and yet there are billposters up about it all over Kingston.

Friday, March 13, 1992: Nothing too terrible occurred today, despite it being the dreaded 13th. Didn't feel well today and had to stay at home, but I just wish I had gone or that Mum would be home. Maybe I left myself somewhere and don't know where to find me or start picking up the pieces.

Friday, March 20, 1992: Mum is really annoying me at present and I found it really frustrating that she wants a catch up day when the church party return from Israel, so I am to stay with Auntie another day. At least I get to do work experience at the hospital where she works and with her gone, I will be a person in my own right, not just "Mave's daughter." Our time at the care home went well and the staff are very kind to Mel and me. My cleaning for Dennis went well this afternoon and he is so kind to continue to pay me a good wage. It was so nice to feel affirmed in Cornerstone this evening. Grow up, girl! Do you need compliments to make you feel mature?

Tuesday, March 24, 1992: Squash today was really hard work. I get so out of breath, and I know I have another chest infection. I really need to decide if it's worth paying for a court. I've enjoyed a variety of sports over the years but am wondering how much longer I can play games that cause this much exertion.

April, 1992

Monday, April 6, 1992: Help! Is it really April already? All I have jotted in my diary are intermittent entries. Dear Journal, I am sorry for neglecting you so. Sometimes Mondays are too difficult to handle so it was an added bonus to see Faye at the bus stop this morning, when I felt so vulnerable with the task ahead. I was really nervous of doing the school assembly talk on CF with one of our teachers, Dr T., though I must say I enjoyed it and hopefully everyone would have benefitted from learning about such a common hereditary disease. I didn't give enough eye contact to the audience, but I got through it, which was the main thing. It was really nice when Ndullee told me today that I am one of her best friends. I'm so confused about Christianity at present because we are back to doing more on Science versus Creation in class and also looking at this in Christian Union, but I don't think we can emphasise the Christian perspective too much when that is the reason we are Christians. It's like a political party being apologetic for what they believe. There are so many issues that I need to be aware of as a Christian.

Wednesday, April 8, 1992: I attended Sussex Open Day but wasn't impressed with it as I thought I would be. (Sorry, Sussex!) So I have crossed that off my list. I enjoyed Easter vacation as it was a change to getting up early, but have had to do loads of coursework. We have all been moaning at the amount we have to do. Hard done by are we!

Thursday, April 9, 1992: It was good to see Jo today and read out different parts of my diary to her. We had a good laugh and there was so much to talk about. I also had a lovely time with Hannah and Rachel before they go to Caister. My friends are so precious to me.

Friday, April 10, 1992: Off to Belgium to see my family there. I was a bundle of nerves travelling on the coach to Dover and then getting on the ferry, but it was all okay.

Friday April 17, 1992: I enjoyed my time in Brussels and relaxed a lot. For some reason, coming home hasn't been so heart-wrenching as usual. Maybe because Auntie Lesley is coming to England next week. It's good to be back in my own home, own room and, you've guessed it, my own bed. This evening I talked to Mum as in three months I will start driving lessons and it's been agreed I can drive the family car and not an old banger.

Monday, April 20, 1992: Easter Monday. I must have slept soundly, as I feel so much better this morning. Maybe that is my problem. I get so used to coughing and waking myself up and thus sleep is not restful enough.

Wednesday, April 29, 1992: Back to school for the summer term today and Ndullee and Rebecca in good spirits. I've said in past years, I know, but today again I could *smell* the summer coming as I walked into the back garden after school; to get the waft of the fragrant flowers and lawn. My mum is in a bad mood with me for some reason. I can't think what it is, but never mind. Maybe it is because I fell asleep this afternoon from too many late nights instead of revising. Sometimes I dig my own potholes.

May, 1992

Sunday, May 2, 1992: To Epsom Downs with Cornerstone but it is now 1:05 a.m., so we are very late back. I believe the older we get and the nearer to us all going off to uni, I want to cling on to the past I am familiar with and the people I know; literally to stay in a time warp, however paradoxically. I am very realistic that can't happen. Rachel and I are trying to encourage others to be baptised. I really enjoyed speaking to Jo, because she kind of keeps my feet on the solid ground. Nostalgia.

Monday, May 4, 1992: Mum was really mad at me today and in such a bad mood now. I feel so guilty about what I had done because I found it hard to sleep. I have been out late four nights in a row, but it has motivated me to really crack on with things now. Staying on the phone for so long was a mistake and I know that my friends' parents are not keen for us to be wasting so much time phoning each other when we see one another at church so often. I must remember that I should be a witness to everyone and if I am a stumbling block to others then I am accountable and need to ask forgiveness when I am wrong.

Thursday, May 7, 1992: I went to Bath Uni open day today. Our form tutor has said it's best to dip in to as many open days as we have time for, because that will give us both a feel for the university and the courses they offer.

Friday, May 8, 1992: Nothing too terrible occurred today. I even quite enjoyed school and going to yet another party this evening with a host of school friends, super to chat to everyone in a relaxed atmosphere and out of school. The discussion about sex before marriage was difficult to handle and I found it hard to argue why we should keep our bodies as the living sacrifice that God intended and why, in the States, there are so many lobbying for chastity. As one of my friends said, "That's your view, Claire, because you are a Christian, but I'm not, so I feel at liberty to do what I want." That certainly put me in my place.

Monday, May 18, 1992: LVI exam leave starts today. It will be weird not seeing my school chums except for when we meet up to sit our exams, but the least said about them, the better! The boys came round this evening and we all had a good chat. Mum was cross that I stayed on the phone again for so long and didn't get my homework finished. So much to do, so little time to do it in and this is why I must discipline my social activities on week evenings.

Thursday, May 28, 1992: This is definitely the one for me, but can I get good enough grades? Kent Open Day. Wow, I just loved it. If only I could gain a place here I would be over the moon!

Friday, May 29, 1992: Half term.

June 1992

Monday, June 1, 1992: LVI exams begin. I was actually looking forward to going to school today and I quite enjoyed it, despite the awful exams. I've stopped crying about them now (maybe it's just my age, who knows?) and feel more relaxed concerning them. It was a good atmosphere and am glad we are all basically friends and it will be so sad when we have to part and say goodbye in the upper 6th form. I hope we will never forget about each other and invite everyone in the class to our weddings. It's going to be hard going with school work in the next year, but if we hold on and stick together we will get through it okay. The English exam was okay; there was a question on the use of irony in "My Country's Good" by T. Wertenbaker.

Tuesday, June 2, 1992: Thankfully no exam today, as I've been quite unwell overnight and sick too. This morning I have just slept and slept as I feel so tired. Have managed a bath, but still feel clammy. I don't want another long line for antibiotics at present. I want to be well enough to do my exam tomorrow.

Thursday, June 11, 1992: Today I had an argument with Mum because I was in the shower for far too long; it was my fault. I am feeling better and exams continue.

Monday, June 22, 1992: A really lovely day. I couldn't do without all my friends. We received some exam marks already today and luckily mine weren't as bad as I had anticipated. Having said that, I didn't do too well in the English exam and I got a lower mark than the average. Mum wasn't too pleased with my English result, but neither was I for that matter. She suggested I spend less time on the phone and more time on the computer. Well, she is right. Someone has failed Sociology again and the average mark was only 51% (phew, I managed to get a bit above that), but yet again the school is not pleased. Faye came to the church youth group this evening, then we had a sleepover at hers and watched a good video. Life does have its positive sides.

Tuesday, June 23, 1992: After breakfast, the two of us went up to the Kings Road today; it was a good atmosphere and people appearing happy with buying their designer clothes, though I doubt they are really happy inside of themselves; outward things don't last. For some reason Mum was in a really bad mood when I got home (probably because I was late).

Wednesday, June 24, 1992: It was open home for students at our house again today. We had a great time and I do like hearing how they are getting on at uni; it will be me one day! I want to be spiritual, but my ambitions never seem to be fulfilled. I don't want to rely on material possessions to give me contentment. I don't know why I feel at such a low pressure; it just seems all the air is sucked out of me and placed in the unknown. I guess I need to stop being cruel to myself. I am not an only child who is spoilt. Family have made sure of that and I am pleased. I find it hard to accept that not everyone goes to Heaven, but that is typical of me and I know I need to witness more to my friends. I did well in English Literature, so the self-fulfilling prophecy of, "You're a failure," sometimes comes up short! I hope I said the right words to someone who was very upset today. It's so important to cry with those who weep.

July, 1992

Thursday, July 2, 1992: The weather was dreary today. How very English of me to complain about the weather! The scripture truth that came to mind was that we love God because He first loved us. I don't think I could have got through today without God; He helped me a great deal. I needed help and people were there to help me. This made me feel better inside. School was not only good but I actually did enjoy it and if truth be told, it was brilliant. A nice ride home in the car and I was extremely grateful for the lift.

Saturday, July 4, 1992: American Independence Day today. I'm in love with America and Canada and want to live and work there right now. I want to pretend I'm an American high school student with loads of friends. I want to be popular and just be myself, just totally, 100% myself and no one else. I am over my word count in my extended essay.

Monday, July 6, 1992: It felt strange going back to school today – the day seemed tiresome, but I am getting to sound very much like my mother! I saw someone on the bus today that I felt really sorry for; to not fit in at all must be so hard. The buses were all askew today so I was late for school and my prefect duty. M.D. is anorexic (rather worrying when we are a year away from our A level exams) and the person I know that had this problem had another attempt at taking her life, so scary. It was, as usual, good to be back and to chat with everyone, nonetheless, especially the finals at Wimbledon, now over for another year.

I actually won at tennis today; wonders will never cease! I spoke at length to a teacher today regarding some of my concerns and she was really sweet, assuring me my feelings were not at all unusual. Christian Union was fine, but I am not that good at leading it and I wish we could take it in turns more.

Monday, July 13, 1992: My friends are so supportive and kind, especially when I feel so unwell and go back and forth to hospital. I felt guilty about not doing P.E. today, but just didn't have the breath. The hospital this after-noon was very officious. Blood tests are not my favourite past time and sometimes they really hurt. My veins are becoming more of a problem, so such tests will continue to be a challenge. I had just about put on a pound in weight, but as far as they were concerned it wasn't nearly enough. And yet I saw someone who only weighed 34 kilos and I felt guilty that I was so healthy compared to her.

Friday, July 17, 1992: Not many people turned up for lessons today which I thought was disrespectful, although we didn't do much work, it being the last week of school. There were so many offers from classmates to spend days with them over the summer vacation, but I had to turn some down, which I felt bad about.

Monday, July 20, 1992: It's my birthday in ten days' time and whilst I am excited, I don't want to be seventeen, let alone older. Oh to stay nice and young, free and happy. I am quite scared of what the future holds and there are so many things troubling me.

Thursday, July 23, 1992: The last day of the LVIth and I have now been at Tiffin for six years. The upper sixth form had their last day of school today and so many agreed that these had been the best days of their lives. It feels weird to realise that this time next year it will be our last day. Beth and Kate came into school to see us today; as usual Richmond College breaks up before Tiffin. Faye came round this evening and we did a Bible reading together. My mum is going out on my birthday next week so that I and my friends can have the house to ourselves.

We had our school reports, so starts my proverbial photocopying to stick the pages in this journal.

Lower sixth, Mr. H. wrote: "Claire has made a positive start to her A level studies. She is a sincere and conscientious young lady and participates fully in the life of the school. She is a prefect, leader of the Christian Union, and makes many other valuable contributions to various activities."

In English, Mrs. P. wrote: "Claire has made a good start to this course. Her class preparation work is thorough and perceptive and she shows an excellent knowledge of the text. Her written work is good, but she needs to keep the momentum going and not tail off towards the end of the essay."

Religious Studies, Mrs. K.: "Claire has worked with determination and a keen interest. She has made some worthwhile contributions to discussions. She must now develop her written style in order to improve the quality of her essays. She is always willing to ask questions and put forward her views. Her biblical knowledge is good."

Sociology, Mr. R.: "Claire's work is neatly presented and of a consistently high standard. She has achieved high grades for every piece of work and obviously has an aptitude for this subject."

August 1992

Saturday, August 8, 1992: Beach Mission ended today, but I thoroughly enjoyed myself; it was fantastic and brilliant, despite so much to do as a team. The atmosphere among all us Christians was great and spilled off to the kids and their parents on the beach. I guess you get out what you put into it and at the moment I think I'm on a spiritual high, so I hope it will last a long time.

Monday, August 10, 1992: It was the first day of the summer day camps today and all of a sudden I feel thrust back into the work of my church.

Tuesday, August 18, 1992: Who am I to judge, especially because most of my friends are a bit older than me, but I think that some parents don't have a grip on what their kids are doing. I really want my mum to strike up friendships with some other mums for this last year of school, but to give her her due, she does know quite a few from being on the parent/teacher committee.

Friday, August 18, 1992: The last day of Holiday Bible Club and I wonder why I am so tired. Burning the candle at both ends for so many weeks is not very intelligent. Mum took me out driving in the Escort this afternoon, which was quite fun. Mum got really panicked, though, and I don't blame her.

September 1992

Thursday, September 3, 1992: First day in the UVI, but I wish it was the fourth year all over again. I can't quite believe that I will (hopefully) be going to uni in 1993!

Tuesday, September 22, 1992: Driving lesson 2:30pm but first at 11:20, driving medical that Mum took me to. What a load of rubbish! Just because I have CF doesn't mean I can't drive, nor will I be a risk to other people using the roads.

Thursday, September 24, 1992: So sad to say bye to those a year older than us in Cornerstone who are off to uni.

Friday, September 25, 1992: Today was the Beach Mission reunion. I won't be doing it next year, so it will be the last chance to say, "Cheerio," to all the fab people I met in the summer.

Sunday, September 27, 1992: Harvest today and seeing the children go up with their produce brought back memories of when I was their age.

October, 1992

Friday, October 9, 1992: The joint C.U. meeting with Tiffin boys went really well again. But why do I have a cold, need to blow my nose and cough so much today of all days? It was so good to be appreciated: Lewis thanked me for the minutes, Nigel remembered my name and Wayne or Adam (unsure exactly who) called across the playground to say, "Cheerio." Sam asked me if I was okay holding a bundle of things and Josh let me go first into the room. I want to put my mark on this world; put something into it but also get something out of it before I blow up and evaporate into a cloudless bubble.

Friday, October 30, 1992: For a couple of days in half term we went to Belgium to see Auntie Lesley. I am so pleased we did, because very sadly Auntie Lesley died in the early hours of this morning. We will return for the funeral next week. I feel so, so sad for my uncle and my cousins.

November, 1992

Thursday, November 5, 1992: Auntie Lesley was buried yesterday in a beautiful cemetery on the outskirts of Boisfort forest. It was a very sorrowful day. How I wish that Adam and Eve had not sinned; then there would be no death, but conversely, there would be no Cross either.

Tuesday, November 10, 1992: I have to go into hospital next Monday and I haven't got time for this! It was good to chat to Caroline today and make arrangements for later in the week.

Monday, November 23, 1992: I need to commit all my concerns to God. Who am I without Him? Watching TV this evening in *Home and Away*, Meg died. One day I will go up far into the sky and see the beauty of the world. In that day I will be truly happy and secure, but until then, life goes on and nothing stays static. As a Christian I should be much more positive about my life and everything and I should be more cheerful. Mum says I should forget the things that aren't important and she is exactly right, but it's so hard to do. I'm not taking enough responsibility for my health either. I am blessed with so many truly loyal and supportive friends.

Thursday, November 26, 1992: The home care nurse came from the hospital today to follow up on my progress since leaving hospital. Lewis gave me a lift home, which I was very grateful for. If I am a Christian, why am I so bitter about life? And why don't I commit everything, even the hard things to God in prayer? I do believe I am growing stronger as a Christian, and yet I fail so often. My friends need me to support them and X. came to confide in me in the Common Room at school yesterday, so I feel friendships are definitely about supporting each other. When one is sad, the other helps and vice versa.

December, 1992

Sunday, December 6, 1992: The thing that prompts me to write now is that four of my lovely friends have their interviews for Oxbridge and we are all behind them. Met up with Catherine et al on her birthday today to celebrate with her.

Tuesday, December 8, 1992: The fact that Caroline is a Christian is really wonderful and I pray that other friends will follow suit. I drove round Kingston's one way system today. Was proud of myself, but it was scary. I have to send off for my test soon. How come that, when Elijah called out to God, He answered in such a quick and profound way? Maybe I'm just a doubting Thomas. Sue is worried she won't get into the university of her choice, so to some degree we all have doubts. Sometimes when I feel things are really unfair, God surprises me with His goodness. Despite the way I regale myself, today was very manageable.

Thursday, December 17, 1992: As we reflect on our final C.U. meeting this year, I hope we have been an encouragement to all those that attend. We sang:

"We shall stand with our feet on the Rock
Whatever men will say, we'll lift your name on high.
We shall walk through the darkest night
Setting our faces like flint
We'll walk into the light."[30]

---

[30]   Graham Kendrick © 1988 Make Way Music. www.grahamkendrick.co.uk.

(**A**s an aside, Claire, little did you or any of us know then that you would indeed walk through the blackest of all times, set your face as flint and yet, thankfully as the hymn says, walk into God's light and presence.)

Thursday December 17, 1992: Tomorrow will be our last ever final day before Christmas in school, but nonetheless I'm looking forward to it, then to hosting the joint C.U. meeting at mine on Saturday. I am so, so tired. F. phoned to say he thought I had a real vision for God, but I basically set the record straight on that one.

Saturday, December 26, 1992: Christmas Day and Boxing Day have been good family days, but my thoughts were so often with my uncle and cousins in Belgium.

Thursday, December 31, 1992: A new year on the horizon and thus a new beginning to focus on the future. These are some of my new year resolutions – rather a list!

To be selfless rather than selfish and think of others' needs

To seek peace, especially at home/think before I speak

To look after myself better by taking my antibiotics, etc. on a regular basis and undertake regular physio

Not to lie or cover up the truth

Not to use bad language, either spoken or in my mind

To be pleasant to people, even if I don't feel like it

Not to be false, but rather sincere in my intentions

To include those people who may be on the side-lines

To put extra work into my A level studies and do the background reading

To see school friends out of school and witness more often

Not be creepy and false to teachers

To do my prefect duties well

Not to say things I don't mean

To admit I am wrong when I am at fault

To tithe

My precious Claire, as we entered into 1993, your final year of senior school, I could tell you were both ready to begin preparing to leave the nest for university, while also not wanting your circle of friends to change, nor to leave anyone behind. Things do change, as we well know, but at least we are promised all things work together for good for those who love the Lord, and are called according to His purpose (Romans 8.28). That is my comfort above all else; that you are with Him. As your journals show, 1993 was a big year for you. You were blossoming into a young adult, and as always you embraced the change with more bravery and enthusiasm than anyone I've ever known.

Chapter Nine

Preparing for University – 1993's Journals

January 1993

Friday, January 1, 1993: Last night with Cornerstone was okay. Some of my school friends have got into Oxbridge, so I am really pleased and proud for/ of them. I also spoke to Grandma and Granddad and said, "I have a boy-friend," but that's not looking too good at the moment. Lewis telephoned me to say I had been invited to Sam's so I asked about F. Then I rang him; he seemed cheerful enough, but it's me whose done all of the telephoning recently, which is a bit difficult. At Sam's I had hoped we could have com-municated better, but he's not being very easy to talk to and I must admit I have not been too helpful in that area. I got a lift home with Lewis. The usual group from Tiffin Boys' and Tiffin Girls' were all there.

Saturday, January 2, 1993: I wish today had just been one big nightmare. I totally ruined everyone's day. F. got a letter from L. on Christmas Eve asking what would happen between the two of them when she got back. He says that all week long he's been thinking about her. Anyway, basically he dumped me for good. He's obviously thought about it a lot and realised that he cares about L. too much. All I remember him saying is, "Sorry." I certainly was very unkind to him. I told him that I didn't care about what he felt about L. and that I just wanted him to honour what he had said about our relationship. I asked him what I was supposed to say to my friends and family. He said that it wasn't my fault at all; it was all his fault. He said that his feelings for me hadn't changed; I said they must have because he wouldn't be telling me that about L. Then I said that I hoped he realised how much he'd messed my life up and I hope that he suffered for it. Then I telephoned everyone in tears. Rosanne was really helpful. Everyone was so nice to me. All the family must have known that something was wrong. Then I stupidly went to Rosanne's party, but I really needed to see her. She was great, and so was Sam. They prayed with me and it was great. As Sam said: "Don't get bitter, get better. Keep close to God."

Sunday, January 3, 1993: "When I met with storm and trial[31] and my heart was filled with fear
When there was no one around to speak a word of help and cheer,
Then the Lord Himself stood by me and I had no cause fear,
All was changed when He drew near.
When my earthly friends forsook me and they all misunderstood
When my words they took for evil and I meant them all for good
When I walked the vale of sorrow and my heart was aching so
When I faced a dark tomorrow with no ray of hope before. . .
Then the Lord Himself stood by me and I had no cause to fear
All was changed when He drew near."[32]

---

[31]   Author unknown

[32]   Author unknown

I cried in junior church today; I cried in church this evening. Poor J., I always cry on him. He laughed when I told him it had only been 1.5 weeks. Maybe it's all just a big excuse. I cried on Rachel and Jo and really embarrassed myself, but such is life really. I need to depend on God a lot more rather than my feelings because He is far more important,

Monday, January 4, 1993: Well, F. is fully out of my life now. We spoke today but made no arrangements to see or speak to each other again. We talked for 1.5 hours. I haven't cried in the past few hours, so I think that I'm getting over it.

Tuesday, January 5, 1993: I feel so hurt and I really need my friends around me, but I'm not going back to school properly for the next 2.5 weeks because of our mocks. I feel embarrassed because I really thought it was going to work out. If L.'s letter had not arrived, would we still be going out now?

Wednesday, January 6, 1993: Joni Eareckson Tada in *Glorious Intruder: God's Presence in Life's Chaos* says:

"Ah, be encouraged, friend. Even though your name may not roll off the tip of many tongues, God truly remembers who you are. He not only knows your name. . . ., He knows the exact number of hairs that grace the top of your head. He knows your heart, your worries, your dreams and your deepest longings. As the Lord told Israel: Your name is inscribed on the palm of My hands.

"Furthermore, there's no 'what's his name' or 'who's that' written down in the Lamb's Book of Life. That's your name written there. A name well known in heaven and well loved."[33]

"When Christians suffer with grace under pressure, people who observe even casually are forced to consider the fact of a God able to inspire such loyalty.

"The way you and I handle our big and little trials makes the world pause in its frantic, headlong pursuits. . . . The unbeliever can no longer refuse to face the reality of our faith."[34]

It helped so much talking to Caroline today as she was such an encouragement.

Thursday, January 7, 1993: When I called D.'s today, his mum answered. She was the one who glared at me during my exam in the 5th form and then afterwards told me to suck cough sweets instead of disturbing other people. By that time I had had enough and just burst into tears. I expect more than this from a teacher; if a person with CF could stop coughing by sucking cough sweets, then we would never cough again; fat chance! One of these days I may well have a nervous breakdown. Mocks started today but I felt so ill I could hardly walk downstairs. Mum told me not to go, but I couldn't not, so she took me in and was waiting for me when the exam was over to drive me straight up to the hospital.

---

[33] Joni Eareckson Tada, Glorious Intruder: God's Presence in Life's Chaos, pg 209 (Multnomah Books, 1989)

[34] Joni Eareckson Tada, Glorious Intruder: God's Presence in Life's Chaos, pg 211 (Multnomah Books, 1989)

Friday, January 8, 1993: The last day of people being at Cornerstone before they head back to uni and we parted on good terms.

Saturday, January 9, 1993: The locum doctor took blood from me today then put another long line in for yet another course of intravenous antibiotics.

Sunday, January 10, 1993: Today is the anniversary of my grandma's (my mum's mum, who died even before my mum was married) death and we went to see her name in the Book of Remembrance at Kingston Crematorium. It is 24 years today since she went to Heaven.

Monday, January 11, 1993: F. is going to be sorry I slipped through his fingers and the sooner he knows that, the better. He used me; he was selfish and made it clear that he'd had enough girlfriends without adding me to the list. He played with my heart as if it was a toy. People in general think he is immature. My long line came out today; it was so painful when Mum tried to put the IVABs through and my arm is so tender and swollen now. I got a conditional offer from Cheltenham and Gloucester Uni today.

Tuesday, January 12, 1993: Another long line inserted today, this time in the other arm.

Wednesday, January 13, 1993: Lewis came round this evening. He said that he hopes F. has learned his lesson. I think Stuart might fancy me, but that doesn't worry me too much at the moment. Lewis coming round, Catherine ringing, Chris writing proves that I do have friends that care.

Thursday, January 14, 1993: I've been thinking of all the flings I've had. Well, there was Rupert in the second year; Chris, Julius and Russell in the 3rd year; Robert in the 4th year; Edgar in the 5th year; F. in the UVIth. My driving test date is February 3rd.

Wednesday, January 20, 1993: It was sad saying goodbye to Mrs. White, my piano teacher, especially after so long, but it was okay. I don't think that I thanked her enough; she has been so kind to me all along and I guess that I should repay her in some small way for this. Rachel told me on the phone this evening that I am going to be her bridesmaid along with her sister, Sharon. It will be a great honour for me. Sometimes I behave so immaturely and disrespectful as a Christian and I need to ask forgiveness and live as I should. I need to maintain a good witness at all costs. Some couples, not only among my school friends but also at church, are splitting up and maybe it's because girls show their feelings more openly than boys, but it always seems to be the females who are really upset. I drove round Richmond Park and also Bushy Park today in preparation for my driving test.

Tuesday, January 26, 1993: Ndullee's 18th birthday today and we all had a whale of a time to celebrate. Cardiff has made me an offer, so now I have four. I just need to see what my grades are in the summer.

Saturday, January 30, 1993: I went out with Jo and Rachel today to Richmond and had a good time. Mum is getting extremely annoying at the moment and it's hard to tolerate. She said I wasted a lot of time in the lower sixth form and she is absolutely right. F. spoke to Sam as to whether he should ring me or not, so he is still thinking about our relationship.

February 1993

Monday, February 8, 1993: In retrospect I realise that I haven't been cross with F. but at myself and life in general. By the time he came along I was looking for some happiness, a little bit of security and excitement in my life. Then he took away what little hope I had. So although to a certain extent I was mad at him, I was also mad at my situation in life. Two weeks today until my driving test and I am dreading it. My life's theme is dread, fear, insecurity, lack of Christian values, no time, embarrassment and that's just for starters.

Sunday, February 14, 1993: *Love is a Many-Splendored Thing*[35] (a 1955 film). 5 Valentine's cards, so beat that!

Monday, February 15, 1993: The Villa in Spain for our summer holiday with Faye looks nice and I'm really looking forward to it. It will be good fun with lots to do and I can't wait until then. Time continues to go so quickly. In Religious Studies we haven't finished John's Gospel yet, so we are way behind.

Monday, February 22, 1993: Half term and I passed my driving test today first time, yippee. I've got three congrats cards already. We also received our final school reports; mine read (and yes, this is the last time I need to use the photocopier to glue said reports into my journal):

Sociology, Mr. R. wrote: "Claire's exam results were just above the average. Her work is well presented and of a good standard. She has a

---

[35] Love Is A Many-Splendored Thing, (Twentieth Century Fox Film Corporation, 1955)

positive attitude towards her work, always handing in her homework on time. She should read more widely and include more detail in her essays."

English, Mrs P.: "Claire's exam mark was above average and she has worked well throughout the year. She did a particularly good piece of work on *Pride and Prejudice* and showed she is capable of good grade A work.'

Religious Studies, Mrs. K.: "Claire's examination mark was pleasingly above the average. She is working with interest and enthusiasm. She has researched efficiently for her "Evolution versus Creation" assignment. Claire needs to now concentrate more on the Isaiah text. She must have a critical approach to the questions and do more background reading."

In summing them up, my form tutor, Mr. H. wrote: "This is a very good set of reports for Claire. She is a conscientious and hardworking student who can always be relied upon to give her full effort to everything she attempts. Claire is a sensitive and caring person and it has been a pleasure having her as a member of the form."

Thursday, February 25, 1993: I need to do my physio more regularly. Sue bumped her car yesterday and is a bit worried about telling her Mum. I have too high an opinion of myself and I really need to be more of a role model to the 4th and 5th years in C.U. at school. F. has let L. down and is going out with a 3rd girl in as many months. He seems to have made a fool out of himself and is totally selfish; so much so for his Christian faith.

March 1993

Thursday, March 4, 1993: We received our exam time-tables today. Mine will all be over by the 21st June and already I can't wait. It will be brilliant to have them over with, go on holiday and get a good sun tan and feel totally relaxed.

Tuesday, March 9, 1993: The physio at the hospital wasn't very nice to me today and unfortunately when the nurse did my blood test, she dropped the blood, so it had to be done again, ouch! To make matters worse, my mum was very domineering. Amy is quite a sweet person, but she isn't going to any of her lectures at uni and she calls her parents by their Christian names, which is rather weird, or so I thought.

Friday, March 12, 1993: "I will survive,"[36] sung by Gloria Gaynor 1979. It's a song that talks about moving on with life after a bad relationship.

Sunday, March 14, 1993: This evening the sermon mentioned death so much that it got me thinking about my funeral, which was quite depressing. I was trying to think who would be there and, depending on the people that came, would mean that they loved me or cared about me. But God knows what's going to happen in the immediate future and in the distant too.

Mave: As an aside, Claire, there were nearly 200 people at your Cremation Service and over 400 at your Thanksgiving Service!

Wednesday, March 17, 1993: I went up to see Bangor Uni today as their Psychology course is meant to be good. North Wales is so pretty, especially the Snowdonia area. Seeing the sheep grazing on the hillside is picturesque

---

[36] 'I Will Survive' performed by Gloria Gaynor, released in October 1978, written by Freddie Perren and Dino Fekaris. From the album: Love Tracks.

and there are so few people there; however I can see it will be very harsh in the winter.

Friday, March 19, 1993: Spectrum and Cornerstone were excellent this evening and I hadn't enjoyed either so much for ages.

Saturday, March 20, 1993: In ten years, lots of us will be married. Will I be? I hope so; if not married, hopefully engaged. But I somehow doubt it, but I can dream at least. We only have a few years of this life to prove ourselves. So few years, so much to contribute.

Sunday, March 21, 1993: Nothing, nothing is going well at present. I don't really understand why I'm so tired because I slept for so long yesterday. I complain about my mum too much, which is totally unfair and bitchy of me, especially after all she does for me.

Monday, March 22, 1993: I wish my diary could answer me back, and give me some suggestions as to how to get on in life, but I guess it's asking too much of such an inanimate object.

Tuesday, March 23, 1993: Terrorism strikes again. When is all this violence going to end, and especially against innocent children? Why does God allow it to continue? I guess it boils down to the parable of the wheat and the tares in Matthew's Gospel chapter 13; let both grow until the harvest, when God will separate them. My heart literally aches for every person who suffers unnecessarily in such hateful and cowardly warfare. A Christian friend confided in me today that he can't get close to people because of something that happened in his past. Oh, I do pray he will be able to talk to me or someone else about it again and feel some release and healing from the situation.

Saturday, March 27, 1993: Proverbs 16:3: "Commit to the Lord whatever you do and he will establish your plans." Faye and I had a real heart to heart at break in the common room yesterday. At least I have something to live for. At least I know what's happening in the world. At least I am secure and happy in my church and in a lot of my relationships.

Monday, March 29, 1993: Ten weeks today until the end of term and I am already dreading it. We had the photo done today, the last one with us all together and it was quite sad. It will be the last time, too, that we are all together as we'll all be coming in at different times for the exams.

Tuesday, March 30, 1993: Blocking the most important things out of my life, like the choice of which university I am going to go to. Reading Uni has now made me an offer, but Kent is offering a new Social Psychology course, which sounds better for a career in Social Work than the one I was first interested in.

Wednesday, March 31, 1993: One girl lower down the school confided that she has taken an overdose twice. Wow, and I think I have problems. It's to do with her exams and that she doesn't think she is doing well enough. Thankfully her mum knows about it, so that is a relief. I really didn't know what to say to encourage her, but ended up saying that she is important to so many people; that she is loved by so many and that exams will be a thing of the past soon. I could have shaken myself. If only I could have thought of more to say to reassure her.

April 1993

Thursday, April 1, 1993: It was Rebecca's 18th birthday today and we celebrated with her. We're off school tomorrow. Caroline passed her driving test today, so one by one we are all getting through first time round. I wonder what it will be like to drive a new car. Mum says that it's not as powerful, which is a bit of a shame but we'll see what it's like.

Monday, April 5, 1993: It helped me not see anyone today as I needed to speak sternly to myself: Claire, this is a warning, be careful what you say. Your tongue is dangerous and can hurt and harm people. Just think how many people have hurt you and then think of the reverse.

Thursday, April 8, 1993: Sue was upset today and she phoned me to talk about it. I'm so pleased she did. It seems that we are all supportive to one another; when one is down, the other one helps out and that's what friendship is all about. To receive such lovely Easter cards meant so much to me.

Monday, April 26, 1993: Back to school today after the Easter holidays. I was really annoyed with my mum and took my frustrations out on her; she doesn't think I am doing enough work and I must say I totally agree with her. She is in a well bad mood with me for some reason. I can't think what it is, but never mind. Maybe it is because I fell asleep this afternoon from too many late nights instead of revising. Once again I dig my own potholes. I asked God to speak to me through my Bible study this evening and He did.

May 1993

Monday, May 3, 1993: Five weeks exactly to my exams and I've hardly done any work this weekend, which is totally my own fault; I have got to start working much harder. The strong, independent woman I am turns to jelly sometimes. It's no good pretending I am studying when I am doing nothing of the kind.

Wednesday, May 5, 1993: As a Christian I should be much more positive about my life and everything and I should be more cheerful.

Tuesday, May 11, 1993: I got the dress for the school ball today which I really like. It's long, black and not too expensive. I can't wait until I wear it on 25th June.

Saturday, May 15, 1993: Ali wrote out the words to "Everybody Hurts"[37] (by R. E. M, 1992) for me, which is really good of her.

Sunday, May 16, 1993: In John chapter 16 v33, Jesus says that He has over-come the world. This was the key verse we looked at today.

Monday, May 17, 1993: Panic! Only 3 weeks to go and only 5 until they are all over. I missed my last ever senior C.U. meeting and I'm really sad to think this is the last ever normal Monday of school. I'm going to miss everyone so much. Now I'm not particularly looking forward to Friday. I can tell you it's going to be such a nightmare. I should have bought a different size dress, but I am so vain. What would I have done without Ndullee helping

---

[37]   R.E.M. , Everybody Hurts, Automatic For The People (Warner Bros, 1992)

with my folder today? L. asked after me! Quite a few of us are panicking and there are some who are on anti-depressants. You would think we were the first cohort to ever take A levels!

June 1993

Wednesday, June 10, 1993: I like writing out secular songs, Christian songs and Bible verses. Life is so hurtful. We don't have fire drill that often at school, so I guess today's was the last ever that our form will experience all these final things.

Tuesday, June 18, 1993: My hair is really greasy and I hate it when it's like this. It doesn't seem that many boys (especially not Tiffin boys) are coming to the 6th Form Ball, but I guess that's the problem of going to an all girls' school.

Monday, June 21, 1993: The less I write about them, the better; they are over and I never need sit another A level paper. To celebrate I went to Wimbledon tennis today with Melanie; a great day and so many famous tennis players willing to give their autographs. What an enjoyable and fun time. Claire E. got into Chester to do midwifery, which is really great news. It was sad saying goodbye to everyone at C.U. today. I gave hugs to Narin, Ruth and Claire and everyone, including Laura. We were all crying. Another end of an era.

Wednesday, June 23, 1993: We were told in school today about those who will be receiving prizes; for me the Mary Williams prize for Progress and

Commitment. The pupil who got this last year achieved 3 A levels, but will I get my 3 As to live up to the previous recipient?

Friday, June 25, 1993: Everyone looked so nice this evening at the ball. We all enjoyed ourselves and it was great to go to Rebecca's first. The evening was a lovely way to celebrate together and the blokes were good fun. (Well, some of them were, some of the time!) We discussed the yearbook.

Wednesday, June 30, 1993: Hannah passed her driving test first time. Brilliant. Ali's Exhibition went really well. One month until I am eighteen!

July 1993

Thursday, July 1 to Sunday July 4 1993: I drove to the caravan with my school mates; it was hair-raising for me to be driving for nearly 2 hours, but I managed it. Highcliffe in the evening. New Forest and Southbourne the following day, including Christchurch and Hurst Castle on Saturday and home Sunday. It was great to relax, chill, and hang out together.

Thursday, July 8 to Thursday, July 22 1993: To Spain's Costa del Sol with Faye for two weeks. We are spending quite a few days on Nerja beach, including rides on a pedalo and banana boat. I am not feeling great and the heat is irritating my cough. I'm in love with the man who did my portrait! We went to Granada and back down the mountain roads. Off to Gibraltar tomorrow. Hard going around the Alhambra Palace due to the heat. It has been great to relax after the last few months we've had before returning to the UK.

Friday, July 23, 1993: Last day of school, which was really sad and depressing; not as much tearfulness as I thought there would be. However, my school friends, both in the 5th and 6th forms have been brilliant and none of us really wanted them to end. I am so pleased we all feel the same way, but some more upset than others. At the end of the day, we have all been through so much together. I am sure there is something about groups psyching themselves up to leave, kind of distancing themselves from each other whilst wanting desperately to cling on to the familiar. Others have said how weird it will be making new friends at uni.

We all received the 1992-3 Upper Sixth Yearbook with the highlights of our years at Tiffin. There is a super photo of Ndullee and me when we first started at the school, some great ones of various friends, like Beth and Catherine, Claire E., Rebecca, etc. There was a photo of each of us in our last year, and our fellow class members had written about us in a caption under the photo, humorous as well as some more serious comments. Mine read:

"Claire is one of the most sensitive people I've ever met. Having said that she is also one of the most gullible; examples follow: Thalia has had her ankles surgically removed and Ndullee regularly offers her body for extra pocket money. Claire's been worried since the first year about whether she's going to have a date for the 6th Form Ball. Will her childhood sweetheart turn up on that white steed? We think not. Neurosis from first year to present day includes saying, "I'm too fat," every three seconds. If you ignore it, it goes away. A self-proclaimed 'tart' in the third year, nothing could be further from the truth! Claire is everyone's friend and always there when you need a shoulder to cry on. Lots of love xxx."

Aaahh!

We again exchanged our hymnbooks for each other to write in. Mine included:

Alice: "You've been a brilliant friend. X."

Melissa: "You can't leave the school. You're the only one who keeps every-thing nice and polite. Thanks for everything, especially all the 'Thank-Yous!'"

Catherine: "I'll never forget all the traumas we've been through together. Take care. X"

Sarah: "Haven't the years gone by quickly –whoosh! Thank you for being a very, very, very good friend to me."

Kate: "Life wouldn't have been as good if I hadn't met you. Much love."

My Drama teacher: "I will always feel guilty about leaving your name off the programme in 'Rebels.' Thank you for sharing so much commitment and sensitivity to the subject in spite of my oversight! Keep life dramatic – it was a pleasure to have taught you."

Kate G.: "I hope one day you get to be famous. Thanks for always being there for me."

Gemma: "Stop worrying about other people. Take care of yourself; you're too nice to be spread so thin."

Caroline: "There's no need to say 'good luck' cos [sic] you don't need it; you'll pass with flying colours."

Naureen: "I've only known you for two years but I think you're brilliant and a really good friend."

Sarah: "Dear Claire, you are the nicest person in the form. Lots of love and luck. X."

Helen: "Glad you stayed in the VIth form – you were too nice to go. X."

Thursday, July 29, 1993: Well, the party with my friends to celebrate my eighteenth wasn't brilliant, but all the same I think people enjoyed it. (As you know by now, Diary, I am forever the pessimist.) Matt and Claire came as Mr. and Mrs. Dracula and Mark as a Mummy; Graham as a dinosaur, which was really funny, and Faye as a movie star. Michelle and also Lewis came, plus Jo and David as Rachel and Michael! Beth and Ndullee came with Thalia and Naureen, Jacquetta and Eileen. Rebecca was brilliant and so was Caroline.

Friday, July 30, 1993: My 18th birthday. Who am I going to vote for? I've had a brilliant day and really enjoyed it. I had a letter and stuff from Mum and a book containing a potted version of my life, it read:

"30th July, 1975. Shortly after midnight you are born – your low birth rate classed you as 'premature.' I thought you were going to be a boy, you gave so much anxiety, but looking at your tiny, though perfect body in the Special Care Baby Unit, no one in the family would change you for a football team of males!

"In October, you are dedicated at Hook evangelical Church. You are God's special gift. You have so many pretty dresses and outfits, it's a job to choose what you should wear. Your first Christmas you have pneumonia, but you manage to smile and gurgle as usual. Your first winter, Grampsie is in Surbiton hospital, and we trudge through the snow (you in the pram) to go and visit him every day; you bring some reality to his confused life.

"On your first birthday Uncle Keith, with the help of your cousins Kevin and Gary, hang you up on the washing line! You have meals in the garden. You learn to feed yourself (you are such a messy pup that I strip you off and

then hose you down afterwards). Friends say they hope you don't grow up to strip off and bathe every time you have a meal!

"You have your second holiday in Bournemouth and you tear around the caravan in your walker on wheels. You like your cousins' dog Beauty and we also go to Belgium to see the other side of your family. Uncle Keith is still living in the area, so he looks after you while I work occasionally. You have lots of little friends from the neighbourhood and church that you play with.

"Your second Christmas you are old enough to get excited and over-whelmed with all your toys. In the New Year I am ill and spend six weeks recovering from surgery in hospital. You are looked after by family and friends. When I come out of hospital we have moved to Surbiton and Margaret M. looks after both of us.

"1977, now you are two. Your second birthday is a party in the garden. We continue our walks, etc. Although the summer is not as hot, holidays at the caravan continue. At Christmas you enjoy loads of toys and clothes. At two and a half you start Sunday school and playgroup at church. You get to say a short verse in Sunday school and lots of your class win first prize for 'excellent attendance.'

"1978, third birthday; you have lots of friends for tea and love your first bike. In September you start nursery school at Surbiton Hill, alongside Daniel, Louise, Vicky and Sarah. (You also go to ballet lessons with Sarah and Gail, which you really enjoy. There's a photo in the Surrey Comet to prove it!) You enjoy lots of outings with Auntie Pat and Uncle Pete. Around Christmas you have your first experience of deep snow and enjoy playing in it. You take part in the Sunday school Nativity as an angel. Jo, Bev and Sam are your buddies in this. At three and a half, for Christmas you have

Paddington Bear and love his wellington boots best. Along with Daniel N., you win a swimming certificate for completing a length of the pool.

"Fifth birthday, 1980. Your birthday is attended by nursery school, church and neighbourhood friends. You go to your first wedding. You look so pretty with your hat, too! You start school at St. Mary's, alongside Jack, Daniel and Laura.

"You have another bad bout of pneumonia and have to go into hospital for your first course of intra-venous antibiotics (IVABs.) We meet Dr. S. and little realise how often we will see her in the future! You are diagnosed with cystic fibrosis. In Psalm 23, God promises to walk through the valley with us. We realised how short childhood is and wanted you to enjoy it while you can; 'to have memories of a little girl playing, laughing, happy as the sky is blue,'[38] to ensure you loved life and also God. You are bridesmaid for the first time. We go and visit your cousins for New Year in Belgium.

"When you are five and a half it's my turn to go into hospital (for a second operation) and you are cared for by lots of nice people. At school you enjoy sports, and also learning to read, etc. Later Mrs. O. teaches you the basics of playing the guitar. You also have your first piano lesson, one of many and you love your time with Mrs. W. You get very upset as you think you have caused me to be ill. We explain that it is nothing to do with what you have done, or not done.

"Aged six and Grampsie is so pleased that you have brought such joy to an old man. This year you also have a new cousin, Lee. Holidays include fun in a dinghy and on a li-lo. In the evenings you enjoy crabbing at Mudeford Quay. At church, you start Junos (a uniformed Christian movement) and Young Searcher's League (where you learn verses from the Bible).

---

[38]   Source unknown

"1981, seven and your interest in Cindy dolls reaches its peak. As usual either Auntie Pat or Auntie Anita bake you a cake. You change schools this year to St. Mary's (middle) school. [Mrs S. is your first teacher, and right up until your death, you had a soft spot for her and kept in touch, visiting her in her own home, sometimes with Jo.] You have lots of school friends such as the two Daniels, Laura, Kirsten, Josephine, Caroline, Michelle, Emma, Sarah and Stephanie. We continue to enjoy summer outings to Ewell Court Farm. (Grampsie likes this best because he can sit and watch you on the swings, or see you catching tadpoles.)

"At eight years old, it is sadly Grampsie's last Christmas with us. You come to visit him in hospital to say goodbye. You are now into rabbits, and Snowflake and Fluffy give you lots of baby bunnies. You take part in church swims and go off to church camps. You get a distinction in the Scripture Exam. You enjoy seeing your Belgian cousins again at Christmas.

"Nine and you gain awards for gymnastics and also obtain your Cycling Proficiency certificate. You go to Florida! So exciting to think you're the first person in the family to have travelled that far! The Surrey Comet and other local newspapers photograph you. Uncle Keith moves to Dartmouth in Devon and we start enjoying long weekends and holidays down there.

"1985, At ten you take up horse riding and win first prize. You go to Switzerland to visit Sara. You have your first long-line for intra-venous anti-biotics so that you can have these at home, rather than staying in hospital.

"1986, At eleven, you are bridesmaid to Steve and Louise. You don't think much of senior school at the start (it's so huge and you don't know anyone), but by the time you leave at 18 you absolutely loved the experience and the friends you've made). You've progressed from appearing in the local papers to appearing on National TV for a few brief seconds at prime news time in a Tiffin school item.

"1987, Twelve years old, quite a young lady and very pedantic about clothes! You travel each day on the bus to school with Claire, Louise and Melissa.

"1988, Thirteen, years old, a teenager and you are in to loads of friends and class mates at Tiffin.

Mave: As another aside, Claire, many you were still in touch with, right up until the time of your last illness, and so many attended your funeral and Thanksgiving service.

"You take part in the Kingston Young Poet's competition and you go with classmates to present your poems at the Guildhall. You have more mature birthday parties, either in the garden, or at the local skating rink or swimming pool. You also take part in the school play, "The Rebels of Old Bridge Street," and love acting.

"1989, Fourteen and you celebrate in San Francisco. We are on our first family holiday abroad outside of Europe. You are the proud owner of your first job, working in a care home after school one evening a week. You are not impressed but determined to stick it out! You also do our neighbour Dennis' cleaning. You visit Uncle Keith with Jo, then Hannah. You help with the church's holiday Bible club for kids and a club for handicapped children. You write and get published your first article on Cystic Fibrosis.

"1990, Your 15th party is quite an occasion with all your buddies from Tiffin. Your actual birthday you spend with Hannah on the Isle of Wight. You start helping regularly in Spectrum, one of the church's youth groups. You are also doing your GCSE school exams. Additionally you work at another nursing home and also gain work experience in a Social Services Department in Walton on Thames.

"Sixteen and school exams finished for a short while. We go off again with Auntie Pat to America and Canada. On return to England, you go on your first Beach Mission. You return to school to start your advanced level courses. In October you are baptised with Rachel J.

"1992, Seventeen, and you want me out of the way while you have your birthday party. You also start driving lessons. You take your A levels and are also awarded the Mary William's prize for Commitment and Progress.

"1993, Eighteen, key of the door year, independence! Good riddance, to your rules, Mum. Yes, Claire, far from perfect, you drove me to distraction at times; your indomitable will, your stubborn nature when you were determined to go to school, to work, to go out socially when you could hardly stand up, and yet so many people have said that this is what kept you going. Soon you'll be off to university to read Social Psychology, in readiness for your social work training. I am so proud of you and very thankful to God for these eighteen years. 'Father God, on the day I was born, you were there, cared and loved me. Throughout school you were there, cared and loved me. There is not a moment in this life of mine when you will not be there, caring for and loving me.'[39]

Mum has been really brilliant and the weather wasn't bad at all; so we've done really well. I had loads of cards and I've done so well with presents, too, which has been really exciting. People's kindness has been colossal. I was really chuffed with seeing friends again today; it's been so nice and refreshing. I don't want to be 18; I don't want to be anything at all. What my birthday has really taught me is that material things don't matter; what does matter are our relationships, the love we share with each other, etc. I'm an adult now, so change.

---

[39]   Source unknown

August 1993

Sunday, August 1 to Friday August 6, 1993: Spending a week in Warrington to help with a mission in a local church up there.

Thursday, August 19, 1993: We got our A level results from school; it was a real anti-climax, as if we are all past caring on the one hand, but realising the huge importance of them as they would be our pass card to the university of our choice. I need to phone Kent. Will my grades get me in?

Friday, August 20, 1993: We celebrated by going to a U2 Concert, but before going I had to stay in and phone the universities. The switchboards were jammed with all us A level students up and down the country trying to get through.

Saturday, August 21, 1993: Kent has accepted me! PTL!

Monday, August 23, 1993: Telephoned Reading and Sussex to ask if they would release me as I had made the decision to accept Kent.

Wednesday, August 25, 1993: I met Dawn today in London; it was great to see her. We talked lots of our memories in Florida as 9 year old kids. She looked really well but may have to have a Port-a-cath. Dr. Butler confirmed my place at Kent and said he would not take it away from me. I'll be so pleased when I see it in writing. My feelings of life being unfair have been turned on their head.

September 1993

Wednesday, September 1, 1993: It's the last day I'll see Claire E. before she goes up to Chester to start her Midwifery training; 7 years of great friendship, of meeting at the bus stop; of being at school together, so many brilliant memories. I can't believe that we won't be going back to school again, ever. Sometimes I feel I am flung on a lonely sea, holding on to distant memories and that hurts me so much more than it shows; so much more than it should.

Friday, September 3, 1993: Had a call from Dr. Butler in the Admissions office. I've had my formal acceptance from Kent and have a place on campus! Really thrilling. There's so much to think about and prepare now. Just a month away and I'll be a fresher in a world of strangers. The University of Kent at Canterbury; the view of the superb Cathedral, that's where I'll be studying for the next 3 years! I love Canterbury and Auntie Shirley says it's going back to the family's roots. Post war, my mum, aunts and uncle lived in Kent with their parents, very close to Canterbury.

Saturday, September 4, 1993: "Much Ado About Nothing" was a great performance. We got our bridesmaids' dresses today, jade green, such a super shade and so exciting to start planning for next June! Rachel looked beautiful when she tried on her wedding dress; absolutely gorgeous.

Wednesday, September 8, 1993: Another friend who has flown the nest. Faye has gone to Bristol to commence her physio training; one by one we are all disappearing off into the sunset; only to return at the end of each term to hopefully start again where we left off. My church membership interview was a nightmare, but I survived!

Thursday, September 16, 1993: Returning to school today to hand over stuff for C.U. was fine, but why do I worry so? Good to catch up with Roseanne. She said she missed me! 18 out of the 24 regulars turned up. F. said hi.

Tuesday, September 21, 1993: Saw Catherine and Ndullee. Eek! We will all be biting the dust soon and disappearing in different directions.

Wednesday, September 22, 1993: School Speech Day and walking up onto that platform with others to collect our prizes was scary. Ali and I said *au-revoir* to each other today. She was really sweet to me and I so appreciated her.

Friday, September 24, 1993: I totally messed everything up at the joint schools' C.U. meeting today by walking out and crying; very unlike me. Nigel is going to Canterbury next year, which is brilliant. He said he was really pleased to be going as I would be there! Sam gave me a hug. Simon is, of course, going to Canterbury this year too, but so sad saying goodbye to Roseanne.

Sunday, September 26, 1993: Admitted into church membership this evening on my last Sunday at Hook prior to uni. Rachel and Sharon were crying. Jim said that he was getting emotional. Maria was lovely; but I don't think I thanked everyone enough (though Mum said I did). It's exciting what plans God has for us all.

Thursday, September 30, 1993: Final goodbyes to all my best school mates this evening. Will we be forever friends?

October 1993

Saturday, October 2, 1993: What am I doing? How did I come to get this far? I'm going to university tomorrow. I know that I can't rely on myself; I have to rely completely on God. I am in His hands and this is so vital:

"Dear God, I just pray that You would keep me safe and secure in Your hands. I know that I can't trust myself; all I can do is trust You. I ask that You would be with me now and forever. Thank You for all that You have done for me in the past and all that you will do for me in the future. Thank You especially for sending Your Son down to earth to die to save us from our sins. With lots of love and thanks for all You've done for me."

Sunday, October 3, 1993: To UKC and a new life; please help me dear God, to be a good witness, a good friend and to stay close to You.

Claire, as you left for university you were so excited, yet the trepidation in your eyes was evident too. Despite the many things on your mind, your sweet, beautiful nature shone through yet again; you left a lovely card of a Native American Indian that read:

"You are on mind and in my heart. Thank you so much for all you've done for me in the past. Thank you so much for the time, effort and sacrifice that you have endured to make it possible for me to go to university. I don't know what I'd do without you, I love you so much."

No, Claire, it was no sacrifice; it was my absolute pleasure to see you go off and fulfil your dream of going to university. It was a joy to see you serve God with your fellow students from C.U. and gain a degree. It was you that sacrificed for me; living at home when I was not the nicest person to be with. So often in your teen years you dealt with my gremlins and skeletons in the cupboard when I should have put you first, but I didn't. I was the parent, but you so often behaved like the adult. I was in awe of you then and I still am. I know God provides grace for us when we need it however, and I suppose I've realized you were my grace so many times. These memories of your love and care are not sad at all; no, they're beautiful and precious mementos of a person so uniquely strong and wonderful, God may have allowed you to have CF so that physically you struggled so much, but He also created you with an awesome personality and true resolve of character.

Chapter Ten

University Years – 1993, The Adventure Begins

Dear Claire,

So started your university years. It is a curious mix of emotions only a parent knows when your child who, only yesterday it seems, was starting school, and now she is young adult, brimming with energy and enthusiasm, ready to fly far and clear of the nest. Pride and wistfulness swirl around the soul like oil and water, both healthy in their own right, but restless together. You began reading Social Psychology in preparation for your intended career in social work. In your chapter, "Life is an Adventure – Dare It," you say that Kent was the university for you and you loved it; and indeed, love it you did. Although I expected nothing less, I was still so glad you were accepted into the university of your choice.

As you closed the chapter on high school, you received "Wishing you well" messages from your many friends. Some of these read:

"Dear Claire as you go to University, we just wanted to send you love and prayers for:

Health,

Friendship,

Academic success

And for the most fun 3 years of your life!

That you will grow even closer to Him. You are a shining light of His love and faithfulness. Julie and Nevin."

"I'm going to really, really miss you. Who's going to wash up after Cornerstone? Who's going to ask the questions and contribute to the discussions?! Everyone's going to miss you loads. Thank you for everything when we were younger, my teenage years were brilliant. Thanks for everything with Mark and school and helping me spiritually. Hannah G."

"You'll be greatly missed as you go off to uni. Your great concern for everyone has been so tangible. Friday nights at Spectrum and Discovery won't be the same; you've been such a great help and encouragement. Bev and Graham."

Steve and Louise, Cornerstone leaders wrote: *"Hold to what you know to be the truth. You are a gentle, 'unpushy' person who has a great influence for good, together with your quiet conscientiousness and cheerfulness. You will be a great asset to Kent Uni, but a great loss to us."*

Your focus and excitement, yet also the stress of your unique challenges were evident as you prepared to embark on your great adventure. Perhaps this was only to me, though. Your thoughts and feelings were well reflected in section three of "Life is an Adventure – Dare It."

Life is an Adventure – Dare It

University – A New Life Experience

I completed my A levels exams and in 1993 started at the University of Kent at Canterbury to read Social Psychology. I found the statistics part of the course incredibly difficult. Not being a mathematical person at all, I hated maths with a passion and still do. However, I surprised myself by passing the stats exam and confess to being quite proud of the achievement! I enjoyed university tremendously. I loved student life and being away from home. But my health started to deteriorate during the first year at university and my CF became more apparent. No one can particularly see there is anything wrong with me. I'm not very tall, which may or may not be linked to CF, but apart from that I can pass as an average person in the street. Once I started to tell people, the news spread, so I didn't have to tell all my friends; it was like being diagnosed all over again, explaining things to people. The Christian union was very supportive, as was my church in praying for me, particularly when I was unwell. Their love and concern has always meant a lot to me.

I had some great friends in my College Hall of Residence who always looked out for me and encouraged me to eat when I didn't particularly feel like it. My next door neighbours were a great support, and one evening one of them knocked on my door to ask me if I wanted help with my intravenous antibiotics. But instead of saying, "Do you want help with your IVs?" she asked me if I wanted help with my IQ! However, she was a bit tipsy and in no way fit to help; we still laugh about that incident. At the end of my first year at university I became quite ill. I had lost weight and contracted a bad chest infection; the day after I was bridesmaid for a good friend at church (I think I just made it up the aisle in one piece) I was taken into hospital.

In cystic fibrosis, as more areas of the lung become "fibrosed" due to the repeated chest infections, so breathing becomes more of a problem, which impacts on how much exercise you can do. Even walking up one flight of stairs becomes difficult for some people with CF. A few years ago scientists isolated the defective gene in the DNA and this has added to their knowledge in treating the disease. It is anticipated in a few years' time gene therapy, a technique to correct the faulty gene will halt some of the damage to the lungs that frequent infections cause. Although gene therapy can prevent ongoing damage, it cannot correct the fibrosis that has already occurred; but it is the nearest thing to a cure, and when it becomes available, patients should benefit.

Antibiotics are taken in a combination of oral, nebulised (through an aerosol) and, when infections really get a hold, intravenous injections. It is not uncommon for people with CF to have two or three different bacteria at one time, so long term antibiotic therapy is normal. As chest infections take a hold, maintaining adequate food intake is a problem. Feeling one (or a few) degrees under occurs frequently with people who have CF and it can be difficult to maintain body weight; therefore high calorie drinks are required as well as high protein food.

For many people, the digestive system is also affected, leading to difficulty digesting food. This is another reason why people with CF are low in weight. Pancreatic enzymes, that help digestion, are required before each meal. Sometimes people with CF need to be fed by a tube inserted into their stomach. People with CF can become diabetic because of the effect on their pancreas. Thankfully my digestive system is not affected yet and hopefully this won't develop in the future. However, CF is not just confined to the lungs and digestive tract, it is a multi-system disease that affects the liver and other organs. One new finding is that osteoporosis (the bone thinning that is common especially among the older population) is found at a much younger age in people with CF, so this is another area that needs regular follow-up. Cystic fibrosis is a chronic condition that can deteriorate each time a new chest infection is present.

My precious Claire,

When you arrived, we helped you unpack in your room at Darwin College Halls of Residence and met your fellow dorm corridor students. In a flash, you were off to the fresher's welcome that evening, not wanting to miss the initial social event, of course. I thanked the Lord that when you were settled in, you soon met up with fellow Christians from the Christian Union, and seemed to be in your element. Given your spirit of adventure, homesickness would have no hold on you; straight into university life and the treasures it would unfold. How thankful I continue to be for your diaries, where I have gleaned so much about your experiences; even to the point of learning more about, and some might say, gaining a fuller vision of who you really are.

That first week you enjoyed attending Fresher's Fayre events, presentations on Kent University itself, as well as a library tour and several events particular to your course. Your first week was also when you met Dr. Abrams, your lead tutor. By Wednesday you had already befriended others in the Christian Union, and attended your first meeting that Friday. I remember you buying a street map of Canterbury to read all you could about the city, always wanting to become well oriented with your surroundings in order to best explore, discover and investigate. Being ever bright and resourceful, you also soon discovered the friendly porters in Darwin were a wealth of information and assistance.

True to form, it didn't take you long to get involved in voluntary work either; the Monday of that second week you were in Canterbury participating in the Soup

Run for the homeless and an Amnesty International meeting the day after. As if that wasn't enough, you signed up to help at the Canterbury Day Centre, which was affiliated with the Soup Run. Some might have thought these commitments could be flashes in the pan, but I knew better. You continued to be involved in Soup Run right up until your last term. The only reason you stopped volunteering was your deteriorating health meant you could no longer walk the long distance from your dorm to catch the transport into town. Thankfully, Amnesty International events took place on campus (although there were regular street collections in town too, which you attended when you could).

Despite your busy schedule, in your first few days you even remembered to send Jo R. a card for her birthday! Your kind heart always made the right priorities for you. Ten days into uni and you were meeting with other Christian Union (C.U.) members for your first prayer meeting. Of course, uni wouldn't be uni without the ever present parties that continued to feature regularly, but it was comforting that you knew how to enjoy yourself while keeping your spiritual priorities in order too. A mother really cannot ask for much more.

In all this hustle and bustle of your first couple of weeks, I was relieved when you made a point to visit the sick bay and meet Dr. Norman, who administered your flu jab, and wrote your prescription for oral antibiotics. Liz, the home care nurse from the hospital in London, even visited you and met with the sick bay nurses. I'll admit it was very reassuring for me to know they were keeping a close eye on you. That visit was also when you saw Ali Browne again, and you were able to swap health updates and share a sense of camaraderie. It was only later you were individually advised by the hospital you should not be in close contact with one another, for fear of passing on infections. This would be one of those periodic ambushes of reality; grim reminders of the unpleasant challenges and hindrances of CF.

Thankfully, your friends from home were there to support you as well, however. Rachel J. wrote:

"How are you? Auntie Pat told me you had met some other students from your halls. Also that the church you went to was good. I was so pleased. I know it will be some time before you really settle, but I'm glad you weren't left all alone. It was nice that we could all see you off. Anyway, Claire, I really miss you already but am comforted to know that you have made some friends, and knowing that God is with you."

You soon made a new circle of friends; namely Ele, Lisa, Karen, Hollie and Sally, to mention but a few. You all became good dorm mates and Ele's family kindly invited you and Lisa to holiday in their villa in Sardinia at the end of your first year. Other names I came to recognise and later meet up with were Isla, Becky, Lynn, Rachael and Keleigh. Sarah (your soon-to-be prayer partner) featured, too. Being in such close proximity to the English Channel, the university had strong links with overseas students and featured many international student exchanges, adding to the richness of university life.

You were two weeks in when the local church you had decided to attend hosted a student lunch. (Why does food always attract students?!) Oh Claire, why am I not surprised to read in your diaries that you were soon teaching Sunday school there? The Student Union also hosted a variety of social events and the first you attended was an evening of classical music. You really were going to receive an all-round education! It seemed from your diary notes that the C.U. was studying the book of Job within the "Flip" (Fellowship) groups that were scattered around the campus. I thought it interesting that Job's sufferings, including poor health, were the subject of these studies. I knew you'd understand the book better than most. Of course, not long into your time at Kent, you were co-leading one of these groups with Rachael.

By that time Faye, one of your friends from school, had already visited, and so had a group of friends from your home church. This really encouraged you, and I think made the change seem not so permanent in its separation of your childhood friends. Hannah wrote:

"I just wanted to tell you what a great time I had yesterday and I know Jo, Ali and Mark felt the same too. I didn't realise how much I had missed you until I saw you! It was so weird seeing you living on campus and not in Surrey and then leaving you there. It's weird, too, not having you at church and Cornerstone. Your new friends seemed really nice but I can't wait until you come home for Christmas and we can have a good catch-up! Take really good care of yourself, eat like a pig, and dress up like an Eskimo; it's so cold! Miss you loads."

By the third week you attended a Niteline Training Day and regularly took your turn on the rota, manning the phone overnight, much to my concern. Your health status, however, continued to be monitored both by the sick bay on campus and hospital appointments in London, so I tried not to worry too much.

Much to my delight, you would sometimes come up on the train and I would meet you in London for your hospital appointments. Any excuse to see you! By the beginning of November you were already handing in large amounts of coursework and had borrowed a plethora of library books. Despite your newfound friendships and course work, however, you regularly kept in touch with your school friends dotted around the country's universities. You exchanged phone numbers (in 1994 it was still mostly land lines) and subsequently letters. One friend, Sarah M., wrote from Oxford:

"Life's a ball, but oh I miss you, Claire, and the others from TGS."

Ndullee, also at Oxford, wrote:

"Although I have some good friends here, Claire, we don't know each other well enough to have the heart to hearts we have clocked up over time."

I smiled when I read this Claire because, even though you are a fiercely loyal person, I knew you were beginning to understand just how valuable lifelong relationships are.

After your first six weeks, you gave a thrilled Pat and me permission to visit you. It was good to see how you had adapted to this new life like a duck to water, unlike some freshers who seemed to really struggle initially to put down roots. We had such a lovely time, and I couldn't have been prouder of my beautiful, strong Claire. After our visit you wrote:

"Thanks for coming to see me at the weekend and bringing my bike down. Even if I don't use it, I know my friends will! Thanks also for the parcel that arrived today. I've already had some milkshake as extra calories. Could you perhaps cook some Yorkshire puddings, Mum, for the 29th? x."

Ever the responsible one, you ensured you spent your money wisely for food, for socializing and for travel around town as much as you could.

You and your fellow course students had conducted your first Psychology experiment by then and the mind boggles as to what it was. This had to be written up as an essay and handed in the following week. Your Psychology stats and practical, together with other mathematical coursework, were due in for marking too. Just as with your English coursework at school, I was enamoured with both the topics of some of your course lectures and essay titles, your first one being on Individual Differences and Cognition. It was such a joy to see you spreading your wings to fulfil your greatest potential.

Thus your first semester at uni sped by, and before you all trundled home for Christmas, the last evening found many students walking down the hill towards Canterbury Cathedral for a memorable carol service (one of the many plusses of being in a city). Kim, your uni friend with whom you and Rach shared accommodation during your last year on campus, wrote recently:

"I remember years ago when we had all made the trek down from uni to the Cathedral in Canterbury and Claire wasn't particularly well. Nothing ever stopped her from living the life she wanted to lead. I'd often wonder why she didn't take things more slowly, but the more I got to know her, the more I understood."

Karen, Sally's friend, wrote on her Christmas card to you:

"I hope you have a wonderful Christmas with your family, Claire. Thank you for being so nice."

From Jennie, who was off to visit her parents in Hong Kong:

"I thought I'd add to your massive amount of post! Thanks for your phone number, but fortunately no problems at Heathrow. See you soon, Xx."

Justin wrote:

"Season's greetings! Thank you for the times you've asked me how I am doing over this last term and lending a listening ear. It makes all the difference."

The Christian Union prayer sheet for Michaelmas term read:

"Pray that God would be preparing hearts this coming summer, for those who will be awaiting results from clearing. Pray for a Christian on each corridor in halls, who would reach out to their peers in Fresher's Week. Pray that as a C.U we will be approachable and not cliquey; that we'll be committed to looking out for new freshers, checking they're okay and generally being there for them. We need to ensure that Christians can be found in every group and society throughout uni so that there is a notice-able Christian influence."

I was so moved by this Claire. It's an unspeakably joyful gift to know your child is walking with Godly companions. I am sure many Christians at uni prayed similar prayers, but what a vision you all had in seeking to reach out with the Gospel.

That concluded 1993; for you, a milestone year. The changes you underwent were dramatic and good, and I was and still am so proud of you, Claire. I could try to explain this wonderful transformation, but I think your diaries can do the perfect job of that.

Chapter Eleven

University Years – 1994's Journals

As soon as you were back home for the holidays, you and all your childhood friends lost no time catching up with each other; school and church friends alike. According to your diaries our home, as always and much to my enjoyment, was host to many gatherings (some of which I cannot remember even taking place!). I can, however, remember that you were on the phone so much I gave up, either expecting or making calls. One of your C.U. friends, Melissa, lived locally and you met up with her during the Christmas vacation too, which was a nice link to your uni life. Your new friend, Ele, came to us on Boxing Day that year, too.

Whilst recognising it was your life; that you were now an adult and living away from home, I was nevertheless worried about the huge extracurricular commitments you had made at uni. You came home very unwell and I wrote to you when you returned for your second semester, some of which is too personal to share, but it contained:

"Be assured that this home is always your home, despite you going off to uni and your intention to live independently afterwards. Remember 1 Corinthians 13: Love is kind, patient and keeps no record of wrong. It is not contrary to Christianity to love yourself, and peace is looking in the mirror

and accepting who you see there, CF and all. I encourage you to stop and smell the roses too, and maybe we can stop and occasionally smell them together. I am reminded that I used to sing "This is My Song"[40] to you at bedtime when you were very young (I know you thought in later years that I sang completely out of tune!)"

The song explains the writer's feelings towards the love of his life in meeting a special person; that his heart is lighter, the stars brighter, the sky with a special hue. He continues that his song is a serenade to that special person in his life; that as long as she was in the world, nothing could really be a problem, and she is all he needs.

"I know this dates me Claire, written a decade before you were even born, but we all have our favourites, old or new. As part of the Crusade for World Revival (Waverley Abbey) counselling course that I am undertaking, we have to be in counselling ourselves, so that we can empathise with what it feels like. The counsellor that I saw picked up very quickly that you were my main reason for living. Only you and I know what I mean when I say you have been worth all the sadness and you have brought me so much happiness that I would have never experienced had I not had you in my life. So thank you a million for being the lovely daughter you are and for putting up, not only with all my foibles, but my downright unkindness so often too. With all my love and prayers, Mum. Xx"

I was not alone in my pleas; Pat had written (January, 19th, 1994):

"Glad you have got your new coat, and eat well and do your physio!"

---

[40] Written by Charlie Chaplin in 1966 and performed by Petula Clark

Your friend Rachel J. also wrote:

"Please look after yourself. Wear a coat when you go out in winter and do your physio, at least every other day. Sorry to be a nag, but you are too precious to get ill!"

Rachel had a vested interest in you keeping well, for you were to be bridesmaid to her, alongside her sister Sharon. She would be wedding her fiancé Michael in the summer and when you tried your dress on, it showed you had already lost weight during your first, frantic semester.

During your second semester, Pat again wrote:

"Thanks for your letter, I was so pleased to get it. I guess it will be some time before you settle down again and get in to your second term at uni, but I also expect it was nice to see your buddies again. Mum said you rang last Sunday at 11:30 pm, and were concerned about your house share this coming autumn. I expect you have to make up your mind soon, so will be praying you will all make a good decision."

You and your friends had such a camaraderie with each other, helping out when any of you needed it. Your note to Sally read:

"Hope you had a good time. Sorry I'm not here. Your clothes and file are in the shower room opposite. I've kept your cheque in my room. See you tomorrow. Love Claire."

Sally promptly responded:

"Thank you, Claire. I love your piggy paper. Love S."

Not that any of our suggestions that you look after your health had any effect, Claire. Sally also cajoled you:

"Remember to relax during the vacations, Claire. We know what you are like; you never give a moment to yourself!"

Nevertheless, at Easter following your second term you were helping out with the Fellowship of Independent Evangelical Churches' (FIEC) youth work on their annual assembly. To hear first-hand your personal experiences in this year, here are some excerpts from your diary in 1994:

January 1994

Sunday, January 2, 1994: "Christ in me is to live and to die is gain," Philippians 1:21. They are such powerful words, but do I really mean them? The answer is sadly no. My home church took on a new meaning this evening; we didn't have a proper sermon, but rather a discussion about this morning's sermon and it proved a good move from the norm. So many people pairing off; it's hard. One Christian friend felt I acted out of character yesterday, and I need to repent and be the witness I should be.

Sunday, January 9, 1994: There's so much to pray for. I'm a bit nervous about going back now, but hopefully it will be okay in the end.

Wednesday, January 12, 1994: Well, here I am back again after our first vacations at home; it's been really great to see everyone and share experiences. The things of this life aren't important, so why am I worried about them? I've had lots of offers to share a house next year; Karen and Sally said I could move in with them, so I need to consider this carefully. I went to aerobics this evening and feel quite proud of myself. X. is leaving; she can't hack the course and that is so sad. Nervous breakdowns are not uncommon at university and she feels the stress and homesickness is too much.

Thursday, January 13, 1994: What a nice hello from Ashley.

Friday, January 14, 1994: "And in His presence, our problems disappear." How true that is, as someone prayed that this evening. The meeting was very powerful tonight, and even I sat in the front row and felt better for it. I'm a bit concerned that we're really good in these meetings and full of prayer and praise; but when we wake up the next day, it's a different story. Relationships! I don't know what God is trying to teach me, but there was a look that encouraged me.

Wednesday, January 19, 1994: Very difficult evening with Niteline. Manipulative caller, which was very unnerving, so I phoned my supervisor for advice.

February 1994

Thursday, February 3, 1994: I'm so tired and it's my own fault. The day centre was such hard work.

Tuesday, February 8, 1994: Stats were not great today, but as long as I get through my exam, that's all I care about.

Wednesday, February 9, 1994: C.U. topic this evening was on Relationships, that we get hurt, but we need to forgive. I learned that people who I thought were annoyed with me are not and that's a huge relief.

Friday, February 18, 1994: Claire, learn to control your tongue. I need to learn to be more confident.

Tuesday, February 22, 1994: What a busy day, I was so tired! Rachael and I had such a good laugh.

Sunday, February 27, 1994: He came round today and great to chat, but dream on Claire, you've got no chance whatsoever and when it comes down to it, it's not what you want, it's what God wants.

Monday, February 28, 1994: I messed up Soup Run and I prayed to impress, not from the heart.

March 1994

Tuesday, March 8, 1994: I was asked to be a Darwin College Rep for C.U. Oh, that will be fun!

Wednesday, March 9, 1994: We've been burgled at home again and Mum is quite upset. She says now an intruder alarm is essential. Good to spend time with Rachael and Ele today. Dinner with Master in College was an experience.

Thursday, March 10, 1994: Sooooo stressed, it's untrue. I am feeling ill. J. feels rejected by her mum as her mum feels she should be free to live her own life now. She also feels neglected by her friends. The song come to mind again: "Everybody hurts."[41]

April 1994

Saturday, April 9, 1994: Mum really challenged me in a letter today and I'll have to sort myself out.

Sunday, April 10, 1994: Got upset, as I'll probably have to go into hospital.

Wednesday, April 20, 1994: Back to uni, felt a bit homesick.

Claire, although your health status afforded you campus living for the three years of your course, you wanted to be off-site with your friends. You wrote to your grandparents:

"It's been nice to come back to university and I have really enjoyed seeing my friends again. We are busy house-hunting for our middle year starting October. I've found out what being an adult is really about. Oh to be ten years old again! Some of the houses we have seen are absolutely awful, others really posh and expensive. The weather has been gorgeous, consid-

---

41 R.E.M., Everybody Hurts, Automatic for the People (Warner Bros, 1992)

ering it is only April; the sun shines everywhere and students lay sunbathing, scattered all over the grass.

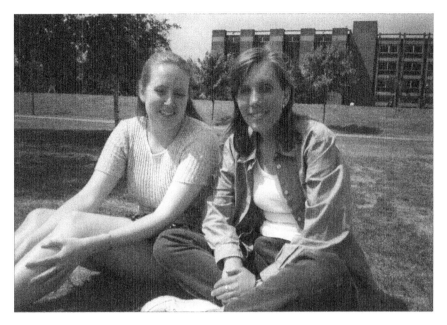

Outside Halls of Residence, University of Kent at Canterbury

"P.S. Thanks very much for the cakes, fruit and money; the only thing I haven't eaten is the money! Also, I forgot to say that the Student Union shop was selling this photo of Darwin College so I thought I'd send you a little reminder of what my halls of residence are like! With love, Claire."

I don't believe I was overly protective of you, Claire, when I read a comment by one of your friends: 'Plans of living out for my second year, took a lot of persuasive reasoning on my part to my parents.'

Your diaries continued:

Friday, April 22, 1994: Jennie, Ele and Lisa were all so good to me today and it was great that they waited for me.

Monday, April 23, 1994: Saw three houses today for living off site next year, but they were all too expensive. Long talk about housing and how do we know what God wants us to do?

Thursday, April 28, 1994: Stress! The house we were after fell through.

May 1994

Sunday, May 1, 1994: Philippians 2 v3, "Do nothing from selfish ambition or conceit, but in humility count others more significant than yourselves."

Monday, May 9, 1994: Was so humbled this evening about what people said about me as I genuinely didn't know they cared.

Wednesday, May 11, 1994: Timed essay today. Had chat to X. I think he's very lonely, but he's got a lot of depth to him.

Monday, May 16, 1994: I really boasted in Soup Run this evening and I need to pray against that. It should be God, God, God; not Claire, Claire, Claire. Rob popped in on my return.

Thursday, May 19, 1994: Went into Canterbury today, but was absolutely shattered as this chest infection just isn't going away. Miss Popularity, D., feels let down by her friends. So many of us have such low self-esteem.

Monday, May 23, 1994: Chris came to my rescue in Soup Run, thank you! I must rid myself of pride, bitterness and self-pity.

Thursday, May 26, 1994: Niteline and the worst night of my entire life. I was so scared. The phone calls were absolutely terrible and the door knocker freaky. I hated it so much.

Friday, May 27, 1994: Trying to recover from last night; Ele and Lisa were so supportive again, and again, and again.

Claire, knowing you were planning to go Inter-Railing round Europe with a group of fellow students in 1995, I wrote:

"The new nebuliser has arrived and looks very compact, so I hope it won't be too heavy. We just need to find out how you can re-freeze the ice blocks to carry your medication. Looking forward to seeing you. Pastor is very interested to hear about C.U. and wants you to do a report back to the church when you return."

You returned home for Rachel and Michael's wedding, but everyone could see how much weight you had lost. You managed to cope with being bridesmaid, but Sunday found you (as you so clearly relate to in your *Horizons of Hope* chapter) at the hospital needing intravenous antibiotics (IVABs). After sitting your first year exams, you had to return to hospital for insertion of your first port-a-cath, as referred to below.

June 1994

Sunday, June 5, 1994: Hospital all day, very unwell, doctors took literally hours to find a vein for intravenous antibiotics. Return to uni this evening ready for exams this coming week.

In June Dr S., your paediatric consultant wrote:

"I get a copy of the GP's letters so I know what your medical side is doing but I am as interested in your social side. I see you are at Kent University reading Social Psychology so hope they are not working you too hard!"

Monday, June 6, 1994: Drove Rachael mad talking about my health. Didn't go to Soup Run as too unwell. Matt called round but I was out. Don't quite feel in the mood for exams this week.

Tuesday, June 7, 1994: Guess when I have to go into hospital? Typical, I will miss the uni social event of the year, but hey, I'm all cried out now. He came to meet me from my exam, ahh. We're all going to miss these guys soooooo much. They've been there to see us through our first year at both uni in general and C.U. in particular.

Saturday, June 11, 1994: So many of my friends have popped round to my room this week to see how I am.

Monday, June 13, 1994: Soup Run presented us with a tough situation which was hard to deal with. D. is dead, he was found in the Thames (alcohol related). The other men were so upset. Chris was great not only with them, but with looking out for me, too.

Claire, as I drove you up to London for your first port-a-cath operation, no less than four of your favourite songs (at that time) played on the car radio. (The reason I remember it so well was because I wanted to talk to you and you kept telling me to be quiet!) I'll never forget those songs, as they played: Wet, Wet,

Wet's hit song "Love is all Around," "You Fill up My Senses" by John Denver, "Lady in Red" by Chris de Burgh and last, but definitely not least, "Take My Breath Away" by the band Berlin. (This was the love song from the blockbuster, *Top Gun*.)

I was feeling particularly emotional because ahead of you that day was this significant op, and whilst to you they were merely popular love songs that any teenager would swoon over, to me they all contained words that summed up my love for you (at least as far as secular music went.)

With the operation behind you, your diaries continued:

Tuesday, June 21, 1994: I haven't felt this much pain saying goodbye to people in 2 years; I guess it's different from school because we have all been living on campus together (mostly, anyway) and our lives have been joined at the hip in ways us first years hadn't experienced before. Next year, living off campus will be so different; this is the only year that has been so very special.

Wednesday, June 22, 1994: Last day of our first year at uni. Very tearful day as it was so sad saying bye to Ele, Lisa, and Rachael especially, plus my room, my home away from home for a whole year of this new life called uni. It just won't be the same again, especially when we have to start cooking for ourselves as we house-share next year. It was also sad saying goodbye to the Darwin College porters and everyone. I'm going to miss them all. Emotional pain is so much harder than physical pain because there's no cure. All our families came to fill the cars with our stuff and then final farewells and the drive home. I love uni; I don't want to be back here. I want to go back and live my first year all over again. I wish, eh! It's gone so quickly and I just can't believe it or get over it. Where has the time gone? I just don't understand; it is so weird.

Thursday, June 23, 1994: I want to go back, please! In the words of Shelby in *Steel Magnolias*,[42] "I would rather have thirty minutes of wonderful than a life time of nothing special." What I should be looking to do is speaking to God. I thank God that….. ever came my way. I should feel honoured that these people ever entered my life. Thank You, Lord. One of my greatest fears is falling in love with someone and they don't feel the same.

And thus, Claire, your first year at uni came to a close, and you returned home at the end of June to play catch up with all your friends once more. If any reader of this diary thought that after your port-a-cath operation you were going to spend the summer on a beach somewhere, I have to say this would not be the case. August found us heading up to London on the train, complete with your case and sleeping bag ready for you to spend two weeks with the London City Mission. As if this wasn't enough, it was followed by helping at a Holiday Bible Club for young children. No, my dear Claire, "Taking it easy" were not words in your agenda!

You and Ali both worked in the Civil Service crèche in Hinchley Wood. (These offices were eventually demolished and a housing development built. I find it interesting this was where you moved to in 2011.) You worked for Auntie Pat in Chessington Computer Centre. This would be where you met Gary, as you both held temporary jobs over the summer. You spent some time in hospital over the summer vacation but you also went to Wimbledon fortnight with Uncle Keith and some friends, standing in line to get into the tennis. We only lived twenty minutes away and I loved dropping you and your friends off to save you the walk from the train station. (Your elation at going to Wimbledon was always great to witness.) Indeed, Rachael and Ruth had jobs there that summer and staying at our home meant they only had a short ride on the train to arrive for their early shifts. We

---

[42]   Steel Magnolias, 1988, Robert Harling, Dramatists Play Service Inc.

were still making trips to see your family in Belgium, however, but the highlight was your holiday in Sardinia!

The details of the aforementioned adventures are reflected in your continued diaries:

July 1994

Friday, July 1, 1994: Three months till I'm back at uni. Got the job at Ali's Nursery and start next week. Relief or what! Cornerstone was good, but I need to sort out my prayer life a great deal.

Saturday, July 2, 1994: Mum really spoilt me when we went shopping today, which was nice. We've been having quite a good time so that's okay, no worries there. I earned £13.00 this morning which is better than nothing, so I ought to be proud that I've found a job. Received a letter from Isla and spoke to Lynn on the phone, which was nice.

Friday, July 29, 1994: My birthday tomorrow. Usually when it's this time of year I'm all nostalgic and I think of life and all that's happened in the past year, the blokes I've fancied. It's so strange that you think they are the answer to life's problems but that's not strictly true. Then starting uni has been quite an experience for me; the old school/church friendships and the new uni friends; realising that all of them do love and care for me, which is a great comfort. I saw Ndullee and other school friends, another great highlight of today. One year left till I'm twenty – now that's freaky!

Saturday, July 30, 1994: Nineteen today is a weird concept. I did really well with pressies and was quite chuffed. I was so touched. I got loads of money, clothes and flowers. So many people remembered my birthday. All the people came to my gathering, which was brilliant and stuff. Auntie made me a really nice cake. This evening I saw church friends. Change, Claire, or else!

Sunday, July 31, 1994: I'm really dreading tomorrow. Oh, Lord, really be with me I ask and give me, I pray, the confidence to make friends. I need You now more than ever. I'm in my 20th year. Ahh!

August 1994

Monday, August 1, 1994 to Saturday, August 13, 1994: My fortnight with London City Mission that I was dreading so much is over. It was really sad saying bye to everyone, so many an inspiration and all very sweet.

As an aside, Claire, you survived, as you always did, but I felt so often that you punished yourself and put your body through so much. You certainly used your vacations from uni to the hilt, so that when you were not working or holidaying, you were found in a variety of Christian service opportunities.

Sunday, August 14, 1994: I really appreciate Mark and Hannah's friendship.

Wednesday, August 19, 1994: Long talk with our pastor, Brian Edwards; he has sussed me and very well at that! He said I do evangelism because I feel it is the right thing to do. He certainly has a point and I need to learn a lot from it. I have to learn to live with the fact that I'm a nineteen year old with Cystic Fibrosis and therefore limitations to what I can do. He was very gracious and went about it exactly the right way. This was supposed to happen, I believe, although I was in tears. I love Jo so much; she's brilliant and it was so good to talk to her.

Thursday, August 25, 1994: I'm so tired. It's been a hectic day, but at least I have everything done now. I'm so looking forward to going to sleep. I have to be careful what I say to Mum. Some of my uni friends have problems they need to resolve and I must pray for them particularly.

Tuesday, August 27, 1994: I know I must desire a relationship with God before earthly relationships; of course they are important and necessary, but ultimately it is God who matters. Some friends feel that their self-esteem hasn't been improved by their past relationships and there is so much healing that is required.

Friday, August 30, 1994: The hospital visit was okay, but I just need to put on weight.

October 1994

By your second year, you were well established in the C.U. and helped with preparing Fresher's Week in advance from home before travelling to Canterbury for the start of term. You then participated in leaflet dropping with other C.U members around all the halls of residence.

Your journal entry from early October read:

Sunday, October 1, 1994: To 93 Downs Road, up a bit of a steep hill to uni, but the exercise will do me good. It's great to see Isla, Ruth, Lynn and Becky and fantastic that we are house-sharing this year. Good to catch up with Ele and Rach, plus everyone else too. One of our friends failed uni again and is back home working. I think she is quite down.

You continued to work with the Eating Disorders Group and this led to you choosing your extended essay on the topic. As is the experience of every student, your social life was forever full, attending picnics, university balls and generally hanging out with friends (including those who had lived in close proximity to you in Darwin College). Oh, yes, and the *raison d'etre* for going to uni in the first place, i.e. to obtain a degree, did figure in your life as your wall calendar demonstrated. Your journal entries continued:

Wednesday, October 5, 1994: Mad day, met my allocated Freshers, nine of them (eight were girls). It was really good to meet them. It seems weird to be second year students!

Thursday, October 6, 1994: Four people to coffee; four people needing a shoulder to cry on.

Wednesday, October 12, 1994: First C.U. meeting of this term and many freshers came, PTL.

Saturday, October 15, 1994: Rachel and Mish came for pasta with the rest of us. Mum came and I'm feeling a lot happier about the situation, so that's okay.

Claire, around this time you also created a poster that read:

"On Monday evenings the C.U head up Soup Run for the homeless down in the town.

We meet at 7:30pm at 93 Downs Rd. If anyone is interested in helping out (or praying while the team runs the evening), please see Claire Salter or e-mail her.

Thank you."

Monday, October 17, 1994: Jo's 21st birthday today! I'm not being me and I need to stop being fake. I'm not doing things in God's strength, so am falling flat on my face.

Wednesday, October 19, 1994: My new jeans were stolen from the washing line and I'm miffed about that. If that wasn't enough, I ruined my new £25.00 top with the naff iron. Present Personality Seminar and write up afterwards, deadline one week.

Friday, October 21, 1994: Our house is known as Hug Central and we had our first party, which went okay. Freshers came and I feel I'm getting to know them a bit more.

Monday, October 24, 1994: I'm so exhausted, I just want to fall into bed and sleep. I want to go home for some TLC. Rachael has loaned my bike. Soup Run was hard today. Isaiah chapter 41 v 13:

"For I, the Lord your God, hold your right hand; it is I who say to you, 'Fear not, I am the one who helps you.'"

Life seems to have truly broken me.

November 1994

Wednesday, November 2, 1994: Spoke to Sarah, Ele and Mish this morning and was reminded that God can give me so much more than others and that we are to learn to call him our Bridegroom. God may have been saving me from something terrible that could happen in the future. Sarah thought A. was quite immature in relationships. Sarah also said it's not a sin to get angry with God and let him know of your frustrations, as He knows anyway.

Thursday, November 3, 1994: Had such a lovely lunch with Ele and Lisa today. I'm spending money like water as the house is really eating it at present. Everyone has been so good to me.

Friday, November 4, 1994: I'm being so damn selfish and nasty to everyone and they must be getting really fed up with me. I was rude to Mum on the phone. You've made many false starts, Claire; it's time you started focusing on God. Yes, of course I need to go to Him daily, but my recurring sins must stop.

Monday, November 7, 1994: My Seminar Presentation is over and I'm so pleased to get that behind me.

Tuesday, November 8, 1994: Am shattered and all I want to do is go to bed!

Monday, November 21, 1994: I should know by now to continually take things to God in prayer, but why do I not?

Saturday, November 26, 1994: Lost most of my work on the computer so note to self: save it, save it, save it. Then I managed to jam the printer. Niteline no better; a call from a male doing his Ph.D wanting to talk about his relationship problems. I'll definitely have to take that one to Supervision!

Monday, November 28, 1994: Well, Claire, how often does "bad day" come in to my diary? Seems another one today with Soup Run, and then essay prep didn't go well.

December 1994

Saturday, December 3, 1994: Things are doing my head in now. I can't wait to go home. Everyone in the house is so kind to me.

Thursday, December 8, 1994: Really good to see Auntie. She brought Mum's debit card so that I could change a top in Debenham's. (Whoops, she told me not to tell anyone!) Good chat to house mates re: putting my faith more in God.

You had pasted in your diary a note from Lynn:

"Hi Claire, I am the only one in this evening and the phone hasn't stopped ringing and all calls for you! So here goes (I've had to make a new list on a larger sheet of paper!): Kate, Ele and Caroline rang. Liz B from the hospital rang about flushing your port, so please phone her back with a date for her to come down from London. Vicky rang about a hen night. Maz rang. Rach rang. Last but not least, phone your Mum! Xx."

Thursday, December 15, 1994: Met up with some mates at Woodie's Pub on campus and I am aware that everyone has problems. Indeed, life is about suffering and that's that.

Friday, December 16, 1994: End of term today. First term completed living off campus. No jobs available, so I'll do some cleaning for Ray and Maria, my previous youth group leaders.

Tuesday, December 20, 1994: Met loads of school friends at the Pub. Got an "Okay" regarding my health from the hospital.

Sunday, December 25, 1994: Christmas Day and good time with family.

Tuesday, December 27, 1994: Saw Rob and his friend Geoff and we all went to Leicester Square, Covent Garden, National Gallery and Westminster Abbey.

Wednesday, December 28, 1994: Had a really lazy day at home and enjoyed it.

Thursday, December 29, 1994: D. phoned from uni; she's had a bad time with her parents over Christmas.

Claire, I think 1994 was a year of tremendous growth for you. I would have thought it would be the most growth you'd experience initially, but I was wrong. As we moved into 1995, your beautiful metamorphosis kept amazing me.

Chapter Twelve

University Years 1995

Research naturally featured strongly in your course and at an open day for future undergraduates wanting to also read Social Psychology, your class had the job of demonstrating some of the projects in which you were involved. As already said, it wasn't all education and voluntary work; you also had time to socialise and, with a cinema on site, the films were some light relief. You often met friends for coffee in the Gulbenkian Café; however, despite the food outlets on campus, it was not unusual for you all to cook for one another in your rooms. This extended to those living off campus as you got to know others and the rich variety of friendships you cultivated really began blooming. I believe this was due, in large part, to the C.U. not being insular; you all wanted to reach out to others. One significant way you did this was running "Just Looking" evenings for those interested. I think that did a great deal for those who had questions, and could enquire in a non-threatening way. It also greatly diversified your group and fostered a culture of openness, which was vital, in my humble opinion.

Lastly, never to neglect your need for exercise, some of you attended "keep fit" and ballroom dancing evenings, which both resulted in some spectacular results. As we'll see directly from you diaries, however, 1995 brought both challenges and abundant rewards:

January 1995

Sunday, January 1, 1995: My twentieth year. It didn't start off as smoothly as was planned, though I did get a hug from Bros. Feelings I thought were buried have come up in quite a big way.

Wednesday, January 4, 1995: Very powerful mid-week church meeting with people sharing testimony. Report on Cornerstone: G& G came into membership. Hannah said thanks for having her to tea. I was so encouraged by the day! Spoke to Catherine on the phone; it was great to chat.

Saturday, January 7, 1995: Met up with uni friends in Trafalgar Square: Matt, Alan, Flora, William and Rachel, though felt guilty that I didn't invite others, but it was so last-minute. We hadn't seen Matt for a while and he told us he missed Canterbury and thinks he may go back to uni. His dream is to invent something. He asked mine; I said to see the potential in everyone. Remember, think twice: when you are halfway up, you're also halfway down.

Tuesday, January 10, 1995: Good to see people from school today. I get so jealous of others at times and need to guard this like the plague.

Wednesday, January 11, 1995: Back to uni and back to 93 Downs Road. (Mum couldn't bring me back, but we came down a few days earlier with loads of my clothes and things. Then she paid for a taxi to the station our end, and money for another one this end.) Ele is such a good friend to me. William wasn't here and I could have done with a chat.

Received our time table for this semester:

Personality and Child Development

Interpersonal and Group Behaviour

Maths/Stats and Practical

Computing

Cognition and Language

Social Legislation and Welfare

Psychology and Law

Clinical Psychology

Sociology of Learning

Regular writing up of experiments

Do Psychology Experiment

Claire, I want to add that another note in the back of your diary reads:

"Here I return again

Tired, numb and totally dissatisfied

Yet again I feel so down

I had such respect, admiration

All now has been crushed

I loved, heart, soul and mind.

For a minute

I married you and had your children

Although a week

In my mind you were in my arms

Just a night

You're an image, perfect, untouchable, for-ever.

What makes you so popular?

Is it your confidence?

Superficial kindness

Face value?"[43]

Thursday, January 12, 1995: Mum has organised the hospital to keep an eye on me while she is away. Also Dorothy and Ivan and Ray and Maria are my surrogate parents for the next few weeks!

Saturday, January 14, 1995: Spent an hour in the Psychology Unit today catching up with things. Finished my practical; luverly *[sic]*! Ele is so good and really looking out for me, taking me shopping, etc. so I don't have to struggle on the bus with it. X. is having a hard time with his parents.

Saturday, January 21, 1995: I had a really good time at the Abba concert. Well, not Abba exactly but a foursome that took them off to a T – look alike/sing alike. Out with the old Darwin crowd tonight was really excellent. Does God want me to be single? It's a big question for me at the moment.

Thursday, January 26, 1995: Ele said my health depended a lot on doing all my treatment, nebuliser included and I know she is right. Isla is absolutely amazing too; so helpful, so sweet and kind, as Lynn is. It was good to see William and Justin and also Hollie today. Another of our friends is suicidal.

Sunday, January 29, 1995: Steve A. good in church today as very helpful preaching.

---

[43]   Source unknown

Monday, January 30, 1995: Five hours of pure hard work! Got a good mark for my presentation, so that was okay. Dr. Abrams wants most of us to re-do our essay (Not so good!)

February 1995

Monday, February 6, 1995: Needed to kick Satan into touch today and that's where he's gonna stay! Went out for coffee with J. – was it a date or not? Lost my purse but everyone was so lovely helping me hunt for it; makes me feel special when this happens. My cold is no better and definitely is a chest infection, so out come the extra antibiotics.

Friday, February 10, 1995: I so want to be a good witness to my friends, but don't want to have to twist their arm; need to find a happy medium. Had a bit of a hassle at C.U. over an admirer. Interesting how those I like seem not to like me and those I don't do!

Saturday, February 11, 1995: Help! Asked out again for Tuesday but declined. Hope I did it in a kind way.

Sunday, February 12, 1995: Ele's 21st birthday today. Was told that I have matured in friendship evangelism. I'm not going to put a halo on my own head, but this meant a lot to me, because I have tried so hard in this area.

Tuesday, February 14, 1995: Valentine's Day and without boasting, did okay! But if only the one who breaks my heart was the one who loved me!

Wednesday, February 15, 1995: The fall after a good day. Very upset; can't understand God. Very tired. Feel empty and hollow – what is the point of life? But it was so good to talk to X., who basically brought me back to God and said that we have to see Him as the Lover of our soul and put all our trust and confidence in Him. stuff I've, of course heard before, but so true. She said she had the same feelings over Y. as I had over . . . and often we busy ourselves in lots of things to deny the sad feelings.

March 1995

Wednesday, March 1, 1995: Frightening to think that we are two months into the New Year and us second years are half way through our uni course. I guess it's the mid-term blues or something. Really enjoyed the Eating Disorders Support Group and more people have joined as helpers, so it takes the pressure off the rest of us.

Sunday, March 5, 1995: Mum and Auntie came down so had lovely lunch out and lots of pressies. I felt so at home. I am tired and just can't get my head round this next essay.

Saturday, March 11, 1995: Although I didn't get my essay completed, it was a good day. I had a load of mail and had a good laugh and lunch with everyone in the garden. Not bad for March!

Your friends, Claire, ever looking out for you, put the following notice in Downs Road kitchen. I was highly amused they called your nebuliser by this friendly term:

"Appointment with Mr. Neb: After Breakfast, Before Dinner, Before going to Bed."

Monday, March 13, 1995: Bad day at Soup Run; so much in-fighting between the homeless and we are having to call the police more frequently.

Wednesday, March 22, 1995: Very good C.U. meeting which made me cry; God's purpose and all that.

Friday, March 24, 1995: End of term, it's so good to be home! But nobody understands how I feel; nobody.

Thursday, March 30, 1995: I had the car today, so collected Melissa for dinner, met up with Ele and collected Mum from work. Saw baby Joshua today and he's lovely. Usual phone calls to all my friends each evening.

April 1995

Saturday, April 1, 1995: Rebecca's 20th today and such a great time. Spoke to Caroline.

Monday, April 3, 1995: Meal out with Ali and Jo. Ali and Russell engaged!

Friday, April 14, 1995: Good Friday. Half day of prayer with Cornerstone. Stayed night at Auntie's, but I think I confided in her too much.

Tuesday, April 18, 1995: Return to uni. I never thought I'd say this but really don't want to be back here again; this term's lectures are going to be a nightmare, with exams at the end of it. I feel really ill today.

Claire, I was very touched to see a long list of Bible verses printed inside your 1995 diary. No doubt these been circulated by the Christian Union. I have kept them, Claire, and am determined to learn some of them, as I am sure you did also back then. Your normal pursuits continued: Voluntary work, C.U, meetings, socialising, and with your own well-equipped kitchen it afforded more space to cook for yourselves and invite others back to eat too. Not forgetting, of course, your lectures, essay preparation and seminar presentations.

Unfortunately, it was necessary for a further hospital admission and on your return to the house the girls had written:

"We love Claire (big hugs) Lynn, Isla, Becky and Ruth."

They made you a 'chocolate' wrapper poster with their welcome back notes attached to it. The flip side contained newspaper cuttings of men! Whilst on the subject of men, I know you were very upset many other times in your life regarding your love for members of the opposite sex who did not feel the same way about you. You kept a letter from one of your female friends who wrote to say that so many females found themselves in the same position, not that she was judging your emotion of sadness, but just trying to support you in it. I prayed so much for you on this front.

I was so thankful for your housemates at No. 93, who were a great at encouragement and were constantly looking out for you:

"Thank you for the use of your concordance. Lots of hugs, Isla."

They were always taking messages for you, such as:

"Sally phoned about the D-block reunion and she'll phone back later. Ruthie."

"Claire, pleeeeeze call Ele up until midnight x."

"Claire, D. called about an essay she's finding difficulty with. Will call back later."

"Dear Claire, when you come in from Soup Run, could you spare me a few minutes? I've been put in a rather difficult spot and need some advice! Ruthie x."

I realised this wonderful group of house mates was always looking out for you, and that not only did they have to be Heaven-sent, I wasn't the only one to be concerned about your health. Your friends wrote:

Claire's Routine:

1. *Go to gym*
2. *Medication*
3. *Physio*
4. *Three proper meals a day and loads of high calorie food including chocolate, yum, yum*
5. *Rest*
6. *Admit when you're feeling ill and learn to say no!*

God always has His messengers, I suppose. Your diaries continued:

Wednesday, April 26, 1995: C.U. really good this evening. . . . X. opened up about problematic life with abuse, etc. But despite all this, God does and did intervene, which was amazing. At the heart of so many people's problems is the need to be loved. I wish we weren't so concerned about other people's opinions. I feel I am mediating in so many relationships. Still no resolution to Inter Railing plans.

May 1995

Saturday, May 6, 1995: My house mates are such an encouragement to me and I thank God for the great time we have had this year.

Sunday, May 7, 1995: Home just for the day. So many people at church asked about my CF today, so maybe they heard I haven't been great lately. It was super to meet up with Sally and Karen on my return.

Monday, May 15, 1995: I've just realised I could be alone next year in Parkwood. I've had an awful day at Soup Run; we could have been in the middle of a really bad accident as S. got hold of an iron bar, so scary.

Wednesday, May 17, 1995: Bad day today. Cried in front of a guest. All of my whites are pink! I will jolly well show everyone I can pass these exams with flying colours.

Forever trying to encourage you too, I wrote:

"Remember Claire, God wouldn't have placed you at uni if He didn't want you to do the degree you are doing because it all fell into place so well, so He must have a purpose in it. You have so much going on and that's no doubt contributing to how you feel. Val A. and others at church yesterday

told me how lovely you are, what a strong character you have so others think well of you and maybe this will help you think well of yourself. Just thank God for the lovely Christian He has made you and all the good things in your life (not the bad!) and remember the Holy Spirit lives in you. Be kind to yourself especially over these next few weeks of exams and if I can help, you know I'm only at the end of a phone. I hope revision is going okay and hope you're managing to do some sun-bathing too!"

Thursday, May 18, 1995: Good day and met up with Hollie. I know I need to get my relationship with God more on track. Matt rang. It was good to speak to him, especially as he's okay to come Inter Railing with us, which is brilliant. He will ring Rach for exam timetables to pray.

Monday, May 22, 1995: I've done more than okay in my coursework so can scrape through on minimal exam marks if I have to. So good to pray with Ruthie.

Friday, May 26, 1995: Despite a very stressed day, it was also really good. What wasn't so great was that Dr. Norman at the uni sick bay wrote a letter to my tutor, Dr. Abrams, saying I was coughing up a fair amount of blood. Dr. Norman says I should be resting more and doesn't want me attending lectures, but I said I needed to for the last minute revision before exams.

Sunday, May 28, 1995: One of my teen friends from my home church, Carrie, has died. She was only seventeen. She was in a car accident in the States and was very badly brain-damaged and they had to turn the life-support machine off. I don't know what to feel. I wonder how her lovely family is; they must be absolutely broken-hearted. We should tell each other how we feel about one another; we should get out there and witness to our friends instead of sitting on our backsides and being cliquey and introverted. I just can't believe it. I don't know how such a thing could happen. When the family was living in England, we used to walk across the field together in the summer. One evening she wore a white T-shirt and green shorts; another she had a lovely flowery skirt. It's strange how such images come to mind. We had a party to say goodbye to her when she left England. Carrie had such a lovely American accent. Rest in Peace, Carrie. See you in Heaven.

Monday, May 29, 1995: Bad day as kept thinking of Carrie.

June 1995

Thursday, June 1, 1995: I can't believe it's June and soon we'll all be heading home for the summer vacs.

Monday, June 5, 1995: Cognition and Language 9:30am exam and only one more to go!

Tuesday, June 6, 1995 to Wednesday, June 7, 1995: To Oxford to visit Ndullee and Sarah and 'twas really good. (Am so proud of my friends who made it to these prestigious unis, with Rebecca at Cambridge, too.)

Saturday, June 10, 1995: Felt so upset today despite my Mum being supportive.

Sunday, June 11, 1995: Cooked my first proper roast dinner today. I say proper because I cooked chicken for everyone, despite me being veggie. Very good talk on Suffering at CU. Very tearful today, thinking a lot about Carrie and her family.

Tuesday, June 12, 1995: Excellent party and was waltzed by two young men!

Friday, June 16, 1995: Taking Dr. Norman up on his suggestion of resting, so went to Broadstairs with Ruthie.

Friday, June 23, 1995: Hey, I got to go to the end of year ball and have photos to prove it!

Claire, this Friday in June the C.U group wrote encouragements to one another and so many wrote of their respect for you, though I am sure you also reciprocated these:

"Where do I start, I could write an essay! Claire, I love you so much; you're so precious. Your support, love, care, consideration is so apparent. Your faithfulness is 100%. You are a living sacrifice for Him, you radiate Jesus and point many to Him. 2 Sam. 22. To the faithful you show yourself faithful. Claire, God will honour you for your faithfulness. You are always such a brick for everyone else. Your gentleness, compassion understanding and, as Will said, your servant heart is so evident. God seems to be preparing you for a special role in the future, just as you have a special role at Canterbury. Know that you are loved so much by me and others. Rach."

"Well mate, let's thank the Lord for our beautiful friendship. Claire, you have been such an encouragement and I pray that this will only strengthen. Keleigh x."

"I'll always remember how kind and understanding you were in my first few weeks here when I was having trouble finding my feet and I really want to thank you for that. I love the way you are so caring, sincere and sensitive and that you always have time for people. It has been a real honour to know you. Thank you. Natalie."

"To the gorgeous, lovely sweet and blessed Claire, you are such a wonderful friend to have. Thank you for all your time, encouragement and prayer. I'll never forget all those times we sat talking about men! It's all in the Lord's hands, as are our lives. God has so much blessing to pour out on you. Love you, Ruth."

"Hey Claire, thanks for all the great chats and for always encouraging me so much. You've been such a sweet friend —always coming to my room to see if I am okay. Much love, Patricia."

Saturday, June 24, 1995: It was a really emotional day today, yet again the end of an era when we had to say goodbye to everyone. I cried a lot and so did others. I saw loads of people; they have all meant so much to me (I don't see how I can ever repay them) and we have got each other through some difficult times. Rach is coming home with me, whilst Isla and Becky head for home tomorrow.

Thursday, June 29, 1995: To Wimbledon tennis, which is an annual foray. Enjoyable catch-up with school friends, so great we all keep in touch. We met in Fortunes, a coffee bar in Surbiton. I'm doing a bit of cleaning for our neighbour Dennis over the summer and will work at the computer centre again as all this cash helps to fund my InterRailing trip!

Friday, June 30, 1995: Rob left; I cried/sobbed and generally embarrassed myself at Wimbledon station. What a nice man. I love him dearly as a brother. Ruth was such a support. After all the drama, had to ring my tutor re: my abstract.

July 1995

Tuesday, July 11, 1995: Am working in Auntie's office. Myself and another student, Gary, have been taken on again as summer workers. He's really nice and looks out for me.

Thursday, July 12, 1995: I asked God for a 2.2 and I got it in my second year exams; not bad seeing my chest infection just didn't shift. He really did bless me and I am so pleased. Thank You God. What a relief!

Mum was really sweet making dinner for Ele today, but she knows how good my buddy has been to me in our two years at uni.

Monday, July 17, 1995: Good day at work, although I think Gary and I talk too much; he makes me laugh. He feels I give 100% in relationships and that's sweet. He suggested we celebrate our exam success together. He gives me confidence.

Tuesday, July 18, 1995: Okay Claire, get a grip. Don't compromise your faith.

Tuesday, July 25, 1995: I felt I defended no sex before marriage very well today but must acknowledge that people have their own views. God is so faithful.

Friday, July 28, 1995: Hospital appointment today and they had a right go at me about a lot of stuff. School friends here this evening: Ndullee, Mel, Naureen, Faye and Ruth.

On 31st July, Claire, you headed off for two weeks to the Czech Republic with a group from your home church. Emma S., one of your travelling companions, wrote a report on your return that read:

"On 31st July a group of twelve young people from Hook Evangelical Church plus Rev. Brian and Barbara E. and the W. family set off on an expedition that was to cover 2,500 miles and take us through the sun-scorched maize fields of France, Belgium, Holland, Germany and on to our final destination, the Czech Republic. The visit was made at the invitation of the Czech Council of Brethren churches. Our first stop was a youth hostel just outside Prague. The showers were worse than freezing but the hospitality was warm. The excursion to the stunning city of Prague gave us several opportunities to place some of our 200 copies of Ultimate Questions in Czech around the city. All our young people gave testimony through translation and we sang as a newly-formed choir! We returned on 12th August, thankful to God for all his provision."

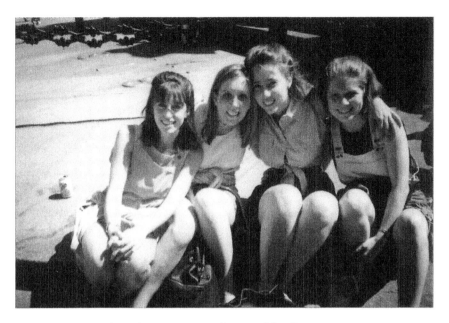

Church trip to Czech Republic from L-R:

Claire N, Claire S, Helen C, Emma S

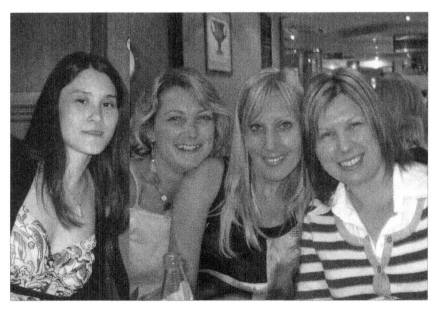

Church and Uni friends: Kim, Nicola and Natalie

August 1995

Wednesday, August 16, 1995: I've just been reading about my feelings for that person at uni; who would have thought that my feelings would have transformed so quickly!

September 1995

Friday, September 1, 1995: Before heading up to the hospital this afternoon, Gary took my address today and said I was virtually "one of the family," aah. He said I haven't got any problems and even having CF was not a problem. He said I get too hung up about how I feel about myself and how I come across to others.

Saturday, September 2, 1995: Felt really ill all day. Mum had to pack my rucksack while I supervised her as I just couldn't get out of bed; every time I tried, I just had to give up. Will I be well enough tomorrow?

Little did we know at the time, Claire, that your port was infected and flushing it meant the infection travelled around your body. However, we were not to discover this until your next admission at Easter in 1996.

Sunday, September 3, 1995: Good job am feeling better today, or just couldn't have carried my heavy rucksack.

Inter-Railing September 1995

Monday, September 3, 1995: Having been dropped off at South Kensington station, I met Will at Kings Cross, feeling very upset, apprehensive and tired. I guess that I was really going to miss everyone a lot. Told Will about my health scare yesterday and that my Mum had to pack my rucksack as I was in bed ill all day. I'd had my port flushed the day before, in readiness to be in Europe for this trip but then was running a very high temperature and felt so ill I thought I was going to die! That got him scared; however he said he wouldn't be upset if I died. Cheers, mate! Met up later with Rach and her parents and good to see them. Arrived at Felixstowe very nervous. Matt arrived with orange hair and his parents! Got kissed goodbye by both dads! Walked to ferry, got seats, had a laugh, wrote in Rach's diary. Me and Rach slept on floor; well kind of. Rach slept okay, but the rest of us didn't.

Monday, September 4, 1995: Washed hair on the boat, but I really scared a little boy with my nebuliser. His parents said he'd never seen a nebuliser before. Walked to Zeebrugge station to get train to Bruges, which was a real success. Had a waffle in the Square, then walked to the river before getting on the train to Brussels. Got lost in Brussels, because we came out of the station the wrong way and we had to ring various hostels before we found the right one. We carried our rucksacks around all day, which was a complete nightmare. But still we saw the sights and then caught the Metro to the Grand Place, saw the famous (or infamous!) Manneken Pis, then we made our way to the youth hostel, although we didn't really know where we were going. However, Matt sorted it. It was a really lovely place with showers in the room. We were so shattered, so tired, that we just went to bed and slept, getting up later for dinner. Couldn't find anywhere and I was

319

getting really dehydrated, so snapped at Matt that I needed water. Well done, Claire, good way to start a holiday! Went back to the hostel and I was feeling quite ill due to staying in bed on Saturday. Matt and Will really went out of their way to look out for us. Thanks, guys.

Tuesday, September 5, 1995: Matt and I didn't sleep very well at all, we found out when comparing notes this morning. Top bunks and I kept thinking I would fall out. Matt, bless him, kept waiting for me as we walked to the station, then got the train to Amsterdam (known as "the Venice of the North"). Went to shopping centre then walked round Ann Frank's house. Rach and I took a waterbus. We went for an Italian meal before catching the overnight train to Germany.

Wednesday, September 6, 1995: To Berlin Zoo, but we were all so tired, not having slept on the train. It was great to experience the Berlin Wall and we walked back and forth until we were too tired to do anymore. We stopped at the supermarket for dinner, then went to the youth hostel to sleep.

Thursday, September 7, 1995: Onwards to Prague. We knew this would be a long trip ahead of us on the train, but it was very beautiful. On arrival, we had a good apartment off Wenceslas Square. Off to the supermarket for food, then off to see the sights, but got lost 2 miles away from Charles Bridge. We dashed up the Tower while we had the time and energy.

Friday, September 8, 1995: Walked to station that proved quite a distance. On the way stopped at the Hard Rock Café for Matt to buy T-shirts for his sisters.

We met up with Alan, one of our uni friends who was working in Prague. Too tired to write up dairy for over a week!

Sunday, September 17, 1995: I really missed not worshipping at church today. Will and Rach astound me in their desire to know Scripture.

Rach, Will and I continued on our Inter-Railing experience and on to Rome (Matt had to leave early to return to the UK). We had spaghetti for lunch in this really nice café, then on to see the Coliseum; very spectacular. Loved Venice. God really challenged me today through Will. Will I put God's or people's view of me first? Good music in Square. Nikita, etc.

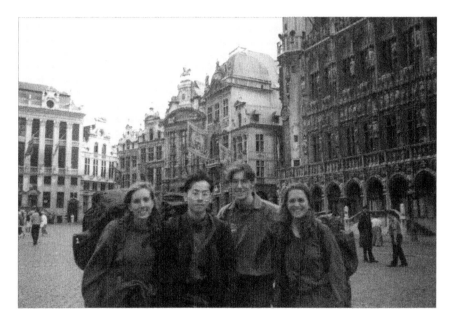

Inter-railing around Europe with University mates:

L-R Claire, William, Matt, Rach

Rach and Will don't think I'll make it to Budapest. I'm annoyed because they're too much like my mum and I'm stubborn! Rang Mum. My large wall-mounted bookcase fell down on my bed in the middle of last night, so maybe I am supposed to be here. Living so closely to each other and being so tired from all our travelling, I know I am getting impatient and ready for home. I need God's forgiveness when I am behaving like this.

Monday, September 18, 1995: It was good to have a good chat to Rach this morning. Went to Sienna, which is really beautiful. Had lunch on the steps, then found the square and sunbathed for a while. It was so small and quiet compared to Rome; less tourists, very simple and lots of potential for good photos and I really recommend it. Back on the train travelling through Tuscany area, which is really beautiful. I felt there was nothing like it anywhere and it was just like the postcards!

Tuesday, September 19, 1995: Went out early to get breakfast; a long queue in the shop but it was worth it as the bread was wonderful. Then to Florence and after a bit of a rushed visit, on to Bologna, changed trains for Verona. Saw Juliet's balcony and one could really picture the scene there. Loads of people had drawn graffiti of their undying love for each other, so we were not impressed. Then a cup of coffee and chat about relationships and that sort of thing. I realise I am not the best travelling companion as I am tired and feeling ill. Upward and onward to the castle with lovely views of the river. Once more on the train, and had a good chat about different versions of the Bible. Spoke to Elke, what a blessing, but it's going to take us ages to get to her in Munich.

Wednesday, September 20, 1995: Weird night as we didn't get much sleep at all, although we were able to spread out over the seats. Had to walk a long distance to get to the other train, but once on it we saw beautiful scenery of the Austrian Alps. Arrived in Salzburg and had the most wonderful breakfast I had ever had. Then walked to youth hostel, but they wouldn't let us in, so we left our rucksacks and walked into town. Wonderful sights, but we were really tired. Shopped in supermarket for tonight's meal; back to youth hostel for a much needed shower. Wanted to sleep, but it was so cold and we were all hungry as we were told we couldn't use the kitchen, so it was off to McDonalds. (Good job they do bean burgers!)

Thursday, September 21, 1995: We travelled most of the day from Munich to Kassel and then to Marburg; very beautiful, old and I thought similar to Canterbury. We rang Elke and her cousin was staying, so we felt bad. However, we go the bus and the house was lovely, typically German. Had pasta and then went to the pub.

Friday, September 22, 1995: Woke up early, had shower and good chat with Elke. What a woman, she really affirms me so much. I think we identify with each other, which I appreciate. We tried to speak to Simon, also in Germany, but he wasn't in. We were able to do some laundry, get it dry and then back on the train to Frankfurt. We rang the youth hostel and changed some money, although it was a very dodgy area; red light district and there were quite a few people about. Really big youth hostel, but brought back memories of school canteen, where we had dinner. Rang Debra, she came to the youth hostel to see us and had really good chat; so good to see each other. Hopefully, we'll keep in touch.

Saturday, September 23, 1995: Got the train to Basel and then it was only an hour to Bern. Bern was lovely; there was a carnival going on, part of which was an evangelistic meeting. Had a McDonalds and then bought the most gorgeous bread ever! The youth hostel was by the houses of Parliament, a lovely setting but spoilt by the experience of seeing someone mainlining in public. To bed at 9:00 as we were so tired.

Sunday, September 24, 1995: Woke up and attempted the walk up the hill to the station. Yuk! Bread was our staple breakfast, but it tasted good. Really beautiful train ride to Interlaken. The mountains were absolutely fantastic, as were the lakes. Our next train journey was to Geneva, another really lovely ride. Mountains and lakes en-route and Lausanne looked really beautiful, too. Nice hostel, but quite expensive. Went to Pizza Hut and to chat about our travels! We walked into town, discussed how much money to get on our Visa debit cards, and then to sleep!

Monday, September 25, 1995: Realised I had left my poster somewhere. How annoying when I had carried it for so long. Really good breakfast again and then to station, only to find the French trains were on strike and we couldn't get the train to Marseilles! Panic! However, we were able to catch the Lyon train and from there train to Marseilles and some more sight-seeing. Dinner was great (we cut out lunch so often to survive on the money we had, and thus breakfasts and dinners were eaten with great appreciation, even having a Haagen-Dazs after this meal). As usual, so tired and fell into bed.

Tuesday, September 26, 1995: Bought croissants from just down the road. Then, after a lie-in, went to the station and all the way up the steps with our rucksacks – ugh! We had planned to leave our rucksacks in the lockers, but because of the bomb scares couldn't do so, thus decided to go on to Aix en Provence. Of course, typically very French and just how I imagined it, tree lined avenues but no locker space there either! Thus we lugged our stuff all around town and bought loads of croissants again to feed ourselves with. The rare lunch treat was a luxury! The park was very beautiful with an amazing array of flowers and trees. Slept on the grass for ages, then went to find the train times. Haagen-Dazs time again before yet another train journey. Meeting fellow travellers on trains was great for exchange of ideas and experiences. Then from Calais, ferry to England. Over three weeks away from home, visited so many countries and experienced so many train journeys, youth hostels and cultural exchanges. Another ten days or so and we would be back at uni for our final year.

So your thrilling inter-railing experience drew to a close, Claire. You kept all the tickets and maps related to your trip. I had forgotten that you met Alan, who was working out in Prague, and that Matt had to return to UK about a week earlier than you others. To think that being ill the day before you travelled almost prevented you from this rich experience. A postcard from when you were inter-railing read:

"I hope you are okay. We are having a good time, and have just spent the day in Rome. There is so much to see and we didn't quite manage it all, but never mind! I come home on Wednesday! Until then, take care and give my love to everyone."

Wednesday, September 27, 1995: Really enjoyed these past 3.5 weeks' experience, but so good to be home. I just feel so at home and felt great to be at Hook with everyone this evening.

What a blessed people we are. We sang "What Kind of Love is This?"[44] a hymn that describes the amazing love of Christ; that although it's me/us who are guilty, by His death and sacrifice, we bear no penalty for our sin.

---

[44]   Written by Bryn & Sally Haworth. Performed by Sarah Lacy (*© 1983 Kingsway Thankyou Music*)

Thursday, September 28, 1995: Went to Ray and Maria's after being treated by Mum and spending lots of money on clothes for my return to uni; it was really good to see them. Maria says I don't have to prove myself to anyone. I shouldn't wind Mum up by doing so much. I should look after my health. Hmm, I do, I do. Maria encouraged me to place all the difficulties in God's hands and I couldn't agree more. Had big row with Mum. She needs to butt out of my life.

October 1995

Sunday, October 1, 1995: Returned to uni to live back on campus for our third year, sharing a house with Kim and Rach. (Others are in the complex too, but our rooms are located down the same corridor.) Great to see everyone again, who came to check out our new accommodation.

Claire, as an aside, Elke, Isla and Simon each had a year abroad and you continued to keep in touch with them. Going through your correspondence, I got to recognise people's handwriting on the envelopes, but they were personal to you. However, I was grateful for the occasional postcard. Simon wrote:

"You are a great friend, Claire, and I'm really glad that I know you. Please keep me informed about UKC life as one feels rather distant when our course takes us abroad for our studies, even though we are still in Europe. Please look after Lynn."

Monday, October 2, 1995: I didn't really want to go on Wednesday but I am. (Won't tell Mum!) The men cooked this evening. Felt sad as a Malaysian girl had to say goodbye to her mum and oops, we were right in the hall when this was happening. Her mum asked us to take care of her daughter for her and we said of course we will.

Tuesday, October 3, 1995: Had second day of training and then put posters up for freshers. Had good chat with Ali; brilliant, brilliant day.

Wednesday, October 4, 1995: Went to Calais. Phew, got back without Mum finding out! Mum has asked me to request Dr. Norman if he could write regarding a disabled badge; even I know I need one now.

Saturday, October 7, 1995: Still feeling ill. Hectic time at the Fresher's Bazaar. Had my hair cut. Please, Lord, help me not to feel jealous of people. (How many times have I had to pray that?)

Monday, October 9, 1995: Lectures started today, but guess who got the time muddled and arrived 30 minutes late? I completed my options wrongly. Help. Learn to concentrate, Claire. So good to catch up with: Ele, Hollie, 2 x Simons, Claire, Rach. This evening we all felt so bad as we forgot to collect A. for the Cinema. I know how rejected I felt when this happened to me, and it was a big lesson learned tonight.

Saturday, October 14, 1995: Met up with Sally, and then Lynn and after that Mish. So good to chill with my friends.

Sunday, October 15, 1995: Met up with someone from the Eating Disorders Group for counselling. I couldn't believe this person had an eating disorder and was desperate. What kind of a counsellor am I? What not to do: never show shock! Sunday school was hard work today.

Friday, October 20, 1995: The computer crashed and I lost most of my work, so I just cried. I'm going to have to work so hard to get this dissertation ready in time.

Saturday, October 21, 1995: I am so tired. Spent 4.5 hours on the computer this morning catching up, then saw friends.

Sunday, October 22, 1995: I hate to admit it again, but when will this darn tiredness go? Good day at church but spoilt by my stress re: being so far behind with my research project. Will brought my photos from InterRailing round, such great memories.

Monday, October 23, 1995: Presented my research project today. I hate it when all the attention is on me, so embarrassing.

Monday, October 30, 1995: This tiredness continues. . . .chest infection continues. . . .need to get to bed earlier but late to bed after talking to Chris.

Tuesday, October 31, 1995: Another of our Social Psychology group can't hack the course and is leaving. Such a shame when we only have just over 2 terms to go.

November 1995

Friday, November 3, 1995: Managed to get enough breath to cycle from Parkwood to the Psychology Department to meet with Julie, my tutor. She is pleased with my "Embarrassibility" research project so far. Now I just have to write my letters to local primary schools asking if I can try my theory out on 5 year olds. Help! (I don't much like this title, and would prefer to have called it "Self Esteem in Young Children," but hey, does it really matter as long as the outcome is the same?)

Sunday, November 5, 1995: Felt very upset today and the devil really knows how to catch me out with my non-Christian friends. I just need God to fill the gaps in my life so that I don't fall flat.

Tuesday, November 7, 1995: I got my social work course application through although they stipulate applicants should have "two years life-experience post University," so that rather rules me out, but *moi*, I'm going to apply anyway. . .while there's life and all that. . .I'm not really enjoying being on the C.U. Executive Committee, but maybe I need to learn more of how I can contribute.

Wednesday, November 8, 1995: Julie, my tutor, said my stories for the primary school children are excellent. I haven't been praised so much in ages and it made me feel good. But as if that wasn't enough, when the computer went wrong, she offered to type it all up for me. Praise the Lord again. Rach and Kim really look after me a lot and I'm so grateful. I hate to say this (how dare I, but I will): some of the blokes have a lot of growing up to do!

Monday, November 13, 1995: This stupid tiredness continues, so I went to the doctor today. I have flu and he confirmed why I was feeling so ill for so long. Strict orders to rest, so I spent the evening in bed watching TV.

Wednesday, November 15, 1995: I'm really worried and frustrated that being ill has prevented me from doing all my work.

Sunday, November 19, 1995: So Claire, your philosophy is that you want to live a life that honours God but unfortunately it's not true. Your witness is completely down the drain, so what are you gonna do, eh? My friends are still visiting me to make sure I am okay health-wise. I go on and on about it, but I am so tired; that, along with this infection just not shifting makes me so moody, or is this just an excuse? I need to witness more to the people in the house. Sharing a kitchen between us all is a good venue. E. is really passionate about spiritual things. Caught up with Lisa and Ele. Still feeling ill.

Saturday, November 25, 1995: Mum brought Uncle Gilbert down today. Helen, her cousin and the only one in the family apart from me who has CF, has sadly died. She did so well, living to the age of fifty-two. I don't know how I feel. I could have killed Mum for telling me the way she did. Well done, Mum. So much for your counselling skills. I want to join a support group for CF and help those who are worse than me.

Monday, November 27, 1995: Spent my first day in school today, testing my questionnaire in the reception class. I so enjoyed working with them.

December 1995

Monday, December 4, 1995: Going in to school again today was a day well spent, and I feel the children are now getting used to seeing me. It was good to relax this evening and unwind from the weekend. Lynn was so helpful to me in our discussion. Had an acknowledgement that my Social Work Course application had been received. I won't mention the "T" word again, but you know what I mean!

Tuesday, December 5, 1995: Bad day and coughed so much in lectures that the tutor asked if I had flu. Replied I had had it but no more. I didn't know whether to tell her about CF or not. I don't like too many people knowing, so didn't.

Wednesday, December 6, 1995: Really good night with friends. Felt spoilt and was chuffed about that. God's been good to me; I'm feeling a lot better, praise the Lord. Thank You! Thank You!

Thursday, December 7, 1995: Keep talking about my health as it's a major problem in my life at present, especially as I feel I've struggled to get all the work completed these past few weeks when I haven't been well enough to attend all the lectures. Think I'll go home next Friday as I'm really t. . . . (sssh, don't say the word again!) Felt pleased with the way I have caught up with my work. Roll on Christmas, as I can't wait for a rest!

Friday, December 8, 1995: What is faith all about then? All this term I have been carried and there's been nothing that I have done to help others. End of term Cabaret was excellent; uni is such a good time to study, to enjoy social events, as well as the opportunity for us Christians to grow together.

Monday, December 11, 1995: I need to go into school again this week to complete the research project, then write it up over the Christmas vacs. Felt much better today. Didn't throw up while coughing this morning; now that's improvement.

I cannot remember what option you were so desperate to take Claire, but I do know it was a particularly popular one, so you were extremely grateful that Lynn came running to tell you that you had got on to the course of your choice. She brought the piece of paper that said:

"Second and Final year Psychology students: a list of students accepted for the Clinical Psychology Course is posted on the Psychology notice board in Keynes College. If you are not accepted onto this course, you will need to choose another course from the Part 2 Handbook."

Praise the Lord you were successful! Forever remembering to be grateful, you wrote:

"Thanks for the lovely weekend spent at home; I really appreciated having some lovely food, my laundry done and clean sheets plus driven back to uni with all my things. Not long till Christmas now, I can't wait!"

In response, I wrote:

"Dear Claire, hope your research in the primary school has gone okay and that you kept dry in all this rain. You said it should be the last time you need to go as your tutor thinks you have enough material now; I do hope so. Love, Mum."

Tuesday, December 12, 1995: "I Am Blessed," written by Mark Mueller and Marsha Malamet, explains the powerful feeling of knowing nothing in the world could really be that wrong, or keep you feeling sad because one is so blessed. I love this song.

Good chat to Hazel, my previous dorm cleaner, who actually asked me about suffering. Her son's wife is being cared for. So many people lost in the

Zeebrugge ferry disaster of 1987 and Hazel's son was one of the crew. She lost another son, so desperately sad.

Friday, December 15, 1995: Mum came down early and really helped with photocopying the children's responses to my stories. Then home to Surbiton. It was so good to be at home after all. She said she would help with the typing up of my research project. What a relief, phew!

As an aside, Claire, I found some of my scrappy handwriting on a bundle of references from your third year at Kent and I vaguely remember coming down on another occasion to help you find some books for your research project on "Embarassibility in Children," and also your dissertation. Between the two of us, when you had been on intravenous antibiotics and couldn't carry heavy books and we needed to get the catalogue numbers from the University library, I guess you looked them up in the drawers and I wrote them down so that we could then go to the shelves and find them. What a shame Google wasn't as prolific as it is now! Why am I not surprised that thumbing through your uni keepsakes, I found your Templeman Library pass!

Recently I re-read your dissertation and again, was so impressed with it. For someone who didn't like Maths, you presented the quantitative research in a very professional way. I was thoroughly fascinated with your statistical work, but then, of course, I am biased! I must admit, though, I didn't understand much of it as Stats was not my strong point either!

Equally, Claire, I re-read your final essay submission on "Anorexia Nervosa." Whilst, of course, I always wrote from a nursing perspective, you obviously wrote from a socio-psychological one, and the research that went into this paper was absolutely amazing. You tackled it from every angle, arguing your points so well. I know many parents are proud of their children, Claire, but these two final pieces of work for your degree make me especially proud of you.

Saturday, December 16, 1995: Felt very much the centre of attention at home in our church youth group. I feel very loved and accepted here; maybe it's just because I'm not around very often.

Claire, before returning home for Christmas your diary notes that for your health's sake you decided to forego Soup Run. Dave wrote:

"Dear Claire, any unbiased reading of the gospels affirms the heart of God for the poor, the homeless, the refugee. Thank you so much for labouring with us, we're sorry to see you leave Soup Run but entirely understand your reasons – you've done a brilliant job!"

I believe this statement was an apt summary of who you are, Claire; you gave so much to others that you were willing, at times, to even risk your own health to ensure the less privileged had a greater degree of comfort in this life. You did it with warmth and love and loyalty to your friends as well. I know you only wanted to enjoy every minute of life you possibly could, as even from a child you had a very real sense of your own mortality. In that way, Claire, I suppose you again left us with more than we could imagine at the time of your passing. We need to live this life to the fullest, in the emulation of our Lord Jesus, for that is where true riches lie.

As you entered 1996, you became increasingly busy, and your diary entries became more sparse, but there was still a record of what you accomplished; friends, professors and fellow students all could not help but notice what a special person you were.

Chapter Thirteen

Your Troubled teen Years

Dear Claire,

In this chapter, the year before your university graduation as you became an exceptional, functioning adult, I wanted to reflect for a moment on how difficult your teen years were; how you may have wobbled at times, but also how you always returned to your Saviour, and did so by accomplishing so very much as an adult.

The recurring themes in your journals are how ill you felt at times (and this went hand in hand with the difference you think was portrayed that set you aside from your peers) and also how alone and apprehensive you felt about life. However, paradoxically, you were so very popular, loved, valued, affirmed and this was confirmed by the huge number of people, from all walks of your life that attended your funeral and Thanksgiving services (as observed by your childhood pastor, Brian in his address) as well as all the correspondence you received throughout your life, again affirming the senders' love and respect for you.

Reading your teen diaries, Claire, all these years after they were written, haunt me. The dashed hopes, the despair, the pain, the betrayal of male friendships that were never to be, despite your longing for them. You portray what many adolescents feel and you write intuitively. Your words are thought-provoking, representing a picture that few would expose or admit to. Nicky K., one of my work colleagues wrote:

"Don't be hard on yourself, Mave, I agree all teens have low self-esteem. I think teen years are horrible actually. I don't remember enjoying mine much at all."'

Our friend Jane T. wrote:

"We are all frail species of humanity and can only cope with the here and now or, in our cases, the 'then and now.' It is all very well to look back and admit the mistakes you made, but at the time we are in the midst of it and it overwhelms. I am sad you feel so disheartened, for the truth is that you did your utmost at the time to keep a happy family life. Claire would have understood that as she matured. I share with you something Claire said. I'm sure it will make you sad but it shows how well, even as a child, that Claire understood her condition. It may be useful to you in your writing. I hope it does not grieve you further.

When Claire came on an outing with us, Edward (who as you are aware is younger than her) asked how old she was. She replied, 'I'm 8, then I'll be 9, then 10, then 11, then I'll probably die.' I did not know how to respond to that. It goes through my head often when I think of Claire."

For someone who appeared so apprehensive in your adolescence (I wondered then, and still do, whether the situation in the family home caused you such angst, spilling over into your life in general), let me remind you of all you accomplished (some of which I wrote to you about on your thirty-fifth birthday, but also reminded you often before then). Of course, many of these one attains during one's rite of passage through life but not all, and I believe you achieved more in your thirty-six years than others who live much longer, as many of your friends have said of you, so it is not just me.

As a young child you went away from home for holidays and this is no mean feat considering you had to fend for yourself emotionally, as all children have to in those circumstances, but you with the added effects of a long term illness (witness Jane's disclosure previously). You had to contend with hospital admissions when parents were not permitted to stay overnight.

You participated in a variety of projects and presentations; for example saying verses at church for anniversary occasions, being a Young Searcher of the Bible, entering the scripture exam and doing so well. Other projects included being selected to read your poems (together with some of your peers) at the Guildhall in Kingston on two occasions for the Young Poet's Competition. As I recently re-read your poems, including those you and Beth composed, you depict the emotions of so many love-smitten youngsters and I cry, I sob for what was not yours; and I cry not just for you, but for the millions of others who trusted that life would turn out differently than it has. Like Desdemona in Shakespeare's "Othello," we put our hope in what this world offers, but that God-shaped hole will never be filled until Eternity and you know that now. You experience it; you are part of it.

You won first prize at a horse-riding course when you were eleven. You loved performing in the play "The Rebels of Old Bridge Street" at senior school. You were a Christian Union leader at school and Caroline gives testimony to you being influential in her conversion. Similarly, Faye's mum wrote to you:

"To dear Claire, you are the angel that led my darling Faye to God, and for that I shall always be thankful."

You participated in a school assembly where you spoke about CF (so brave when you dreaded drawing attention to yourself in this way).

At uni you participated in seminar presentations alongside your peers. God used you in bringing people to know Him, whilst I know of only a couple on whom I have had the same effect. You stayed the course when you undertook some voluntary work at London City Mission during one of your uni vacations. Oh, of course many people have done all the things listed above, but with your ill-health you could have made an excuse to not do anything, but you did not. You lived life as if you had no life-threatening disease. A couple of your Tiffin peers failed their first year exams – no doubt partying too hard rather than not hacking it academically – but you passed yours. I'm not saying this to blow your trumpet, but you always felt you were not quite good enough. Balderdash! You did so well. Even one of your school friends wrote at that time:

"I hate my course as it's far too difficult for me and everyone else is extremely intelligent."

Also at school you were a prefect and a form associate (which meant you were responsible for a 3rd year form). Your prefect duties included Parents' Open Evening duties. You were a form leader and form captain for games, doing well in many sports, despite your breathlessness and low lung capacity.

You became one of the leaders in "Flip Group," part of the University Christian Union small gatherings. You were one of the Niteline Listening Service members, holding the phone overnight for those students who were lonely, had problems or just wanted to talk. You were a helper in the Eating Disorders Group, an active member reaching out to the homeless of Canterbury, assisting in their day centre and the weekly Soup Run.

You did not tell me the half of what went on at uni (and why should you?), but you always led me to believe that Soup Run was held in a hall in town until in the car one day visiting Canterbury when you had long left, you said to Auntie, "That's where we did the Soup Run, under that bridge!" So there I was thinking you were in a nice, warm hall when in reality you were out in the cold night air. What is more you stuck to your course at uni when others did not, or were asked to leave.

Some of your friends, the brightest academically, wrestled with their emotions. I can remember how self-conscious I was as a teenager about having so much old-fashioned furniture in our house; of being embarrassed when my friends came home. Pat and I hated it, just as we did the ex-army catalogue shoes our dad bought us for our senior school years, so much so that we wore them out the house each morning until we were out of sight, then exchanged them for the shoes we kept in a plastic bag, hidden in the bushes down the road!

Your "gap year" was spent with the Schools' Work Christian Trust and again, this meant taking lessons and leading Christian Unions. As a student on your Masters in Social Work Course one of your placements was within an education unit for those not attending school; you gave presentations to mentors of those teens and one said that you were a natural.

You ran both self-esteem groups for adolescent boys and domestic abuse groups. You excelled in your social work career, attaining a string of qualifications that eventually led to a management position. Whilst still at school you actively sought and gained employment, both after school one evening a week, together with a short term employment when you had completed your GCSEs. Your work experience was spent firstly in a busy London hospital and secondly in a Social Services department, when you were asked to undertake a project at the sharp end of the community.

I tried to support you, to share in what I knew of your feelings at the time, although reading your journals now has given me a fuller insight as to how you felt. I can remember you coming down the stairs sobbing that fateful day of 2nd January in 1993 and wrote in a card to you:

"I know that 'breaking up is so very hard to do,' especially when it's only just begun. I know a little of how you must be feeling and what a mess you may feel just at the beginning of a new year, and such an important one with A level exams and university looming. Please know that I am praying for you and while God is fully able to know, love, care and understand, I am also trying to hold you in my arms and my prayers. It is not you that is the failure."

Your upper sixth form tutor wrote:

"It has been a pleasure to support Claire in the sixth form; she has been courteous and undemanding, as well as so brave concerning her ill-health."

I found evidence we had kept from the hospital regarding the time you took both your GCSE and A level public exams, stating you had three different bacteria causing chest infections on each occasion and were on IVABs.

From your head mistress, this time on leaving the school in the upper sixth:

"We have all been impressed by Claire's calmness, courage and determination. She is a lovely girl and has played an important part in the life of the school. We will miss her."

You may not have been the most academic in the class, but you were at a grammar school where there was lots of competition. Equally, Claire, I take responsibility for the behaviour you learned from me regarding my lack of self-worth.

Whilst I am in the mode of praising you, I think of those very frightening last weeks of your life when you felt so out of control and the amazing courage you demonstrated.

I think it was rather like a self-fulfilling prophecy with you, in that you didn't believe you were clever or good at things, so you might as well not show yourself to be. However, I also believe that God used the difficulties you underwent to assist you in all the abundant ways that He did as an adult. Your continual theme of sadness at saying goodbye, knowing from a very early age that yours would not be a long life, had such a profound effect on you and I am so very sorry that I was so busy handling my own emotional issues/abuse that I did not give you the full support you needed. However, in one of Bobby Warrenburg's sermons, he mentions Lori Gottlieb's (a clinical psychologist) article: "How to Land Your Kid in Therapy."[45] Bobby refers to her work regarding a variety of young people who came for therapy in their mid-to-late twenties. Gottlieb's research found that their parents had not neglected them nor that they were uncared for, but that actually they were over-protected and over-sheltered, thus never faced the reality of their own failure and guilt. Bobby linked this to what John Calvin said regarding the importance of knowing oneself and knowing God and that until we know God in all His holiness and love, we will never really know ourselves. Rightly or wrongly, Claire, and whilst not making excuses for my parenting of you, this gave me a glimmer of hope that I hadn't failed you completely. How I have loved you over the years, but I am also so conscious, Claire, that I have not lived up to the godly ideals I had when I first became a mother. All I can do is ask your forgiveness again (I did this so often in your life, but I need to do this post-humously, too) for the rules and restrictions I imposed, albeit in your best interest as far as your CF is concerned. You are not responsible for the pain I have caused you. You blamed yourself for many things that were not of your making, neither your responsibility.

---

[45]　Lori Goottlieb, How to Land Your Kid in Therapy, The Atlantic, June 7 2011

You accomplished so much in life that you should have never, ever felt that you failed to achieve, when actually you achieved so much. I used to say to you often, "Well done," and I meant it. Well done for keeping going when life was made so hard due to CF; well done for achieving so much when so much was against you; well done for being you – for the joy you brought so many, for the way you did far more than anyone else who has lived twice as long. Well done from the bottom of my heart for all you accomplished; well done for doing so much that terrified you and for going outside your comfort zone again and again. I just can't praise you enough and I hope and pray you felt that praise when you were alive.

As you mourn each rite of passage, as you say goodbye to many experiences, friends and situations, I'm crying with you, Claire, for the wonderfully sensitive, loving and endearing soul you were, so very sad that you did not live a long life. As in the words of a song sung by Elvis Presley, I did not treat you as you so deserved but now it is too late. However, you remain forever "'On my Mind"[46] and in my heart.

Rest assured, that what you endured gave you the capacity to empathise with others, as one of your close friends gives voice:

"There was a young girl crying in the playground. We didn't know her but Claire went over and put her arm around her and asked if she was okay. She was always doing sweet, kind things like that. Ndullee xxxx."

I want you to know that now you are gone, I daily regret the times I failed you. Not just the type of regret I feel when I forget an important item of shopping, so need to retrace my steps to purchase it, but the heart-breaking remorse, guilt and repentance, shamefulness and sorrow that only God can deal with in me.

---

[46] You Are Always On My Mind, Songwriters: Johnny Christopher, Wayne Carson, Mark James, , published by Lyrics © EMI Music Publishing

Wanting to be of service in the church, I wonder if I put other, even legitimate things before you. I do wish I had stored up more memories of you – documented them, recorded those special events – but there was never time. However paradoxically, between us we created a lot of memories. I am reminded that Auntie Lesley and Uncle Gilbert were ill, which meant we travelled back and forth to Belgium often during your adolescent years. Of course we were pleased to do it and we were sad, particularly, for your cousins when both parents died of cancer. To be bereft of two parents when they were still so young was particularly hard. The same year that Uncle Gilbert died, your other Granddad did also. Illness was a real marker in your teen years. This, together with your CF, took up an inordinate amount of time.

Yet, Claire, as you were growing up and especially in your teen years, I am so sorry that I didn't express to you often enough just how much I valued you, saluted you, emphasised how much I admired you for all you coped with. I knew it in my head, Claire, how as a Christian mother I should be role-modelling Jesus to you, but so often the busyness of life with CF (yes, and a million other things that led to a lifetime of rushing) took over and it did not happen. I shouted, I lost my temper, I was not the mother I should have been. Now I have to live with that, but it is cold comfort.

All I can say, without abdicating from my accountability, is that I believe that God goes ahead of us and behind us. He makes up for my mistakes. Parenting is so hard and God provides grace to help us. If only I could have those years over again, but they are gone. Again, I am not making excuses, but I remember seeing a counsellor when you were away at uni because of family problems when your Granddad was ill, and she asked how you were coping. Whenever I have talked about you (which of course was often), whether at work, in the counselling course I did, or to whoever, I was always animated, singing your praises, and the counsellor replied that you had spunk, and that was what got you through life. (Well, that, and as we know, God too!) So it is not to say that we did not have happy times and times when we got on really well, but know also that I meant every word of remorse.

Returning to the theme of permitting children to learn without parents being over-protective, Mogel suggests that sometimes it is all right for your children to hate you and to realise that families are not always perfect.[47] I was so relieved to read this, and yet I am not trying to let myself off the hook when I blatantly did not follow God's teaching on parenting; when my own agenda and emotions got in the way and a thousand other things of which I have been guilty. There were times, as your diaries bear witness, when I argued with you and I shouldn't have done, when I insisted you do things when you would have learned so much more by deciding for yourself and the list can go on and on. . .all I can do this side of Heaven is ask your forgiveness, knowing that one never knows what one has until it is gone; and Claire, I never appreciated you so much as when you were no longer here.

Again, I am so grateful to my heroine, Meg Woodson who also regretted the times she failed as a mother. One specific incident she relates in depth in her book[48]: Peggie told her mum that she did not understand how she could get upset over such little things. Meg retaliated that equally she did not comprehend why Peggie was so picky over so many things. Meg told Peggie she was sorry and would try not to shout at her again, but that she was under a lot of stress and hoped her daughter would understand. Meg asked herself why, as Peg's mum, she could not use this last chance to make up for her past failures, but she felt God did not care why. He wanted Meg to be real and for them to go easy on each other. God knew the huge grief Meg was about to suffer when she lost her second child to CF too.

God uses all our experiences to mould us into the people He wants us to be. Your teen diaries, and indeed your life, demonstrated that you worked through

---

[47]   Wendy Mogel, Ph.D, *The Blessing of a Skinned Knee: Using Jewish Teachings To Raise Self-Reliant Children* 2001, Scribner

[48]   Meg Woodson, *Turn It Into Glory,* 1991 Hodder and Stoughton

your emotions head on and that is such a compliment with all you had to bear in having CF. You never drank to excess, smoked, or took drugs. We know people do these things to dull their senses, but you were courageous enough, like so many good living people, to not be tempted by them. You were worried about what people thought of you so often and never heard the numerous positive comments made (and of course this is a natural part of being a teenager). I wish, Claire, added to all these, that you could hear what people have said about your life after your death. You would be humbled and yet, I hope proud too. It is okay to be proud of what God has accomplished in our lives; to give the glory to Him.

Again, I am not defending my parenting, but as John White suggests in his *Parents in Pain:* "We can neither take all the credit for our children when they turn out well nor all the blame when they turn out badly."[49] (Not of course that you turned out badly; you were the epitome of grace.)

Ron Dunn says: "Dear Lord, I made many mistakes, but it was in my heart to be the best father I could be."[50]

He continues on page 172: "We dreamed that . . . . .our marriages would be perfect, and our children exemplary. When things do not turn out that way, we feel like failures."

How grateful I am to God, Claire (and also to you), that you became the well-rounded, resilient person you were. In an attempt to fight back my tears following these last few pages, I want to end on a more positive tone: This is note you left for me one evening during your school years. It still makes me smile:

"Too scared to phone library as book very overdue. Realise parents are useful for this type of thing. Please see inside of book for details. Thank you, love Claire. P.S. Please be kind to me tomorrow. Xxx."

---

[49]   John White, Parents in Pain, p36 (Downers Grove: Intervarsity Press, 1979)

[50]   Ron Dunn, When Heaven is Silent, p171 (Thomas Nelson Inc, Nashville, 1994)

Chapter Fourteen

2012 – The Beginning of the Decline

"Life is not measured by the number of breaths you take but by the people, places and moments that take your breath away."[51]

Claire, I wanted to begin this chapter with a particularly pointed insight for our guest readers. Unless someone has experienced firsthand not only the infections, lethargy and general "unwellness" that Cystic Fibrosis inflicts on a person, but the continuous disruption to daily life, it is very difficult to fathom the strength it took for you to not only complete your degree in standard time, but also to volunteer as much as you did. You could never, ever have been accused of failing to live life to the full just because you did not want to die. I have said all this before, so I thought a better presentation of this reality is captured in the next section of your essay, "Life is an Adventure – "Dare It" – Needles, Needles and More Needles:

---

[51] Anonymous, quoted in 1000 Places To See Before You Die, by Patricia Schultz. (2010, Workman Publishing 2010)

Life is an Adventure – Dare It

Needles, Needles and More Needles

Ending up in hospital on a bright Sunday morning was inconvenient; I had an exam to sit the next day! But CF is often inconvenient – it interferes with my plans, which annoys me. The doctors wanted to give me intravenous antibiotics to treat the infection I had, but unfortunately my veins had completely collapsed. After four hours of trying (including attempts at the veins in my feet and neck) they decided to give up. By this time my arms and feet had been soaking in hot water for ages. This supposedly "warms" the veins and makes them more prominent. The doctors were really frustrated; there was blood everywhere from their aborted attempts. They finally decided I would need to have a port-a-cath (a surgical implant that makes it easier to administer intravenous medication). They recommended this approach as it would save a lot of trauma in the future. I had had the "port-a-cath talk" prior to this because it is a much easier way of giving intravenous medication.

The talk emphasises all the positive sides of immediate access to the veins, and I was introduced to other patients who have one and I listened to them promote it. However, I had only had minor surgery before and although it is a small operation, I didn't want scars on my body, especially at eighteen! A port-a-cath is a metal-coated device that is inserted in the chest wall. The size and shape of a ten pence coin, it is inserted surgically under the skin of the chest wall, giving access to a central vein. The fine tube, or "line" attached to the device, is tunnelled under the skin, the end of which lies at the tip of the right side of the heart. It works wonders because it is permanent, avoiding the need for the sometimes painful and messy search for a vein. (Port-a-caths are often used for cancer patients when they have chemotherapy.) Now, when I have intravenous antibiotics, the port is accessed by a special hooked needle and there is immediate access to the vein. When I was younger I had horrible experiences when the doctors put little venflons (needles) or even long lines up the veins in my arms; they took hours to put in because my veins are so small and fragile from years of intravenous antibiotics.

Before the port-a-cath operation I had to return to university to complete my exams. When I arrived that evening my friends were there to make tea, run errands and one even promised to walk me to the exam the following day. They were so good to me, especially as I was feeling quite fragile and very grumpy at the time. After the exam I had to return to hospital for the port-a-cath operation.

Like most people I hate needles, but they are a major part of my treatment. I have a lot of bad memories about needles and blood tests as I've had so many, but I realise I have nothing to complain about when so many people live lives of continual pain. When the port (for short) was first mentioned, I must admit I wasn't keen to have surgery. I don't like anaesthetics, and the operation had to be done as soon as possible, giving little time to prepare myself for it. Four years after the operation I now think it's wonderful compared to all the hurt before. I consider myself extremely fortunate to have it. One drawback is that the port protrudes from under the skin. I didn't want it just below my neck because I thought that if I wear V-necked T-shirts for instance, people would notice, so I had it inserted lower down next to my ribs, so nobody can see and my clothes cover it. I have got a scar just below my collarbone, but it's quite small and I can cover it up most of the time.

After the port was inserted I went back to university with intra-venous antibiotics, which I had to administer myself. When I was about sixteen the hospital staff had taught me how to manage my own intravenous drugs

(IVs) because it gave me more independence and I didn't have to spend so much time in hospital. Instead I live a busy life and continue with my treatment at home. However, to do my own IVs away from hospital and home is a big responsibility. I always prefer to have someone around when I'm injecting myself just in case anything goes wrong. I'm very choosy about who helps me with my injections. I feel vulnerable to germs when I am on IVs and am always washing my hands when preparing the injections. I think this is because my port did become infected once, necessitating further surgery.

Most people with CF have two different antibiotics as part of the course. These cannot be given straight after one another but have to be flushed through with a saline solution to ensure they don't mix once they are in the veins. One evening at 11:00pm, while drawing up my drugs and talking to a friend on the phone, I forgot to flush. Fortunately nothing happened but I got my mum to ring the hospital immediately. I really panicked as I thought I was going to die, with only minutes to live. I asked my auntie, who was with me at the time, to hold my hand as I was sure any minute my heart would stop beating. We sat rigid for a few minutes until I realised I was okay. I felt so stupid afterwards, but I frightened myself enough to take better care in the future. I admit that I do get a little bit lazy with my intravenous medication and sometimes I don't take enough time over them as I should. They interfere with my social life, and my family is always nagging me about my carelessness, but I know they are right.

January 2012

Following your return to work after Christmas, Claire, you had a new manager start work on the January 10. I was somewhat dismayed that, despite your recent bout of illness, you began to work so very, very late. You even went back to helping with the church youth group again, frequently going straight from work and only eating when you arrived home after 10:00 at night. That was your heart, Claire; you sacrificed so much for your friends, for God's work and your Social Services job, but also for me.

As always, you so very kindly took the day off on my birthday and from memory, I swept the garage out (a job the builders had still not done) while you showered and dressed. Your lovely new black rattan garden furniture was being delivered that day and we needed a clean space to store it. I remember we went to see *The Iron Lady* at Esher Cinema, and then went home for round two, watching a DVD and dining on Indian take away.

As part of your Christmas present, I bought a hotel voucher for us to visit Canterbury in February. Little did we know it would be your final visit; your final stay in a hotel; a final weekend away. People always talk about cherishing every moment you have with someone, as we simply have no idea what the future holds, and I realise now those seemingly cliché quotes were begun by someone with deep, and heartbreaking experiences. Again, Claire, I am so very sorry I got cross because you were not ready on time. I did not realise what an effort it was for you to just get yourself up and out, even at the weekend. As love's intentions are so often ironic, it is just that you so wanted to have Sunday lunch in the hotel with the bespoke Chef, I was really worried you would miss out on it. You were unwell again and we had to come home early. In hindsight, I can see you hid your true, desperate plight, even from me.

Although I was not privy to them at the time, of course, some of your text messages demonstrated your concerns regarding your health. To your friend Yasmine you wrote:

"Decisions to make regarding my health and work; things quite difficult."

You texted Chris F., another person with CF, on 19th February:

"Love my new house, it's great but haven't been doing well since new year, so now infection is really bad; am sure will be better soon xx."

Chris F. responded:

"Thanks hun [sic], that's it for us with CF, ups and downs. Glad you have your new place."

On February 21, you texted another friend:

"Have been put on three weeks of intra-venous antibiotics and signed off for rest of week."

We were never in each other's pockets, however, even then. When you had friends around, I would quite happily either sit in the kitchen with the laptop or go up into the bedroom to watch T.V. or read. In the mornings I would get up and prepare your nebulisers and medication; this included the IVABs that you seemed to be on permanently by then. Then I would prepare your breakfast and packed lunch. We did your treatment in bed as much as possible, so you could rest in preparation for the day ahead. Because I was only working part time during your time at No. 10, I would be able to see you out of the house and ensure you had everything with you. By that point, you were finding it hard to carry your bag/ briefcase, so I would bring them out to the car for you.

At weekends during those last months, while you slept I would creep down into the kitchen and get up to date with the ironing or read or go online. When you awoke, I helped you get ready for the day. During the week you would text me when you were leaving work (as I mentioned, this was often very late as you were so busy at work) and I would have your meal prepared so that, once changed out of your work clothes, you could come and finally relax in the lounge for what was left of the evening.

So often, as your last dose of IVs went through in the evening, we sat on your bed watching T.V. I remember a sci-fi programme you liked called *The Walking Dead.* Personally, I hated it. Perhaps my fear was that you were becoming like one of those people, but people say it is during difficult times the most treasured moments are revealed. It is true, and for me, I truly thank God that we had that time together, just being content in each other's company. I suppose it really is a gift when viewed in the right light.

That same month I received this email from you while you were at work:

"Guess what? Out of my 3 supervision files two are good and one is adequate. I am so pleased!"

Doing well in your career meant so much to you, Claire. Of course it was no surprise to me you were a star in your work as well, despite your health challenges, and I rejoiced with you over every positive report.

On the afternoon of Bernie's party, we went into Kingston to buy the mask you wanted to wear, and that evening you had gone up to London for her fortieth celebrations. Sadly, you returned home very early as you were far from well. In retrospect, I can see the writing was on the wall, and perhaps there was just too much on your plate, but at the time, no one had any idea you would not recover. Whilst babysitting for Bernie and Edwin, however (all their usual babysitters were at the party), I texted you:

"Bernie and Edwin not home yet but wake me if u r unwell in night. Hope rest of eve is ok, we can chill tomorrow eve xx."

Adding to the stress, we unfortunately continued to have problems with the snagging, but you will be pleased to know Claire, I took this up with the new building manager who subsequently wrote a letter of apology, and sent a generous cheque to the hospital in London, whose staff had cared for you throughout your life. I worked a couple of days in March, but left you to finish your morning IVABs. That day, your port-a-cath just would not flush for you, so I vowed never to work again until you were admitted to hospital (we were awaiting a bed to become available.).

I sometimes wonder, if you'd met a Godly man to be your husband, would things have been easier for you? Would you have been less stressed, and put less pressure on yourself, being more content with a good home life? It is idle thinking I suppose, for the past is unchangeable. Why this never happened is not for me to question, but I do believe it would have helped.

That Valentine's Day you decorated your dining table with cards, roses and heart-shaped biscuits and chocolates. There they stayed, Claire, with your Easter eggs, right up until I emptied your home of all your possessions in the summer of that year.

Your friend, Helen M. came to stay the first weekend in March, so I went to my own home to sleep for the couple of nights she was with you. (You only had one spare bed at the time, and anyway, you always preferred to entertain friends without me being present. Who can blame you?) On 7th March, following minor surgery on your back at Kingston hospital, you had texted me at work:

"Thanks for your call, Mum, will need new dressing for needle as virtually all off tonight and new one for back too xx."

Not only did you have to contend with the dressings that covered the port-a-cath's Huber needle, but you also somehow developed a fungus under your toe nail. You became so breathless bending down after your shower each day to treat this that I have to wonder why, when life was so difficult for you anyway, did you have to battle with so much in your last weeks of life?

While it is challenging, I believe God understands when we ask such questions, as long as it doesn't embitter us. At the end of the day, there will always be things we don't understand; things that don't fit into our existential framework and view of God's justice and fairness. It is these things that we need to file away in our, "I don't understand it" file, and perhaps even wait until we graduate to Heaven to receive answers. Trusting that there are indeed answers, I believe, is key to surviving life's difficult questions.

Faye came to stay the third weekend in March and you texted me:

"'On way home now. Mum. Willow delivering my IVABs tomorrow between 9 and 11 at mine, can you stay in for that? Then on the 10th, had a great time at cinema, u ok Mum?"

Despite your condition, you were always concerned about others. On the March 11, you again texted:

"Love you, Mum x. Off to church with Faye, shall I take IVABs out of fridge?"

On the March 12, you texted:

"Mum, can you call GP for my nail results, ta. X."

Claire, I truly loved it when you asked me to do things for you, as it would be less of a struggle for you. Sadly, this did not seem to have much of an effect on your deteriorating health, as you texted some friends on March 20:

"Mum staying as struggling to breathe."

Reflecting now on those dark days, I see how many friends you had Claire, to visit you, text, email, call and to rally around you as you were feeling more and more unwell. I see now that these relationships and these deep, human connections you made were more than most people would make in a full lifetime. This is truly part of your legacy; your love and kindness impacted so many lives in your shortened stay in this world. Looking at your diaries for 1996, it's easy to see how you did it; how you gathered people to you like cherished collectibles, and thus affecting so many lives for the better.

Chapter Fifteen

Graduation & 1996's Journals

My dear Claire,

As 1996 began, it stood out as a milestone year for adulthood. You graduated university and truly faced your new future with courage and determination. Yes, you had your share of special challenges, as usual, but I think your journals speak for themselves in this regard:

January 1996

> *Tuesday, January 1, 1996:* Happy 1996 Claire. Flip, this is the year that I'm going to be 21. Quite scary!

> *Thursday, January 4, 1996*: Faye told me she was worried I was going to die and I smiled; she had a massive go at me because I should've taken her seriously after my last long bout of illness.

> *Saturday, January 6, 1996*: What has God taught me in the couple of weeks that I have been back in my old youth group is that:

-Gossip can be very harmful

-I need to place my security in God

-My emotions need to be channelled appropriately

-I am a romantic and day dream far too much

-I need to look to God to discern His will. (Hannah really helped me out today in this respect.)

-That some of the guys are lonely and we need to be more inclusive of them.

-Always think positively

-Focus on God

-Ask God to help you understand how other people feel

-Ask God to use you in His work

-Think of everyone else who is worse off than you

-Pray for all the single people in the church

-Look to God to fulfil you

-Place your security in Him

Tuesday, January 9, 1996: Why have I been so introvert over the past 2 years and what am I going to do about it? Hopefully, a lot. Right, I need a mechanism that when I start thinking about myself I need to think about something else. How about, if I can smell the daisies? Each day I want to pray for my friends that are not converted. I want to pray each morning that God will use me for that day and that He will control my tongue. To pray that God will show me the future.

But to pray the above is quite hard – am I saying to God that I don't have enough faith to depend on Him? God will honour me if I honour him. I hope to be strong and faithful enough to know that God is with me and with Him I can face anything, even a lifetime of singleness, because this life is only for a short time anyway. I'm worried about the future, though; worried about what the future holds and it's scary to think about it.

Monday, January 15, 1996: So good to greet people as we walked to lectures today. Spoke to Mum on the phone and she said she was missing me. I need to keep in mind my prayer list that I made whilst at home. There's been such a lot to do today and not enough time, but I hope that will change. Please, God, use me this term.

Tuesday, January 16, 1996: Life is good at the moment, but I know that things aren't always going to be like this; in fact, they are trying to be quite scary. I had my seminar cancelled so I met with some friends for a hot chocolate in the Gulbenkian Café area. I spoke with a friend for two and a half hours today who needed a great deal of help. I really don't know how to deal with this so please help me, Lord, or help me point her in the right direction to speak with someone more professional. I started another essay before having a lazy evening.

Wednesday, January 17, 1996: Felt ill again this evening. Perhaps I'm coming down with another chest infection.

Saturday, January 20, 1996: I get so jealous when C.U. members report having great discussions about Christianity with their non-Christian friends. Going through that chronic tired phase again.

Monday, January 29, 1996: Rach said I have giftings and I need to accept them as from God. Christ-centred; I want to be now and forever.

February 1996

Thursday, February 1, 1996: I was having a good day today until I realised I was running really late for Mel and Ele. I must remember that I just can't walk as fast as I used to so need to leave plenty of time to get to the main campus area. Mel spoke such sound advice;:God sees the end of our life and he sorts it out.

"For I know the plans I have for you, declares the Lord; plants to prosper you and not to harm you; plans to give you a hope and a future. Then you will call upon me and come and pray to me and I will listen to you. You will seek me and find me when you seek me with all your heart," Jeremiah 29 v11-13.

I need to guard against spending too much time with my Christian friends and thus neglect my other buddies. I'm so tired that I am going to go to sleep soon, but my nebuliser is playing up and I really need to get these antibiotics into me.

Friday, February 2, 1996: Back into school today and hopefully for the last time. Julie, my tutor, still seems to be pleased with my project. It was really good to speak to Mum on the phone. I don't think she fully understood what I was going through; I feel quite alone right now.

Tuesday, February 6, 1996: Cold is now fully blown (excuse the pun!). Wrote today:

"Dear Mum, thanks so much for sending me all the stuff. Here's my form, long overdue. Do you think it is okay? How are you? I hope work is okay. I'm really fed up with everything now and am really looking forward end

of term (yes, already!). Maybe we can go out for a meal over the vacation. Thanks so much for all you have done helping with the Master's degree application and my move back to Chessington. It's meant so much when I feel really ill."

As an aside, Claire, your final year back on campus was in accommodation well off the beaten track, which meant you had to walk long distances to get to the hub of the university site. I knew the deterioration in mobility in your last year meant this was such an effort for you. Hence, any way I may have helped was an honour.

Wednesday, February 7, 1996: I felt really at peace during the social work interview today; the type of questions I had thought of all came up, for example: types of discrimination; what was meant by anti-oppressive practice; give some examples of child abuse; what made me want to do social work; what kind of a family background I came from; what were my values in life, how I felt I worked within a team, etc.

However, and this was the crunch point, at the end of the interview they told me they had already allocated the twenty places (Why they didn't tell me before? I just don't know, so annoying) but that if I took a year out and got some "life experience" they would put me on the fast track placement list for next year, i.e. I would be interviewed one of the first and get an allocated place. Mum was disappointed for me, but said, "You're not meant to be there for another two years."

Thursday, February 8, 1996: Sometimes I feel so obsolete; I ask God: Why isn't He using me? I want to be used by Him before I drop down dead. All my mates have been supportive regarding the social work interview and I feel honoured they have behaved in such a way. I feel much better that I can move on to what I would like to do with my year "out" next year. My tiredness from last term continues.

As a further aside, Claire, Rach wrote to me recently:

"Claire was always the one to reach out to people at university, especially the difficult characters. I can remember a few people who Claire would find demanding and trying, but she would still meet up with them, cook pasta and be available to help. Even when she was very aware of their issues or found their perspective on life contrary to hers or selfish, Claire never let that show. She really showed grace to people. She put others' needs before hers and rarely let on her frustrations with people. Claire had such a pastoral and loving heart."

Saturday, February 17, 1996: Slept badly last night, maybe just home too late or maybe coughing so much kept me awake again. Mum was very supportive about my plans for next year.

Monday, February 19, 1996: Woke up to loads of snow today. Help, how do I get through it all to lectures? We had a group of people from C.U. for dinner and it was a good time.

Tuesday, February 20, 1996: Got a really encouraging letter from Mum re: schools work. It read:

"I admire you following your convictions re: Christian Schools' Work. Pursue it and if God closes doors, fine, but if He doesn't then it's His will. I'm praying He'll show you what to do. I also admire your willingness to serve Him."

On the downside I really tried to witness round the coffee table in the Gulbenkian, but just felt mocked!

Thursday, February 22, 1996: I can't wait to go home. (Yes, very unlike me but I am so fed up and dog-beat-tired and yes, I know the same record is wearing out and not exactly creative in my diary jottings.) I got £50.00 from the Accommodation Office as an overpayment, which was brill. Our clinical went well today. Phew, that was a surprise and also a relief.

Tuesday, February 27, 1996: Granddad has had a stroke. Poor Mum must be fed up all the time with so much family illness through the years. She is staying with Grandma at present. Rach and Kim were really kind to me this evening.

Wednesday, February 28, 1996: Felt really ill again today and back to throwing up with so much coughing. Granddad's stroke hasn't affected his mobility, but he can't speak and the doctors say his thought processes are affected. Interestingly, we covered cerebral vascular accidents in Neurology today, so it was quite timely.

March 1996

Saturday, March 2, 1996: I have felt so unwell for two terms now, and the infections make me lacking in energy and I can't help but moan. I know this sounds horrible, but I challenge anyone to feel they can't get rid of the flu for five plus months and see how they cope with life. Being off my food certainly hasn't helped my weight, but hey, I can't eat and then throw up (sorry, Diary, to continually mention this) and then eat again before morning lectures start. However, I have kept supper down, so feel a bit better.

Tuesday, March 5, 1996: Another bad day as can hardly put one leg in front of another. Mum has sent money to get lifts or pay for a taxi to main campus area to preserve some of my energy. I still don't know what God wants me to do when uni finishes and time is fast going by. Rach and Kim have been real rocks these past few days, but I think I take the people closest to me for granted.

Monday, March 11, 1996: Stats were a bit of a nightmare today and someone just walked out, couldn't hack it (I don't know why I always use that word but it seems most appropriate); can't say I blamed her. I should have gone after her. If I am wanting God to use me, then I should be sensitive to other people's pain. Can't stop thinking about Schools' Work for my year out and I do feel God is leading me in that direction. I'm so excited, but want to make sure it's for the right reasons. Lisa is planning to go to Australia for 6 months, brill.

Saturday, March 16, 1996: The feeling "I" and feeling "T" words are so much part of my vocabulary for this second term of our third year, that it must be so boring for those that listen to me. I just need to get home, get up to the hospital for a good overhaul and get some good nights' sleep. Maybe that will make me feel better.

Thursday, March 21, 1996: What? Couldn't believe it when my tutor lost my work today and so near to end of term. Not my responsibility, she'd better find it!

Term ended on the 22ⁿᵈ March and I wonder how you felt, you who hated goodbyes, that you only had one term left at uni.

You wrote to me:

"Just to say I'm really looking forward to coming home and seeing you at the weekend. Thank you for sending all the articles for me to read (I just didn't have enough breath to get to the library this week)."

Friday, March 29, 1996: They must all think I'm a complete emotional wreck at Cornerstone. I just cried in front of everyone and said I was so lonely. When Geoff heard my tutor had lost my work, he offered to type it up for me and help input my Stats too (maybe they know what a difficult two terms I've had and with Granddad with his stroke on top of it all).

April 1996

Tuesday, April 2, 1996: Some people have told me that I would be perfect for the Schools' Work post, but I remain so nervous, yet excited about it. However, I'm really looking forward to the interview. Life is young, free and vibrant so we should enjoy it; it's not worth all the angst. God has my life all sorted. He knows what's going on. Praise God; He is in control.

Friday, April 5, 1996: Good Friday. Phew! Saw Ian at the joint church service and he asked if I was still interested. I said that of course I was. He said the Committee is keen to have me and that two guys would also working as year outers.

You returned to Uni for your last term on the 17th and wrote:

"Tues 23rd. This is our last term! There's still so much to do and not enough time to do it in."

Friday, April 26, 1996: Mum has spent all week typing up my essay and I feel bad about it. It's so unfair on her but I'm tired already and I haven't been back a week yet!

Monday, April 29, 1996: Had Eating Disorders Support Group training today and looked at the circle of abuse. Four weeks exactly until the exams.

I wrote to you as you approached your finals:

"I hope your cold doesn't come too much and that you get on well revising. Not long before the exams! Try and do what you can, but do come home if you want to and aim for some early nights."

May 1996

Tuesday, May 7, 1996: Feeling much better about my predicted degree results now; my tutor, Dr. Abrams, said I should be confident. He is really such a nice man. To lighten the revision period, Lynn wrote:

"Once an addict always an addict. Addictive behaviours have been recognised as one of the world's greatest social/health problems. McAllister (1996) has reported the rapid worldwide spread of addiction to chocolate, which is believed to have started in 19 Lypeat Court, on the university campus in Canterbury!"

Rach went home to her Gran's funeral. I have been so sad for her. I get lonely when I am here without others, but such is life. I need to realise that we are all vulnerable. D. cried so much today over a broken relationship. I'm just wondering if I miss the opportunities of relationships. Should I go out with the men who ask me out just to test the water? Am I slow on the uptake? However, I want to meet the right person if this is in God's plan for me. I'm so tired I want to go to bed now forever. I dislike my hair cut intensely. I want my long, blond hair back!

Friday, May 17, 1996: I had such an ideal opportunity with the Gospel this evening, but I completely flunked it. I need to ask for forgiveness. I can't believe I let that chance slip through my fingers. Please, Lord, give me another opportunity. I'm not eating (a sure sign another chest infection is on the way) and subsequently losing weight.

Tuesday, May 21, 1996: I'm so tired today and I need some sleep so am going to put that to rights now. I've got a temperature and I feel ill (not good timing with exams now immediate, but a week today and they'll all be over). Thank the Lord, I had another opportunity to witness and took it.

Friday, May 24, 1996: I really thought I'd messed the exam up today and just cried; only time will tell. Kim and Rach were such an encouragement. Please Lord, keep me focused not on my health, not on my fear of failure, but on Your great love.

Monday, May 27, 1996: Revised all day for exams tomorrow.

Wednesday, May 29, 1996: Went home today for Christian Schools' Work Trust interview tomorrow.

Thursday, May 30, 1996: I dressed too smartly but I got the job, PTL. Emma and also Kenny came round for a couple of hours this evening and it was great to see them.

June 1996

Tuesday, June 4, 1996: Back to uni. Said goodbye to loads of people who are heading home before the results come out. Felt very lonely.

Friday, June 14, 1996: Keleigh, Justin, Patricia, Ali, Jo, Lynn, Isla and loads of other people came around. So many of us acknowledged that life sucks and you just have to get off your *derriere* and live life. That's all one can do, we can't be thinking, "What if" forever. Holiness is the balance between my disposition and the law of God as expressed in Jesus Christ' so said this evening's speaker.

Just as in my home church youth group, so in uni we studied the Bible together and saw that the God of the Old and New Testament people was indeed the same God of today, such a liberating message. I wrote some reflections in my diary of the worst scenario life could present:

-Acceptance that one day you will have to be cared for

-Coming to terms with no longevity of life

-Physical self image changes as CF worsens

-Impact of CF on relationships and marriage

-6 hours of physio, what quality of life

-Can't hold down full time job

Keleigh has just given me a book on stress; she knows how much I need it.

Thursday, June 20, 1996: As I come to the end of uni, I want to have been seen as an encourager and what I crave is God to be in my life and for people to see I desire Him. I'm going to find leaving UKC so hard. It's been hard, actually, these last few days, the finale.

Tuesday, June 25, 1996: Exam results were posted at 5:00pm. I got a 2.2! Mel just held me up for the last little bit. I was crying before I got there as I thought I'd done badly in one exam. It was such a rush to get the results and you can't see your name at all, which is really, really concerning.

The following people also got a 2.2: Justin, Becky, Sam, Andy, Ele, Kate and loads of other people from our Psychology course, too.

The rest got a 2.1. There were no 3rds. Phew! Hol, Kim, Jane, Karen, Rach, etc on other courses all get 2.1s so all in all it was really great. Simon got a 1st. He looks great with his new hair-cut. Rob came round; so did Keleigh and her sisters. I rang Mum, anxiously waiting at home to hear. The Psychology group had a party in Woodies and everyone happy with exam results.

Wednesday, June 26, 1996: To Woodies bar again; Gem, Kate, Natasha, Will, Emma and Justin came to dinner. Missed C.U. but said bye to Grant, Jon, Big J, Justin, Will, and Jon. I got really upset saying bye to Justin. I'm going to miss him a lot.

Thursday, June 27, 1996: Said my goodbyes to sick bay. Goodbye to Dr. Abrams too; as usual, he was so nice. We cleared our rooms and had our last evening meal together.

Saturday, June 29, 1996: Everyone had to be out of their rooms and off site today; we eked it out to the very last and left at 10:00am. Rach came back home with me; I doubt I could have coped if I was leaving uni for the last time alone.

Words on my card to you read:

"Welcome home, even if it is only temporary. I can't believe you have a degree and are a graduate. We are so very proud of you because you've battled against ill-health to get this far."

Keleigh, Jemma and Jade following your results sent a card:

"Congratulations and all the best for your wonderful, exciting future. Don't forget to keep in touch!"

Keep in touch you all did, Claire; the three intrepid sisters from Leicestershire either came to visit you regularly or you went up to meet with them. Since your sad death, they have come south each year to meet up on your birthday for picnics in Richmond Park.

All those friendships you forged at uni did not end there; you kept in touch with many, many of your peers and indeed even before your graduation Elke wrote:

"God has got such a good life for you. Don't think that when God was dishing out happiness in life He skipped you. I know you have had it tough, more than the rest of us, though we are so wrapped up in our own lives, we don't even see your struggles and you are too nice to tell anyone! He walks everywhere where you go, and when you cry, He is sitting there holding you. Generosity is His nature."

Flora wrote:

"God is silently faithful and all He requires is to put our faith and trust in Him."

From a friend at uni:

"Dear Claire, I want to thank you for being such an awesome friend. I praise God for bringing us together. You have listened to me when I needed to cry out to someone; you have comforted me when I've been upset. You have warmed my spirit when I have felt so far away; you have offered unconditional friendship and your prayer support. What more could anyone ask for in a friend? Thank you, Claire for taking the time to be there for me. I owe you so much."

Only a couple of months ago, Claire, I was tidying out your special box of keepsakes where I found much of the correspondence I have used within this diary (but only that to and from your friends written on cards; I did not read any letters as they were personal between you and them). I thank God for allowing me to be your mum; what a joy you have been to me and to God, too. I can remember Steve W. saying how lovely your permed hair looked when you were a fourteen year old and what a credit you were in every way. I just want you to know that if I could have your life over again, things would be so different.

Your journal continued:

Rob came back to ours to stay and then wrote:

"Thanks so much for taking me into your family home these past few days. I can't express really how much your friendship means to me; you are a young woman with such a tender heart for others. I shall miss you so much when I return from my university year in England to San Diego."

July 1996

Interestingly, Claire, in particularly difficult or emotional times in your life, your diary was glaringly empty; it was almost as if you had no words to describe your feelings. One example was the resolution of your university years at Kent. It was no secret how much you had enjoyed them, despite your health taking a downward spiral. God created us to metaphorically fly; to soar above the earth in joy and praise and I believe some of your experiences at Kent enabled you to do just that. Maybe at other times you even experienced the Lord carrying you, as so eloquently described in the "Footprints" poem.

On Friday, July 5, 1996, a few days after your final year at university your diary recorded:

I'm probably one of the luckiest people alive, I have loads of support, yet I'm still so flipping selfish. I felt really inadequate today as if I didn't belong, as if my life is a mess and I have no control over it. What is God trying to teach me? Everyone seems so established and together, yet I'm not at all. I still need to trust God with all my problems. Things in Cornerstone aren't the same as how I left three years ago, but I guess that is to be expected; I've changed so much in that time span, as I am sure so many others have too.

One thing I strongly believe, Claire, is you were way too hard on yourself much of the time. Yes, it is important we recognise sin in our lives, but as Brian your pastor reminded you in 1994, you were a young woman battling cystic fibrosis. Also, you did have your life together; you had just completed a degree, having undergone many months of ill health, and you'd been appointed to a Schools' Work position. What's more is you were even living away from your family home with Auntie Pat, having set your sights firmly on independence.

As if you had not had enough studying, the summer you finished at Kent, you embarked on a week's basic Counselling Course with *Crusade for World Revival* (CWR[52]) at Waverley Abbey in Farnham. You must have been excited, because your diaries sprang to life again:

Tuesday, July 9, 1996: Felt very intimidated by the group. Oh, they were kindness itself but I felt very young; some of them will make wonderful counsellors.

Wednesday, July 10, 1996: The older pastor is a really lovely man and I want to take him home with me to help me – aah, he is so sweet. Counselling is so much harder than I thought. God has raised up a good Christian friend just when I needed this person.

Thursday, July 11, 1996: It has been a really good day in terms of being encouraged. I think they're brilliant and I don't want to leave the place or the people; they are just so good. Our utter dependency must be in God

[52]   www.cwr.org.uk

and I've given it all to Him and in a way I expect Him to deal with it all now. I don't ever want to forget the good time I've had here at Waverley. He certainly has blessed me this week and I have to pray that He chooses to again. I can't explain myself very well though, which really frustrates me. I need to rely, not so much on people, but on God.

Friday, July 12, 1996: It was a really brilliant Communion service. It was lovely to pray in small groups with Cath and Rachel. Great picture of an athlete and different sports and God saying: "I'm going to make you strong in all areas." Praise Him and phew. Felt really like I wanted to spend an hour with Him in my quiet time. This week was a glimpse of heaven.

You clearly met with God in a new way on that course, and this is what you wrote to yourself in response to questions you were all asked:

"Dear Me, you have spent a year focussing on yourself and not giving God a look in. Please change."

Similarly, a questionnaire that you completed:

How will the fact that your body is the temple of the Holy Spirit affect your lifestyle?

Everything I do affects God

Are you more eager to be in favour with men than with God?

Yes, I am ashamed to say.

How can you be devoted to Him?

By focusing on Him and thinking less of myself.

How will you avoid 1. Materialism and 2. Sex outside marriage being barriers to Christian growth?

By asking the Lord for help and being strong in self-discipline.

If you died at 17 like my friend Paul, would you be ready for it?

I hope so, but not as ready as I'd like.

Is the baton of the Good News being passed on by you?

I try to do this in my daily life, but I know I fail so often.

Predictably, wherever you went, Claire, you again touched people's lives, as the following excerpts illustrate. These snippets are responses from the people you met on the counselling course, when you were each asked to comment on each other's strengths (I have included just a few):

"I haven't changed my opinion of you since the first day; I really like and admire you. Xx."

"I like your kind and effective attitude. You're respectful and dedicated, a safe practitioner."

"Quiet, calm and very sensitive."

"Your quiet strength."

"You are lovely, generous, warm and exude a sense of contentment. Love Caro."

"A very sensitive, warm, caring person."

Your diaries then continued:

Tuesday, July 16, 1996: This is our Graduation Day in Canterbury Cathedral. It must be one of the best days of my life so far! We had trouble parking but managed to have lunch and get gowned up. Saw Will, Ele and Hollie. Then the procession, ahh! In line with Nicola. It was a really good atmosphere, checking out the gowns and hats.

I kept asking people to check my hat as I had to take it off loads of times for some reason (kept smiling though). When my name was called I went up, shook hands and the Chancellor said, "Congratulations," I then followed the person in front, walking down the aisle of the Cathedral. Once the whole ceremony was over, it was outside on the Cathedral lawns for many photos. Just amazing. Ele, Lynn, Ali, Sally, Hazel, Peggy and Sam all part of the day. It was great. Then we went in for tea, and then time for more professional photos. Saw Karen, Ali, Claire and Claire, Simon, Kim and Dom. It was really fantastic just seeing everyone and saying hi. Then we went up to UKC to get Will, a whole hour late, and phew, he was still waiting patiently for us! Had a really lovely meal at Chestfield Barn. I was really spoilt with so many cards and gifts and such great friends. You don't know what you've got until you lose it.

Following your graduation, Claire, I so admired your independence in sticking to your guns, being determined not to return home to live. Having tasted freedom, that was it for you, despite your struggles with CF. You maintained your indomitable spirit to get by without returning home. However, to afford your year's voluntary work, you ended up staying with Auntie Pat which, from my perspective, was the perfect transition from the nest to complete independence.

Thursday, July 18, 1996: Went to see "Miss Saigon" with Emma; Mum was really good buying ice cream, etc. We got a taxi there and walked back, but it went really well.

Friday, July 19, 1996: I went to the hospital for my annual assessment to be told that I've kept up the same stability for 4 years. They said I was bound to be tired, chronically tired, especially over my finals year at university, as that's due to the disease. I didn't let on that I felt really ill today.

Sunday, July 21, 1996: Down to the caravan with Rach and Will and was so tired. We went to Lansdowne Baptist Church and saw Ali. The chronic tiredness from uni hasn't dissipated.

Monday, July 22, 1996: Went shopping and then went out to a lake, but it was too hot so we came back to sleep. We were so tired that physically I couldn't have woken up if Alan had not come. It was like a force that couldn't help me, truly awful being so whacked. It was so good to see him. We had dinner and watched: *A Room with a View*. Brilliant, we really enjoyed it.

Tuesday, July 23, 1996: Today we went to the beach after getting up late and then returned for lunch before meeting Claire in Boscombe, proceeding to Bournemouth where we met up with Ali and Debbie. I had an awful headache. I've realised I've been really selfish these past few days because I haven't put my trust in God. My security is not in Him and I have, thus, got problems. The day finished with cake and pressies a week in advance of my birthday. I was spoilt!

Wednesday, July 24, 1996: Rachel B. came today. It was good to see her after so long. We had our usual outing to the beach, back for lunch, which we had outside in the sun. Said goodbye to Alan, which was a real shame. It was good to hear about the Czech Republic. Then Ali, Deb, Natasha and her friend came for tea. It's the last time we'll see Nat before she goes away.

Tuesday, July 30, 1996: My twenty-first birthday and I've had the most brilliant day. People have been so good, so friendly and I've been saying, "I'm a Spoilt brat," with a capital S! I've had some really lovely presents, especially one from Faye which I'm really happy about. Phew! Mum gave me loads and loads of stuff and I'm just so blessed. The day really surpassed my expectations. Then I came home for a break as I was just so tired and worn out; really tired, but I'll soon sort myself. Although my proper party will be the Barn Dance in September (when everyone is back from their holidays), quite a few people came round this evening, about twenty-two people in all. It's been a great day. Rach rang to say Kim's dad so very sadly died. I am blessed a thousand x ten thousand.

What a super twenty-first Barn Dance you had, Claire. Your friends attended from every walk of life, and from far and wide. Kim reminded me recently that lots of your uni friends stayed overnight, sleeping in the church hall. I truly believe they would have done anything for you, Claire. Ele gave you a lovely album to commemorate your years at Kent, full of photos taken there. I thought her summary of your time at Kent, included in the album, was wonderful:

"In your first year at the University of Kent at Canterbury you meet many people you will keep in touch with, some of whom will have a great impact on your life, like Alison, all your Christian Union friends and roommates in Darwin. During the year you participate in the C.U., do soup runs and work on the Niteline Listening Service. At the end of this year, just before your exams, you get very ill and undergo an operation which will facilitate the

intake of antibiotics, making life a little easier for you in terms of intrave-nous medication. That was tough, but you were stronger than all of us. We all thought you were a real trooper. To recover, you go to sunny Sardinia with some roommates.

"Your second year goes relatively smoothly health wise. Your course starts taking you on the path towards your career ambitions and you pass the year in flying colours.

"Your third year is a year of encounters, achievements, highs and lows. You live on site in Park Wood, leading an independent student life style. You graduate alongside all your mates and the parting of the ways for us all is very nostalgic."

Your journals, Claire, fall silent in September of 1996 and you only record action items you were required to remember. This might have been due to your shift toward adult, professional life, using your diary almost as a planner, instead of a memoir recorder. These action items typically included standard stuff like where you needed to be each day, and which friends you were meeting. Friendships continued to feature hugely in your years following uni, of course, and these continued to be from all walks of life. One such entry recording a day full of busy activity that was just "so *you*" made me smile: "Catherine Y. lunch, cinema with Ndullee. Claire E. outside local parade of shops." I could list a host of names you had mentioned as well, but your friends knew who they were and how often you all met up together. .

One of the first steps you took into your career was acceptance for Schools' Work. Pastor Trevor A., the chairman of the charity wrote to you:

"On behalf of the General Council of the Trust, I am delighted to confirm our acceptance of your application to spend an academic year as a 'year out'

worker. The council were unanimous in their desire to have you work for the Trust and the prospect of Tony and Jonathan working together with you as a small team was one which we believe will really strengthen the work in the Christian Unions as well as expand the evangelistic opportunities. The Council were enormously impressed by your approach and attitude and we are very grateful to the Lord for bringing you to us for this year.

"We would reiterate the concern I mentioned today on the 'phone over your health. The council are insistent that you must not over stretch yourself to the detriment of your health. Thus we would want you to take time out whenever it was necessary and not overburden or overtire yourself. . ."

That September saw you commence your voluntary "gap/year out" with the Christian Schools' Work Trust, working with Jon A. and Tony W. On the evening of your induction to the work at their annual meeting, each of you recounted how you came to be in Schools' Work. Your story included:

I would like to introduce myself and to explain why I'm working this year with the Trust. This summer I completed my studies in Psychology at Kent University in Canterbury, where I have been based for 3 years. Before my student days I was brought up in Surbiton and attended Tiffin Girls' School, where I first worked alongside Ian (and I've still come back for more!). I remember being at the Schools' Work anniversary last year and wondering, "Could I be a Year-Outer?" I believe God has firmly helped and guided me since then and here I am!

At the age of 8 I became a Christian at a youth camp organised by my church (Hook Evangelical in Surbiton), but my Christian growth was slow until I became involved with both the youth work at Hook and leading the C.U. in the sixth form at school. University was also a great experience for me as I helped out again in the Christian Union there and the local church. Because of these responsibilities I had to lean heavily on the Lord, and I am grateful for the opportunity this coming year presents.

Hand in hand with Schools' Work went the Genesis training project that local churches ran on Saturday mornings, over a two year period. It was expected that year out workers attend this training and at the end of the course, having completed all the assignments, participants received a diploma.

Whilst you were at school, co-leading the C.U., this was just confined to Tiffin Girls' and Tiffin Boys'. This year, however, you gained wide experience in the work as a whole across the entire Royal Borough of Kingston, in both junior and senior schools within the Christian Unions. What is more is that Awareness Weeks were held at the beginning of the school year for interested pupils. Thus your time was spent attending lessons (progressing, predictably, to giving some) and assemblies, as well as work in training and equipping C.U. leaders in their own faith, and learning to defend it in the schools.

Christian pupils were taught how to run effective C.U.s by way of a Plumb Line course. This originated from Amos 7:7 (NIV): "This is what he showed me: The Lord was standing by a wall that had been built true to plumb, with a plumb line in his hand." Much of the work was effectively getting alongside pupils and encouraging them, and Christian teachers were, of course, an important resource to tap into. This was one way of getting into the schools to impart Christian beliefs and values to the students on a wide range of topics that included: relationships, self-image and substance abuse.

You would all meet often at Ian and Nina's home for prayer and I remember them being such a tremendous encouragement to you three. Additionally, you were each assigned a mentor. Maggie S. was assigned as yours, and she was real encouragement to you.

At the same time, you continued to be involved in the youth work at your home church; however your voluntary work coincided with another infection in your port. This required another admission to hospital for removal of it, and that necessitated dressings to the affected area by the district nurse. Just another day in the life of a girl who lived with CF, I suppose.

With your first term behind you, you were ready to thoroughly enjoy Christmas, which you did true to form with plenty of socialising and reverie. In the New Year you headed off to meet uni friends in London for some resourceful fun. Your friend, Matt D. told me in an email me following your death that, "We'd say something like, 'Wear blue,' so we could find each other in the crowd. . ."

I also found a card that Emma N. had written to you that read:

"Dear Claire, it was lovely to speak to you the other day. It's good to know you are still out there wearing blue! Please let me know when you plan to visit campus this year. Lots of love, Emma."

Thus another year drew to a close, my precious Claire. Thankfully, 1997 would continue in the happy spirit with which it began. Yes, there would be challenges, as there always are for anyone stricken with CF, but far be it from Claire Salter to let mere challenges get her down.

Chapter Sixteen

University Years – 1997-1999

1997

So dawned 1997, my dearest Claire, as you continued weaving the richest tapestry of life, daring to live, even then, the bravest adventure. My heart is so joyful to find your 1997 diary includes a list, in true Claire fashion, of people and events for which to pray. Your report for the Schools' prayer diary (after two terms in the above work) read:

> *"It seems impossible that it is the summer term already as the time has gone so quickly. I have enjoyed working for the Trust as well as learning a lot from everyone, too. All three of us year outers have been involved in the Christian Unions and have been able to form good relationships with many pupils and the more we can get to know them, the more we can help them spiritually. We have also assisted Ian in lessons, and have taken three assemblies, which were nerve-wracking, but gave us valuable experience to share the gospel. Thank you so much for your support over the year."*

As the school year drew to an end on 18ᵗʰ July it was, as in all your goodbyes, another nostalgic event, but nonetheless a year you enjoyed immensely. You had attended a plethora of peers' weddings and, as Susan G. records in Surrey Social Services' "Tribute to Claire Salter," you were bridesmaid to people like Caroline, Melanie, Faye, Jo C., Lynn, Nat and Rach, to name but a few. I know your own desire to meet a godly man and be married was heavy on your heart at these times, and I was praying for the same.

In the summer you flew, with some Christian friends (Kiwi and Rachael, among others), to Turkey. I was so thrilled you were able to experience a land rich in so many Biblical treasures, where you retraced the steps of much of St. Paul's third missionary journey. You stayed on the Aegean coast, camping just outside Izmir, an ideal base for you to explore the seven churches listed in the book of Revelation (Thyatira, Pergamos, Sardis, Philadelphia, Ephesus, Smyrna and lastly Laodicea). As a change to camping, you spent two nights in a hotel and subsequently visited the famous Cotton Castles. I wondered what these were when you wrote about them in your holiday diary, and had to search online to discover they are a natural site in south-western Turkey containing hot springs in travertine pools. The pools are stacked as terraces, when carbonate minerals are left by the flowing water. The pools, or "castles," are absolutely beautiful, and it must have been tremendously fun and rejuvenating to swim in them. After the Cotton Castles you wound your trip down with some time at a beautiful resort in Kemer.

Claire, I think in your shortened yet busy and beautiful life, you did so much to further the gospel, and I am so proud of all you accomplished. I can be proud, because you truly did live your adventure, pushing yourself and risking your health each time you lived your dreams. Living under canvas and catching a D&V bug did not do the CF any good and on your return your G.P. was very concerned at the amount of weight you had lost. Thankfully, back in a cooler England, with a third lot of intravenous antibiotics that year and with some T.L.C., you recovered. That

September you enrolled in a secular, one-year Certificated Counselling Course that would require two evenings a week. You certainly did not let the grass grow under your feet!

You kept in mind the advice received in 1996 from your social work course tutor while at the University of Kent, when she told you she preferred students to get some life experience prior to commencing training. As such, you applied for a teaching assistant post to aid a senior pupil with cerebral palsy, and alongside this part-time work you gained additional employment at a local Christian bookshop.

As the year rounded out, you were so excited to begin 1998 with new goals and focus. As ever, Claire, for the challenges you faced, you sure gave back to life twice as much in energy and passion.

1998

The front of your diaries continued to feature New Year resolutions, 1998 being no exception:

-Pray for. . . .each day

-Pray for each member of Cornerstone once a week

-Read, read, read

-Work hard

-Learn to accept myself and be more confident

-Don't be consumed by superficial things

-Be who I am and be sincere

-Have one night in a week

-Forget about people's problems and give their burdens to God.

Ever ambitious, January saw you apply to Reading University to pursue a Master's degree in Social Work. You had completed the long application form, however, and it was there I found a note you had written to me that read: "Please read through, Mum, and can we check we both interpret this correctly?" Of course you were accepted and were also blessed enough to receive a bursary to undertake these studies which would commence in the autumn.

Your life experience had paid off and you were excitedly on your way to social work training. Nobody could ever say that you did not live life to the max, nor that you trod water. Truly, the amount of paperwork you had to complete for your social work application was a feat in itself. I am testament to that, having just emptied your file. The amount of work any university course requires can be quite staggering, as I'm sure many people will agree, and for you, Claire, this was before you even started your treatment for the day. Indeed, the rich life skills you had accomplished since school – volunteering with educationally challenged children, working in two care homes, visiting in a third and working for our older neighbour, Dennis, together with your voluntary work at the University of Kent and temporary vacation jobs – all worked to set you up nicely with a very strong résumé. As I said, nothing held you back.

Ian F. provided you with a reference:

"Claire Salter worked for the Royal Borough of Kingston Schools' Christian Trust from September 1996 until July 1997 inclusive. During this time Claire gained wide experience working with secondary aged children from a wide range of social and cultural backgrounds.

"Claire was part of a team of three post-graduates working for the Trust. She has a genuinely caring and sensitive disposition and was a pleasure to work with. Her ability to defuse any tensions in the team was a notable and welcome asset. Her relational skills meant that Claire also quickly gained the confidence and trust of the young people. She was able to empathise without being patronising and give advice and support to them.

"Claire undertook an extended assignment as well as following a structured reading course. Her self-discipline and conscientiousness were prominent in the way she conducted her studies. There was no difficulty in motivating her enquiring mind.

"Claire has Cystic Fibrosis but never allowed this to interfere with her work. She had very little time off with illness. Her character, determination and skills are highly commendable and I sincerely hope that she will gain a place on the course. Signed: Ian F."

In July I wanted to treat you to a proper holiday before you started your course, so we headed off to San Diego's beautiful beaches for Rob and Diana's wedding! Then we were on to sunny Cancún before heading for a stunning cruise of the Caribbean! Rach wrote before you travelled:

"I wish you could hear the lovely comments about you that I hear and how special you are. I will be praying for you as you travel to the wedding. Rob loved Jim Elliot when he was in England and no doubt still does, so I started reading Elizabeth Elliot's books. Jim's favourite verse was from Psalm 91: 'He who dwells in the shelter of the most high will rest in the shadow of the Almighty.' (I find this so nostalgic, Claire, bearing in mind it was this Psalm, specifically verse 4 that featured significantly during your last hospital admission.)"

I recently browsed through the San Diego guide you bought, which reminded me of the beautiful view of the Pacific from our hotel. One forgets some things like that without context, but thankfully you were always thinking and acquiring the memoirs which would someday allow me to relive our epic times together. In addition to our gorgeous view, we had ourselves a true adventure with visits to

Seaport Village, Balboa Park, Mission Bay and La Jolla, as well as the renowned San Diego Zoo.

Your holidays so often contained significant cultural elements to them as well. It did not suffice just to enjoy the sun, the sea, and the beach – you were careful to gain as many enriching experiences as you could. This was again true when you insisted we visit *Chichen Itza* on the Yucatan Peninsula, the famous pre-Columbian city built by the Mayans, with the great *El Castillo* step-pyramid dominating the landscape. It was a fascinating experience, to say the least.

When we cruised with the Royal Caribbean cruise company, I'll never forget the live band playing a song that was new to us, yet summed up that great holiday so well: "Summer, eating on the side walk, summer, walking in the park."[53] Music always generates such strong memories. Wanting to record your trip, as became your habit, Claire, you kept information on The Crane Hotel in Barbados. I still have a beautiful photo of you lounging on the terrace, overlooking the famous Crane Beach. Indulging your curious mind, you bought a map of the Gulf, Caribbean and also the Atlantic Coast area so you could happily follow our route as we holidayed. It fills me with joy to think you had such wonderful experiences amidst your daily challenges. As always, the amount of medical equipment we had to take for you was extensive, but relying on our detailed lists ensured we did not forget anything.

After that holiday, being rested and relaxed, it was back to business and you were ready to tackle the next step in your life's adventure. Having had such an awesome experience of the University of Kent, and I suppose having matured greatly so that the University experience was no longer novel, you appeared to view Reading more as a means to an end to obtain a career-related qualification. Given you would spend a large amount of the course on placement, neither did any of you have the daily support of colleagues. You would not be you however,

---

[53]   Author unknown

if you did not form at least a few lasting friendships, namely with Jo C., Ruth W. and Charlie.

Reading was an entirely different experience, it seemed, and there were only a few of you living on campus. As Reading had different campus localities, you were unable to meet up much, either. Hence, having spent the previous two years back home in Chessington, and renewed your co-leadership role in the church youth work, you were anxious to return each weekend. I can still picture your room in Bulmershe Court; it was the first one in the block and you had to pass the kitchen to reach it. The disabled bay was right outside, so you never had any trouble getting a car space.

In November of that year, I was so proud when you drove to London's Hilton Hotel to accept your CF Achiever's Award. I have no recollection of your plan to drive back to Reading in the evening, but I remember so well receiving a phone call from you in the early hours of the morning as you were having great difficulty breathing. I jumped in the car and raced to your campus, and did some low flying to get you to the Royal Berks Hospital A&E. They rushed to give you some oxygen and thankfully, before very long, your saturations came back up. After a brief period of observation I drove you back to uni, and Claire, how you got up for lectures the next day, I do not know. I suppose how you achieved so much in life, though, I also cannot fathom.

1999

1999 saw your adventures continue; you and Pat holidayed in stunning South Africa, enjoying Cape Town and the picturesque Garden Route. You even visited a game reserve and saw all manner of wild animals. As if that wasn't enough to satiate your explorer's thirst, you travelled with some Christian friends on an Oak Hall (Christian) holiday to Israel and Egypt. In a letter you wrote to me:

"Hope you are okay. Have been to Jerusalem and Cairo. Love Egypt, so much more than Israel. There's so much to see. Hotel a bit sparse in Israel, but nice one in Egypt. Been on the Nile, too. Can't wait for an English cuppa!"

I asked Rach about your trip to Israel and Egypt and she replied:

"We laughed a lot on that holiday; saw so many places and did things that Claire wanted to do; the Dead Sea, the Wailing Wall, the via Dolorosa and Garden of Gethsemane."

Again, I'm so thankful you were able to experience more than most people do with a full lifetime, and visiting the sites your Saviour walked was so important to you.

On your return you continued your quest to fit as much into life as possible, and were able to find time to return to Schools' Work for a couple of sessions each week, working with Camilla E. (the Trust was not taking on year outers that year, so they were very happy to use you both). Your report for the Schools' Work Trust read:

"I am helping with Tolworth Girls' C.U this year which meets on a Monday lunch time (Juniors) and Wednesday lunch time (Seniors).

"Juniors: We have had a very encouraging number of girls, approximately 35 attending each week. At the moment we are teaching them about the life of David and the girls are listening well. One really encouraging aspect is the number of Christian girls who are bringing their friends. Another is the involvement of the senior girls in running the quiz before the talk. Camilla and I would really value your prayers as we take on the talks from Ian, who hopes to visit two other CUs that meet on the same day.

"Seniors: There are about a dozen who attend. The majority are Christians, but there are some who we are uncertain about. We are studying the first 8 chapters of Romans, using Scripture under Scrutiny (SUS). Thank you for your prayers and continued support. The girls are really keen and enthusiastic to share their faith. Camilla and me have been jointly running the 'Plumb line' group for Tolworth Girls. Seven girls attend on a two weekly basis and the aim is to give them some basic training for running a C.U. or small group. All of this has been really encouraging. On 6th December, male students of the Secondary Schools in Kingston are joining for a Christian Unions' event to share what has been happening in their individual C.U.s."

What really made me see you were growing up, Claire, was when you knew you would not be returning to our family home to live, and realising that you could not outstay your welcome sharing Auntie Pat's home (despite her never giving that impression!), you wanted to plan ahead for your new world of work. So in the autumn of 1999, you began house-hunting. It was a relatively easy decision, considering your modest budget, and soon the formalities of conveyance were over. Just before Christmas, and with all the pride that goes with being a home owner for the first time, you collected the keys from the estate agent and stood in your empty home once term had ended at uni.

That was how 1999 wrapped up Claire. At this point, you were almost ready to enter true adult life, having been well primed for full-time work by your diligent preparation. You were so eager, so ready to face the world of full time employment and bravely carve out your niche. Like your first year at Kent in 1993, the year 2000 would appear to bring another new beginning.

March 2012

As the New Year of 2012 paced on, despite your ailing health you shopped online steadily, meticulously searching for the remaining items required for your home. By Easter, you were still searching out and purchasing these items prior to your hospital stay. You always amazed me with your head for bargains; never paying full price if you could get away with finding reduced items. Indeed, you waited patiently for your Laura Ashley mirror in the kitchen to be reduced twice in the sale, before buying it. Then there was the Next *Love Your Home* picture, which was sadly never hung. The computer chair at the desk in the small bedroom and the lantern in the hall were also but fleeting memories for you. You had asked Auntie Pat to shop for a new vacuum cleaner, and I only used it a couple of times before you went into hospital. Uncle Keith came over to hang two mirrors, but you were not at home long enough to use them. You never did see the lovely silver blinds you ordered for the en-suite bedroom, nor did you see the bed in there I made up with such love and care. Your new duvet covers you had purchased from House of Fraser were so elegantly dazzling. You found the lovely pale-pink throw, and the two pink cushions for the small bedroom, which I gave to your goddaughter Asha after your death. Rach and Saj were so thankful, knowing that pink is Asha's favourite colour and you had bought those with a view to your god-daughter coming to stay when she was older.

I can't quite believe, Claire, when you were so ill we still managed to fit in ballets. I had forgotten we went to see *The Nutcracker* at the Royal Opera House in the New Year, so much was your courage and perseverance. Throughout your life you faced multiple hospital admissions, with all the painful procedures you had to endure and then, once back home, you continued to battle through physiotherapy, medication, nebulisers, intra-venous antibiotics and the like.

We both pursued our own interests and careers, and as adults we even went to different churches. We did share an amazing bond, however, and thus I thank God for this. We were both free to be what we wanted to be. As Brian Edwards said at your Committal Service, you had CF for a reason, and that reason enabled God to be glorified through it all. Furthermore, I am so grateful I wrote to you each birthday and Christmas to tell you how very special you are.

Yes, we fell out at times; we may have disagreed with each other's decisions, but at the end of the day our relationship was special, and I hope you agree. How grateful I am that, however much I would have loved you to live on, we did not always presume we had tomorrow to make things different. I believe even in this way alone, we always had something other mothers and daughters *could* have, but often do not. Indeed, we were very aware of Jeremiah chapter 29 v 11 (ESV): "For I know the plans I have for you, declares the Lord, plans for welfare and not for evil, to give you a future and a hope." Similar was your first ever Sunday school poem, learned when you were three: "God loves me, says the snowdrop white, that's why He makes me grow, when all the other flowers are gone beneath the frost and snow." Little did we realise then, Claire, how much God's love would be shown in your life, despite all the "frost and snow."

By late March, you desperately needed to be hospitalized but there was no available bed when you had gone to the clinic the week before. It was taking longer to get a bed over the previous months because every CF patient needed to have a single room due to the risks of cross-infection. It became necessary for you to be on intravenous antibiotics at home, as had been the situation so very many times before in your life. You were finding it more and more difficult to shower however, and get yourself ready in the mornings, and looking back I realized you had been struggling badly for months.

I found some emails from the prior autumn when you moved house, where I was telling friends that asked after you that you felt as if the swine-flu was back, and that you had forgotten what it felt like to be well. You always thought you had a mild form of CF because you were not finally diagnosed until pre-school, but I always knew that was not the case. Your aunt had lived with CF to fifty-two, so I can't fully understand why you were so ill at barely past thirty-five. You always chose how to live your life, however, and as hard it was to let you do it your way, you were your own person and I needed to respect that. I also recognize that you wouldn't have let me interfere anyway, and I say that with a sad smile.

It was the little things that began to tip me off to how grave your condition was, Claire. You mentioned earlier that year you did not know how on earth I could keep the cleaning under control in your new home. I knew you were struggling so much to have said that, wanting to help and almost envying my energy. Equally, when I came to meet you at Morden station a few months before when you returned from a weekend away and we saw a young mum on the tube with three small children, you remarked that you did not know how she had the energy to cope with them. These little comments showed me how frail you were, even then. We would go into Kingston to shop so often, and I can remember the way you would drive home, or direct me to the route we should take, and yet even on those trips you often held on to my arm for support. It shows how feeble you felt, yet just how much sheer determination you had to keep going when you were so very ill.

At the time you were under the care of the hospital in London, on treatment, and I remember one of the consultants said you were having intravenous antibiotics every four-to-six weeks, which was more often than normal. So, looking back, we were not throwing caution to the wind, yet your condition continued to worsen. Other indicators were when in October 2011, following your return from Tenerife, you had the week off and remained in bed most of the time. We sat on your bed and watched T.V. and I am so very glad I took that time out with you. November brought your goddaughter Asha's second birthday and you drove to Wandsworth to celebrate with her family. The next day we packed up the last items in your house, ready for your move.

Not only did you keep going after the move, when I was certain you would collapse and be admitted to hospital, but Claire, you did all your Christmas cards and gift shopping. I have to wonder if, subconsciously, you knew it would be your last Christmas. You even kept going through those dark evenings in January when a new manager joined your team, and you worked so late trying to catch up with the backlog of work that was inevitably the case with so many grossly overworked social workers and team managers. How often you did this in your condition, Claire, and I am amazed you had the capacity to do so. Your tenacity, courage, indomitable spirit and God's help must have kept you going. In a research paper given at a CF conference by Dr. Gilljam, M. et al (2004) titled "Manifestations of Cystic Fibrosis Among Patients with Diagnosis in Adulthood," she summed up how CF people feel so often, regarding accepting their deteriorating health and the battle between wanting to hide your condition from others, but needing acknowledgement. People with CF often appear okay on the outside, but the reality is they feel so very ill.

How often in your adult years, particularly, we worked so hard at overcoming some of your health problems that seemed to take up an inordinate amount of your time. You had such difficulty swallowing your medication, but that was only a fraction of the huge treatment programme necessary throughout your life to combat CF. The times those tablets would get stuck in your throat, all the nebulisers each morning and evening, the intravenous line becoming infected and needing to be flushed. . . It wasn't so much that you were busy making other plans that life sped by (as Beatle's star, John Lennon, 1940-1980, famously said) but that there was *so* much to do.[54]

---

[54] John Lennon, "Beautiful Boy," in *Double Fantasy* (Geffen, 1980)

Frequently CF took our lives hostage, and finding time to do the ordinary, everyday things sometimes did not happen. I must confess I sometimes feel guilty when I remember the times I became frustrated with the long waits in the hospital. Then there was the drive home, always in rush-hour traffic, always trying to beat the clock to get home in time for your next IVAB, once we had unpacked all the medications and refrigerated them, sorted the ancillary packs of needles, syringes and the like. We knew each time that we were in for the long haul of yet another course of IVABs and however used to it we were, the time element was always daunting. I found a note in my diary for the summer of 2012 that was to remind us both to enjoy the light evenings and for you to spend time sitting in your lovely new garden. Sadly, that was not to be.

So on the morning of 26th March a bed became available, and you were admitted to hospital. You emailed your friends:

"Morning, just to let you know am being admitted to hospital today as am not responding to these IVABs (5th week now). Please could you pray that I get better on new treatment and have a stronger appetite" (I don't want to even eat chocolate!) Thanks, Claire."

The consultant said more than once that your lovely outward appearance betrayed your diseased body, a trait so common in patients with CF.

During this March admission, you were prescribed the intravenous antibiotic from Germany, Fosfomycin, and also oral steroids. (You were a "named" patient for certain antibiotics because you were allergic to so many and also because the ones you could have often did not have the desired therapeutic effect.) When you progressed to both intravenous steroids and aminophylline, there began a string of occasions when you felt extremely odd and downright unwell as a result of the large doses of medication you had to endure. The day following your admission, you and I texted:

"Will leave soon, Oasis delivery just arrived."
"Ok, feeling poorly Mum x."

A couple of days later, after I had left for the evening, you texted (after having lost both your phone and the TV remote!):

"Found both lost items in bed so good job nurse didn't strip the bed and dispose of my items too. R U OK?"

My sweet Claire, you were always so concerned about me, as I travelled back and forth from London to home.

More text messages followed:

27th March, to Chris F., another CF patient:

"I am sitting in park enjoying the sun in between IVABs."

Then again on the 29th:

"Hi Chris, had a difficult day and now on steroids and oxygen again, but have been to the park, so that's good."

29th March, when Jo and Leah brought you up a toy orang-utan:

"Thanks for my lovely pressie, girlies. I'm going to call him Tufty. Bless his little cottons."

31st and to me:

"Yes am ok, just full of muck from chest. Please could you bring me a clean pair of slippers, ta? Xx."

April 2012

Ages before, you had purchased tickets for the *Swan Lake* ballet for my Ma's day present and in a show of pure willpower, on 1st April, you wangled an evening pass from the hospital so we could go to the ballet. We had a lovely time, despite my concern, and of course the ballet was beautiful, but your company was even better, Claire. We drove straight back to the hospital, and after settling you in bed, you asked me to text you when I arrived home. I did, and your response was: "That's fab, Mum, now go straight to sleep; love you lots and thanks for driving." This text demonstrates nothing, Claire, of the cost to you in terms of your health of that evening out.

On the 6th April, you texted all your friends:

"Morning guys, good news, hoping to leave hospital today or tomorrow, please could you continue to pray for me and Mum as I have to be on exactly the same treatment at home for the next 2 and a half weeks. Mum and I are both pretty exhausted already, so please remember Mum in prayer if you can, and have a lovely Easter. Roll on those Easter eggs. Xx."

Thus you came home on Maundy Thursday and that same evening you were keen to go to Kate's with others from the girls' group and just about managed it. You were so far from well, however, and struggled all weekend, even finding it hard to get ready to go to Marg's for Easter Sunday lunch. You were still determined, though, to get as fit as you could as per the physio's advice, so Good Friday after-noon found us in Bushey Park walking a short distance in the sun. We even saw Bernie and family and Caroline, a school friend who had recently moved back to Surrey, also came to visit you, but it was obvious to all that you were losing ground.

That Sunday, you gave me an Easter card that read:

"So happy to be spending Easter at home with you. Thanks for looking after me and for keeping me strong. All my love, Claire."

Chapter Seventeen

The new Millennium and Your new Adult Life

My dearest Claire,

A s the millennium turned, so your deepest desires of complete independence drew within your grasp. The drive to, perhaps, prove to yourself that you could be entirely self-sufficient, as you so longed for, became just a several mere months of diligent, focused devotion; something you embraced as though it were as necessary as breathing. I have spoken many times of your indomitable spirit, and the sheer fortitude and willpower you displayed to study, become qualified and earn a full-time position, but to this day your resilience is unparalleled in my experience.

As the New Year rolled around, your responsibilities were increasing and changing, and so you were a little sad to be unable to continue your involvement with the Kingston Schools' Work Trust any longer. However, you sent them the most caring and professional notice:

"As of January 2000, I will be working full time and will, unfortunately, be unable to help out with the Schools' Work. I have gained a lot from being part of the team this term and have enjoyed working with the girls

immensely. Thank you so much for your support and prayer and thanks to Ian, Nina and Camilla too, for their support."

The Trust Board Chairperson and then pastor of Hook's sister church in Chessington, Trevor A., wrote to me:

"In the midst of her illness Claire is a shining beacon of loveliness and grace, and you must be immensely proud of her."

While you were studying at Reading, I remember coming down on the odd occasion to accompany you to the library situated on another campus, and to help you trawl through the mammoth amount of books there. Although there was a library situated on the Bulmershe campus, some of the books you needed were located in Whiteknights. When I thought of this it reminded me that even in the late '90s you were finding it difficult to stand for long periods as you poured over the reading list, trying to locate the books on the shelves. As with any university course, the amount of essays and presentations truly seemed unending. Consequently, the amount of ill-health you experienced largely led to your foregoing the dorm room at the university and returning to Chessington to live, where I could assist with your intravenous antibiotics. As so many times in your life, I suppose it was a trade-off between the lesser of two evils: Driving down the M4 each day when you needed to attend modules seemed preferable to managing alone on site.

Thus, in January of 2000, you commenced your second placement with the Admovere Project, and what an answer to prayer as this was based in Chessington. During this placement you also worked for the Social Services Department in Kingston where, having made such an impression, you were offered your first job in social work once you graduated. This, again, appeared to be the hand of God providing for you as you only had to travel about five minutes by car to work. At the end of your placement, Admovere's Project Manager wrote your report that read:

Claire Salter: Report by Joyce H., Project Manager, 24.5.00

Admovere comprises a multidisciplinary team for young people of school age but not in formal education. Young people attending the project do so on a voluntary basis, which is different to the statutory provision that Social Services provide.

I was reluctant to take on a student social worker as the project was coming to an end in March 2000 half way through the placement period. Claire would also have to be long armed by a social work practice teacher, which I could foresee was a complication. Finally, as our work was predominantly informal education teaching I was unsure if the placement would be able to fulfil Claire's criteria for University. Claire's assertiveness, however, persuaded me to have her as a student.

This was a new student placement for the project and Claire worked hard to ascertain her role within the team. It was a learning experience for me to see at first hand the difference in social work training and what is expected of students in their final year. The main thing that stands out is the excessive amount of paper work in comparison to other students I have had. This defers from the hands on work with young people, which I feel is very important. Claire worked very hard to ensure this was addressed and that she had a significant amount of face to face time with the client group. This included helping out on a residential experience where Claire proved herself to be an excellent team player.

We also had to redesign the format of the placement as it was initially anticipated it was not fulfilling Claire's placement needs. I feel that this change was helpful and gave her a clearer insight into the different operational and administration functions of the Admovere Project and the Looked After Team.

Claire was flexible in her approach and was able to adjust well to the change in her placement. This was a positive change, enhancing the placement. Claire challenged anti-discriminatory practice very well and was not afraid to challenge the negative and stereotype views of our client group and some staff.

"Her main roles within the team were to develop relationships with the young people in the Education Unit and organise and deliver Personal Health and Social Education (PHSE) to the group. Her organisation abilities are good and she was able to develop fruitful and meaningful relationships with the young people. Claire shared anxieties regarding presentations; these were unfounded, as her delivery on all her presentations was very good and she confidently absorbed and answered questions presented. She gave a presentation on the Project to some of the Mentors one evening and one wrote to me afterwards to say that she was a natural.

She assertively presents arguments and is non-aggressive in her approach which I feel is an essential skill in working with young people as a team member. I felt that Claire coped very well in a project which is undergoing a lot of transitional change and which is very different to social work professional practice. She was able to demonstrate good use of her transferable work skills.

It still warms my heart so tremendously to read these glowing reports, my precious Claire. You were about to leap into the big, wide world of fulltime adulthood and again, as a reference for your first job Sue S., your Freelance Practice teacher on the course, wrote the following commendation:

14.9.2000 To Human Resources, Royal Borough of Kingston upon Thames.
Reference for Claire Salter: Post: Social Worker in a Children and Families Locality Team.

Claire has recently completed a Diploma in Social Work and Master's course at Reading University. I was Claire's Practice Teacher on her second placement (10th January-15th June 2000) which was at the Admovere Project and Looked after team in Kingston.

Claire showed herself to be competent and able and her work was of a high standard. Claire has had a range of experience with working with children, and young people and their families as well as with foster carers. Claire's first placement was in a children and families locality team in Reading, Berkshire. Claire has a working knowledge of the Children Act and of other relevant legislation and guidance. I have observed Claire working with young people and children – she has sound communication skills and conducts interviews in a very appropriate manner.

Claire is able to prioritise and organise her work well. Her assessment skills are sound. Her report and other writing are of a good standard. Claire works well in a team and with other professionals.

I am aware that Claire suffers from Cystic Fibrosis. This did not affect the work Claire did on her placement. She had a couple of days off sick but ensured that she made the time up.

I have no hesitation in recommending Claire for the above post.

Yours sincerely,

S.S'

As a break after your final exams, you and Ele took a long weekend mini-holiday in Stockholm. You must have had a wonderful time, as Ele recently told me you remarked you would have liked to have been born a Swede! Other weekends away that featured in your diary were to Rachel and Michael's and Hannah and Mark's. There is also a lovely photo of a group of you walking on Ilkley Moor on one such visit.

That spring, the book *Horizons of Hope* was published and several people sent you written congratulations for the chapter you wrote in it. Your good friend from school, Catherine D. said:

"I wanted to write and tell you that you are amazing and after reading your chapter in the book twice over the weekend I feel so proud of you and honoured to be your friend. You are such a special person and it was reassuring to see the façade dropped and the thoughts that go through your mind each day come through on paper in such a clear way. You have the love, admiration and support of so many people, so never bottle up your feelings as it will do you more good to get them out in to the open. I hope that you will always call on me if you have the need to talk or share your problems. I know life has been unfair to you Claire, but you are very special and very brave. Xx."

Catherine would prove to be one of those friends, akin to many, who supported you up to and through your final illness.

For the reader, Brian Edwards was Claire's pastor during her younger years and also took the Cremation Service at her funeral. In his role as editor of *Horizons of Hope*[55] Brian wrote, regarding the draft of your chapter:

"Claire, a brilliant start, excellent material and all the right ingredients. My extensive comments are to polish the gem. How are you fixed for time? Another draft ASAP would be great, but you may have a lot on at Uni. Be encouraged, we're going to have a good chapter here."

---

[55]   Horizons of hope' Edwards, B.H. (Day One Publications, 2000, ISBN 1903087 02-3)

Doctor Wright, an elder at your home church for many years, wrote:

"My dear Claire, I was very touched by your lovely chapter, so well written and beautifully put together. You are an inspiration to us all at Hook and we thank God for your bright witness and what you mean to us."

From one of your friends:

"Your honesty will make many people really see the struggles that you go through, but how your faith upholds you even in dark, difficult times. I felt that the strength of the book was showing that when we are weak, 'He is strong.'"

Lastly, From Terry Waite, CBE, May 2000:

"Dear Claire, I was delighted to read the chapter in Horizons of Hope;" it really is very good indeed and I am so pleased that you are making such good progress on so many fronts. I well remember the day we spent in London for the 1998 CF Achievement Award ceremony. I hope that you will keep in touch as I should be delighted to hear how you are getting on. Meanwhile Frances, my wife, joins me in sending you and your family our very best love."

I suppose it wouldn't be appropriate to show these congratulations without providing another section of your chapter from "Life is an Adventure – Dare It." Also appropriately, I believe it is this section that most accurately reflects one of the most real, but overlooked struggles that accompanies CF: the emotional (let alone the physical) trauma from the persistent coughing. You never complained much about this part, but I know you certainly suffered as a result of many people's inability to empathize with your condition, only hearing the coughing, and never truly understanding what CF is. Neither you nor I blamed them, but it saddened me this was one extra factor you had to deal with, regardless.

Life is an Adventure – Dare It

Cough, Cough, Cough

I shared a room with Carol during my last hospital visit, and she just could not stop coughing. The CF cough could be classed as a trademark of the disease, and it certainly gave me an inkling that Ali had CF. As a child, my mum was apparently told more than once by complete strangers that she shouldn't bring me out with such a terrible cough. As I grew older, my cough was frequently mistaken for that of a smoker! Coughing can be as annoying to the person doing the coughing as it is to others. It's really difficult to try and control a CF cough, and most embarrassing when everyone looks at you. One of the amusing things about coughing in public is that it can often be misconstrued. For example, when I am waiting in queues such as a supermarket checkout and I cough, the cashier has interpreted it as my impatience. All people with CF have a cough and it can be quite distinctive. I remember being away with a group I had never met before; I had not mentioned to anyone that I had CF but one of the team members said, "You've got CF, haven't you?" It was my cough that betrayed me.

One of my few downs at senior school was being seated near a window with the sun streaming through all day whilst taking exams. A teacher who did not know of my condition said that I disturbed everyone by my coughing and that in future I must sit my exams in a room alone. Since then, even throughout university, I have sat in isolation for my exams, but I prefer that, as I hate having to disturb other people.

Ele, one of my good friends on the course at university, met up with another girl on the course whom I did not know. Ele happened to say that she was meeting me later that day; the response was, "Oh, is that the girl who coughs all the time?" It's funny how other people notice things that are so familiar to me that I forget I'm doing it. People who know me well can always tell if I'm in church, or in lectures, because my cough is very distinctive.

As the year marched on, your Master's dissertation loomed nearer, and you subsequently chose "Depression in Adolescents" as your topic. You performed a thoroughly qualitative work of research, and you also included detailed stats on the risk of suicide in this vulnerable age group. Unsurprisingly, your dissertation was received extremely well, and on 29th June, 2000 the class of '98 proudly graduated! This included, of course, Jo and Ruth, fellow students with which you had made firm friends. Sadly, your friend Charlie had to defer graduation to the following year following a family bereavement, but she very kindly and bravely came to the graduation ceremony and is seen in several photos with you all. A truly great time was had, taking photos after the ceremony in the lovely grounds, after which we journeyed back to Surrey later to have a meal at a wonderful Italian restaurant.

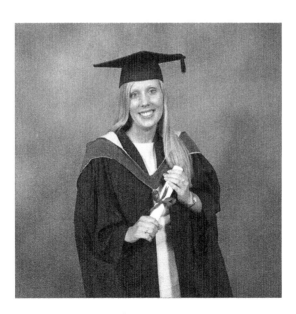

Official photo: Master's in Social Work Degree, 2000

But there was no real rest for you over the summer; having bought your very own first home the previous December, and wisely renting it out for the first six months to pay the mortgage, the tenant left towards the latter part of July, just in time for you to renovate it. On what was really a student's budget, it was not a palace but was certainly a great first home. (You even had friends a few houses up the road, namely: Tasha, Vicky and Victoria, followed by Natalie and then Rachel.)

Victoria became your prayer partner those early years in Ranyard Close until she returned to her family home Scotland, then to Canada to live when she married Ethan but still remaining very much in touch with you. Natalie, still living locally, also remained a close friend up until your death. You all would come to have great times drinking coffee with each other, and enjoying your neighbourhood together.

The house needed a good amount of work after your tenant left, so as part of a graduation gift, Uncle Keith came up from Devon and together with others in three weeks we managed to remove the carpets, make alterations, decorate and re-carpet every room upstairs. Uncle Keith also installed a brand new kitchen, and laid wood flooring throughout the ground floor.

On your twenty-fifth birthday I had posted loads of posters round the family home congratulating you on your Master's, but true to form you never wanted to brag, so they were all removed before your guests arrived! Your friends' love was so apparent, and Hannah and Mark wrote:

"Wishing you a very happy 25th birthday. Now that you've got your Master's under your belt and a job in the offing, you have such an exciting year ahead of you, especially as you move into your very own home next month. Thanks for being a star friend, we love you loads."

Of course, as reported in other places in this diary, your birthdays were always celebrated in utmost style. (A note in one of your packing boxes read you needed to book a table for thirty-five people one year!) I had put a note in with your birthday card that read:

"You loved the bitter-sweet film Steel Magnolias and being sorry to leave the Magnolia in the grounds of our family home, a Magnolia tree will be planted in your garden in the autumn."

We just about managed to get the garden in order for the tree to embed. However, to backtrack to your twenty-fifth, you invited all your friends on a lovely summer's day to a barbeque, whilst Keith (with a little help from me) laid the floor in your new home.

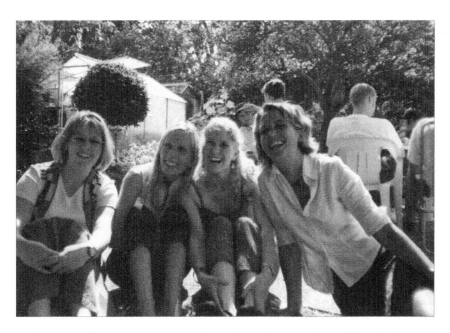

Relaxing with Kent University friends in the garden of family home:
L-R Isla, Claire, Ruth, Rach

Then, birthday celebrations over, it was time to retrace your steps to continue to help with your home renovations. Andy C. completed the kitchen by applying wall tiles whilst you and I managed to clean everywhere, put up curtains and move your furniture in just in time for your house mate, Anna, to move in around 7th August. I remember the long action plan we had devised earlier in July to ensure you had bought the shower, chosen the carpets and paint, etc. Pete put in additional electrical plugs and the last job was to make the back garden presentable (after we had used it as a dumping ground for the rollers and paint). The front garden contained a skip for the old carpets, kitchen and wood that had been removed in the renovations, so it too required some necessary restoring. It was a mammoth job, Claire, but you fully deserved all the help, considering how hard you had worked on your degree, and the fact you would be starting full-time social work in the autumn!

Hence, it was *au-revoir* and "Thank you" to Auntie Pat for having you to live with her for four years, and she joined in telling you how proud we were at your final step to proper independence.

My Move from Surbiton to Chessington

In 2001, a year after you were settled in your own home, I moved from our family home in Surbiton to a much smaller house in Chessington, a few roads away from you. This meant that, although not living on your doorstep, I could be round to you within a couple of minutes in an emergency. This is one of those bittersweet memories, as I am so glad I moved because of how necessary this became as your CF continued to affect you with every passing year. You gave me a new home card which was so apt; it had a picture of a packing box labelled: "The moving on company." Only you really understand the deep significance of those words, my precious daughter.

It wasn't long before you found that managing the plethora of treatment alone in the morning was simply too time-consuming, since you had to fit in breakfast and still pack a lunch. This was particularly so when you were on IVABs, so we both agreed that I should call round each morning on my way to work to assist. Your days started at various times, so it became normal practice for us to check with each other when you needed me. I'd text:

"Dear Claire, I'll be to you at 7:45 tomorrow morning, unless you phone and tell me otherwise. Love Mum."

Your response said:

"Okay, but will have to start intravenous antibiotics dead on 7:45, so maybe come at 7:30 please."

Other ways Pat and your friends and I tried to make life a little easier for you was by accompanying you on shopping trips (grocery and non-grocery alike) in order to carry the bags and also drop you off as near to the shops as humanly (and legally) possible, then we could go and park the car appropriately. Even by that point, I could walk at least twice as fast as you. Never one to take a back seat and leave others to take the strain, however, when we repainted your kitchen in a different colour, there you were, paint brush and roller at the ready. (That fortitude again!)

Thus it was that, up until about the summer of 2000, and despite being in hospital so often and feeling ill far too many times, you were relatively able to cope with life. I say relatively because, reading your diaries and witnessing first-hand your struggles, it is very apparent there were long periods of time when you were just unable to do so; the ravages of CF just wreaked havoc on your body.

It was your first Contagious Camp as a leader in August 2000 that you had to come home early due to ill-health. You sat out in your less than organised garden, a picture of delicate, if frail, loveliness; the sun shining on your beautiful face, yet those dreadful intravenous antibiotics plugged in and in full swing. (When were you *not* on IVs?)

The summer cooled and turned into autumn and you began working full time in your first social work position (which was your choice, as you were never one to give in without a fight). I, and others, could clearly see this taking its toll on you. You were just so determined to continue that you kept this ultra-devoted professional life right up until you went into hospital for the final time. My sweet Claire, you always just wanted to be as normal as possible, whilst battling a killer disease. With studying behind you (at least for a while), a few of you young women from church got together for "girly" Bible studies which soon became tremendously uplifting for you. Later, these Bible studies were converted to a triplet group where you, Nicola and Maz met to pray together, later joined by Natalie.

As we entered December of that year and all the Christmas cheer was in full swing, you began a tradition that your home had to be sparkling clean for Christmas, and kept that up each passing year. Of course, one deep clean a year was not enough, and as time allowed, we did this every quarter. You sure knew how to stay busy Claire, doing your best to enjoy every moment of life! You even continued to help with the church's youth work, but as time went by it became more of a struggle.

That is my daughter; never one to let a moment pass her by. I still firmly believe you lived more than most people do in a full life-time, and left a legacy that is rarely matched. I can still see you sitting in your garden, adorned in the prettiest summer dress with the sun's rays backlighting your exquisite, long hair. I am certain you are far more radiant now, my love, illuminated by the Son's glory, and someday we will hug again, and perhaps you can help me decorate *my* mansion as we decorated your first home together.

Until then, I have more to tell about your treasured years with your family and friends on Earth, so let's take a look at what came in 2001.

Chapter Eighteen

2001 to 2004 – Bittersweet
is Better than Simply Bitter

Dear Claire,

When you commenced your career in social work in October 2000, joining a team with predominantly young social workers, it meant the demands of the job had to be balanced with the fun times you had outside of work. This caused an interesting twist in your life; specifically, this meant your closest relationships became closer, and as a result you remained firm friends with three work colleagues right up until your death, namely Bernie P., Helen M. and Yasmine M. The three of you would come to entwine your lives in beautiful ways, and most importantly, be there for each other through good times and bad.

By the time 2001 arrived you had begun post-qualifying courses with Kingston University, which most social workers take to further their career options and gain additional expertise. Indeed, these courses continued year on year, and you would typically undertake them on a day release basis.

I remember during this time you particularly enjoyed working with Young Asylum Seekers but with your primary focus being on Child Protection. As I have written elsewhere in this diary, I firmly believe God used your difficult teen years to mould you into the person you became; a person who could not only empathise with troubled teens, but offer them authentic guidance they would trust and receive. In your portfolio, whilst undertaking the Child Care Award, you wrote:

"Self Esteem Group for boys aged 9-12 years: this group was set up to work with boys within a setting that encouraged them to build on relationships with each other in order to feel more confident in themselves. The group is currently running for eight weeks and includes both activities in the family centre to tackle self-esteem issues and outdoor pursuits. One role of social workers is to undertake life story work with children who are moving on to their 'forever' home."

You were commended for your artistic approach while, at the same time, per-mitting each child to make it his or her own personal story.

Another great find I came across was the Team Building Day that included all of you describing each other's assets by completing the following sentence: "I really like the way you. . ."

- are so genuinely interested and caring for others
- smile, no matter what
- try really hard with difficult clients
- Similarly, you were all requested to complete the following statement: "I think one of your greatest strengths is. . ."
- very sensitive to others' feelings
- how you carry on when you are feeling really unwell
- listening carefully and remaining focussed
- ability to be calm and supportive with young people you work with

You had long desired to experience the Far East, so at the beginning of 2001 I offered to accompany you on a trip and in February we simply made it happen. What an amazing holiday that was; after a long flight we landed in Hong Kong and experienced the sights, scenery and sounds. Next we moved on to Vietnam, then after spending a couple of days in Bangkok, Thailand, we had a wonderfully relaxing beach holiday in Phuket but first, of course, it meant packing all your medications, equipment, supplies, etc. As ever, you loved every new experience despite having me as a travelling companion. It was not unusual for you to be ill, even on holiday, so by the time we arrived on the last leg of the journey, I worried you may not enjoy the beach experience. Thankfully you did, as it meant you could relax and not be concerned about sight-seeing. We had a truly memorable time, and I was so pleased you were able to rest somewhat.

The year whizzed by with your now adult routine of work, including course modules, completing assignments and all that these entailed. Soon it was time for your birthday again, always a festive occasion! That July you threw a large party in your home, and of course as your mum I wasn't allowed to attend, but you were diligent to show me photos of friends everywhere! (So many friends in fact, you spilled out into the garden as the house wasn't large enough to contain you all.) As if on cue, the day was filled with brilliant sunshine.

It was not, however, all about your friends; you also gave time to your cousins, both those in England and also in Belgium, and to me and Pat, together with the wider family. You always wanted to help us celebrate these special occasions with you as well, so we usually enjoyed meals out, cinema and theatre treats, especially on our birthdays. Equally, we also helped you celebrate special times in your life.

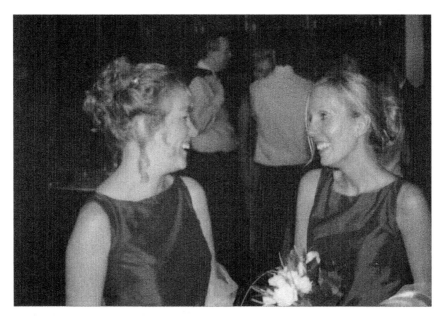

Ali Sa and Claire, bridesmaids to Natalie, all great friends from church

2002

2002 was off to another great start and found you visiting Rachel, one of your church friends working among the street children in Belem, Brazil, where you were blessed to experience the mighty Amazon. You also stopped in Rio de Janeiro and on your postcard wrote:

"Dear Auntie and Mum, having a great time. I can't wait to show you all of the photos when we're back. We went up Sugarloaf Mountain this week and saw this view! Hope you're both okay. Can't wait to see you soon. Lots of love, Claire."

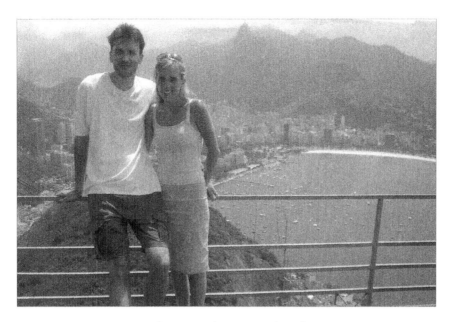

Visiting Rach T in Belem, Brazil with Gary too

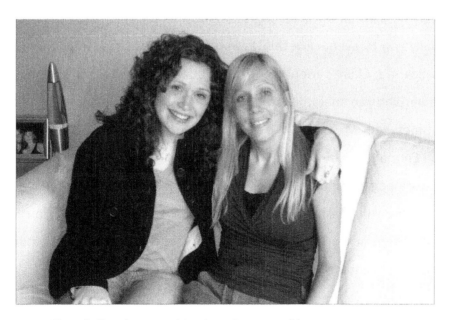

In Claire's first home with Victoria, one of her prayer partners

Back home one of your friends, Victoria from up the road, wrote:

"Just wanted to say how great it's been to get to know you over the last couple of years. I'm so thankful to have been your neighbour and prayer partner. I've been really blessed to have you as a friend. Thank you for all the love and support. Will phone soon for our next prayer time. Xx."

You and your friends were ever keen to support each other and this was especially evidenced when various people ran marathons in aid of CF. We would always do our best to get sponsors for them and, in return, you often attended special events they hosted. Of special note was one of Rich B.'s photographic exhibitions, full of beautiful photography. Rich also told you about the Landscape Photography Exhibition which we attended at the National Theatre in London in 2011, followed by a lovely meal, then a walk along the South Bank. I was really so honoured to accompany you to events like this. I am really worried I may forget some names (and forgive me, Claire's friends, if I have) but from memory these are some of the people who ran marathons/breakfast runs to support the CF cause, some several times: Rob M., Bruce M., Mark W., Matt and Claire N., Phil and Jane S., Matt and Emma S.

You were beginning to become seasoned in social work, so you began to see some heartbreaking cases. Ever wondering how you were getting on in these unique situations at work but at the same time knowing the huge confidentiality you needed to maintain, I emailed: *"Wonder how things are."'*

Your response was:

"Fine, thanks, I am back from Court and all went well. Mother not permitted to see children alone and must have supervised contact. X."

2003

2003 started with yet another international excursion as one of your uni friends, Ruth H., was working in Australia and invited you out for a holiday! As was so often the case prior to holidays, you had a course of intravenous antibiotics to stand you in good stead while you were away. These times were often trying, as it was one of the more immediate reminders of your condition, and I suppose I was wearing my concern somewhat visibly as one of my colleagues emailed me at work to ask how you were. This was my response:

"Thanks for asking, she is at home now continuing her intravenous antibiotics, but although she is allergic to so many (so we have an Epipen, intravenous hydrocortisone standing by and she is on steroids and Piriton), she is responding well."

You wanted to see as much of God's wonderful world as you could and thought absolutely nothing of making the long trek down under on your own. I am unsure if you ran out of energy or stamps, but I came across a postcard that you wrote but did not post; it bore a picture of the Great Ocean Road and was addressed to Hannah and Mark, and read:

"Am loving it here, it's so huge and beautiful. People are really friendly and kind. Have seen all the sights on the front of this p.c. Saw a kola bear today! I'm off to Sydney on Tuesday for a few days. Hope all okay with you two; speak soon."

One of your highlights was seeing the Southern Cross in the night sky. Geelong beach also matched as a favourite, as did the Gippsland lakes in Victoria, together with the red rock (dormant volcano) at Colac.

You also wrote me a note from Victoria:

"Dear Mum, hope you are okay. I am having a great time in Oz and am loving the scenery. I have seen all the sights on the front of this card from the Great Ocean Road. I saw a wallaby today, which was great. Have been out on a boat on the lakes, which I really loved. See you soon. Lots of love, Claire."

Excerpts from your holiday notes read (obviously from a notice board in the National Park!):

"Through Otway National Park, to Appollo Bay, then along the coast road. The Great Otway National Park stretches from Torquay through Princetown and up through the Otways hinterland towards Colic. The park features rugged coastlines, sandy beaches, rock platforms and windswept heath-land. In the north, the park features tall forests, ferny gullies, magnificent waterfalls and tranquil lakes."

During this trip you saw Mount Defiance and the Erskine Falls, then on to Sale, part of the Gippsland Lakes region. Throughout your visit, Ruth arranged for you both to stay with some of her many friends. This included a visit to a sheep farm, which was a novel change of pace for you! Your visit to Sydney to see the Opera House was special too, and when you wrote to Ruth on your return to England to thank her for the truly lovely time you had, she replied that she was equally thrilled to show you around.

Upon your return, after a brilliant but somewhat physically taxing trip, you continued to help out with the church youth work while also regularly attending your midweek home group meeting. You became more adept at balancing your busy work life with regular play time, including a weekend in Paris with friends. You just loved these short city breaks, and later travelled with Yasmine to Madrid, too. You regularly went with Jo R. and others to the Ideal Home Exhibition in London. You also found many other similar events to attend, and when you were too short of breath to catch the Tube, it was my great pleasure to transport you, Jo et al in the car. I am sure, Claire, that you knew your condition was deteriorating year on year. This short quote I found in your diary for that year certainly implies it:

"Yesterday is history

Tomorrow is mystery

Today is a gift (i.e. the present)."[56]

On some occasions your job required you to travel to other parts of the country to see potential foster families for the at-risk children with whom you worked. One trip included the city of Hull, where you were also able to visit Alison and Graham S., who worked there at the time. On another occasion you travelled to Northern Ireland to interview a kinship family regarding their wish to foster their niece's young child. I can remember coming to Heathrow to meet you from the latter in winter and was so pleased I had made it through the snow in time for your plane to land. Despite the information board stating your flight had landed, however, I waited and waited for over an hour. Others awaiting this flight could not understand the delay either, so when you eventually walked through the gate, you explained the information board had been incorrect, and the plane had been

---

[56]   Origin uncertain

circling for ages as the snow prevented landing! (I think it was probably better I did not know this beforehand!)

Then there were the spot checks you were required to do at weekends and in the evenings to ensure that children were safe in their homes and that their mothers were not entertaining a boyfriend or partner (or vice-versa if the child was in the custody of the father) who was banned from seeing the youngsters. I remember one such check you particularly hated doing and one day you asked me to accompany you. I carefully parked the car around the corner of the residence so I could not be seen, but I made you leave the house number with me so that I could phone the police if you did not re-appear! I was thrilled you were working in a field you loved so much, but times like this really wreaked havoc on my nerves. I also remember a few times I bailed you out of problems, like the time your car had a flat tyre while you and Bernie were on the way to court. Of course, as always it was my pleasure to help in all these crises, although I did wonder how the entire department managed to cope with their own crises.

Adding to the other concerns, I worried about your health too, but thankfully we were not without help. Whilst I was still working full-time, if I was on a late shift Auntie Pat was so good at having you call in on your way home from work for a vegetarian roast dinner. I wonder at times if some readers may feel I exaggerate on your health status, but anyone who saw how breathless you were the majority of the time would know, if anything, I was understating your condition and would only feel empathy for you. Many times I would drop you right outside your hair-dresser's shop in Epsom or Cobham so that you were saved the walk, especially on cold, dark winter evenings.

There were also many more times I felt you were overtaxing yourself, when perhaps it might have been better to simply skip some festivities, but that was not ever an option for you. Well, the one time it was when you were going to Catherine and Steve D.'s wedding and you just about made it on time because you weren't paying attention and had muddled up the church! Another time, however, you were discharged from hospital on the morning you had been invited to attend Naureen's wedding, and Faye and Iain were delayed in traffic coming down from Stafford. You and I jumped in the car and I drove you up to Battersea Park, again just about making the service on time. Of course there were also all the drop off and pickup trips to and from the airport that Pat and I made, but if my assistance meant you were more able to live some semblance of a normal life, I was more than happy to do it.

The crises were also not just over work; on two occasions we averted *major* drug errors. Once at the hospital, a nurse came into your room with the wrong antibiotic, actually bringing one to which you were severely allergic. Thanks to our Heavenly Father I just managed to stop her from injecting it, having noticed the labelling did not reflect the antibiotic you were supposed to receive. The other time was when the pharmacy sent us home with the wrong one, too. Again, in our exhaustion I could have easily automatically drawn this up into the syringes, but the visual oversight caught my attention, and once again we avoided disaster. How grateful we were that God enabled us to keep our wits about us on these occasions.

That July, you celebrated your twenty-eighth birthday and while enjoying joint celebrations with a friend, Vicky, who shared your birth date, you phoned me very distressed. You had received a call from the hospital stating you needed to be admitted immediately. You had been complaining of a fast heart rate since the reinsertion of yet another port-a-cath that had actually split inside your body. Christine, the home care nurse who had visited the previous day to take blood, called and reported the doctor was very concerned about the blood samples, but you were anxious not to have to go in on your birthday. I spoke to the doctor and assured him I would stay overnight with you and bring you up to the hospital the next day.

You spent an uneventful night and I thought it would be okay for us both to pop into work first to clear our desks to ready ourselves for this admission. How very wrong I was! The doctor called me wondering where you were, and when I explained we had made a brief stop, he told me quite sternly that your heart could stop at any moment, and I was to bring you in immediately. So I rushed over to collect you and up we went.

On hearing this your pastor, Paul, and your group elder, Steve, dropped everything and drove up too. You were admitted to the High Dependency Unit (HDU) and I was permitted to stay in the next bed to you. (The Unit consisted of four beds and if it was not full, relatives were able to stay on the ward, rather than in relative's accommodation along the corridor.) The doctor eventually discharged you, but the problem persisted, so back you went to HDU, not twice, but three times. It often seemed as though problems begat problems. The diagnosis was eventually confirmed to be the fact that the port they had implanted a couple of weeks previously had dropped from the right atrium into the ventricle of the heart and was causing the fast heart rate. I have to say it was an extremely worrying time until the cause was identified; but again it was bittersweet as so many times before, because it meant yet a further operation to pull the port tube back until it was resting nicely on the tip of your heart.

During this trying time, church notices read:

"Please pray for Claire who has had to be re-admitted to hospital with complications arising from recent surgery related to her treatment for CF; there is concern that her heart may have been affected by the treatment to re-insert a line into her chest that facilitates the drugs she receives."

My card to you read:

"Welcome home, again. (Please stop going into hospital, and especially into the High Dependency Unit!) Have missed you loads. Love you loads."

One autumn evening found you and Barbara S. speaking at your church's Natter and Nosh; this was an evening ladies' outreach that was held on a monthly basis. A variety of topics were covered and on this night Barbara, who had been a foster carer, spoke from her perspective, after which you followed up with the joys and heartaches of a social worker. The response was tremendous and the subsequent write up for Hook Evangelical Church's magazine read:

"We enjoyed one of our best evenings yet in September, when Barbara S. and Claire S. talked about their work in foster care and social work respectively. Nearly forty ladies were present and, following refreshments, Barbara and Claire were interviewed. Their stories, although quite different, were a testimony to the way God has helped them in their lives and vocations."

After you spoke, someone remarked to me privately that you were always ready to see the fun side of life, and repeated stories you felt helped the children you were caring for too. One friend wrote:

"Dear Claire, you'd left before I had a chance to say how much I appreciated your talk yesterday evening. You were really excellent in what you had to say and you came across as being totally yourself – very open and honest. My Spanish friend was very struck by your professionalism and commitment. So thank you for your contribution to what I thought was a first class

evening all round. Remember to never apologise for tears; they show a warm and sensitive heart! God bless you, with lots of love, Linda S."

Despite your health challenges, you were certainly born to help others, and dare I say, born to do social work! This took a decent amount of continuing studies as I've mentioned, and through all the years even as you undertook courses you would occasionally ask me to buy you a *Sunday Telegraph* or *Sunday Times* so you could catch up with not only current affairs, but also the latest in education. You were always striving for perfection, even when you could have easily slid by with mere average results. A testament to your professionalism was even when you were no longer able to get through all your treatment in time to go to church on Sunday mornings, you would sit in bed and read, telling me it was the height of luxury! Then, by the time Monday morning rolled around, your work diaries had a neat list of all your action items for the day, and by Monday evening these items had a bold tick against what you accomplished. You were so organised, Claire; much more so than me.

Of course, these setbacks did not slow you down for long; you had arranged to meet Rach in Zanzibar in November (she was working in East Africa at the time) and it was touch-and-go as to whether you would be able to travel or not because of the recent surgery. Praise the Lord the insurance company said that, as they had already agreed to insure you, they would honour this but if you did become ill whilst travelling, you would have to pay a £500.00 excess. Knowing how difficult it was to get insurance in your latter years, this was a real bonus, in that it was not any more expensive. Thank the Lord you stayed well, however, and we did not need to pay anything. How I esteemed you, when you went all that way by yourself when you knew you could become unwell so easily, and so far from home.

2004

In autumn 2004, as your health continued in its downward spiral I wrote to you:

"Dear Claire, I wanted to write to add my congratulations on all you have accomplished this year in your career as a social worker and to tell you how much I have learned from you, not only in your above role, but in so many areas of your life. Manning suggests that on the road to heaven we inevitably meet hurting people and we need to be as Christ to them. I want to acknowledge again that I understand a little of the difficulty you have of living with CF and the cumulative effect it has had on your daily life. I cannot fully stand in your shoes, but seeing you suffer so much, perhaps I can stand in similar ones, if that is not an offence to you. There are so many people who ask after you, pray for you and admire you. All your suffering has made you the wonderful person you are. There are times in our lives, whether we suffer a draining illness or a broken relationship, when we doubt God's love, and yet I have directed so many urgent prayers to God, telling him about your hurt, pain and disappointment and your struggles amid your sheer will-power to continue to live as normal a life as possible. It is not for a mother to interfere with God's plan for you by attempting to arrange things in my own strength, because you don't need that and anyway, Manning also reminds us that as we travel to heaven, God's grip on us is firm; he does not let us go.[57]

So the paradox has been the ecstatic joy you have brought to me life, but also that my heart breaks for you; words are never enough, for if you could read my heart as well as the hearts of many others, then maybe you could understand a little of how your family and friends want to be with you

[57] Brennan Manning, Abba's Child (NavPress, Colorado, 2011)

in your battling with CF and so many other things. If I could stem your flow of tears, take away your sadness, make your dreams come true, I would have done so a thousand times over. Manning's book Abba's Child: The cry of the heart for intimate belonging,[58] had a profound effect on you and I want to remind you again of what he says; that God hasn't got it in for us, as some austere Person, but that He is for us.

If God should spare you and take me, remember that we need not be afraid of saying goodbye, or afraid of the surgeon's knife or the CF prognosis because your life is in God's hand. He may not cure you or take away the daily disappointments, but He promises to be with us. One day, whether it be you or me first, we will have to depart this world. There may be a longing to stay but knowing we must go. At the time, just as Jesus got into a boat with His disciples at night, He will invite us into the boat also, to put our trust in Him. We may feel out of our depth and so frightened, but He invites us to Himself. It is a letting go of this world and trusting Him as we make this final journey heavenward. If it is me that goes first, please remind me of this and if it is you, I will endeavour to equally remind you. The extent of the sadness of losing you, or of your longing to stay, will need to be entrusted to God, for it is only when we are ready to go willingly that we can say goodbye to all this life holds and journey to Heaven. I pray that you and I will be ready when it is our time. Remember that we intuitively make our way when we are ready. The choice, as we know, is not whether or not we die, but more so how we die.[59] With all my love, Mum.

Your friends missed you at church too, and in that same year (2004) Jenny and Pete, whom you worked alongside in the youth work, wrote:

---

[58]   Brennan Manning, Abba's Child (NavPress, Colorado, 2011)

[59]   Michael Kearney, Mortally Wounded: Stories of Soul Pain, Death and Healing, (Touchstone Books, an imprint of Simon and Schuster 1997)

"We really hope these antibiotics kick in soon and do their job, without making you feel too dizzy. We missed your quiet 'getting alongside' qualities at Impact on Friday, but of course understand why, being in hospital, you couldn't make it."

The autumn of 2004 saw you take another trip with Rach, holidaying together in Sri Lanka this time. Unfortunately, it was not the best time to go, as the weather was poor, and I think the trip was not as adventurous as many of the others you had taken. The year was to close with more sad tidings, as within a couple of weeks of you returning, your social services team manager died suddenly on a football pitch. It was such a shock to everyone, and attending his funeral was a really heart-rending affair for you all.

Elaine H. was especially good to you around this time, as the abject sadness of you all really worried me. After I had discussed my concerns with your pastor, Paul P., he wrote these wise words to me:

"We parents always want to do more for our children, but really there is only so much we can do. I think she is right when she said that no one can take away the sorrow they all feel. It is something she will have to learn to live with; but we can help her bear it and carry it with her so that she doesn't carry it alone."

Then again, on Boxing Day that same year, the most devastating tsunami in recorded history struck the Far East. We joined the world in the utter shock of such an occurrence, in disbelief over the hundreds of thousands who had lost their lives, let alone the grieving people left behind.

As I look back over the years, so often you were off work, so often unwell and yet more than unwell, downright ill. Christmas was always a hugely busy time, so

I ensured I did my preparation over the summer so that it was all completed by October, with enough postage stamps bought for the two of us. That way, I had the rest of the time to concentrate on assisting you. Except, of course, you hated doing things too much in advance, so there always seemed to be a last minute rush to get everything done. We quickly learned to buy gift bags in the preceding year's sales, so you weren't wrapping presents on Christmas Eve, but could instead just pop your gifts into the bags! The bed in the spare room had mountains of Christmas presents carefully labelled so that those going to family, work, friends or church were quickly and easily identified. Perhaps it was just my maternal instinct, and your (possibly subconscious) resistance to the idea of needing to be cared for, but I was certainly one for preparation, and you were undoubtedly spontaneous. I have to say Claire, we are similar in many ways, but also different in several ways. As such, I heaved a genuine sigh of relief when the presents had all been distributed, so I could focus on you again.

2004 had been a good year, as I am thankful for every year I had with you (and every year the Lord blessed me with). However, 2004 was truly a bittersweet year in many, unrelated ways. Thankfully, although it brought challenges of its own, 2005 would be a year where I believe many people in the world would begin to express their love for one another, and appreciate their loved ones in light of the increasing devastation around the world. This would be beautifully reflected in the many hopeful, special notes and messages you received, as we'll see in the next chapter.

Chapter Nineteen

2005-2006 – Through Suffering, True Strength

2005

Dear Claire, for some reason some of your diaries were missing from among your boxes. Since 2000 you had used the same diary each year to list your work commitments as well as social events. This ensured you could cross through each line item with an indelible marker once you had recorded your social work notes to your work's software on the computer. All I can conclude is, despite this system working so well for you and protecting client confidentiality, you social workers were required to hand in your diaries occasionally for audit purposes, thus I don't have them available for reference.

I can remember two highlights of 2005, though I am sure there were many more. The first was Jo and Jon C.'s wedding when you and Ruth W., alongside others chosen by Jo, were bridesmaids; you did not permit me to go down to Hampshire for the service, but afterwards I saw the stunning photos of the bridal party. What a vision you all were. Over the years you were bridesmaid to a number of friends and attended many weddings as well. With each wedding, I could sense the deep, underlying desire you had to meet a godly man and be married yourself. Again, it is one of those things we do not understand, but I know the Lord has answers, which you now know, and I someday will. You did have lots and lots of fun, though; I remember travelling all across London one year to get you a matching jacket for a dress. You decided the one you had bought from Next was too big, so armed with the location of half a dozen stores (and before the advent of online shopping), I did the rounds hoping they did indeed have the correct size available that they promised me beforehand. Sure enough, I did accomplish that mission!

Then there was your thirtieth birthday in July. What an event that was. It is such a pity I do not have your diary notes from this event and only my memories, because you enjoyed a huge party at a swanky hotel with a great number of friends. You really were born to socialize and build relationships, Claire, and it was fantastic to witness how all your various friendship groups merged into one on this special occasion. One thing I am so pleased we had recorded from this event was when Rach organised a birthday book in which all those attending could write. These following are just a few of the entries:

"It's a pleasure to call you my friend. You are such a beautiful, lovely, generous person it's amazing you're real. You can really make me laugh and you are great fun to be around. Sally S."

"My memories of you, Claire, are of you always with a smile and with what had to be the busiest social diary of all of us! I always admired you for keeping up and for never quite running out of energy. Love Melissa, Uni of Kent."

"You're a role model to us all – thanks for your support and listening over the years. Lots of love, Andrew S."

"How good of God that He should choose to give you to me as a friend. That out of all the people in the world, He should have caused our paths to cross, our circumstances to intertwine, our minds to spark against each other – so that when we talk, there are so often fresh ways of thinking, new insights into love and life and faith.[60] Lots of love, Keleigh."

"Travelling to Caroline T.'s surprise birthday party in Bedford, speeding round the M25 in her car with windows wide open and the wind in her long blonde hair, only to see the directions go flying out the window." (From Faye)

Another very special entry (each line beginning with a letter of your name) was also included, but I could not see who wrote it:

Claire was born 30 years ago, she was a "prem" baby, starting out in life in Epsom Hospital's Special Care Baby Unit.

Later, as she grew up, she has displayed certain qualities, some to the point of stubbornness, partly due to her health situation, which she has contended with over the years.

Appreciation of the gift of life, both for herself and those around her, has been her trademark.

Intelligent to a degree (in actual fact, two) you would really have though she would have learnt her lesson the first time, but even as an adult, she felt she just had to go back to school!

Really the reason was taking a year out with the Christian Schools' Work Trust, to help the pupils and Christian Unions.

60   Marion Stroud, The Gift of Friends (Lion Hudson Plc, 1995)

Enthusiastic and encouraging, a good and faithful friend, Claire is far more concerned in finding out about you and your news than telling you about herself.

Seemingly impervious to the cold, Claire habitually dresses for winter in a T-shirt and short skirt, much to the concern of her mum and Auntie Pat.

A warm sense of humour and fun; Claire always seems to be smiling.

Lateness is her hallmark, but to be honest, her treatment regime takes hours each day.

Tendency to play down her health concerns and carry on, regardless.

Ever the optimist, Claire shows perseverance and fortitude.

Remaining positive in adversity (especially when receiving potentially embarrassing homilies), we wish Claire well and thank God for her.

In this same box I found the following card from Isla:

"Dear Claire, Happy birthday.

I've had lots of fun thinking of very fond memories of our year spent together at 93 Downs Road whilst we were at Uni:-

Is the phone free –it's surely still not engaged!

Will someone turn off the smoke alarm – whose toast was that?

When will that person vacate the shower?

I have a neuropsychology lecture today – can anyone sit in on it so I don't have to?

Seriously, you are a wonderful friend and source of inspiration. I'm so glad we've stayed in touch and know we'll continue to (even if I always speak to Auntie Pat or the answerphone!). Do you remember that cocktail party, visits to Broadstairs, day trips to Chilham, and there was me thinking we went to Uni to study! Claire, enjoy your birthday, I'm delighted to celebrate it with you.

Lots of love, Isla.

Yet another one was signed. "Anonymous":

"Claire has brought many treasured times to my life. Her ability to smile through a struggle often impressed me. There have been times I made her laugh just to hear that contagious giggle. One such occasion stands out clearly in my memory; when Pete W. made a prank call to her mobile. As a result she was persuaded that her Oak Hall trip to Israel had been cancelled, the alternative being a white water rafting holiday with men only. This brought home to me Claire's ability to cope in the most tricky of situations. Claire, you're loved so much and always bring a laugh with you. You are a trustworthy and excellent friend."

Of course, there was also one from Auntie Pat:

"Dearest Claire,

As a baby, you were so beautiful and good and I looked after you from time to time.

As a little girl you were beautiful, good and stubborn, and I looked after you from time to time.

These times included a holiday – remember the trampoline?

Now as a young woman you are still beautiful, good, stubborn and caring and it's been a bonus for me to have you share my home these last couple or so years.

One last thing – I'm looking forward to when you look after me from time to time!"

Then, on this momentous day I wrote you a letter, as was (and it appears, still is) my custom:

"Dear Claire, congratulations on your thirtieth birthday. Herewith a cheque towards a new car. (Ulterior motive is that I need your old one!)

At thirty, remember that there is more to life than increasing its speed, so don't lose the 'now' moments. Life is precarious and life is precious— none of us can assume on tomorrow. No longer in your twenties, you have such a wealth of qualifications, experience and hard work under your belt, besides loads of travel and friends. You have a lovely home, the interior of which you have designed yourself, and you always look stunning despite the effort each day. I am so very, very proud of you.

However, I am very aware that the good times have also been saddened by the bad, by so many disappointments, ill health and problems/hassle that you could have done without. As I have said so often, I don't know why God has allowed you to suffer year on year, but I do know that one day He will give you beauty for ashes. . .[61]

I have often said that if I could take away your pain I would gladly do so, but I cannot. God made you to be you and we have that promise (Romans 8v28) that He will work all things for our good. Hard, oh, so very hard to accept. However, I must be content with the following:

'And shall I pray Thee change Thy will, my Father,

Until it be according unto mine?

But, no, Lord, no, that never shall be, rather

I pray Thee blend my human will with Thine.' [62]

---

[61] Crystal Lewis, Beauty for Ashes, on Beauty for Ashes (CD released by Metro One Inc, September 23, 1996)

[62] Amy Carmichael, Gold Cord: The Story of a Fellowship, (© 1932 by the Dohnavur Fellowship. Used by permission of CLC Publications) May not be further produced. All rights reserved

So enjoy today, and this thirtieth year, despite the toughness of life and remember what Grampsie said in your 8th birthday card: 'To a little darling, who has made an old man so happy.' And as your mum I can only echo that, knowing how many people's lives you have touched as well as mine.

As a child you began to show some of the wonderful characteristics that you have now started to develop into a career as a social worker and involving your love for God and people. I could write so much, as I have done on many of your birthdays in the past, but will curtail this letter to a few paras [sic]!

So happy special birthday. Some years ago I started a 'gems' memory box where I put mementos and songs/quotes, so that when you become really ill there may be opportunity to reflect on God's love in your life. I thought I would mention it on this your 30th, and to say I will continue to add to it as the years go by, although praying that we will not need to use it for many years to come. With all my love to my loveliest and best daughter. May God richly bless you in this new phase in your life.

Some Times Remembered

The time you forgot to let go of the car as I drove off and you ran up part of Mandeville Drive at Olympic speed – that was a heart stopper.

The day we set off from Highcliffe beach in a rubber dingy and landed at Friars cliff just up the coast.

And then there was the day we went white water rafting for real in Montana – the expression on your face said it all.

The hotly contested photo you took at Mojarve point in the Grand Canyon. It was the best.

Those lunch times when you hoped it would be sunny so we could sit al fresco and enjoy the warmth. . .and many, many more.

Mum."

I don't want to belabour the fact that you suffered; indeed, you know it, I know it and our readers know it. I do, however, wish to be sure the reader recognizes a deep, underlying spiritual theme that appears in the *midst* of suffering – that is the deep strength that is forged from difficult times.

Together in a box you had labelled "2005 and all that," I found some scrappy jottings in a notepad you had kept from Joni Eareckson-Tada's visit to the King's Centre on October 5th, 2005. These are your few excerpts of that talk. You had written that life is full of suffering; that God hates it, but that He uses it to do something amazing in our lives. Like me and thousands of other mothers, Claire, you recorded that Joni's mum was always thinking of her, fighting the cross-town traffic each day to get to the hospital and binding herself to Joni in so many empathic ways, I guess heart-broken that she could not do more for her daughter. Oh, how this reminds me of the times we also fought the London traffic to either visit you or transport you to and from the hospital. You recorded that Joni felt God closed doors but that she found an open window giving a much better view. How good God is, even in dire circumstances.

Although you didn't have the same gruelling routine for over forty years, even so you undoubtedly faced your share of real suffering; many, many hospital admissions, with all the painful procedures that accompany those admissions. Once back home you continued to battle through difficult physiotherapy, a plethora of medications, nebulisers, intravenous antibiotics and on and on. While others arrived early at work to complete their day in a timely fashion, your day started about at dawn too, but ended even later. After an exhausting day you would drop into bed with your enormous routine still looming over you, only to begin again the next morning. Like Joni, you certainly knew what it was like to ask if you could borrow God's smile. I suppose, it is my turn now, Claire, to learn as you and Joni had that it is not alone sufficient to accept God's will, but that I also need to embrace it.

Ever wanting to encourage you, I wrote that autumn:

"Well done in completing your Post Qualifying course in Social Work and getting such an excellent report. This qualification under your belt as well as promotion, all in your 30th year deserves congratulations."

The words of the hymn, "Above the Voices of the World Around Me"[63] meant a lot to you at that time, and I believe reflect you slowly coming to terms with your mortality, while knowing you were eternally safe with your Creator. You were learning to trust Him in a way so many may never experience. You knew your health could deteriorate, once for good, any day, so you had to learn to trust and abide in your Saviour as though. . .well, as though your life depended on it, because it truly did. Most people never realise that about their own lives, so again, in your suffering and in a strange way, you were deeply blessed.

I remember many special occasions you attended, and it warms my heart that you and our friends were always there for each other. Around this time you and Rach developed a penchant for enjoying the occasional luxury meal out in various London restaurants. On one such occasion Rach was not feeling great and you certainly were not. It was quite normal for you to ask Auntie Pat or myself to transport you to the station. This time, I had come to take you but could immediately see you were so short of breath, but true to form, you would not hear of not going.

As it turned out, we had to get the lift up to the platform and I waited anxiously until you were safely on the train. I was not at all surprised (in fact, I was somewhat relieved) to get a call a couple of hours later to come and collect you! When you wrote in your chapter for *Horizons of Hope* that you should make the effort to do this or that when you have arranged to do things with your friends, you certainly meant it. Of course, your tenacity was sometimes to your detriment, and also

---

63   Timothy Dudley-Smith, Above the Voices of the World, (1987)

often required great effort from all other parties involved. But that is what made you *you*, Claire. Your indomitable spirit is one of the most remarkable aspects of your high standard of character.

2006

In January 2006, I responded to Brian E.'s email:

"Thanks so much for remembering us last week; it was a great birthday organised by Claire, despite her being so unwell with a D&V bug she caught from me. We had to call Thames doc out at midnight and they didn't come until 3:40am, then we had our second visit to hospital in a week on Friday as her Huber needle fell out because she was vomiting so much. However she is improving slowly, which is what's important."

To which he replied:

"Thanks, Mave. Poor Claire, she is a great girl and I admire her so much. So glad your day was not all taken up with hospitals."

That spring found you adventuring again on an exciting holiday in India with Ruth W. Despite your globetrotting undoubtedly taking its toll on your health, you loved sight-seeing and experiencing other cultures so much, I really felt you were fulfilling your dreams of travel. Besides it was your life, and you felt it was all worth it, so how could I argue? Later that spring, however, your lung function was chronically low and the doctors ordered you to not leave the country under any circumstances.

The next milestone of that year came in the autumn when we spent a weekend in Paris, travelling by Eurostar. The weather was warm, sunny, and exactly what the doctor ordered. We enjoyed walking in the gorgeous Parisian gardens, and along the classically picturesque *Champs Elysees*. I really look back with such fond memories of times like this that you invited me to share with you, particularly as that was a time when you seemed to be having a better spell of health.

When we closed the year out on Christmas of 2006, your dreams and hopes continued to burn brightly while your determination to live life as normally as possible (or super-normally is perhaps a better description of your style). In my Christmas card to you I wrote:

"Another year of achievements and yet also another year of complex health problems. May He grant you some dreams that will come true in 2007. With all my love and prayers this Christmas."

Indeed, the Lord had granted you one dream to come true that year; you began going out with a young man named Kev at the time, and you two would share some very special occasions together the next year.

Chapter Twenty

2007 – A Turning Point

My precious Claire,

Y ou were always so very thoughtful in arranging special birthday treats for me each year in January, and as 2007 dawned you especially outdid yourself. You treated Pat and me to a meal out at Brown's restaurant, then on to see the *Jersey Boys* musical. However, although there were not many stairs, you had such difficulty managing these with your gross shortness of breath at the time. . .another occasion when you sacrificed for your family. You were in high spirits as the year kicked off, and one of the first things you did, together with Rach, was to have some professional photos done. I am unsure why you did not have these taken for your thirtieth, but maybe one of your frequent bouts of ill health and/or hospitalisation prevented that.

As I look back, I noticed in hindsight certain things simply dropped off your action list, due to your busyness. One such list item in particular was sending birthday cards to your cousins in Belgium; reflecting on this now, I see you simply could not keep up the pace you had set yourself over the years. The sad part is no one had told us specifically things were deteriorating; indeed the hospital wrote to your Occupational Health Department to say "fortunately" you could continue to work full time. It was only our own observations that told us you were losing ground.

Of course, later in the year you were suddenly told you needed to start considering a lung transplant. By this time I had reduced my hours from full-time to part-time employment to happily attend to your health. Knowing you were apprehensive at the thought of a transplant, I asked what I could do to support you further; you responded you would like me to give up work altogether, which I gladly did. We were both wearing pretty thin, but doing our best to remain strong. I had emailed praying friends at various times throughout the year:

"Bad day with Claire's intravenous antibiotics, which just emotionally tired us both out, so many problems time and again."

Time flew by and I emailed again:

"Claire at the hospital yesterday and started on three weeks of home intravenous antibiotics yet again. It's the beginning of a long haul for both of us. We have to go back again on Friday and should know more about the treatment programme."

The health difficulties I alluded to were two-fold: the side effects of a specific antibiotic that caused vasculitis (a condition where blood vessel changes occur resulting in scarring and blood flow restriction) causing a widespread rash on your legs. When the consultant took you off of that medication she had to find another, which proved to be no easy task when you were allergic to so many. The second problem was the use of aminoglycoside antibiotics that caused you vertigo, lasting many weeks.

One day when you were feeling particularly unwell you asked me outright: "Do you wish I'd die so that you didn't have all this?"

Of course the answer was, is and always will be a resounding, "No!" Claire. Never, ever has such a thought even entered my head and I responded with what I told you so often through your life: "I've had the time of my life having you as a daughter."

Many of our friends were powerful, spiritual allies, though. Freda wrote:

"Dear Mave, my heart goes out to Claire with her vasculitis caused by her antibiotics. I coped okay when I.'s health took a turn for the worse, but when they gave him some antibiotic which burnt his skin, I asked 'Why, God? Hasn't he suffered enough?' So I feel for Claire. Why did the surgeon have to be on his hols this week? I pray when he comes back he'll make Claire a priority for her op. Freda S."

So many people asked after you, Claire, and I am so grateful we were supported by all those who loved and cared for you deeply. I responded to Julie, the Foster Care Chairperson, in 2007 when I was doing respite fostering some weekends:

"Thanks for asking; Claire is still working full-time but needs lots of support in the mornings before she goes into work (has huge regime of medication taken via a nebuliser that seems to take forever, and of course physio too). However, she can't take part in the CF Gene Therapy trials as a patient's lung function must be above 40% and Claire's is below 30%. I can't help but admire her, existing on less than a third of her lung capacity!"

Admire you I truly did, Claire.

It is such a heavy burden you and countless others with serious illness bear, and yet each of you who have overcome and conquered is to be praised. I only pray the thankfulness so many of us feel is apparent, because those of you who have suffered so profoundly must know you have equally enriched our lives just as deeply by your determination.

I cannot, however, help but feel sorrow for the many who still bear that terrible burden, the day-in and day-out struggle to somehow survive against all the odds and the ever-present anxiety such illness provokes. Yes, Claire, sometimes that anxiety is founded in dreadful reality as in 2007 your lung function became chronically low and never picked up again. (It was this dark milestone that caused you to need oxygen on long haul flights.)

You had walked so often in the darkness, Claire, and life had been so tough for you but your commitment to God and your endurance in the faith in the face of huge difficulties are inspiring to say the least. In this spirit I wrote to Val A.:

"Claire has had this week off as annual leave and has been resting. Annual review at the hospital last Friday was not a good report as she was told it was a special favour to allow her home and not keep her in but in future want her under their wing. She's not well, Val, very breathless – takes ages to do everything. Had heart problems on Monday that lasted four and a half hours, and then she gets very panicky and wants me with her all the time as she remembers how frightened she felt when the doctor told her in 2003 that her heart could stop at any time. Felt better when her heart arrhythmia returned to normal pattern. We are awaiting a test result from the hospital, but apart from that we just carry on as before and go back up to London in a couple of weeks. I have just returned from a three hour lunch break, as her intravenous infusion takes so long to go through."

Of course, as we know, just because you had CF it did not exempt you from other problems. In fact, it often only complicated matters. I remember in this year (2007) when we had had a particularly long day at the hospital, the doctor had written the wrong name (another patient's name) on your intra-venous medications for us to give at home. We spent ages into the evening wondering why your prescription could not be traced by the hospital pharmacy, and by the time we arrived home it was extremely late, and we still had to unpack all your antibiotics, together with your ancillary packs and draw up your medication into syringes for that night. We were both exhausted and, again, you said to me, "I expect you can't wait for me to die."

My precious Claire, I know you were likely feeling guilty, and yes we lived in very close proximity to each other so I can understand those thoughts crossing your mind, but no, Claire. Never, never could any normal mother ever think anything like that, no matter what she had to do for her child. I assure you it was not even present in my mind, and now you are gone, I want to scream, "All I want is to have you back!"

I know you felt useless at times, Claire, or that you were a burden, but no, you were never that, and if the person that should have been helping us had been then we would not have been so dog-tired. God made you, Claire; Psalm 139 tells us how He knit us together in our mothers' wombs, and you were always of value in God's sight as you were in mine and so very many others. Despite your illness, it was so evident God was with you, and there were times of tremendously special encouragement. In March, you interviewed for the post of Assistant Team Manager, and on 23.3.2007 I received this subsequent email from you:

"I got the job! My salary will be increased to £xxxx, not bad eh!"

I emailed back:

"Am just so thrilled for you. I have bought a congrats card and will pop it through your door on my way home."

However Claire, despite earning the promotion, as ever, you hated saying goodbye to your current team in readiness to move on to your new one. I emailed you:

"As you move offices, as you clear your desk and empty your drawers and locker, say your goodbyes, painful as it is, the end of another era, please know that God is in this because His purposes for us are to give us a future and a hope. Congratulations again on this achievement. With all my love, Mum.

P.S. Steve W. did his usual check on your car today; how grateful we are for help in these practical tasks."

As was your style, you put your nose to the grind, and the months flew by. By the time summer rolled around, I was pleased to make an appearance in a letter you wrote to one university friend about visiting your old campus at Kent:

"My Mum and I went to Ali Browne's tenth anniversary service in Herne Bay, then back to her house for refreshments. On the way home we drove through the University of Kent campus to see all our old haunts (including driving past Downs Road where we spent our year living out). Such memories!"

I had made one of my rare notes to remind me of this occasion and put it in your "Gems" folder:

"On campus, we drove past Darwin College, where Claire spent her first year, also Rutherford (where Claire used to eat at weekends and get hot bread too) and Eliot (where Rach B. was in halls their first year). We drove past the library, past the psychology block and also past Parkwood, where Claire spent her final year with Rach and Kim. It was really nostalgic, and a trip down memory lane, especially as we saw Canterbury Cathedral from the vantage point of Eliot, just like old days for Claire! So good to see the university again and to think of Claire's superb years spent there. We then went into Canterbury, saw the city walled gate and tower and thought about Claire doing soup runs, etc. We walked up the main street and had dessert and coffee in a café. We saw the Cathedral, the river running through the town, all the shops that Claire used to frequent, and really enjoyed the atmosphere. Walking through the High Street, we saw the Abode hotel and purposed to spend a weekend there one day."

After that lovely trip down memory lane (and reflecting on how far you had come), July was soon upon us, and we were again celebrating your birthday by going to the theatre with Kev to see *Billy Elliot*. A couple of days later you had your usual birthday meal with your friends, and I think it totalled thirty-three people. So many of your friends still tell me how much they miss these gatherings. Paul P. made mention of the New Year's Eve parties you would attend; going the rounds of them was always both special and very typical of you. I remember you had two particularly lovely jackets: a silver sequined one, as well as a black one. You would wear one or the other under your short fur coat, always dressing the part. In fact, it is something I miss greatly about you.

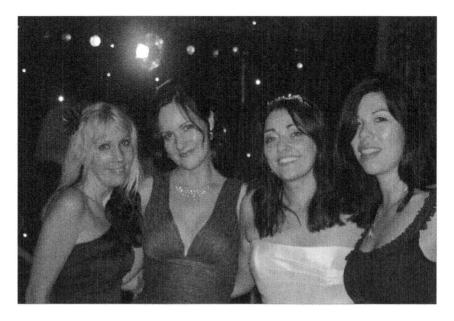

Helen, Yasmine (and Penny), best friends from RBK social work team

I never told you about this little incident, however: You had bought a stunning long purple dress and matching bolero to wear to Helen and Rob's wedding, and on your return, asked me to wash the bolero, which I did. Little did I know that, when I found a supermarket bag to put it in, the bag had *bleach in it*! When I retrieved the garment from the bag, it had a huge white stain on it, and my heart nearly stopped! I did not dare tell you for, despite being the epic bargain-hunter and buying so many of your items of clothing and furnishing in sales, I knew you would not take kindly to me spoiling this lovely bolero after only one wash. I frantically phoned countless Karen Millen stores before I found one in our area that still had the same size (being a sale item meant they had all sold out quickly) and I spent the next day unstitching them both until I could sew the good parts together to make one garment as new! I was on tenterhooks the next time you wore it, in case you noticed my stitching, but you did not notice, and all was okay. (How I thanked God that it was acceptable.)

Yet still health problems took their toll. Freda S., who was a faithful prayer partner and also a social worker, emailed me:

"Thanks for your honesty in home group last evening. It's so hard for Claire; she is a lovely young person with so much drive to do things for God. I know colleagues speak highly of her. I pray her illness will draw her closer to Him and not be a barrier."

The trials with your health continued though, Claire, and that month you had yet another hospital admission. It often seemed as though you would have an admission for some reason before a scheduled trip (especially holidays). This hospital admission was no different, and came before one such memorable trip. In a letter, Rach B. wrote:

"Me cooking for you and Claire is the least I can do with her having had more surgery and I'm glad to help. Claire is such a blessing and inspiration to me so I'm really much more in her debt. Really hope you can both relax in Croatia."

Yes, we were destined for sunny Croatia, so off we went for five full days so you could convalesce from yet another port-a-cath operation. The weather was superb and how we loved going into Split in the evenings, but I believe one of your all-time favourite days out was to the island of Cvar. You were wearing the most elegant sun-dress you bought en-route at the airport, and like so many holiday photos, you looked simply gorgeous. That was a week that really stands out for me, and I will always treasure that holiday; the time out for you to relax gave me much comfort, for I never felt that you ever really took time to recuperate. You always worked yourself so hard.

Yet again, however, struggles often appeared relentless and as a result, I found a card I had written to you:

"I am so very sorry and sad you're having such a tough time of it, for you truly don't deserve it. But, what an encouragement to get an 'A' grade for your coursework, you must be thrilled. I may not be able to fix your health or make other dreams come true, but I can give you all the TLC you so much deserve and help you financially, so this is towards your home improvements."

Ever the artistic one, you had designed your own bathroom a couple of years previously and now were having your bedroom re-decorated after seven years. You chose your furniture so painstakingly, carefully measuring the room to ensure it all fit. Still, despite your own struggles, your selflessness shone through in a sympathy card to me in that same year, when one of my friends Joy R., Philip's wife, died:

"I am so sorry for you, having lost Joy. I know she wouldn't have asked for a better friend and I'm sure she would have felt very happy knowing you would be doing her Tribute. I'm so glad you have many happy memories of both her and Philip. At least they are together once again, now with God. I'm sad that you're sad, Mum."

Of course this was not to negate the huge loss that her family, particularly her son, Kevin and her daughter, Louise felt. The death of parents is always a big sadness but to stand with them in their grief was an honour.

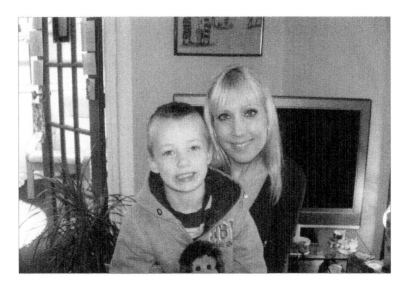

With nephew, Tyler

As you took up your new position in Fairmount House, your manager, Sue W. from St. Faith's wrote:

"Thank you for being such a skillful ATM and a lovely person to have as part of the Mole Valley team. Thanks so much for your thoughtful gifts to the team, and equally, our gifts to you, as you progress to your next post, are to say how much we appreciate your sweet and generous nature."

Your colleague Barbara also wrote:

"Wishing you all success and everything you would wish for in your new job. Thank you for all your support, help and guidance. Shall miss this, together with your saucy smile and laugh."

From your old team, as you left they gave a card to say:

"Don't leave! Don't go! Oh, please don't go! Stay!"

I hoped, as Christmas approached, that you could take some rest and enjoy a bit of downtime with your friends. Alas, you rarely did. I wrote in your card:

"Dear Claire, yet another great year of achievements but coupled with so many problems and ill-health. I could write a book [Reader, little did I know then, that I would indeed write a book regarding Claire's life] on how much I love you; how proud I am of you, how absolutely beautiful you look in your professional photos, but suffice to say that whatever the future holds, God wrote the biography of your life long before you were born and He is not caught unaware.[64] I look forward to more happy times in the future. Happy Christmas and my prayers for 2008. All my love, Mum."

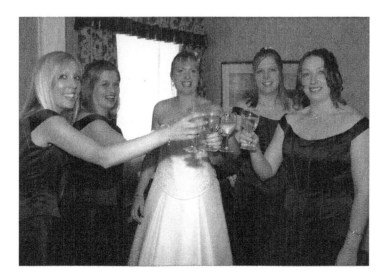

Bridesmaid to Jo C(Claire, Jo and Ruth are good friends from Reading University Social Work course. L-R: Claire, Ruth, Meg, Jo and Jackie

---

[64]   Author unknown

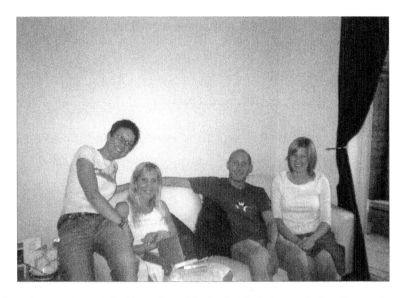

A welcome break before the thirtieth birthday celebrations start,

with Hannah, Mark and Natalie

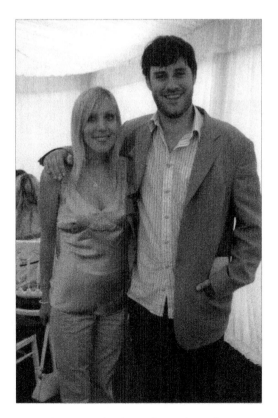

Claire with close friend, Rich B

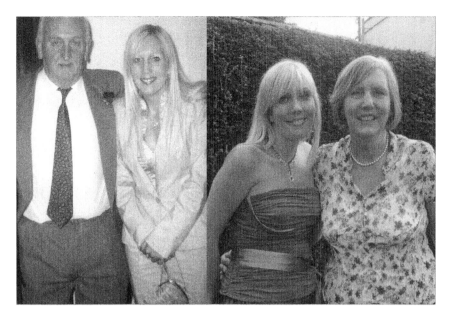

Two family weddings, left: with Uncle Keith and right: with Mum (Mave)

So yes, Claire, 2007 was a bittersweet year, and a downward turning point in your health. It was also a year of astonishing successes, and even more extraordinary tenacity. I was so praying and hoping 2008 would be a better year for you, health-wise, Claire, and I wish I could say it was. I have already told the reader your lung condition was not to improve, so there is no sense in concealing the fact that 2008 would be increasingly difficult for you in that regard. Nevertheless where there is suffering, there is always grace and so 2008 would be a year, much to my amazement, where you would see several more of your famous adventures crossed off your growing, and very remarkable list. Some of these included holidays in Europe, first with Jo R. and then an expanding group: Kate, Leah and Zoe.

Chapter Twenty-One

2008-2009 – Dark Days, a Stronger Spirit

2008

As the new year began the birthday celebrations you planned for me were, as always, so delightfully thoughtful. You arranged to take me and your two aunts for dinner at The Petersham in Richmond, with its fantastic view of the river Thames, slowly meandering its way down to Hampton Court and up to London. That night was so memorable, as everything was absolutely superb. Well, almost everything. . .when we returned from our lovely dinner, your car was only a few feet away from the car parked opposite yours, and it looked so odd straddled across the road.

At first we all thought you had parked badly, but we soon realised you would never have parked in such a position as to prevent another vehicle from exiting. It was only in retrospect we grasped the reason – in your frail state you found it difficult to pull up the handbrake, especially so soon after a port operation. You had not secured the brake enough and the car had rolled back. Despite the averted disaster, we laughed at the car's new placement! (Afterwards, of course, we had the brake adjusted so it wasn't so stiff.) After yet another wonderful birthday evening by your hand, I always wrote a thank you card to demonstrate how grateful I was for the thought you put in to these special occasions.

As always, life carried on, and you continued to do well at work, although you were becoming significantly weaker. That year Surrey Social Services had an Office for Standards in Education, Children's Services and Skills inspection, or better known as "OfSted." You seemed to not be too enthused about the inspection, so I emailed:

"Thinking of and praying for you during your Ofsted Inspection."

A couple of weeks later, I emailed you again:

"I was so pleased to hear of your great report from Beverley. I hope this has really encouraged you, especially when you've been so unwell."

I so wished you would take some time off to rest but that was just not your way, Claire. Ever wanting to tick more countries off your list, your next adventure was to visit the orang-utans in their natural habitat in Borneo. If I could not dissuade you, I had to accompany you so I could at least be there to help. By this point, as mentioned in the previous chapter, it was necessary for you to purchase oxygen for the flights. I was always impressed with the exotic choices you made for your travels, and this had been recommended by Dave and Ruth W. The orang-utans were such beautiful, seemingly wise creatures.

After another wonderful time of building lifelong memories, we broke our return journey in Kuala Lumpur. I can remember reading one of your book group novels on this trip: *Half of a Yellow Sun.*[65]

---

[65] Chimamanda Ngozi Adichie, Half of a Yellow Sun (2007, Random House, LLC)

You so loved your monthly book group meetings with Ndullee, Rebecca, Sarah and later Caroline, and it was my pleasure to contribute by ordering your books from Amazon; a task I really enjoyed as it kept me updated with the titles you were all reading, whilst it was one less small job for you to do.

Life was becoming increasingly difficult, and still you kept working full-time, so I tried to do as much as possible. Not only had you been very unwell on this holiday, but the return journey was no better. You felt so ill in fact, upon landing you needed to be seen at the hospital immediately and because I had a migraine, you had to drive yourself up with me as a passenger. How we both got through that day at the hospital, I just do not know, but as always, God sustained us and we were ever grateful.

Later that year I emailed Val A.:

"Thanks for prayers. Pat is up at the hospital with her now, as I had a nine-hour wait for the doctors to come and see her. Claire was blue-lighted to Kingston A&E on Monday tea time as it was thought she had a collapsed lung; she had phoned the hospital and the doctor could tell she was very breathless (Claire and I are so used to her breathlessness now that we don't always realise how bad it is), and because of severe chest pain, coughing up lots of blood (again we are used to this) he said she must call an ambulance as he wanted her to be seen urgently. However, on arrival, X-ray and ultrasound was okay. We came home for the night, then directly up to the hospital yesterday.

Likely diagnoses were: 1. Pulmonary embolism from long haul flight. 2. Cracked ribs from so much coughing (hasn't stopped for 6 weeks), or 3. Pain caused by infection that has been a feature for weeks now. The hospital aborted the CT scan to rule out pulmonary embolism today as they couldn't find a vein for dye, and the blood test yesterday suggested the likelihood of this diagnosis was minimal. So it is either cracked ribs or just severe pain from infection. They have started her on a third intra-venous antibiotic as she has so much infection on board. She is really fed up and we have made a deal with them that she will be home in next few days and continue treatment at home. We are both exhausted and quite down."

I never liked to share too much about your state, never needing sympathy, but by this point in time, the support of our social network became critical. The writing was starting to appear on the wall, and I think deep down it terrified me. The problem was it was all so exhausting, both from simply the hospital waiting rooms, to the far more emotionally exhausting anxiety of watching a beloved daughter suffer. You always amazed me, Claire, with your resolve to fight back so hard. In September you managed to obtain tickets for the very special *Last Night at the Proms* evening. It was one of my dreams to go and how you got tickets remains a mystery. Every year I watch as many evenings as time allows; the grandeur of the Royal Albert Hall as the camera sweeps around and the atmosphere within it never cease to stir me.

As I have said elsewhere in this diary, your social life was not just about friends; you selflessly gave time to family, too. We both enjoyed the entirely charming classical performance and I wrote you my usual thank you card after any event you hosted. Of course, we had to drive up to London as it was too far for you to walk from the underground station, and we knew trying to get a taxi afterwards with the crowds swarming out would be well-nigh impossible.

Parking became a problem and soon we were running late. As was our routine (I love that we had a routine for such outings), I dropped you off at the steps outside the Royal Albert Hall, then went in search of a parking space. Much to our relief, after some stress, I managed to use your disabled badge to find a spot. I think we were just about the last two to take our seats, and we had to rush so much just to make it in before the doors closed. It was an evening I will never, ever forget though, and although I cannot deny that tears are evoked while remembering our visit, each year the *Proms* are televised, I always watch as much of them as I can.

Christmas rolled around again, and 2008 had been such a difficult year I felt it necessary to write the following in your card:

> *"I couldn't find a card that was appropriate or summed up my feelings for the beautiful and lovely daughter you are. I don't know why you have to suffer so much in all areas of life, and I pray that the God of reversal and the God of the impossible (my pastor, John T., preached on this recently) will bring you happiness and lots to look forward to in this coming year. You're beautiful in every way. I know it is you that has to do all the hard work of being ill, etc., but I want you to know how proud I am of you, that despite CF you have achieved so much. You may have CF, but up to now, it has not had you."*

I wish I could say 2008 wasn't so bad, but to be honest, it was so miserable your previous pastor Brian E. wrote the following note to you. Thank the Lord for such people in your life, Claire, and the blessing they were:

> *"Dear Claire, I am writing to encourage you, for none of us can fully grasp how wearisome must be your daily round of physio, your too regular emergency trips to the hospital, and your constant supply of antibiotics. Yet through it all you maintain a dogged determination to get on with life and to the full. Add to this your firm hold on the Lord who loves you and saved you and you are a magnificent example to us all of the constancy of faith under trial. Claire, did I ever explain to you how it was a comment made by you at a spring camp when, as a young girl, you wanted to commit your life to*

Christ, that led us to devise the Young Disciples classes at Hook Evangelical Church? Well, be encouraged; you are greatly loved and respected at Hook and a blessing to us all."

2009

2009 began exceptionally well. We holidayed in sunny South Africa as you visited two of your friends. Whilst you continued to enjoy European holidays with various friends, I mostly accompanied you on long-haul because of your need for oxygen. However, to give you your independence, I stayed in a couple of hotels and did my own exploring while you stayed with Patricia and Tom in Cape Town, and then with Helen and Stuart in Durban before travelling to see the Victoria Falls in Zambia. It was a very good trip, and I do believe you actually rested a bit. We met a couple of fellow travellers at Victoria Falls, Betty and Cathy, and kept in touch with them; they were so sad to hear of your passing.

When we arrived home, it was life and work as usual, but it was becoming very evident your health was continuously deteriorating. I so much wanted 2009 to be a much better year than 2008, but sadly it was not to be. By the time summer arrived, you were feeling so ill, I was thrilled when you decided to take another holiday to Greece with Jo R. and the girls. Your immune system was so weakened, however, I could not believe it when you contracted swine flu on a flight back.

A couple of days after you arrived home we went up to London to the hospital. You were offered the opportunity to go home on IVABs if you were. "Well enough," as they did not really want you as an in-patient if they could help it. You were so determined to have your birthday at home, which you did followed by the meal for all your mates as usual, but you became so sick you needed to go up to the hospital the following day for further treatment. You were given the usual blood test that measured the amount of infection in your body, and we were told your

C-reactive protein (CRP) level was 199. Little did we know, in actual fact, it was 399 and never had it been that high before. Why you were permitted to leave the hospital with such a high reading, I will never know. We did not realise this until you had to be admitted again on the following Tuesday.

One of the clinical nurse specialists visited you at home on the Monday and could instantly see how ill you were. She wanted you in hospital right away and a bed became available the following day. I admit I cried when she said you needed to be hospitalised, because I was truly fearful of what would become of you at home, and the reality of the situation suddenly overwhelmed me. On the day before her visit, I slept in your bed with you overnight as I was extremely worried about you. The night you were admitted you were diagnosed with a septic inflammatory crisis and at 2:00 a.m. the on-call physio immediately put you on the "Bird" machine to try and relieve some of the copious amount of mucous in your lungs.

Yes, Claire, it breaks my heart that 2009 was yet another year so dominated by how ill you were. All I wanted was a break in the clouds for you, but it just seemed like one thing after another. The realisation that you had swine flu and could easily have died from it reminded me of the refrain to the song, "Say What You Want"[66] by Texas; that I could indeed not hide, no longer deny your crucial state of health.

Those days you suffered from the swine flu were severely difficult for you, Claire. I can remember Dr. Dev explaining your lungs were like a "pus factory." Because of the infection risk, all staff entering your room had to gown up every time and of course you were not permitted to leave your room. Once you began improving (although improvement was relative, in that you had multiple admissions over the ensuing months), I was able to take you out in the wheelchair, oxygen in tow, to give you some time away from your tiny hospital room. We were not allowed to

---

[66] Say What You Want by Texas, Album: White on Blonde, 1997 ,Songwriters: McElphone, John, Spiteri, Sharleen, Smith, Clifford. © EMI Music Publishing, Sony/ATV Music Publishing LLC, Warner/Chappell Music, Inc., Universal Music Publishing Group, BMG RIGHTS MANAGEMENT US, LLC

linger in the corridor, however, so once out of your room we made straight for the open air, away from other vulnerable patients. Short trips to the Kings Road and also to Battersea Park, together with eating out at Pizza Hut brought some normalcy to those awful weeks. We also ate al fresco at Chelsea Farmer's Market, as well as visiting the Chelsea Gardener. Another highlight was when you bought clothes from Warehouse with a 20% voucher, ever with a bargain in mind. I just loved that red raincoat. The TV programme *Made in Chelsea* is too racy for me to watch, but I see the opening credits (sound muted) showing the familiar sites around the hospital that became part of the fabric of our lives.

I think the intravenous aminophylline, together with the intravenous steroids you were prescribed, just added to the claustrophobia you felt in such a confined space. Pat and I did our best to advocate for you in requesting a larger room, but our pleas went unnoticed. When you finally were released and made it home weeks later, I eventually felt you were okay to be left at night. However I received a call from you at 2:00 a.m. one morning to say you had been sitting on the loo, constipated for over two hours and just did not have enough strength to get yourself back to bed. How I chided you for not calling me sooner, but oh, how I chastised myself more for not staying with you. It was always a struggle for me as you were so desperate to be independent, and in all truth, you loved your own home and the freedom it brought to your life, which made you happy and always feel better.

I wish I could interject a positive note for our readers, but sadly they were few and far between in 2009. Your struggles did not end there as you were admitted to hospital time and again as the flu ravaged your body. When we thought there was a window of opportunity, you, Jo and I had an overnight stay at Chewton Glen Hotel (one of your favourites). I had promised you and Jo I would take you both, as she had been so good to you during this time, but the following day proved to be yet another admission to hospital. You met Ele in Richmond after you were discharged, hoping for some joy and distraction from the pain, but you were so breathless that she had to support you as you walked.

As detailed above, over that summer you spent weeks and weeks in hospital and when you were permitted to have some hours out of the confines of your room, we met Auntie Pat and Uncle Keith in Richmond Park, a halfway stop between the hospital and home. I believe these little trips really kept your morale up, which was one of my major concerns. I would also take you out to Richmond town or to the park.

Three months after the first flu struck, in late autumn, you were able to return to work but were so breathless a manager colleague said you really should forego your allegiance to your job and rest at home until you were really well. You would not hear of it though, as I believe feeling useful was a great source of strength for you. That month saw the awful afternoon when Auntie Pat drove you to hospital for more intra-venous antibiotics (while I cleaned your home) and you went into anaphylactic shock. Your port-a-cath again became infected but this time, possibly because you were so weak, your body's reaction was severe. That meant, of course, yet another surgery to have the port removed and, once the infection had cleared, a new one inserted.

Those were the times, Claire, when you were so scared of dying you begged me to sleep in your king-sized bed with you. I just cannot imagine how very hard those horrible, desperate days were for you. Praise to you, Claire (and shame on me). When I wondered why you had to endure so much, your words to me were: "Don't go down the bitterness route, Mum. It's not worth it." Such wisdom is born from suffering; perhaps we can see part of the answer right there. You so desperately missed your own home at this time, however, so on a couple of occasions I took you home for a few hours from the hospital. Nevertheless, it was always necessary to ensure we had enough portable oxygen to last these trips, bearing in mind that if we got stuck in traffic, there was sufficient for such eventualities.

It would be misleading if I said there were no bright spots at all during this time and Paul P. your pastor at that time, gave me notes (after your death) that he had kept during these difficult years of 2008-9. Your friends and loved ones had always been a strong source of support for you, and this time it was especially comforting to see everyone rally around you. The great mystery was why such a wonderful woman, so very determined to just live,, was enduring these awful trials. It certainly did produce the best in so many people, though.

Kate G. was such a star. Being based in London, she visited you in hospital often, and her sense of humour was priceless. A typical example was the post card she sent with a picture of Prince William on that read:

"Dear Claire, One hopes that you are feeling a bit better. Thinking of you love ~~Will~~ Kate!"

Barb and Darrell B., friends visiting from the USA, also came to lunch to see you. When you were so breathless and you could hardly eat, on return to the USA, Barb wrote:

"I am meeting with my Bible study group today and am going to ask them to take Claire on as a continuing prayer concern. I must also thank you for the wonderful Sunday lunch."

Equally, your namesake, the lovely Claire M. wrote:

"Dear Claire, how can I express my thoughts for you today, by just saying you are loved by all who you have touched? God bless and keep you."

To me she wrote:

"Dearest Mave, I have this card before me but I am lost for words. What can I say that you haven't heard before? My thoughts are known to God. He knows best and strange as it seems at this moment He never gives us more than we can bear, so my dear sister in the Lord, please hold fast to your faith as a mother. As a sister my heart goes out to you and to dear Claire. I love you both. God bless and keep you."

Sue C., a colleague that worked in the same building as you, wrote:

"Claire, you have been so much in my thoughts and prayers these past weeks and I hope you continue to improve in health. To Mave, remembering you too as you continue to care and support Claire in all that you do for her. To you both, you are such an inspiration to us all. I so admire the way you both cope with all that life throws at you!"

Eventually, likely due at least in part to the immense support and love of your friends and family, your health began to pick back up. Ever wanting to return to some semblance of walking without being too breathless, you re-joined the gym with Nicola W. as your buddy. You always went all out Claire, and your attitude was that of simply being stronger than your challenges. Your indomitable will most certainly was stronger as you tried so hard to build up your fragile body.

A strong will did not mean that you were never shaken by your trials, however. I think how much you were challenged is the testament to how resilient you were. I hope these words will not cause offence to any readers of this Diary, but I remember when you had swine flu, you once commented some people only had to worry about whether they would have another baby or not, or what school their children would go to, while you wrestled with these life and death issues. How much tougher were you, Claire, as a result? I imagine tougher than most professional boxers, as you were knocked down so many times and just kept getting back up.

I remember the times your gigantic tablets became stuck in your throat and in a panic you struggled to get them down. From then we had to use a pill crusher to split them into smaller pieces. Then when you had allergic reactions to the many various antibiotics you began to be worried the hospital would run out of options for treating you. The myriad prescriptions to collect from the pharmacy, ensuring we had enough dressings for your port-a-cath needle, the list can go on and on. There was always so much to think about, and so much to do.

Things so rarely went well, coupled with the pressures at work, and this is why it was important for you to have some good times by way of holidays and outings. I felt it necessary and thoroughly enjoyed treating you as much as I could while you battled everything life threw at you. Indeed, before you were done with 2009 another significant problem reared its ugly head; a baby that was open to your team, while in the care of his mother died in a freak accident. (I will add this was not confidential as it was reported in the local newspaper.)

It was absolutely no one's fault, but as an Assistant Team Manager, together with the Manager, an investigation was required of your team. Praise the Lord, however, that you were all completely exonerated in the case. I will admit, I even followed this up further after your death, so outraged was I at the way the investigation had been conducted, especially as you had only returned to work three weeks previously from being off the whole of the summer. (I suppose I had some fight in me, too.)

When Christmas finally approached, so did the potential for a better year in 2010. Although you were still weak and we could not say the year had been great, the sights, festivities and joys of Christmastime certainly did feel as though they were bringing some closure to a difficult chapter. Your card from me read:

"You alluded to an 'awful year' already before you were diagnosed with swine flu and I can only imagine that being so ill just added insult to injury. I'm so sorry for the events of the last few days and trust you will know peace re: the situation. Believe in yourself; we all believe in you, so please don't blame yourself. However awful life is, because God knows everything and is everywhere present, we don't have to worry that He has somehow missed something, for nothing can happen that is outside His control. All the sad and awful things will one day be undone. I pray that 2010 will be heaps better than this year. You've brought such meaning and joy to me. I love you more than you'll ever know. All my love."

In the back of your 2009 work diary (that I had to return to your office, along with the latter diaries too) you had written a list of the following significant memories from that year. How sad I was, Claire, that before returning them I had not thought to look in both your 2010 and 2011 work diaries for similar lists:

-Rick Astley, Michael Buble [and other stars]
-Operation [I guess this refers to your port-a-cath op that you had in November that year.]
-V&A Museum
-Kew Gardens
-Impact weekend
-New Job [That is, you joining the Looked After Children's team.]
-Rebecca and Charlotte W. overnight
-Asha babysitting

-CF Trust Support Group, Book Club, Gym

-Vitality show

-Leadership Skills course

-Strictly Come Dancing at the 02 arena

-The Sanctuary Spa in Covent Garden.

-Pantomime [Claire, was this the one when you got there late because of a crisis at work?]

-Hampton Court Flower Show

-Cannizaro Park [Elvis concert with Auntie Pat]

-Planning for Wimbledon 2010

-Horse Riding

-Nobu Restaurant, London

-Bolshoi Ballet [*Spartacus*] and the Royal Opera House

-Weekends away with friends

-Westlife at Sandown Park

-Kevin and Liz host home group so often and we always have lovely cakes when we go. I am so grateful to everyone in my group and the time they give me.

What is most remarkable is you still found time to take Auntie Peggy from church out. Thus among all the awful events of the year, it was dotted with some very positive happenings, too. I suppose it also depends on how we look at them, but thankfully 2010 was a year of, perhaps not fewer challenges, but more victories. Whether it was by premonition or not, one thing was sure: I began to feel a strong determination to show you just how much you had accomplished.

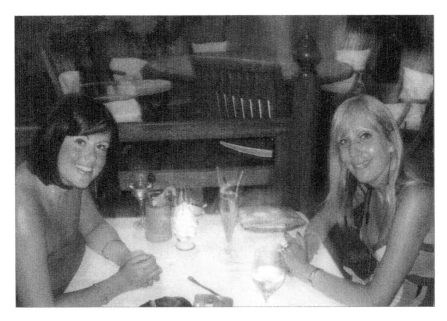

Malta with Jo R, one of Claire's very close, long-standing friends

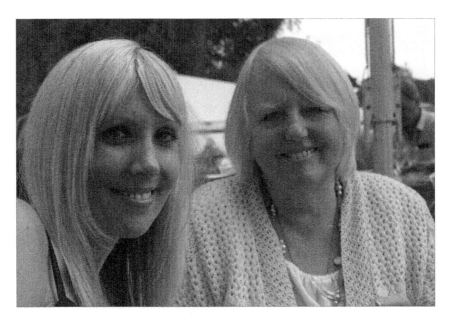

Birthday celebrations with Auntie Pat

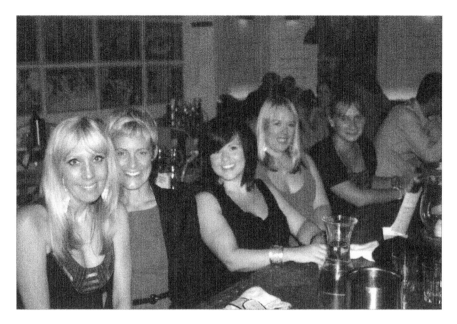

'The girls' group L-R: Claire, Kate, Jo, Zoe and Leah

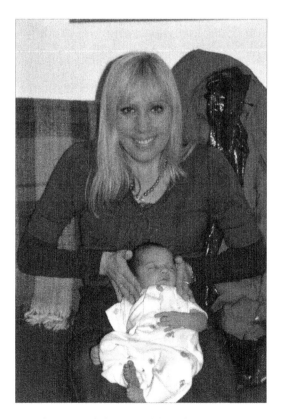

Claire with her goddaughter, Asha

Chapter Twenty-Two

2010-2011 – All We Really Have is each Other

2010

As the year of your thirty-fifth birthday dawned, you were still adamant to get as fit as you could following swine flu, proudly announcing your goal was to get to New Zealand later in the year, which was one of your dream holiday destinations. You were also planning to drop in to Tasmania and see Graham and Ali Sa and their family. To be honest, Claire, I couldn't quite believe this news and it threw me into a sheer panic. How you could even consider travelling so far when you had been so ill was beyond me, but who was I to argue with my adult daughter who lived for taking risks? Indeed, if you had not, I suppose you would never have had that "Life is an adventure – dare it" philosophy.

On Valentine's Day you sent me an email saying you had received a good result from your Individual Performance Review at work. This was such great news after the difficult time your team had endured the previous year, but I did not say, dared not say, "I told you so." You were on a course of IVABs at the time and sent a further message:

"You are such a clever mum. I dropped my flush by mistake and you had a pack all prepared for me to draw up again. Thanks, Mum."

Little did you know how much I so wanted to be the kind of mum you could be proud of. I will never forget (as already alluded to) one particular day in July of that year when you sat crying in the restaurant Giraffe on Gunwharf Quays, I purposed to show you just how much you had accomplished in your life. On your birthday I tied some pink ribbon and wrapped up the following pages like a scroll for you to read at your leisure:

Dear Claire,

The good thing about you being born in 1975 is that it is easy to calculate your age, so happy 35th. I still have bad vibes from a year ago when you were so very seriously ill with swine flu. Little did I realise when you insisted on not going into hospital during your birthday week that we would be driving round Richmond Park in the evenings, car windows fully down, just for you to get some air, and the nights when you felt so ill that you couldn't breathe properly that we could have lost you, but God spared you.

The Hollywood film director Frank Capra was best remembered for his 1946 movie *It's a Wonderful Life.* The film depicts someone who, like you, thought he had accomplished nothing in life, when in reality he had done so much and impacted the lives of others. And the same is exactly true of you, Claire, you have brought such meaning and happiness into so many people's lives so I thought I would try and demonstrate how purposeful your life has been.

You have had so much to cope with in your life and even more so this year (obviously year upon year causes more health problems and your poor body going through so much more; more operations, more treatment, etc.), but you are such a witness to so many and a joy to us all. I read somewhere that "life is downright unfair and God's Son knows this from personal experience,"[67] though I am sure our Lord would not have contextualised it in this way. Forgive the analogy, "but as in a game of cards, so in life, we must play the hand dealt to us and the glory consists not in winning, but in playing a poor hand well."[68]

Although you don't have the physical stamina of someone with good health, I kept a note of what Amy Williams' mum said during a TV inter-view (Amy was the only British Olympian to win a Gold medal in Canada earlier this year) on that occasion: "I am one very proud mother leading the cheering for her. All I can say is 'she's my daughter.'" And I do that every day, Claire, one so very proud mother leading the cheering, not as a physical Olympian, but as a spiritual child of God, going through so much pain and illness to one day win gold. So have a great birthday, all my love and prayers, Mum.

Church work –

Whatever your hand finds to do, do it with all your might, Ecclesiastes 9v10

Work in Spectrum, Impact, Discovery and Cornerstone (not forgetting Contagious)

Year outer for Kingston Schools' Work Trust

Visit to Czech Republic

Genesis course

Visits to former Yugoslavia taking food parcels and encouraging refugees

Articles + Book Chapter

Beach Missions

---

[67]   Author unknown

[68]   Anonymous

Voluntary work / Community Involvement / Social Undertakings –

"Her chapter was a great insight of living with CF" (Professor Hodson)

CF award–Met Terry Waite, etc.

Appearing in local papers and then on national TV news time with Tiffin School.

Helper in school holidays with Learning Disabilities Club

Bridesmaid galore to many friends.

Your own house – designing internally and externally, i.e. garden.

Book Club

Work in nursing homes with older people

CF Fund-Raising Committee + Summer Ball

Family/Leisure –

Ring-fenced time with your cousins, both in England and Belgium

Theatre/Cinema visits with Dennis Gasser

Concerts –including concerts in the park and all musical concerts

Ballet productions

Strictly Come Dancing

Monet art exhibition

Hampton Court and Chelsea Flower Shows

Wimbledon tennis (including front row of Court no. 1)

Last Night of the Proms

School Holidays –

"Claire is a faithful friend to Joanna," (from Joy R.).

Tadpole fishing in Ewell Court Farm Park-with Jo and Sara R., etc.

Caravan and crab fishing on Mudeford Quay – you make friends with Rachel and Rebecca S.

Isle of Wight (+school trip)

Dartmouth

Holidays Abroad + Cultural experiences -

"Claire, you know, is truly amazing; I don't know how she manages day by day." – Jane T.

Chewton Glen Hotel!

Educational –

"School bag in hand, she leaves home in the early morning, waving goodbye with an absent-minded smile. .slipping through my fingers all the time, I try to capture every minute. . ."[69]

Surbiton Hill Nursery School and St. Mary's schools

Tiffin Girls' School Prize

G.C.S.E and 'A' levels

Two degrees (at Bachelor's and Master's Level)

Social Work qualifications

Counselling Course Certificate

Jobs –

Nursing home posts as a teenager/ temporary posts during university vacations/teaching assistant/Christian bookshop/social work posts.

As an aside, Maya Angelou (1928-2014 and author of the book *I Know Why the Caged Bird Sings*, that you read for your English Literature course at school) identified the difference between a person who makes a living, versus someone who makes a life, and you were very much of the latter category, Claire.

---

[69] Slipping Through My Fingers, SONGWRITERS: ANDERSSON, BENNY/ULVAEUS, BJORN by permission of Bocu Music Ltd. Photocopying is illegal without the consent of the Publisher.

Perusing your portfolio I found these; they were some of the comments received during your social work career, mostly from your managers:

22.11.02, From the Director of Children's Services, Royal Borough of Kingston on Thames:

"It was with some relief that I read the Planning Meeting outcome sheet and want to thank everyone who worked so well to safeguard these children and secure the future for them. Thank you again for all your effort."

9.9.03, Mid-Surrey Audit of the 3rd Review Conference re: xxxxx children:

"The above case was recently audited by the audit group and members asked me to write, on their behalf, to thank you for the excellent report and valuable input which was most helpful for conference."

20.10.05, Adoption Panel:

"Everyone involved, including Claire, commended by the team." Mary P., Team Manager.

9.12.05, Core Assessment for each child in large family:

"Claire's report writing skills are as good as ever." Mary P., Team Manager.

7.4.06:

"I should be grateful if you would process Claire's pay progression. Claire is a great asset to this team. She has undertaken considerable training in the last year and increasingly complex work, with good outcomes. She has also taken lead responsibility for some of the project work within the team. Many thanks, Mary P., Team Manager."

Autumn 2006, I just loved this assertive email you sent to one of your managers:

*"I just wanted to raise a few matters regarding my health situation at the present time of change, so that they can be recorded on my personal file. I am aware that there was some concern from a member of staff that I may be passing on a chest infection that I had to them, and thus contributing to their own personal health difficulties. I would like to make it clear that the Cystic Fibrosis Trust has compiled a Fact Sheet for employers (that is already placed in my personal file) which states that 'Employees who do not have Cystic Fibrosis are **not at** risk of contracting an infection from someone with Cystic Fibrosis.' It also states that 'people with Cystic Fibrosis are more susceptible to certain bacterial infections and are at risk from infection from others.' If there are any concerns raised regarding my health, I would like for them to be raised first directly with myself, to ensure that no anxieties are heightened and that also no assumptions are made or alluded to. I am sure that any further consultation, if required, can then occur with the Cystic Fibrosis Trust, the hospital that oversees my care, or Occupational Health if deemed necessary."*

From Dee (a foster carer):

"Thank you so much for all your support, kind words and help with the children. I really enjoyed working with you and hope we can do so again."

12.6. 2007, from Christine A, College Tutor. Re: Reflective Commentary for Social Work course.

"This is a very good piece of work, combining facts, theory, reflection and learning. I really enjoyed reading it and it captures your progression through the placement and your willingness to develop your skills further."

16.7.07, Email from Claire to her Manager:

"Kingston Uni have just called and have recommended me to help with a law lecture next year. I will, of course undertake this in my own time."

6.4.09, from one of your Assistant Team Manager colleagues:

"Dear Claire, wishing you all the success and everything you would wish for in your new job. Thank you for all your support, help and guidance (shall miss this and your saucy smile and laugh!). Very best wishes, Barbara K."

9.6.09,

"J.G-W has been offered secondment for a 6 month period and Claire Salter and B. v d P, the ATMs at Elmbridge will be managing the team until we appoint to this post."

Personal email, 17.9.10:

"Just had my performance review: P. thinks I am an excellent manager, her words, but need to work on my anxiety!"

Claire, when you entrusted me with your professional file (you always said I had more storage space than you!), I stole a look at the above emails, etc and ever wanting to affirm you, I hope you do not mind me including some of these here in my amateur "This is your life" scroll. To conclude, I thought this quotation was so appropriate: "Father God, you cared and loved me even before I was born. There has not been and will not be a moment in this life of mine when you will not be there, caring and loving me."[70]

---

[70] Author unknown

You needed encouragement, Claire, because I could see the ferocity of the disease increasing, and quite honestly it terrified me. You were performing exceptionally, despite your circumstances. No, life was not a bed of roses for you, as I emailed my friend Val on August 11, 2010:

"I left Claire yesterday evening at gone 11:00pm just to 'flush off' her intra venous antibiotics; seven lots of IVs a day again and I need to be up at 06:00 tomorrow to get them out of the fridge, ready to be round at hers for first dose at 07:00. Phone call as I walked in the door. . .Claire very upset to say the least. . .had inadvertently injected her nebuliser drug into her Port-a-cath. Absolutely not sterile and unsure what it would do to her. . .so back round to hers, on phone to hospital and they were so nice, but unfortunately we need to wait, maybe several weeks to see if her central venous line is infected. . .again!

"She is devastated, but these things happen (how, I don't know because we keep her intra-venous syringes in a special, sterile tray and the nebulised drug was in a syringe with no needle and completely separate). I guess she was tired and feeling rotten because of the bad infection."

As someone said to me recently, Claire, happiness is not about getting what we want but enjoying what we have, and despite your struggles, you really tried to enjoy every day. Our happiness, or at least our joy, is contained in Deuteronomy 7:6: The Lord your God has chosen you out of all the people on the face of the earth to be His treasured possession [paraphrased]. In this light, you truly have made this world a better place just by being here. Oh, how gracious God was because the hospital believed the large strength of saline in the syringe for the nebuliser actually prevented the infection in your port! It makes me wonder how many small victories He worked without our realizing it.

I had hoped you might forget about your intended trip to New Zealand, but as the summer months saw you improve, and with Emma as a promised and trusty travelling companion, you asked me to set about devising an itinerary. I think this might have been one of the most complex tasks you ever entrusted to me, Claire, bearing in mind it was yours and Emma's holiday and I was merely the person trying to ensure it met with the approval of you both.

The first job was to enquire what Qantas charged for oxygen on their long-haul flights, and to book travel dates when they could guarantee it would be available. The other problem was that Qantas Airlines did not fly domestic flights within New Zealand; they instead, arranged the flights via other air carriers. Another consideration was that you (understandably) hated very early starts, considering all the treatment you had to complete even before you could start your day. Additionally it was important to be sure shuttle buses from the airport to the hotel, and vice versa, were available, carefully noting where you had to be and at what time to catch these. Your case had to be light enough for you to manoeuvre it, and lastly your carry-on luggage had to be increased under the agreement of each airline, to ensure it contained your nebuliser and medication, in the event of your main luggage going astray.

After countless days of phone calls, emails and juggling, it all somehow came together. With my heart sunken to my feet, on 19th November you and Emma departed on an overnight flight to Singapore. Singapore was a stopover venue for a couple of nights, which you needed to have enough time to enjoy each destination to the full, without rushing from one flight to the next.

From there you flew to Queenstown, which overlooked Lake Wakatipu and the Remarkables mountain range, whilst your hotel was just across the road from the Steam Wharf! God's beauty and majesty surrounded you entirely. Next stop was Christchurch, a vibrant city with the famous, and picturesquely modern-blended-with-historical Cathedral Square. Your real destinations in New Zealand, however, were both Mount Cook and Milford Sound. Mount Cook (also known as Aoraki) is the stunningly scenic tallest mountain in New Zealand, and its series of peaks, glaciers and lakes are a breathtaking sight. Equally gorgeous is Milford Sound, by far the best known (and arguably most beautiful) of the fiords. Emma hired a car so you two could enjoy the sights while driving out there, and perhaps make a few new friends along the way. The area is sparsely populated though, even in the height of the holiday season, and there were very few other cars or coaches on the road.

By the end of that glorious month, you had flown to Sydney. You really seemed to love your second visit there and enjoyed a luxurious evening cruise with Emma before departing the next day for Hobart. It had been a dream at an earlier stage in your adulthood to take a sabbatical from work and live in Australia for a while. Sadly, your health deteriorated and removed that option, so you thus settled for two holidays out there; one in 2003 and a few days' stay in 2010. As recorded elsewhere in this Diary, you were unwell whilst out there and were worried you would have to return early. We kept in constant touch by phone, and I was honestly worried sick myself. Neither of us knew this was to be your last long haul holiday.

The next destination was Tasmania in order to meet up with Graham and Alison Sa, friends you had known from your home church. You and Emma thoroughly enjoyed the time there, but you heard that snow had come relatively early to the Southeast of England, and were concerned I would be unable to get to LHR airport to collect you. You were worrying about me, but you had no idea how I anxious I was about you being the other side of world. It was always such a concern if you took ill abroad, or were involved in any sort of road accident that the medics would know you had a port-a-cath, which would have to be accessed by a special Huber needle. To this end you carried personal information on you, so that it was with you constantly.

I was so relieved and overjoyed when you returned home. Having already bought your Christmas card, I found another when I saw your striking Pandora bracelet you had acquired on the trip. The second card had a diamante ring, and resembled the stones on your bracelet well. With sheer guts and determination, you had managed to remain for the duration of your holiday, and in your Christmas card to me you wrote:

"Dear Mum, just wanted to say and write down how much you mean to me, Mum, and how lovely you are to me when I am poorly. You are a wonderful mum and take care of me so well and in so many ways. You are such a fine example of self-sacrifice and the depth of your love to me seems never ending. I love you so much, Mum, and missed you very much when I was away. Thank you for all you do, the big things and the little things and for all you mean to me by just being there. All my love, Claire. Xxxxxx."

Oh, daughter, reading this now evokes such feelings of guilt (that I also allude to in After Words later) and equally feelings of remorse (that I have recorded earlier in this diary). I was not a good mum; I failed you so often. I became impatient far more times than I dare remember, and yet such was your grace to me to have written this. As Nicholas Wolterstorff so honestly and transparently shares regarding his son: (page 64-65)

What do I do now with my regrets-over the times I neglected to take him along hiking, over the times I placed work ahead of being with him,. . . . over the times I unreasonably got angry with him-over the times I hurt him. . . Over all the times I did not prize the inscape of that image of God in our midst which was he. . . .

When the person is living we can make amends-can say we are sorry. . . . But when the person is dead, what do we do with our regrets?. . . .Putting out of mind is not my way. . . .I believe that God forgives me. I do not doubt that. The matter between God and me is closed. But what about the matter between Eric and me? For my regrets remain. . . .

I shall accept my regrets as part of my life. . . .and intensify the hope for that Great Day coming when we can all throw ourselves into each other's arms and say, "I'm sorry."[71]

Claire, you have absolutely no idea how much I treasure your letter. Probably most of all because I could tell how your spirits had lifted, and you were feeling a good amount of joy again, after your trip. It had been good for you, after all.

Bernie's Christmas card to you read:

"We admire your positive attitude, strength and determination not to let your illness dictate your life. Your ability to be so thoughtful and focus on others' needs is an outstanding quality. We so appreciate you friendship and love."

2010, despite your continued health struggles and the exhausting nature of it all, had turned out to be a wonderful and memorable year.

Reminiscing

In the early 2000s when you were in hospital or feeling unwell at home, you would sit in bed or on the sofa with all your textbooks around you and write by hand an essay, or part of your portfolio for your PQ coursework. You often found

---

[71]   Nicholas Wolterstorf Lament for a Son, Wm. B Eerdmans Publishing Co, 1987

this easier to do than type straight on to the computer, especially as you did not have a wireless PC at the time, and this meant you had to sit in an uncomfortable position on a hard chair upstairs. I would, on occasion, help you out by taking your scribble (which I must admit was 90% better than my writing any day!) and type it up in my home. But woe-betide me if I translated a word incorrectly, or put a reference in the wrong place! Dear me, I would be chastised appropriately.

After having typed your work up as best I could, you would return it to me like any strict teacher (the only difference being you used a black pen, not a red one!) to make alterations. Often these would go to a third or fourth draft, but once the body of the essay was typed, the large percentage of work had already been accomplished and minor amendments, once we got to the final draft, were relatively easy. As I have thumbed through some of your assignments, not a few tears have been shed in reading your revisions and oh, how I wish I could have those days over again. It was my huge pleasure to help you in this way, and my joy to see the perfection in your personality. You so often survived against the odds and I had to help, not being able to bear seeing you suffer with so much ill-health.

Thankfully, Claire, you were able to access disabled bays for your car when on Kingston University campus, but I know when you needed to travel to other office bases throughout Surrey it was not always possible for you to have designated parking, and many times you needed to walk significant distances to the office (or classroom when undertaking in-house training). I can also remember when you were in hospital, yet you needed to get an assignment in on time, I would take it to the Kingston Hill campus where your lectures were held. When I look back, I think we made a great team.

As I continue to rummage through your boxes, it is remarkable how your life jumps out at me so vividly, Claire; you hosted so many CF charity events, kept mementos of the Royal Family—Princess Diana's death, William and Kate's wedding. . . You enjoyed the cinematic production of *The King's Speech* and used to

485

text or email me about the films you had seen, and recommended to me. In 2008 you attended the Gala Charity Summer Ball that you helped organise for CF.

I still even have your tax discs from your car, along with your disability badge. I remember your polite outrage when you parked, put your disabled badge on the windscreen and were met with ridicule from some youngsters who witnessed this. Your calm voice betrayed your true annoyance when you responded with a curt: "Yes, I look well but my lungs are clapped out and I'm waiting to go on the lung transplant list." That promptly ended their untoward remarks! (No, you were never weak, nor slow of wit, my dear daughter.)

It is nostalgic, I know, but I still have your entry tickets from your orang-utan visit in Borneo in 2008. I also have the tickets from the *Harry Potter* films we took Dennis to together, the BBC proms–that special "Last Night" in 2008. I will admit I have kept the tickets from *Strictly Come Dancing*, as well as *Spartacus* at the Royal Opera house for your birthday and then *Cinderella* the same year. West Life, Bros as well as Michael Bubble tickets are also to be found. . .so much, Claire, of your life packed away when you moved from our family home in 1996, and now so much out on display again so that I can remember all that was important in your life.

I have kept some of your school books, including a write up from Tiffin School magazine on "The Rebels of Old Bridge Street," set in 1911, at the time of the school strikes. It depicted one particular significant strike that took place at a Ragged School in Kingston, highlighting the vast social rift between rich and poor. I also have all your Wimbledon Tennis tickets, including the Centre Court game between Maria Sharapova and Sabine Lisicki you attended on 30th June, 2011. I still have your Sealink Calais to Dover crossing pass from your Inter-railing days and your last bus pass from your Tiffin days.

Among my notes was an active one for all your holidays; a reminder to ensure that between the two of us we arranged a hospital letter, listing all the medications you carried, including syringes and needles as well as your nebuliser. As mentioned, we also had to request from the airline additional hand luggage space, and to ensure you had enough medication to last your entire trip. Lastly, the letter had to request refrigeration for your meds whilst in flight, and of course insurance for pre-existing conditions. It was a *mammoth* task to get you all sorted and on the plane, but you so enjoyed your holidays, and it was so good for you, it was always a pleasure to assist with all this.

Other lists with "action by"' dates included renewal of your blue disability badge, your exclusion from congestion charging, plus a myriad of other items that needed appropriate action such as hospital appointments and home care nurse appointments to see how you were doing. Not least, the regular renewal of your Epi-pens in case of a bad allergy reaction to one of your antibiotics. Between the two of us we managed to remember. If it seems as though I miss all of this, Claire, I do. I miss you, and I would do it a trillion times over to have you back. I even miss doing these sorts of daily, seemingly mundane and often exhausting tasks, as I am sure so many, many people do of the person they have lost. That is one of the things I have truly learned from you; life really is an adventure. Dare to appreciate every moment.

Knowing I was forever concerned about my relationship when you were an adolescent, what one of your friends said recently moved me a great deal:

"Mave, I am sure, as I have said before, that Claire saw you as more than a good enough mum. Teenage years are about finding out who you are, breaking the bounds, etc. The strength of the relationship held before is tested then, but if it was strong enough, it remains into adulthood – as yours did and builds upon that as two separate women, joined by birth and an understanding of each other — which seems to grow as time goes on."

Speaking of your friends, Auntie Pat also told me that one of your mates, Helen B., recently brought some people to a church event; one of them saying how great it was. Helen's response was: "I'm only doing what Claire would have done." Isn't that lovely? Your legacy and influence live on to this day. When you were sixteen, you wrote that you wondered where you and your peers would be twenty-five years from then. Little did we know Claire, that you would already be home in Heaven, graduated to glory.

I love remembering your long gone school days, Claire, oh, with such thankfulness as I reminisce over your life. As I reflect on all that represents your life, I am forever grateful that I have discovered so much I did not know about you. When I come across a name I do not recognise, I ask someone who may know; Jo R., Helen G. and Ruth H. have been so good in helping me out, or pointing me in the right direction. They bear with this longing of mine to want to know everything I can that took place in your life. I want to know all about your friends, I want to know all about your holidays, the places you visited, the experiences you have had. You lived such a rich life, it is very comforting and rewarding for me to discover these memories of yours.

As I have said before within these pages, I am crying with you as you say all your goodbyes at school, university, etc. Yes, although you achieved so very much, if I am honest, I am still so very sad you did not live a life full in years. Which mother wouldn't be?

2011

I have already alluded to 2011. You were soon back in the swing of things following your epic trip with Emma, although I knew it was costing you dearly as far as your health was concerned, and the continuing deterioration of it. Nevertheless, you, Claire, were so rich in relationships. You possibly even sacrificed some of your health to build these friendships, and I guess you were wise in doing so. I believe with what was (I am certain), much rumination over your impending death, you understood that all we really have is each other.

In September, just a few months before you were admitted to hospital for the final time, Portia (who also lived in Chessington and whom you knew from the hospital) died. I am sure this was a truly scary event for you, so in another card I wrote:

"I know news of Portia dying from CF is really sad and that it affects you greatly, so I am remembering you especially as you attend her funeral service."

Despite this scary event, you continued to soar. Around this time, you emailed me:

"P., our manager is leaving the team and I am sad. I have just been crying. She thinks I could progress to manager; it is just my health that could hold me back. She says she thinks I'm fantastic. Again, her words, not mine."

With almost a premonition of what was to come, my last Christmas card to you spoke of eternity and thanking you for letting me be part of your life:

"I again pray that the God of reversal and the God of the impossible will make Himself known in a real way this Christmas time. Thanks so much for letting me be a part of your life and for being the fantastic daughter you are. Only Eternity will reveal what a very special and precious child you are to me. As I have said so often, you are my reason for living and I've had the time of my life being your Mum."

Reader, this was my key phrase as no doubt you know by now, but ever wanting to esteem Claire and encourage her (witness her voicing my life would be better if she had died back in 2007), I made every effort to encourage her.

I believe, Claire, that you let so many be part of your life, and sought to be allowed into so many others and that came from your selflessness and compassion, likely born from your suffering. Although in earlier life while you worked out exactly how to manage all of your relationships, especially from your unique situation, you still saw more than most ever will in their life. The section you wrote in your *Horizons of Hope* essay titled "Friends and Family," is the perfect reflection of your awareness of CF as it affected you and others, but also how it reflects your awareness of how critical relationships were despite the obstacles:

Life is an Adventure – Dare It

Friends and Family

I'm a very active person by nature. I want to be going places, doing things, seeing people. One thing I find hard is demanding and expecting too much of myself. There are times when I don't feel well and yet I think that I should make the effort to do this or that when I've arranged to do things with my friends. Then I blame others and myself when life becomes busy and full and I haven't got enough energy to cope.

Perhaps, selfishly on my part, I get frustrated that not many people understand about CF and its implications on daily life. I guess that is the same no matter what illness someone may have. This is one of the reasons why support groups exist. Part of their work is to educate people about certain issues. I remember having 'flu at a time when everyone else was suffering from it; mine went to a chest infection and made me feel quite ill. It didn't help to be told by one of my friends, "We all feel ill when we have flu, Claire." However, I know I'm my own worst enemy. I need to pace myself better because there are some days when I just wish I hadn't arranged to do things in the evenings. After work or a day in lectures, I get so tired and I must learn to say, "No." But that's very hard for me, because my philosophy is that life is to be lived-to the max!

After one of my operations, my friends from the church and university just came and sat with me, and I really appreciated that. One friend particularly, Sam O., understood my need. I didn't feel like talking, but every time I opened my eyes, she was there, jut smiling and being with me; it must have been boring for her just to sit for so long. She was one of the few people who appeared to understand how I was feeling. I am indebted to my friends because they are so good to me. I am never in want for cards, chocolates or visitors when I'm in hospital, or even when I'm unwell at home. I don't have brothers or sisters unfortunately, but God has really showered me with some wonderful friends and without their continued love, care and support, I really don't know where I'd be. They certainly don't allow me to feel sorry for myself, which sometimes is a daily battle. I don't think I began to feel sorry for myself until the last few years when the reality of having CF became a lot more apparent. However, as time progressed I'm ashamed to say I do feel life can be hard. I try not to let it show because that is not constructive, but nevertheless it's a battle when I'm ill.

I know CF has had an effect on my family. They worry about me because I don't worry about myself enough, or at least I don't let them know I worry. They've had to wait to see if I can come home from hospital in time for holidays or Christmas. Christmas with IVs isn't unusual. When I'm ill it's my Mum who knows about me best. She understands the real Claire Salter, because she has seen me at my lowest and my worst both physically and emotionally. I'm sure that if my friends saw me at these times, they wouldn't want to be my friends. She understands best, partly because she's my Mum and partly because she's a nurse. I think she is very strong, especially as she had to cope with so many difficult moments when even the doctors have been concerned.

I know that when I have intravenous antibiotics it puts quite a lot of pressure on my family. I'm grateful that my Mum helps me draw them up into the syringes and sometimes she wakes me up in the morning and gives me my IVS before I have to go to work or lectures, which saves me a lot of time. Mornings are not my favourite time of the day! One thing I do find difficult when I'm on intravenous antibiotics at home is keeping going at work when I feel so drained and when I know that other people can have time off when they're ill; but because I'd already had time off, I feel I have to keep going and when I am exhausted and unable to concentrate I must go into work. When I take time off I feel that CF is winning and I don't like to be defeated.

Sometimes one of the signs of an infection is coughing up blood. I know I have to phone the hospital if I cough up a certain amount, and it's quite frightening not knowing whether it's going to stop. One dilemma I have is that if I tell my family, it worries them, but I feel I want to tell someone because it worries me. Usually I just tell my Mum. She often calms me down and tells me not to worry about things. Being reassured that it doesn't mean I'm necessarily going to be seriously ill makes things feel better. So my family are the ones who do take the brunt of my illness. And they cope with me when I'm in a moaning mood.

When I was first diagnosed with CF, I really enjoyed all the attention but after a while it contributed to me feeling different from other people, so I would downplay my illness because I didn't want to be anyone special. Perhaps adults saw through my façade. However as I got older I realised how much I appreciated and needed the prayer and support of my church, even though I get a lot of attention through this. When I was particularly ill, on one occasion a hundred people met to pray for me. I know many other patients who don't have such a positive back up. However, when I'm feeling ill or down, it's easy to lose sight of these blessings. Hook Evangelical Church has been a tower of strength and encouragement to me. I try not to burden too many people with my problems. When people ask me how I am it's easy to become too introspective, so I generally try to respond to enquiries positively even when I sometimes feel rough, but I am learning more and more to let people know just how it is.[72]

---

[72] B.H.Edwards, Horizons of hope, 2000, Day One Publications

Chapter Twenty-Three

April 2012 – Not Like the Other Hospital Visits

Dear Claire,

In earlier chapters I wrote about the first part of 2012 and now, almost trying to delay the inevitable, I find myself back at this fateful time. As we know, your health continued to spiral out of control from the end of 2011 through the first few months of 2012.

As you grew weaker, one of the saddest things I observed was your decreasing ability to socialize with your beloved circle of friends, (Although, amazingly, you did manage to go out a few times during this time.) You also needed to rest, so while many visited you and checked in on you, you largely began to keep in touch by phone calls and text messages.

One of the first problems that cropped up was when the pump that was supposed to carefully time the infusion rate did not function properly, so we had to calculate the drips per minute as it was critical the antibiotic not be infused too quickly. You texted Rosie P. after she enquired how your IV infusion was going:

"Just running it now, thanks, had to wait a few hours before next dose."

Then to your friend Yasmine:

"Happy Easter; am worried that I'm not getting better and long term implications of that but going to think very positively and take it easy. 7th on Easter Saturday: Went into Kingston with Jo–bought 3 dresses for £34.00! Drugs going nicely without the pump!"

I do not remember this, Claire, but how you managed to shop in Kingston just astounds me. You were far from well, however, and struggled all weekend, even finding it difficult to get ready for Marg's for Easter Sunday lunch. You were finding it oh-so-hard to shower and get dressed in the mornings; indeed in hospital I had been helping you but on your return home, your shortness of breath became so bad you needed help even walking the few steps from the bathroom to the bedroom.

Your Tobramycin levels were too high, so we were told to stop that antibiotic and stop in at the hospital that Friday. You were desperate to go into work just for an hour or so over the three days you were home, as you always worried that you could be made redundant because of your disease. Again, Claire, you demonstrated sheer determination when no one else would have attempted it.

On the 11th April, during the couple of hours you went into work, I texted:

"Are you okay, do you want Debenham's or Laura Ashley duvet set on your bed? Alan from the hospital phoned – I said you would call him."

Your response was:

"Laura Ashley xx."

I am so pleased, Claire, that although you only enjoyed your new bed linen for a couple of nights, at least you chose the set you wanted. It is remarkable how small things like that are such a comfort to me now, knowing I sometimes got things right for you.

During those few days you had at home we sat on the bed together in the evenings, as we had done often over the years. I used to get cross with you wanting a king-sized bed when only you would sleep in it, but on reflection, how wise you were in a myriad of decisions you made. Many was the time when your breathing was so bad, especially during your swine flu days, that I snuck into bed with you overnight just so that I could monitor your shortness of breath and be a presence with you. I also wanted to give reassurance when you so often felt ill watching T.V. while your IVABs went through. I always made sure you had plenty of pillows to prop you up, as this was your most comfortable position. You also needed the windows, curtains and the door left wide open to give you that feeling of space, similar to when you were in your previous house in those awful swine flu days of 2009, and again before you were admitted to hospital. This time, however, the bad nights as well as the difficult days continued until you were readmitted. To lie awake and watch you sleep and to realise how amazingly fragile and precious you were is something I will never, ever forget.

You were always thinking of others, despite your own suffering. On Thursday evening 12th April (the last evening you were home) as you waited for your intravenous infusion to drip through, we sat watching *Sport Relief*. I had gone to the kitchen to make us a cuppa and when I returned you were crying at the injustice of the world. The program featured was a young orphan in Kenya, and you immediately wanted to donate money to make a difference to him and the many like him. Even during the worst of your own pain, your senses were heightened to the sorrow of others; in fact, I believe it made you more aware of their affliction.

This is so reflective of your nature, Claire; when you were so unwell yourself you continued to regularly put the needs of others before your own.

During those final days at home you loved the EDF (Energy supplier) T.V. advert that used Zingy as their mascot, especially loving the song he was based on: "You Walked into My Life," sung by Fern Kinney (1980). It refers to someone coming into our lives and taking over and that's what you did to me the day you were born. I used EDF as my energy supplier, with Zingy as their logo on printed materials, and he amused you so you even had a cut-out of him on display in the kitchen. My heart smiles when I think of that.

On Friday 13th April, you phoned Jo C. (your friend who completed her Social Work degree with you) to say you were needing to go to the hospital to get your Tobramycin levels checked, and you may not be able to make the evening meal you two were planning with Ruth W. I shake my head sadly at the planned events that were delayed, Claire; there would definitely be no meal that evening as, instead of going to the hospital in London, you ended up in the local one. More importantly, the lung transplant we felt sure would become a reality did not happen either, so the person I love most on this Earth could not remain with me either.

It is difficult Claire, when thinking back on these sad times, as I am sure you know. Although I am comforted you are in Heaven with our glorious Father, what do I do when God does not answer the many people's prayers in the way I trusted He would? What do we do when the person we love most is suffering so terribly? What do you do when. . .? The questions go on and on. It reminds me of the quote by Frederick Buechner in his book, *Wishful Thinking:*

"Compassion is the sometimes fatal capacity for feeling what it's like to live inside somebody else's skin. It is the knowledge that there can never really be any peace and joy for me until there is peace and joy finally for you too."[73]

---

[73]   Frederick Buechner, Wishful Thinking, 1993, Harper Collins, used by permission of the Frederick Buechner Literary Assets, LLC

Things came to a dramatic head that Friday morning. You needed help again to shower and get dressed, to attend work again for a short visit. I was mowing your lawn when I received the phone call from one of your work colleagues, Sandra S., to say they were extremely worried about you and an ambulance had been called. You spoke to me on the phone, cool as a cucumber, suggesting I come over. I knew, however, if an ambulance had been called, you had to be direly ill. I arrived barely in time to ride in the ambulance with you to the local hospital and Helen G. kindly followed us in your car. You had been speaking to a senior manager at the time and he had asked if you were okay. It was clear, however, you were not and hence the drama began in your office. When we reached the hospital, you were admitted to that awful Assessment Ward, but thankfully were transferred to the High Dependency Unit that evening; it saddens me you were no stranger to High Dependency Units. That same evening you were given a new antibiotic, which required careful monitoring as you were allergic to so many medications.

Saturday morning found you transferred to yet another ward, but thankfully you were visited by Jo and Leah as well as one of your school friends, Rebecca Mac, who happened to be a doctor at the hospital. You were concerned the nursing staff had not flushed your intravenous line and texted:

"Hi Mum, am worried about my line, nurses didn't flush it earlier or over-night and left the fluids not running and now there is resistance when they tried to flush. Am really worried there is a clot."

I soon arrived, armed with Hepsal (the flushing solution) and sterile equipment to resolve the problem.

Text exchanges with your mates show clearly just how ill you felt:

"Morning, just to let you know I was taken from work by ambulance to Epsom A&E and been in high dependency overnight. Now more stable and being kept at Epsom until there is a bed in London. The infection seems to have really taken a hold and have been feeling quite unwell. Been 8 weeks on IVs and little improvement but hope these new antibiotics help. Being moved to Intensive Care unit for closer observation – feeling very unwell. Xx."

Ever being one to make light of your illness, to another work colleague you wrote:

"Oh, Marianne, you'd have laughed. I came over really faint at work when speaking to one of the Area Managers – tried to hide it but asked to sit down, so he knew I was feeling unwell. He organised an ambulance–he looked concerned. So embarrassing being on office floor with 3 paramedics around me, then poor Helen turned the corner and saw me–her face looked so worried. I am a drama diva so we expect nothing less of course! Hope you have a lovely weekend and we must have coffee soon x."

I think this demonstrates how positive you still felt. Although feeling so unwell, you believed finding the right antibiotic to treat the infection would set you on the road to recovery. The following day, however, saw an ambulance take you up to London, with me accompanying you. Little did we know, as we journeyed up in the ambulance that spring day, we were hurtling toward your worst nightmare. As we left Epsom hospital for London, we had no idea you were now running out of time.

For those couple of weeks in April, your texts continued to plot how unwell you felt. When I left that first day you texted:

"Love you lots-couldn't do this without you."

To which I replied:

"You are my number 1 x."

Your response was:

"Don't forget to give Nicola a ready meal for me to eat later. Feeling a bit weird but not as bad as earlier. Love you lots. Xx."

To other friends:

"I've had a couple of blips and now my pancreas is misbehaving so nil by mouth and on IV fluids; not any improvement in chest infection."

Then to Natalie:

"Morning Nat, my infection is back with a vengeance and when my heart is racing I feel really unwell and weird-quite scary."

Catherine D. texted:

"Hello honeybun, any news?"

To which you replied:

"Had CT scan of my brain today and having a heart scan tomorrow, where they put bubbles in it! Think they are being very thorough in checking everything. Being put on a third IV antibiotic to kill the infection. Thanks so much for asking. How are you both doing?

Hoping to only stay another 7-10 days-thanks for your love and care, it means a lot."

To Sasha you texted:

"Thanks very much for visiting regularly. Echo investigation at 2:30 on Friday. Thank everyone so very much for your prayers, love and care this week; seems that the heart is working very hard due to the lungs not working well and that infection and side effects of drugs are all having an effect on my body. More results next week. Please pray this really eradicates the infection for good, or a few weeks for a bit of a break from feeling so ill. Have a lovely weekend all of you, lots of love, Claire."

On April 26th to Sasha:

"New drug started today; trying not to worry but can't help getting tearful thinking about the future. Being allowed out for an hour. Can I call you later, out at lunch, and then going to Chapel service? Xx."

On the 23rd April Sasha asked:

"And how is the patient today?"

To which you replied:

"The patient is doing better thanks. Ruth and I are in café Romano, just up the road; back at 3:30. x."

On the 25th April you texted to Nat:

"Had bad bleed last night. Loved all my gifts, Nat, you spoil me. Thanks for being there for me. X."

To another friend:

"Starting a new antibiotic that makes me sick so have to have intravenous medication to not make me sick (if that makes sense!)."

To Helen:

"Hi Helen, had a longer sleep, about 7 hours; feeling unwell and can tell the infection is back, but observations stable at moment. Thank you so much for yesterday Helen, am so glad you were here x."

The following day you actually managed a hair appointment and Auntie met us halfway on the ride back, driving you up to hospital through Richmond Park. It was a lovely afternoon and you were really on good form, which encouraged me. It really was a roller coaster, however, as your texts to your friends show, the next day.
April 28th to Helen and Stuart C.:

"So good to have you in England-still in hospital, holiday cancelled for next week, not responding to antibiotics, and feeling poorly."

They replied:

"So good to see you; God is for you, keep fighting like you always have. We send you big hugs and to your Mum too."

To Helen and Rob M. (who later brought their young son Sebastian to see you):

"No change in bloods, it's good levels not up but not down either. On oxygen again. Would so love to be home next weekend. love you all xx."

By the end of April, your pancreatitis returned with a vengeance. To Chris you texted:

"Doctor told me had to be 'nil by mouth' again, due to pancreatitis. Determined to get better this week, so desperate to get back to life, though I think I will be in here a while, was up for two hours in night, heart racing, etc. Feeling poorly and this new antibiotic is not working (I can tell almost immediately what antibiotic will work, and what won't).

Thanks, Chris, can call you tomorrow eve."

He responded:

"Hi Claire, yes any time, would be nice to chat. You are always in my thoughts and my Mum always asks about you. She knows I'm in touch with a special lady called Claire."

Dave M., who also visited you, texted:

"Hey, MBLS [My Beautiful Little Sister], hope you are feeling better today – I hope you don't mind but I shared a little of our time together with the Impact youth group and every one of them prayed for you, Claire. It was really special, just like you. Praying that the Lord will surround you with his love and do a miracle of healing in you. Looking forward to seeing you tomorrow. Sleep well my lovely, and if you ever want to talk I'll keep my phone on all night."

You replied:

"Thanks for your encouragement, Dave – means a lot."

To Patsy, one of your uni friends:

"Thanks, Patsy, feeling weak but going to do my very best to kick this infection into touch! Can't wait till your birthday!"

How little did we know, then, Claire, you would be in Heaven the morning of the 25th May, on Patricia's birthday.

You texted Faye:

"Hi Faye, finding it tough – had pancreatitis as well. Thanks so much for prayers – please pray for right antibiotics and for my body to keep strong along with my mind. Thanks so much."

Her response was:

"Hi Claire, I've got everyone I know praying. I hope you can feel them. Love you. Xx."

To Jo C., one of your social work friends who visited you:

"Hi, Jo, thanks for last night."

By this point, the pancreatitis was making you extremely sick and oral medication was not controlling it, so you were then put on an intravenous antiemetic. Unfortunately you had a bad reaction to that and the crash team was called. Once they left that evening, we practiced breathing techniques the physios had taught you. Although I was becoming terribly concerned, as I'd never seen you take quite so many hits before, this was at least where I could help. It was easy for me with healthy lungs and heart to get into a rhythm, which you were then able to follow.

Your pastor, Paul Pease, had visited you while the medical team was trying to establish what made your heart rate so rapid. At this time, one of the senior house officers had written on the white board in your room all the things that could potentially be wrong. Paul had then texted to say how brave you were, and he told the Wednesday prayer meeting that evening, too.

The next emergency occurred when you attended the Lung Function the following Friday; your oxygen saturation dropped markedly. You then had an enormous bleed which caused three of the doctors to come running when yet another crash call was placed. When they transported you back to the ward, a peripheral line was inserted so there would be another means of intravenous access. That same evening you had a moving text message conversation with Catherine D. who asked:

"Hello, how are you today?"

You responded:

"I would love to say better as so bored of giving same old story, however bit of a drama this eve as crash team were called due to me having a very bad reaction to a drug. How are you two?"

Her reply read:

"Never mind us, you pickle, I've been sitting here staring at my phone going in to panic mode. Sooo good to hear from you but what a very scary evening for you. I am so sorry, you just don't deserve any of this. You are the sweetest person in the world and life just shouldn't be so tough on you."

Several tried to keep you spirit up as you endured things in that time that were truly staggering. You were having blood tests done every day, while the lung transplant talks were still ongoing. They hoped you would make the urgent lung transplant list. Almost a week before you died, the registrar told you that Team Salter had simply hit a brick wall in your marathon, likening it to the worst part of the race, but you were nearing the finishing line of being so unwell, and if you could push through, in a few days you would be feeling better. She did say however, you may have to go home on a ventilator, but she was confident you would get home.

Jo R. came that afternoon, but she realised you were seriously unwell and sensibly did not stay long. Ruth H. had met up with your group of uni friends (you still kept in touch with so many) and brought in a card they had all signed. I still have all your cards, Claire; they demonstrate the love your countless friends had for you and you for them.

Because I visited every day, we did not need to text unless there were specific things you wanted me to bring in etc. Our text exchanges centred mostly around how ill you felt:

April 21st:

"Mum, I found the website with the instructions for the rattan garden furniture so you can get handyman to put it together. Answer to prayer: I walked with Auntie all the way down to Carluccio's at South Kensington station and back without oxygen! Love you so much, Mum, sleep well."

April 24th:

"Love you so much and praying you will feel better."

April 25th:

"Please call. Could you come up later Mum? Just don't feel well xx."

This was the day Yasmine and Bruce visited and I was going to delay a while to give you some time with them; however you were feeling so ill, I came immediately you texted.

April 26th:

Dave M. coming at 11:00, can you call?"

April 30th at 06:22 a.m.

"Really bad, please call."

Then after my whole day spent with you at the hospital, at 8:00 p.m.:

"So bad, Mum, pain so bad. Phone me when you are home."

To which I replied:

"I'm home, ensure oxygen is on 2 litres."

You said:

"Yes, have just checked it. Love you xx."

I said:

"And me you. You are on the church prayer circle. X."

As recorded above, it was a lovely, sunny afternoon when you somehow managed a trip out of hospital for your hair to be done in Cobham. Although we did not have time to call in to No. 10 because your IVABs were due, we circled around the estate in the car and you saw your new home for what would be the last time. We met Pat halfway, and she drove you back to the hospital through Richmond Park (the largest park in London) which was so picturesque on that beautiful afternoon. Little did we know things were about to plummet from bad to worse.

Chapter Twenty-Four

May 2012 – Beginning of the End

My Precious Claire,

May 2012 was to be your last on this Earth, and although I know you are so full of life and joy in our eternal home now, I still grieve as we did not really know they would be your last days. We could have been told, but we were not. Regardless, you faced your challenge with more bravery than any I had personally witnessed in my nursing career. They say courage is not the absence of fear, but the fortitude to move forward in spite of it. In that regard, you are the most courageous person I have ever known; moving forward bravely, even when you knew it was to the end of your time in this world. The fact that you were heroic despite feeling the cold, grey, ghostly fingers of fear is perfectly captured in your section, "The Touch of Fear" in your *Horizons of Hope* essay:

Life is an Adventure – Dare It

The Touch of Fear

Sharing a room with Carol on one hospital visit was a big eye-opener for me. It was quite shocking to see her so ill. Her husband brought their five year old daughter to visit and all the little girl wanted was for her Mummy to play with her, but Carol just couldn't muster the strength to do it. She kept saying to me, "A couple of years ago I was like you, Claire." It was frightening to hear that I could be like Carol in a few years' time. The doctor had just suggested she consider a lung transplant and Carol amazed me how she coped with the news. She was a great source of strength to me; I thought she was so brave. I don't think I could ever be that brave.

Each three monthly outpatient's visit for me means seeing the dietician, the clinical nurse specialist for CF, having blood and lung function tests, chest x-rays, visiting the physiotherapy department, and then waiting to see the doctor. An electro-cardiogram (ECG) once a year is also part of the process, because CF can also affect the heart. Often patients with CF are seriously ill prior to going on the lung transplant list, although survival rates are improving. However, because of the shortage of donors, some patients do not get a suitable donor in time. This is something that really worries me, the thought that I may be put forward for a lung transplant and may not get it, or if I do manage to get a suitable donor, I may be too unwell by that time to go through the operation successfully.

Taking it one step further, if I did have the operation, the new organs may not last long before they would be rejected. In terms of transplantation as well, it is difficult to comprehend what it would be like to have someone else's lungs inside my body. It is possible for "matched" relatives (those whose body-type tissues are a good match with mine) to give part of their lung instead, and whilst I know members of my wider family would be willing to be tested, I'm not sure how I would feel about it all.

My experience of, on the one hand having an incurable illness, but on the other of being able to live life relatively well has meant that when I compare myself with others who have CF or different disabilities, I feel guilty because they may be worse than myself. This is especially so when I am with other CF people and they often look more frail and are, perhaps, coughing more;

I wonder if I am an offence to them because I am comparatively well. At times I hate the fact that life is so unfair to so many others who suffer each day; so the guilt not only incorporates my feelings towards others, but of God too. But I thank God for the relative health He has given me and when I view this life in the light of eternity, I remember that He has a reason for everything. Although I don't understand it fully now, one day I know I will.

Often when I look at other people I wonder, "My goodness, how do they cope?" I have difficult days, but when I see people so much worse than myself, I think that I've got away lightly. However no one can know how you're feeling and I try to avoid using the phrase, "I understand how you feel." I can't fully understand what they are going through, just as no one can fully understand me in my position. There is some common ground, though, when we each experience illness. I believe that sometimes people who have gone through difficult times in their lives are often the best people to talk to because they do understand some of your feelings and experiences. Sometimes I feel very isolated, even from my closest friends and then I get frustrated. I have days when I think just nobody understands, or ever can.

I do struggle and I do find life harsh at times. I'm not pretending that I don't get frustrated with people who can't understand what it's like to be in my shoes. I have to admit that often I don't cope with my illness very well. So it makes me smile when I'm told that I cope well. Sometimes people don't want to know when I'm having a bad day and who can blame them? Often we don't want to hear about each other's troubles because we've got enough troubles of our own. That's when I get frustrated with my situation and with God, because day to day problems come as thick and fast whether one is healthy or ill. But the next person hasn't got CF to cope with, even though the next person has probably many other problems. That's part of the day-to-day struggles of living with a chronic, life-threatening illness. . .getting so tired, needing to take all my medication, do my physio and sort myself out before I leave the house in the morning.

Burghardt, in Horizons of Hope: "In my opinion death is an insult; the stupidest, ugliest thing that can ever happen to a human being."[74]

Brennan Manning, a Christian writer, suggests that the separation from loved ones is too painful to consider. Perhaps for most of us the frenetic pace of life and the immediate claims of the present moment leave no time, except for fleeting reflections at funerals, to contemplate seriously where we came from and where we are going. Saint Benedict offers the sober advice to "keep your own death before your eyes each day." And yet we are not cowed into timidity by death and life. Were we forced to rely on our own shabby resources we would be pitiful people indeed. But the awareness of Christ's presence, risen from the dead, persuades us that we are buoyed up and carried on by a life greater than our own. Hope means that in Christ, by entrusting ourselves to him, we can courageously face evil. . .we can then face death."[75].

Euthanasia is a topic that frightens me and I worry that people won't want me around because I'll be a drain on society in terms of money. Some of my drugs already cost £8,000 per year and I'm worried that if euthanasia becomes legalised, the pressure from society not to "waste" money in this way may be to my detriment. Euthanasia, is of course, such an emotive issue but I know that if it does become legal, there could be problems for those who have long-term incurable illnesses. I don't think society will know where to draw the line even though they may have good intentions, and I believe we will worry about who we can trust and what we say, whilst wanting the best medical advice. It is so important for a patient to have confidence and trust in the medical staff.

---

[74]   (Walter J. Burghardt, 1980 'Tell the next generation', New York Paulist Press, p315).

[75]   Manning, B. 1994 Abba's Child. Navpress, Colorado, p148-150

I do worry about the future – having CF is like having a big, dark cloud hovering over me. I don't notice it all the time but it is always there. I don't know what the future holds; I don't know how long I'm going to live; I don't know which avenue my health will take. I might be reasonably all right for ten or twenty years, or only two or three – life feels very insecure. That's the hardest thing, it's like a time bomb inside you, the clock is ticking but you don't know when time will run out. I get so annoyed when people say they could get run over by a bus tomorrow, because that kind of reasoning doesn't allow me, as a person with a chronic illness, to feel my pain of the uncertainty of my life. It's the fear of the unknown, and perhaps people who don't live with an issue like this do not fully understand.

Because of my worries about my own mortality, I have recently had some very helpful chats with one of the community cystic fibrosis nurses. It has been vital for me to discuss how I feel about certain aspects of CF and how I can come to terms with it. I have found that I can really be open and honest with Liz, partly because she knows what I am talking about and she understands, and also because she is a professional rather than a member of my family or a close friend. All these issues around death and dying made me very tearful. I couldn't talk about this without crying, and Liz reassured me that she would have been worried if I hadn't talked about such important issues and that it was OK and natural to feel this way. I'm a strong believer in counselling and although this is not Christian counselling, I can honestly say that it has helped me speak freely of what I am afraid of. Even as a Christian, it is natural to have these kinds of feelings. What's important is how you work through all this with God.

I don't mind admitting that often I'm very scared. I'm scared of what life may hold and I'm scared of being in pain. I had begun to feel a sense of tremendous anxiety about being away from home and thinking a lot about dying and becoming seriously ill. I was in America at the time, taking a holiday after a friend's wedding there. I was very anxious about going, and just before the return trip I was really worried about not making it home. It was not that I was particularly ill, but I was worried about dying in a country I didn't know, and without my family or friends around me. This was quite frightening, because I suppose I am like everyone else in that I don't want to die alone. My friend Ali had died a year beforehand, surrounded by a loving family and caring friends and her death had affected me a great deal.

Ali's death brought my own mortality a lot closer, and issues that I had blocked out in the past, or did not fully understand, seemed much more apparent. I'm afraid of not being able to cope with my illness, and of being dependent upon other people, or even being wheelchair bound. I'm very concerned with the logistics of how I die. What if I die and leave a husband and young children, or other relatives? There just seems to be so much to think about and there are no answers or guarantees for the future. Before I feel ready to go He may say, "OK Claire, it's time." And I won't want to die. One of my prayers, and it's something I feel strongly that we should all pray, is that God will help me accept my situation and be ready to confront death.

There are times that I get tremendously excited about the thought of heaven and I just can't wait to go. I think it will be amazing to be free from all pain and tears. I cannot fully grasp it, but I guess that if we had a fore-taste of heaven we'd all want to go right now. However, I know God wants to use me while I am here and I hope that, despite myself, I can somehow reach out to other people's hearts and touch their pain. God has been so faithful and loving throughout my life that I know I can and must trust Him for what lies ahead. But it's easy to write that and a lot harder to do. Part of my anger is knowing that God is all powerful and could change my situation if He wanted; yet I know also that in His infinite wisdom He has chosen not to. However, I have very ambiguous feelings. It is frustrating that I can do nothing about my illness, but I try not to let these feelings alter my trust in God, because I know He has everything planned for my ultimate good.

I often think about marrying and having children, even though the opportunity hasn't arisen yet! If I do get married, I wonder if it would be fair to have children. When my health deteriorates, how would my husband cope and respond to major decisions that he would have to make in the future? So is it fair to get married? There are so many questions to consider and I'm not sure how, or if, they will be answered. I guess the hardest thing is just giving it over to God and letting Him control everything.

In writing about my experiences, I feel very exposed. This is all the real Claire Salter. Not the one who so often hides behind a façade that everything is all right.

May 2012

On 1ˢᵗ May, you responded to your Greek friend, Ndullee:

"Thanks for text, feel very weak and tough time since yesterday as I reacted badly to a drug and crash team had to be called – still need the right drug for my chest as infection really taken a hold now. So sorry can't be at book group this evening, let me know if any gossip. Lots of love to you all xx."

On the morning of 2ⁿᵈ May, Auntie Pat had come up so I could do some chores and run some errands; the arrangement was that I would take over from her at lunch time. Pete, our handyman, had come to your home to do a few jobs and then he was to go back to my house to help with some pruning in the garden. I was at the waste disposal site when I received a call from Pat to tell me you had received some serious news regarding your health; all you would say when you came on the phone was that you wanted me at the hospital immediately. When I arrived, you tearfully explained a nurse had come to see you from the pre-ward meeting to say you were very unwell; so much so that you would be fast tracked for a lung transplant. Her sombre warning, however, was you may not get a donor in time as the CF was making you more ill than it ever had in the past.

That evening, the 2nd May the consultant came to see you and we both requested complete honesty and transparency; we made it very clear that we wanted to know exactly when they thought you were deteriorating beyond the point of recovery. We wanted to know because as grave as that news would be, if it became the case, throughout your deterioration I wanted to do all I could for you, remaining at the hospital continuously. We could not have made our request plainer; we could not have made it easier for them to understand; we simply wanted to know your illness trajectory. Thus, the medics promised they would keep us advised at all times. You so deserved it; you deserved even more than I gave. How often through the years your wonderful church stood by you, and that evening of Wednesday 2nd May was no different. Yet not only Hook (your church), but there was so much intercession on your behalf by friends and relatives, up and down the country, and even abroad.

Receiving the awful news of your rapidly deteriorating health on 2nd May was an eventuality I had sort of prepared for; however we had been given assurances by the team that there was lots they could do to bring about improvement. I say "sort of," because even after years of dreading that moment, years of fighting against it and believing you would somehow beat the odds (as you had with swine flu three years earlier, despite us being told how bad your lungs were and how seriously ill you were during that time), there was a sense of dismay that your number might have actually been called. Subsequently, I stayed in your room for eight nights as the doctors tried an assortment of antibiotic cocktails in an attempt to bring your

CRP down. I think by the time they had reached the last, it was about the twelfth or thirteenth different combination of antibiotics.

Somehow, we still managed to get you out in the wheelchair, oxygen in tow, for a cup of coffee with Patricia over at the café. Bernie, Helen and Jo S. also came up that Saturday, where we had cakes in the Humming Bird Café also. Rach came with Asha, your goddaughter, and was so good at bringing you food to tempt your appetite. Over the course of the next couple of weeks you had so many visitors; to name a few: Jo R., Hannah and Mark, Sarah C., Jo C. came up (and with her husband for a second visit as well), Helen G., Marianne T., Susan G. and several other work colleagues. Uni friends included Ruth, Geraldine, Caroline and church friends visited, including Nicola, Nat, Rich B., Emma and Claire. There were so many more too, Claire, and I am worried I will miss many people, who all deserve mention. Emma T. came to enable me to dash home to get some laundry done and she instigated writing Bible texts on the white board in your room to remind you of God's promises.

After the eight nights I stayed with you, I slept at home but called in almost daily to collect items you required and to check all was okay with your empty house. Boxes in the garage were still unpacked, and I knew I would unpack them when I had time, but you were my priority at that point. Almost as one last desperate act of faith, I called Screwdriver to go to your house and put your garden furniture together, hoping and praying you would be able to use it over the summer.

We had enjoyed sitting out in one of the parks close to the hospital one afternoon, when the weather was okay-ish earlier in the year, but it saddened me when you were far too ill to go out when the hot weather came later in May. I pushed you up the Kings Road a couple of times so that you could have a sense of normalcy. We ate pizza and enjoyed a Starbucks, your favourite coffee and always an integral part of your previous hospital rehabilitation programmes.

On previous hospital stays I would nip down the road at lunch time and bring you a latte back, together with a vegetarian panini since you never developed the penchant for hospital food. (Who can blame you?) On one such foray up the Kings Road, we spoke to a wonderful young man in Starbucks who was reading a Christian book. When he offered his help to get the wheelchair and oxygen cylinder down the front step of the shop, you chatted to him and discovered he was indeed a Christian. It reminded us of how God provided these various helps along the way, Claire, just as he did with the hospital's chaplaincy service. One of the consultants involved in your care, also a Christian, came to pray with you when you were too unwell to go to the chapel for the Sunday afternoon service, and you felt very much invigorated by this ministry. They were God's servants, Claire, and it reminded me of the song "Shout to the Lord" by Darlene Zchech, and as the words of this song clearly state, God is our shelter and refuge. How much that lovely young man, unbeknown to him, demonstrated God's love that day.[76]

We bought something towards your birthday present in India Jane, one of the shops you loved. I wanted you to know that there was still a hope, still a future, whether it be on Earth or in Heaven.

Auntie Pat gathered all the phone numbers you had given her when you could no longer speak to friends and relatives yourself. Again, looking at these in your own handwriting is so nostalgic and special to me. Later, Jo R. helped retrieve the mobile numbers from your phone, so we could notify as many as possible of your sad demise, whilst Emma H. retrieved and converted all your text messages into emails for me. Everyone rallied around you, and aside from all the medical care was my minute-by-minute, hour-by-hour care of you in that hospital room, my precious daughter. We bought and used Dettol wet wipes like there was no tomorrow to ensure your room stayed fresh and clean between the hospital domestic daily hygiene visit.

Following the bad news on 2nd May you emailed a handful of friends the following message:

---

[76]   Shout to the Lord, by Darlene Zschech, (Integrity's Hosanna! Music)

"My lovely friends, I'm so sorry to impart this to you by text but it's the best way to communicate and ask for prayer one again. I've been told, in the doctor's words, that I am very, very unwell. I am being fast tracked for transplant although they have had a talk with me about the possibility of that not working and not making it until then. I don't want to scare you or worry you and I will give this all that I have but please, please pray and get others to pray too. You have made my life so wonderful, special, exciting and fun; let's pray there are more times to come. I love you all and wanted the opportunity to say how amazing you are, each and every one of you, and the love and support you have shown me over the years has meant more than words can ever say. I love you all very dearly. Now let's get praying and down to business. Xxxxxxxxxxxxxxxxxxxxxx."

I knew in my heart I would not see you off to work again, but begged God to please help me to see you out with your friends again. Of course, as horrific as it was to watch as a mother, I can only understand a little of how very hard this final road was for you, Claire. I know, however, deep inside you knew God was with you. You spoke of how you felt God may be preparing you to die, and although I did not tell you, at the same time He was preparing me for your untimely death. I make no excuse for numerous references to Meg Woodson, who lost not one, but two children to cystic fibrosis. Her books were my constant companions through your final admission, and continuing in these first three years since your death.

As alluded to in chapter two, I had grabbed a book that morning of 2nd May as I rushed to the hospital; a book I did not recognise and one I certainly had not bought. The book was titled *Turn it into Glory*[77] and was written by an American Christian author. It told the story of her twenty-three year old daughter, Peggie's last weeks of life in hospital when she, too, stayed with her daughter. It detailed the life-upheaving

---

[77]   Turn it into Glory, by Meg Woodson (1991 © Meg Woodson, Hodder and Stoughton)

roller coaster ride they had, similar to ours. She also wrote to her daughter Peggie after she had died, but as if the death of their daughter was not bad enough, she and her pastor husband had already lost a young son, who had died some years earlier from CF. Later I would read the equally heart breaking account of her son's death, titled *Following Joey Home.*[78] During this time, I pleaded with God, Claire, to let us have you just for a short time longer. . .for you to get home (as we had been promised by the hospital you would). . .to sit in your garden that summer. . . .anything, just more time. How often we bargain with God, Claire. At the same time however, I knew I would never, ever be ready to let you go. Yet I knew you were fading when you had no strength left to text and phone people, nor even watch TV those last days.

You received quite a few responses to your landmark email on 2nd May. Some of them read:

"Dearest Claire, please fight this infection. You must feel so overwhelmed by everything. I care about you so much."

More followed the next day, from Rosie P.:

"You are so loved by so many at Hook, stand firm in your faith today. God is for you, not against you."

On 3rd May you replied:

"Been feeling really poorly still had all manner of tests including CT scan-awaiting results."

---

[78]   Following Joey Home, by Meg Woodson (© 1978, Zondervan Publishing House)

From Sandra at work:

"Sitting at my desk having a little weep. Darling, I totally refuse to lose you as my assistant team manager – you know all my secrets! Got all my prayer people praying – keep strong, hun, so many people love you and want you better. Whole of Christ Church Fetcham praying, Naomi sends her love. Kulu is praying for you, Oliver, Scarlet and Julie send their love as indeed everyone does. Keep strong, beautiful lady."

Other texts that week included:

From Sarah C.:

"Both girls prayed for you at breakfast, thinking of you loads."

Other responses to your friends read:

"Infection levels doubled in blood again –please keep praying. Things not good Chris, on emergency viability for transplant. Have been told I'm very ill, will keep fighting. Love to you and your mum."

To Jo C.:

"New IV started yesterday and still not responding. Tough weekend but managed to walk length of ward yesterday with oxygen, hope it's been good weekend for you all."

Helen G. wrote on Friday 4th May:

"Everyone is thinking about you. Stuart said hurry up, get well.

Trish sends her love and will text you. 'Claire is such a special person,' she said.

Joss texted me yesterday and sends her love.

Alex asked me but he walked away when I said you are very unwell. He said, 'No, she can't be, I'm praying for her.'

Carol –Business support –her eyes fill up when she comes to ask me and then she walks away."

So, dear Claire, you had so much love and so many thoughts from everyone around you. You also received beautiful gifts from your colleagues; a basket hamper and also a bay tree. The card accompanying these read:

"Dear Claire, As ever you are in our thoughts and prayers. A little something for your garden in readiness for when you go home. With our love, the North East Teams."

On the 9th May, the day you should have gone to Jordan with Hannah and Mark, you emailed Helen the following. It was the only time when you cancelled a holiday:

"Hi Helen, so poorly, please can you call my auntie for update?"

Other texts over those eight days continued to chart your decline:

"Feel so poorly –gave me 3 new antibiotics. Just so short of breath. Rough weekend but managing to walk length of ward with oxygen. Mum and I just gone out for some fresh air back in 15 x. Of course I am in the wheelchair with oxygen."

A couple of days later you seemed a little better so I left you overnight to come home to sleep. I could not believe how good it felt to be in my own bed after eight solid days and nights in the hospital. It was wonderful but I felt so guilty as I wondered, *What about Claire wanting her own bed, her own home? At least I get to go home, have some normality, even if just to sleep.*

Meg Woodson also experienced this exhaustion; the chronic tiredness I imagine any person goes through knowing they are going to lose someone precious whilst trying to support that loved one. It is not just the physical aspect, but the emotional roller-coaster of the whole experience. Meg told the hospital staff that Joey was always worse at night, during which time Meg, herself, was obviously exhausted too. She, too, guiltily longed for her own bed.

I truly believed, however, that God was watching over you, as the scripture says: "Indeed, he who watches over Israel will neither slumber nor sleep," (Psalm 121:4, NIV). Even at home I dared not delay, for there was so much to do and so little time to do it in and I needed to return to the hospital to care for you.

I suppose, however, some slight respite against the guilt is the notion of being instructed to, "Put on your oxygen mask first," when you fly in a plane. If you are not taking care of yourself to some degree, how can you take care of your child? Still it is difficult, but again, this appears to be a common experience with parents going through the same thing, as Meg Woodson echoes in her account, with her daughter: "How could I take care of Peggie if I could not sleep?"[79]

---

[79]   Turn it into Glory, by Meg Woodson (1991 © Meg Woodson, Hodder and Stoughton)

If you remember, Claire, relatives staying at the hospital was most frowned upon, so I almost had to take a leave for a few days. If the hospital staff had told us how ill you really were, of course, they would have had no option than to let me stay – even encourage it – but I had to ask permission every night I wanted to be with you. As with Meg decades ago, my prayers were in unison with so many of your family and friends up and down the British Isles and beyond. Like Meg, Claire, I had yelled at you, just as she yelled at her son so much in years past, when you did not take care of your health. As if you could have made a difference to it, but we know of course that CF is no respecter of persons, and nothing could ultimately have saved either Meg's children nor you from this cruel disease.

As referred to above, when we were told there was still a possibility you could get home, I put the two new (double) Laura Ashley beds and headboards together that had been delivered to your home, made them up with your new sheets and also tidied the garden. Helen and Janice had planted sweet peas in readiness for your break at home, even if it was going to be just for an afternoon. I had even begun making tentative enquiries about booking a private ambulance to transport you.

Astonishingly (due to your resolute determination again), we did manage a few more trips out, wheelchair and portable oxygen cylinder always in tow. We headed just over the road for coffee in the lovely café where, of course, they loved you to bits and spoiled you. Then we went to Battersea Park for a brief walk around the grounds; I took you in the car, then pushed you in what had become our constant companion on such trips, the ever present wheelchair. I remember the couple of times the oxygen tipped out of the wheelchair while we were going down the kerb though, and hurt your foot! As if you were not suffering enough, Claire, and that was my fault I let it slip. I am so sorry.

You became so desperate, Claire, almost beyond enduring anymore. Meg Woodson remarked concerning her son, that she should have rebelled a long time ago regarding decisions made by the hospital staff.[80] I too should have rebelled. I should have questioned more, and advocated for you more fiercely. Similarly, just as Meg would say to her husband that it could be the day their son died, so you would say to me: "I'm dying Mum, and this could be the day." You would also say, "I wish you would stay tonight," and oh, Claire, I should have, I should have. However, in those dark hospital days when I should have and did not, I know that the Lord Himself stood by you, as He had done so many times before; witness your teen journal when you refer to this (2 Timothy 4:17).

When they put you on the continuous (24/7) IVAB, Aztreonam with yet another aminoglycoside, we tried going across the service road at the back of the hospital just to the local pub. You had egg and chips, but it had become just too much of an effort with the wheelchair, oxygen and now the drip stand. I think that was the start of the real decline, despite your CRP coming down markedly, over the next week. Brian (our pastor when you were a child) once said about his then-wife Barbara's care that the battle was relentless just to survive without anything else going wrong. As with Barbara, so it was with you, Claire, that countless things had indeed gone wrong over the years; your gallstones, your heart murmur, the times in the High Dependency Unit monitoring your heart, the port operations, the months you were ill with swine flu. Indeed the list goes on and you learned not to want, I guess, in order to avoid disappointment.

It is a well-known fact that when we are ill, we want the person closest to us and I cannot tell you, Claire, how much I wanted to be the mum who would care for you perfectly in your last illness. Like all humanity, however, I am imperfect and made so many mistakes. I am only slightly comforted in that Meg Woodson felt the same thing, and told her daughter, Peggie she was sorry she had not been a better mother[81].

---

[80]   Meg Woodson, Following Joey Home, 1978 Zondervan Publishing House

[81]   Meg Woodson, Turn It Into Glory, (Hodder and Stoughton, 1991)

By then, not only were you having daily blood tests but you were also having daily Tinzaparin injections to prevent deep vein thrombosis as you were now spending the majority of time in bed. The problems were escalating exponentially. One day seemed to blur into another as you dipped further into decline; I don't honestly know how you coped, and we still had no feedback from the doctors despite asking numerous times a day. It seemed they would discuss changes of antibiotics with us, tell us you were making progress, but not tell us what we had both pleaded to hear: an honest appraisal as to how you were really doing.

It was not until later in 2012 after I had sent for and read your medical notes, that I discovered on Wednesday the 16th May, two weeks following the news that you were very ill, a "Do Not Attempt Resuscitation" order was written and placed in your notes. Despite this order stating it had been fully discussed with both of us, we were never, ever told. Had I known this, my precious Claire, I would have never have left your hospital room.

In fact, on Friday 18th May, one week before you died, you were given a very positive lung transplant talk, where we were informed fully and formally of the transplant process and that the CF team was proceeding toward this goal. You asked if you could attend Rich and Caroline's wedding, scheduled for December if you were on the list and you were even told you could!

You were in the meantime, however, charted for increased doses of intravenous steroids and that evening you had a large bleed from your lungs as your saturations dropped by 10%. A further intravenous line was inserted so you could start fluids, and you were placed on continuous ventilation via a non-invasive ventilator.

You were fast-approaching the last and worst week of your life, Claire, and all I could do was look on, amazed that, despite all the onslaughts hurled at you, despite barely being able to breathe, you lasted as long as you did. Truthfully it was also the worst week of my life, seeing you suffer in every way, but who am I to complain, when it was you doing the dying?

On Saturday 19th, we received another up-beat talk, this time by the registrar that likened you to running a marathon; stating that you had reached your lowest ebb but that you would get home, even on a ventilator. This talk is actually what caused me to spend time out of the hospital and in your home in preparation for your homecoming. I knew the hospital would need to arrange a generator for the ventilator, plus a myriad of other pieces of medical equipment, and I needed to clear the decks for this to happen. I will never forget you felt so very ill this day and never really recovered past this point. I prepared everything, Claire, but you never came home.

Sunday 20th was another extremely difficult day; I do not recall anything significantly bad happening, it was just another day when you slipped further away. Sheila Hancock, writing of her husband's declining health put it well:

"He is fading; I want to pull him back; force him to stay. I want to scream; don't leave me,[82]" (p20).

Other quotes from Mayfield's book state:

She had so much living to do; she left such a promising, young life. She will never experience x again, she didn't get to make the trip she was planning. The remorse is for words left unsaid and deeds left undone. If last days, last hours or last conversations had been other than we would have wished, we can be left with unfinished business. The words "if only" can drive us mad.

Jer. 51:15, "A voice is heard in Ramah, lamentation and bitter weeping. Rachel weeping for her children, she refused to be comforted for her children, because they are no more," (p 71).

---

[82]   Sheila Hancock, (cited in: Sue Mayfield) Living with Bereavement, 2008, Lion Hudson Plc

(p 87)It's a beautiful, spring day. And I hate it because he can't see it. [83]

I tried to recall the last time you were really yourself on Earth, before the ravages of CF stole your life. You did not live to experience so much of what you wanted but I am comforted that in Heaven you have a far happier life now and for that I must be grateful. Still, it aches that, together with so many others, we thought this was another routine hospitalisation; we had no idea things could get so bad so rapidly and at this point it scared us that we had to admit you were running out of time.

Debby S., who so often emailed/sent cards of encouragement wrote:

"Does hope seem distant? Take a moment to listen to your Shepherd, rather than your fears. Clear your mind of every racing thought and know that these words have been prayed for you: 'May the God of hope fill you with all joy and peace in believing, so that by the power of the Holy Spirit you may abound in hope,' (Romans 15:13 NIV)."

There were so many false hopes, Claire; the promise of you coming home, the false explanation that you had hit a brick wall but that you would overcome this infection. C.S. Lewis faced the same sense of despair concerning prayer during the terminal phase of his wife's illness:

"What chokes every prayer and hope is the memory of the prayers offered and the false hopes we had. Not hopes raised merely by our own wishful thinking; hopes encouraged, even forced upon us, by false diagnoses, by

---

[83] Sue Mayfield, Living with Bereavement, 2008, Lion Hudson Plc

X-ray photographs, by strange remissions; by one temporary recovery that might have been ranked as a miracle."[84]

Meg and her husband, Joe, also experienced this; Joey had eaten six pancakes for breakfast one day and Meg reasoned that if he had such an appetite, how could he be dying?[85]

On Monday the 21st May, we were advised by the consultant that "things were going in the right direction," despite how ill you continued to feel. Sadly I found out later from your medical notes that the hospital knew that things were, indeed, not headed in the right direction. Just looking at you that last Monday, it was extremely clear they were not; you were not going to get well.

On Tuesday the 22nd May, I had been late arriving due to the traffic of the Chelsea Flower Show. Fulham Road and the Kings Road both had road works and it was a daily battle to reach the hospital anyway. You had phoned Auntie sobbing, to say that you could just not do it anymore, that you were feeling so very ill day after day and you could simply not go on. That was when I realised, Claire, you would definitely not come home. The passage from *Streams in the Desert* by Chas. E. Cowman rang in my ears:

"And many a rolling anthem that filled the Father's home, sobbed out its first rehearsal in the shade of a darkened room."[86]

I truly believed, Claire, that God walked with you that morning, despite the depth of the valley you were in, as I know He did each day. . .that despite being

---

[84]   C.S Lewis, A Grief Observed (Faber and Faber, 1961)

[85]   Meg Woodson, Following Joey Home (1978, Zondervan Publishing)

[86]   Chas. E. Cowman, Streams in the Desert May 30, (1961 Cowman Publishing Company, L.A. Copyright by Mrs Chas E Cowman 1925)

alone, humanly speaking, you were in the loving arms of your Heavenly Father, as described in the beautiful hymn by Haldor Lillenas, 1885:

"Jesus will walk with me in life's fair morning and when the shadows of evening must come.

Living or dying He will not forsake me, Jesus will walk with me all the way home.

Jesus will walk with me, He will talk with me. . .

In Joy or in sorrow, today or tomorrow, I know He will walk with me."[87]

I asked to see a doctor immediately upon my arrival but was told, despite me asking for an honest and frank discussion of your condition, that you were clinically improving and if this continued as it was, you would be home in a few weeks. It was inexplicable that I was still not told the truth.

If only we had not been led to believe in false hope that month of May, we could have better been prepared for the awful eventuality. Since that fateful Wednesday, as alluded to previously, although there had been lots of discussions with the doctors regarding your change of antibiotics, not one conversation had been conducted with us to say you were deteriorating beyond recovery. There was absolutely nothing to indicate from the medical team this time that you were losing the battle.

Your intravenous steroids were reduced; another hope that things were improving, only for them to be increased the following day; hopes dashed once more. Your entire body was so oedematous with the larger doses of these steroids, how you managed to keep your ventilator mask over your swollen face in such hot, oppressive weather, I just do not know.

---

[87]   Jesus Will Walk With Me, Haldor Lillenas,

On Wednesday 23rd May, the ward staff suggested you move rooms under the guise that you were improving and having a bigger space would help in this. The deception sadly continued right up until the end; you were diagnosed with T2 Respiratory Failure, but we were never told. Again, I only read this in your notes after your sad demise.

Palliative care medications (patients who are not dying are also prescribed such meds to relieve symptoms, but two days before you died, Claire, I knew you were past saving) commenced to assist your breathing, without any explanation to you as to why, but regardless, I recommenced staying overnight.

Claire, thankfully you are in our eternal home where every tear is wiped away, because even the memory of those final days is difficult to bear.

Chapter Twenty-Five

In Your Father's House

Writing this book is so painful, Claire; yet I am drawn, almost compelled, to it. Considering you, who suffered so much, how dare I complain of emotional sorrow when you underwent such saturating pain for so many years? You suffered physical, spiritual, mental anguish, yet also the very essence of human suffering in a broken heart many times. My dear Claire, how I longed to rescue you from those; when men let you down. . . when a family member disappointed you time and again. How I longed with all my being to make it better; to take away the tears, the heart-wrenching ache consistently present day after day.

Yet that pain was always tempered with the joy you found in life; your smile, the great pleasure you found in friendships, and also simple things like holidays, shopping trips and clothes. You were always a grateful person, Claire, and this trait looms in your memory, since you had much for which you could have been resentful.

This Diary is a recognition I have loved you and still do love you so much. It is a reminder of the Father-heart of God, who loves us with an unconditional love. He did not leave the hospital like I left; He did not abandon you in your need, like I did so often, and so I know He has a purpose and plan for this empty, shallow life of mine even yet.

There were so many mixed messages from the medics. I believed, when they asked Palliative Care to see you, the verdict had already been pronounced. Then the upbeat lung transplant talk that resulted in me texting Val and saying I had read the situation all wrong. Oh, if only, if only I had. A mother knows her child, though.

Ah, but you coped with your illness with such fortitude and grace, finishing strong in the Lord. What struck so many (still people comment on how you touched their lives in this way) was your strength of character and desire to serve God. Not the least was your help with the church youth work in your last weeks at home, but more importantly a trust in God shone through. That was a real example and which many of us are now trying to emulate. From the bottom of my heart, I thank God for you; a challenge and Christian role model to many.

During this terrible time, we were so grateful for those spiritual fathers in the Lord (see Forewords to this Diary) who, together with their wives, prayed for you. I thank God whenever I think of this time for Dave, Paul and Steve who visited and loved you as you so deserved a father's love. In that last week or so, as your oxygen saturation levels continued to drop, you could no longer manage on a continuous oxygen mask, thus requiring the ventilator constantly.

You were the one doing the dying, Claire, yet please believe me when I say I so wanted to take your place; to make it better for you. Thirty-six years old and so much living to do, so much more of "Life is an adventure-dare it." Nevertheless we knew, despite the reverent questions we have, God does not leave us alone; along the road to Heaven, He not only helps, He holds us.[88]

I remember so often seeking to minister to you, but the reverse was always true; it was you who ministered to me, as you did to so many of your friends and colleagues. You trusted God even when you knew there was no chance of your life on Earth being spared. You demonstrated absolute trust in the hardest place of

---

[88]   Brennan Manning, Abba's Child (NavPress, Colorado, 2011)

all; you displayed acceptance and staggering grace. You even expressed care for others; indeed as many have stated, your care for them was exemplary.

I could see in your eyes, however, what hurt you the most in those last days as you hovered between life and death, was the knowledge you would leave behind those you loved most. You knew you were destined for glory with your Saviour, but you knew the core of what matters is relationship, and it still bothered you to leave everyone behind.

I profoundly identify with my mentor and heroine, Meg Woodson, again when she said regarding her son Joey's last hospital admission in her book *Following Joey Home*[89] that time appeared to pass slowly and yet at the same time, go furiously by. Her need to write regarding those last days was her effort to retain the last precious time she had with her son on this Earth.

In the same way, Claire, I had kept a notebook in readiness for your lung transplant, so that I could write a journal of your progress and you also had a notebook ready that your friend Emma gave you one Christmas, but of course, both remain unused. Like Meg Woodson, I bargained with God; like her, I was filled with hope some days, only for those hopes to be dashed. I suppose, like Meg, I also wanted to justify my sheer exhaustion.

How abjectly sad I was to read in your medical notes from May 24th (after your death) of your last attempts to live:

Ventilator not triggering, causing you great distress as unable to breathe.

Still no honesty regarding how ill you were.

". . .Reluctant to sleep because she associates sleep with death. . . . .She worries that people can't hear her worries."

---

[89]   Following Joey Home, by Meg Woodson (© 1978, Zondervan Publishing House)

Dearest Claire, studying your notes later in 2012, the entry directly above was the very saddest information I read. All CF patients are referred to a psychologist because of the very nature and seriousness of the disease and to give you privacy I was never part of these discussions, so never knew that you voiced this fear. Of course you shared with me the very real thoughts you were dying, but as recorded within the pages of this Diary already, we were not told the truth and were given to believe you were improving.

Then at 14:40 hours:

". . .States she is unable to breathe despite being on Non-Invasive Ventilator (NIV). Claire unable to make good seal on mouthpiece. Machine not triggering. Struggling to get on top of Claire's secretion load; observations deteriorating, therefore needs senior PT and medical team review ASAP."

No one could help faulty equipment, but why did this have to happen when so much else had gone wrong? How you felt when you just could not get enough air in your lungs I just do not know; suffice it to say that that record plays so often in my mind. Equally, how you felt when you knew there was no return from this dying process when you had, as the Robert Frost poem so beautifully says, "Promises to keep and miles to go before I sleep.[90]" In that light, I know you so often echoed the sentiments by Ruth Picardi in her book, *Before I Say Goodbye*, when she voiced how much she would miss life.[91]

It became clear in that last week, as you were losing control over so many major areas of your life, in your shrinking world reduced to that sterile, stark room,

[90] Robert Frost 1969, Stopping by Woods on a Snowy Evening. From The Poetry of Robert Frost, edited by Edward Connery Lathem. (Copyright 1923, © 1969 by Henry Holt and Company, Inc., renewed 1951, by Robert Frost.)
[91] Ruth Picardi, Before I Say Goodbye (Penguin, 1998)

it must have been so important you maintained some sense of control. You so desperately hated me to leave you at night, facing that frightening, dark time alone. That is why you always asked me to get you one last glass of milk from the kitchen, or makes sure you had enough water. . .the list goes on.

Even then I knew that God was with you and I have just been reflecting on that lovely hymn:

"I come to the garden alone

While the dew is still on the roses. . .

And He walks with me

And He talks with me

And He tells me I am His own."[92]

I prayed, Claire, after such a difficult night and in all your human loneliness that morning of the 22nd May, that you knew the shadow was safe, because God walked with you (Psalm 23). Yet like Meg, with her Peggie, I who was the first to know you could not be spared, was the last to give up on you being saved.[93]

On Wednesday the 23rd May, they moved you to a larger room as more space was required for the ventilator. We were also told the larger room was a larger space for you to get better in (more lies). When I stayed overnight with you in the smaller room, my put-u-up bed was right up against yours and at right angles, so we could hold hands when you were particularly breathless and unwell. In the larger room, because the bedside table housed the ventilator I had to sleep in the corner, away from you. Oh how I pray, Claire, that you still felt my presence as part of the old you was disappearing before my very eyes with each passing night.

---

[92]   C. Austin Miles (1868-1946)

[93]   Meg woodson, Turn it into Glory, 1991 © Meg Woodson, Hodder and Stoughton

I was amazed on Wednesday, barely thirty-six hours before you died, you got a magazine out to look at and I thought to myself, *What joy, she is rallying!*, only to have those hopes dashed as you sank further into decline. That evening, your breathing became so bad I begged the team to start you on Midazolam and other end-of-life medication as you were in extremis and needed sedating. Auntie Pat remained with you for a couple of hours while I had a bit of break, and then I returned that same evening to stay the next two nights with you.

Again, your hospital notes read:

"Physio-seen 10:00 and 12:00 complaining of feeling agitated, (N.B. a result of intra-venous steroids) very unwell and frustrated, very tired and breath-less. Psychologically is struggling feeling so unwell. Secretions increased in volume and thickness. Refusing Lorazepam as it makes her too sleepy (*see other medical notes-she is scared to sleep in case she dies*). Tolerated physio session well. Liaise with medics."

The day before you died it had taken us hours to get everything sorted; the physios had been coming four times a day since the weekend, and how you man-aged to comply with treatment, I just do not know. You had spunk, Claire, and where you got it from, again I do not know. What I do know is you had masses of determination and will power. I somehow managed a shower for you late that afternoon, and I truly believe you knew it would be your last one and wanted to be prepared. I moaned because it was so very hard trying to manoeuvre a chair for you to sit on into the cramped cubicle space, then to get you in to sit on it, then get the shower to work so that the water temperature was right. All this while you were on a ventilator. These are the things that stand out in one's memory, as we desperately try to resist the urge to mentally self-flagellate. (I say this only to encourage the reader to remain as patient as possible with loved ones, even when you are exhausted.)

The sun shone strongly in the bathroom but there was obviously, for safety reasons, no plug to put a fan in an attempt to cool us both down. Little did I realise, Claire, it was to be my privilege, as Sheila Cassidy wrote in her book, *Good Friday People,* "to wash the feet that will not walk tomorrow."[94] Lovely nurse P. helped us place the bed table housing the ventilator into the bathroom and nurse F. came to brush your very tangled hair, a result of you having the awful mask of that venti-lator constantly strapped tightly round your head.

I fed you mouthfuls of food just for a split second when we took the mask off. You did so very well to synchronise your breathing with the ventilator, something you had to learn to do. That evening, somehow Natalie and Nicola had slipped through the net in us cancelling visitors, so when they knocked on the door of your room, you motioned to me that you did not want to see them with your mask on. Through your mask you said, "I'm dying," but you then allowed them into the room for a while.

As one CF patient said: "I'm not scared of death; I have accepted it, it's just that I'm not ready for it yet." Oh, how we can echo that! You had said so often through your hospital stay that, "I'm dying, Mum and I think today may be the day." Reflecting on your words to Natalie and Nicola, however, I realised you had been saying for those past days not that you were going to die (future tense) but rather, "I'm dying," (present tense).

Yet at the same time I remember the words of that blind preacher, George Matheson who wrote "Oh, Love that will not let me go."[95] God was not going to let you go, Claire. He was taking you with Him, and although I was not going to accompany you and would be left with such grief, paradoxically, He was not going

---

94   Sheila Cassidy, Good Friday People (Darton, Longman and Todd 1991)

95   George Matheson, 1842-1906 (November 7th 1962, Cowman Publishing Company Inc. Los Angeles)

to let me go either. He was simply holding on to both of us, as only He can do, yet leading our paths in different directions.

The night before the morning of Friday the 25th May you had slept very badly and I was up to help you many times. Of course I was pleased to be with you in these, your obviously last nights (even though we did not know for certain when you would pass from death to life abundance).

You finally settled and slept for a while in the early hours of the morning, while the lovely male staff nurse was so great in giving you hourly break-through doses of medication to supplement that which was in your syringe driver. At about 4:00 a.m. you asked to get out to the commode, after which you sat in the chair for a while, finding it so difficult to breathe even sitting upright in bed. Eventually we got you settled and back to sleep at about 4:45 a.m. It was light outside by then and I went to lay on the bed I had in your room, not to sleep but to pray for you, as I listened to that noisy ventilator chugging away every second. I looked over at you time and again, just to be sure you were not needing my help; I had placed a bottle of hand rub near your right hand and you had done well getting my attention by banging it on your table the previous night. Each time I turned to check on you, I continued to pray.

The nurse came in shortly after 6:00 a.m. to administer your medicines. He immediately sensed something was wrong and loudly called, "Claire!" Hearing is the last sense to go. When I heard him, I knew you had already left this Earth, yet I shot out of bed and ran up to your bedside. . .my fears were confirmed. In a tsunami of conflicting emotions, it was almost not fear, but some sense of relief your suffering was over; that you could not have gone on a moment longer in the distressed state in which you were living. The nurse, however, obviously not expecting you to die (how truthful were the medics to even the nurses?) pushed the crash call bell and other staff came rushing in but, of course, it was too late. I would not have wanted you resuscitated then, for you had truly suffered enough.

The one thought that cracked the dam wall of tears was, *If only I could have been there fully for you Claire, to "be" as you so wanted me to, and not to "do."*

I wept and wept.

If only I had been fully prepared for your departure from this world, to have done everything in those last weeks, absolutely perfectly, so that when you died, as inevitably it was going to happen, I would have no regrets. Life is not like that, however much we yearn for it to be in hindsight. I so wanted death with dignity for you, Claire; the deathbed scene written about in novels. In this broken world of sin, however, it evades us.

> After you died I just sat quietly in the room with you, holding you, talking to you, thanking God for you. (I still have the pyjamas you died in; they were the last clothes you wore in this life.) About 7:15 a.m., I phoned Paul P., your pastor, requesting he tell Auntie Pat and Steve W. I telephoned Val A. to ask her to tell Peter H. and Peter C. I also phoned Jo, Helen and Rach; what awful news it was for some of your best friends to hear. Bernie was not answering her phone but Helen phoned her later, and she also told all your managers and work colleagues. Then Pat and Shirl came up, followed one by one of a large number of hospital staff from the ward; the consultant (who had said you had had a "torrid few days." Indeed you had but not just days, weeks and months too), nurses, physios and pharmacy staff.

> You were not there, however. You were already with your Lord and Saviour. I have your baby teeth, I have locks of your baby hair, but God has you, Claire. One particular nurse had said (with the disclaimer that as a professional he should not say it) you were by far one of his favourite patients. "She was so lovely and polite," he said, so sadly. Ruth F. wrote her blog about you that day, and Paul quoted from it at your Thanksgiving service.

"Dear Lord, I want to hear

Your gentle voice

Let other voices

Cease their worrying

And in their stillness

Open my eyes

To your lovely smiling face."[96]

This beautiful song, "Here In This Holy Place," reminds me, Claire, that you would have been welcomed not only by the great King Himself, but by so many known to you who have already passed from death to life. It makes our family so pleased you would have met our mum for the first time (she died before I married, thus you never knew her).

Yet, Claire, I feel your desire to go home to your lovely new home in Soprano Way was transformed into something infinitely more wonderful than that; you were escorted in the grandest fashion to your eternal home, your forever home, one where your body was in perfect health, in a place you would never again have to leave to go into hospital. Yes, Claire, the wonderful truth of the gospel is although we are parted for a season, we will be together eternally. Yes, Claire, although I have so many regrets, one day, when I see your beautiful face again and hug you in the warmest embrace, I will have none.

I believe with all my heart Claire, in that hospital room as you were not long for this world, your Heavenly Father came to meet you for that final journey Home. Indeed, Rach suggested the same thought:

"Even though you were just resting, Mave, when Claire slipped into Eternity, the fact that you didn't hear anything makes me feel that it's as though God just came into the room, took Claire's hand and they quietly slipped out together; there's a

---

kind of peace about it. Claire was particularly outstanding in her sensitivity to the suffering of others and was so good at follow up too. God would not have been less sensitive to her needs as she approached death. We know in part, but then we will know fully."

Claire, blessed are you who mourned that you would not live much longer, mourned that you would not see your friends again, mourned that you would not work again, mourned that you would not see your lovely new home again, for you have inherited Christ's kingdom (Matthew chapter 5). In all your utter vulnerability, you trusted God, in those last weeks and days. You were truly my teacher and again I was the child, not the parent.

My thoughts began to drift to what could have been. . .what *should* have been. You had booked to go to Jordan with Hannah and Mark for early May, but that was not to be. You did not make the Hampton Court Flower Show, or Rosie P.'s birthday. You never managed a spa visit, or your trip to the South of France, nor Wimbledon Tennis, nor even the cinema to see *Salmon Fishing in the Yemen.* You never sat in the sun again, nor on your lovely new garden furniture. . .but you did make Heaven, Claire, and that far outweighs any earthly delights.

Once reality began to settle, the inevitable conflict arose within me, yet the following exchange helped me so much to feel normal, Claire. Oh, not vindicated of the times I hurt you, but just to know that other mums found life hard too. Meg Woodson accused herself of wanting to appear as a perfect mother, but shares her ambivalence of knowing she can do only so much for her son; wanting to respond to his needs, whilst at the same time becoming irritated when he requires her help. Meg is open enough to expose these thoughts in her book, *Following Joey Home.*[97]

Oh, Claire, how glad I am that Meg was honest enough to record her feelings, for they have helped me so much. No, not absolved me of blame, not justified my

---

[97]   Following Joey Home, by Meg Woodson (© 1978, Zondervan Publishing House)

outbursts, but for me to see that like her family, we have also wrestled with CF all your life and that wore, to a far lesser degree, on my soul too. Please forgive me, Claire, just as Meg asked her son to forgive her, for when I should have loved you the most, you who were doing the dying, I was thinking my own selfish thoughts about getting enough sleep.

Even if we did get you home, however, I knew it would only be a matter of days until you were back in hospital again and we would be repeating this. I should have listened both to you and also my gut feeling because I knew there would be no long haul. I could not help myself; I dared to think you might get well, just as Meg dared to think Joey would.

In my naiveté I was also trying to get your garden ready and arrange for the rest of your flat pack garden furniture to be assembled, as you had expressed a wish to have a couple of hours sitting in your lovely new garden. I was investigating how we could get a private ambulance to bring you home for an afternoon. (Helen and Janice had planted some sweet peas while you were in hospital and you were keen to see these, too.) You deserved all this, Claire, and I suppose my thought was it might give you some strength to get well again.

I also have so many regrets about things you never saw: the en-suite bedroom blinds that were delivered while you were in hospital, the guest bedroom fully furnished with the new bed and headboard carefully chosen by you. I know they are not important now; I know your Heavenly home far surpasses any home you had down here, and yet I cannot help but grieve.

That last morning the senior nurse said you had a haemoptysis (meaning you had coughed up blood, as you had often done over the years). I wondered if you were aware of this (I will not in this Diary go into details of what I believe happened), for how could you get my attention if you did know, but perhaps could do nothing with that mask on? You were too weak to remove it yourself and this is something that continued to worry me, so I brought this up with the consultant when I returned to the hospital to see her a few weeks later.

Despite the futility of hindsight, if perhaps only as another caution to the reader, all I would have longed for, had I known your days were so numbered, were to have helped you to die in as dignified and less frightening way that could be afforded you. That in those last hours of darkness when you were so afraid, to have been able to keep watch with you and allayed those fears as much as I may have been able. . .yet that was denied us both. The paradox is, Claire, despite your weariness and despite your shattered hopes, God triumphed as you soared Heavenward.

If a mother is permitted to be proud, Claire, I cannot tell you how proud I was of you clinging to God alone. Sheila Cassidy, in her book *Audacity to Believe* wrote, "I knew, too, that in some strange way the pain which I had suffered was his gift, and that far from being a sign of his lack of care or wrath, it was an unmistakable sign of his love."[98]

To paraphrase the poet, it is not death as we know it if we pass on and leave this entropic world, from a prison-cell body, to instead breath the air of eternity in our Father's home. However much I wanted you back that morning, Claire, I knew you were gone and God had allowed you to go. Still, when I think of the song, "Time of My Life,"[99] this is what you gave me.

Another hymn that I continued to hum that morning was:

The sands of time are sinking, the dawn of Heaven breaks;

The summer morn I've sighed for –the fair, sweet morn awakes;

Dark, dark hath been the midnight

---

[98] (p223 Sheila Cassidy, Audacity to Believe1977, Darton, Longman and Todd Ltd.)

[99] Time of My Life, Composed by Franke Previte, John DeNicola, and Donald Markowitz. Recorded by Bill Medley and Jennifer Warnes (RCA Records Label, September 24, 1987)

(only you truly knew, Claire, just how black it had been those last weeks of
your life)
but dayspring is at hand.
And glory, glory dwelleth in Immanuel's land.[100]

In Deuteronomy 31:3, we see the Lord stating He Himself will go before us, and He followed through on His promise for the Israelites. Beth Moore, in her study book *The Patriarchs*, suggests that God will cross over ahead of us into fearful, unknown places. Claire, without a doubt, God went ahead of you that awful morning when you went to be with Him. I say awful, since it was for us, but once you had crossed over, it was no longer awful for you. God crossed over so you could too, but God not only went ahead of you, He gently came, took you by the hand and tenderly led you all the way to Heaven. The words of the following hymn sum this up so well:

I will glory in my Redeemer Who waits for me at gates of gold
And when He calls me, it will be paradise (verse 3b).[101]

These words from the poem, "Crabbit Old Woman," meant so much to me as I sat in that hospital room, which was sold to us as the environment in which you could get better. This hospital room where your body remained but your soul had departed.

I remember the joy,
I remember the pain and

---

[100]   Anne R. Cousin, in The Christian Treasury.

[101]   Extract taken from the song 'I Will Glory In My Redeemer' by Steve and Vikki Cook Copyright © 2001 Sovereign Grace Praise *Adm. by Capitol CMG Publishing worldwide excl. UK, admin by Integrity Music, part of the David C Cook family, songs@integritymusic.com

I'm loving and living life over again.

I think of the years,

All too few, gone too fast

And accept the stark fact that nothing can last.[102]'

The words from the song "Seasons in the Sun" were desperately poignant

that morning:

Goodbye my friend it's hard to die

When all the birds are singing in the sky.[103]

Oh, Claire, how true this must have been of you, to not just say farewell to one, but many friends. I listened to the dawn chorus, even in the middle of London on that May morning you departed this earth; you, torn with a longing to stay, but knowing that you had to go.[104]

I wept that May morning, for indeed, the piercing azure sky in the middle of London would have been a treat to behold had it not been the day you died. Yet, maybe it was God's sign of welcoming you to Heaven; a royal welcoming home not to be celebrated on a dull winter's day, but on one fitting for so rare and exceedingly lovely a soul. Oh, how you loved gloriously bright days. Even when I ring your mobile and your recorded voicemail plays, your sense of being alive is vivid, as was that May morning resplendent in the radiance of who you were and still are.

I know God came to meet you that morning, Claire, yet I just wish I was there, fully present when you took your last breath. I suppose it was to be a moment between you and He. Psalm 46:4 says there is a river whose stream makes glad the

---

[102] Phyllis McCormack, Crabbit Old Woman (Nursing Mirror, December 1972)

[103] SEASONS IN THE SUN, Adaptation anglaise de Rod McKuen S/les motifs de l'oevre orginale <<LE MORIBOND>> Paroles et Musique de Jacques Brel © Warner Chappell Music France et Editions Jacques Brel. Music and original French lyric by Jacques Brel -English lyric by Rod McKuen © 1961 by INTERSONG PARIS, S.A.-Edward B Marks Music Co: Sole Licensing and Selling Agent for USA, Commonwealth of Nations, including Canada and Australia and New Zealand and Eire - All Rights Reserved -CARLIN MUSIC CORP. London NW1 8BD

[104] Source Unknown

city of God, and whilst I am aware this refers to Jerusalem, verse 5 continues saying God is within Jerusalem. She won't fall; God will help her at the break of day. I like to think, since the apostle Paul says we are of the New Jerusalem (Galatians 4:26), I can use it to refer to you that morning too. Yes, you were always stubborn, Claire, always pushing the boundaries, but these qualities fundamentally made you the feisty, tenacious person you were. I believe these kept you alive for so long.

So now I am no longer a wife Claire, and I am no longer a mother; in fact I guess my status has returned to that of my earlier years before I loved you with every fiber of my being. Yet I do not walk through your loss alone, for I am grateful to your, and my, many friends who mourn too.

While we mourn, we also know you are now experiencing the joy of what Jesus promised, life more abundant. As I have said previously in the pages of this Diary, life may not have been the party you or I had hoped for you, Claire, but your philosophy was, "While I'm here, I might as well dance," and with God's help yours was a dance befitting of a *Ballet d'Claire* at the Royal Opera House. Now you have changed residence, God is the God of reversal; He has already made it as if CF and all its horrible traumas and sadness never happened. Indeed they will never be remembered by you, as your tears have been wiped away.

Yet, while you were still here, you were aware of two people who had died on the ward during your last admission. I realized I had no idea you were so acutely conscious of this, with it affecting you badly. Looking back, it was as if you knew it may be you next. Despite these haunting fears and omens, however, in your last weeks you astounded me with your spiritual maturity, your complicit trust in God. You knew He was in control, and were willing to accept whatever happened. You outdid me in your love for Him, Claire; I am a mere pygmy compared with your trust and inexorable peace despite how ill and frightened you were.

Words can never explain how I feel since your death; I measure time by that before your death and the time after. Again, I am so sorry, Claire, I was not there to support you as I should have done. I have already said it, but I need to say it again. As a nurse, I should have listened to my gut feeling and heard what you were saying, ignoring the doctors. I failed you in your hour of need and I have no excuse for that.

I feel I was too complicit in the hospital, and since reading your medical notes after you died, I wish I had never just accepted things at that time. Yet even when I challenged the medical staff, still there was no honesty regarding your deteriorating condition, and your early demise seemed to go largely unnoticed by me because of the falsehoods they told us. Of course doctors and, indeed, all health care professionals want to cure people, but when that it is not possible truth becomes paramount. Why is it medics find it so hard to tell people they are losing the fight; that they are dying? I later discussed this with a senior work colleague of mine; she said that some medics who knew their patients well and over a long period of time just could not bring themselves to give bad news. I would still rather have had the choice.

A great encouragement, however, was a note your friend Helen M. wrote:

"I know you continue to say that you weren't there for her in those final moments but what I'd like to say is that what I read was that you were very much there; you were always there. Claire knew you were always there and felt very blessed to have an understanding, knowledgeable and loving mother. She often talked about you and I honestly don't believe Claire would have talked fondly about you if she hadn't felt close to you. She wouldn't want you to feel in so much pain and guilt. You got to the hospital as soon as you learned she was deteriorating on that day early in May and you stayed with her for hours on end thereon in. She would have felt your presence – mothers and daughters with your kind of closeness have that special bond."

I can only imagine how awful those weeks were for you; and not only those weeks, but many months before. I can remember you grabbing my hand so often at different times in those months, with such force when you were finding it particularly difficult to breathe. Even so, I must let you go and commit you to God; we can walk no further with you, nor do you need us now.

I needed to continue to repeat scripture and hymns to myself that morning, Claire; God could have made those circumstances different if He had chosen. He could have had the doctors tell us the facts. . .to ensure we both had those precious last weeks, days, hours of your life together. For some reason He did not intervene and that takes great trust on both our parts to trust where we cannot understand.

It is often odd that things we read years ago stay in our minds forever; I remember reading a quote from the devotional Chas E. Cowman's *Streams in the Desert* for February 12: "Even so Father, for so it seemed good in Your sight."[105] That struck a chord with me as I believe one day we will know the reason; though methinks in Heaven you already do.

For now there are so many firsts that we have to experience without you; your empty home, your empty space at work, your friends living life without you. . .me living life without you. It is difficult to think you are never going back to your lovely new home.

After I washed you with the help of one of the nurses, I emptied your locker and found the bookmark Ruth H. had given you. It read:

"In the Shadow of His wings, Psalm 91:4: He will cover you with His feathers and under His wings you will find refuge."

That is where I firmly believed you were, and I do not doubt, for one minute, God's sovereignty in all of this; I am only sorry we did not have more time to

---

prepare. It was enough to know that everything will be okay someday, and that day for you has already come.

From my mentor in all of this, Meg Woodson, whom I only got to know by reading her book in your hospital room (I suppose that was some grace from God), what she went through in not one but both of her children's hospital rooms. She recounts regarding her daughter Peggie her last breath dissolving into the air, and then it was gone. She too, turned to her daughter, and confessed over and over, repenting for all she should have done, or failed to do in Peg's life. She told her departed daughter the countless ways she had been a joy to her, and how privileged she was to have had her. How proud she was that in Peg's mere twenty-three years, she had lived and loved more than most who live many times longer.[106]

Of her son Joey's last days Meg acknowledged her feelings are a contradiction on the matter regarding Joey's impending death, stating she never fully believed it, apart from the few hours when Joey was first hospitalised. She believed the voicing of her fears helped her prepare for the worst scenario, but all along she hoped for a different ending; that, indeed, Joey would live.[107]

After I said my final goodbye to you at the hospital, I went to register your death. I had passed Chelsea Town Hall so many times when we shopped, or when I parked the car, little realising one day I would need to go inside on such an unwelcomed errand. I walked down the road that sunny, warm May afternoon, my natural reaction still being to wonder if I should attempt wheeling you out simply because the day was so beautiful, and you would love it so. It was the most gorgeous day, one I would have made sure you enjoyed if you were still healthy. Yet I had just left your Earthly body in that hospital room, your once beautiful face now marred with the effects of intravenous steroids so that it was virtually unrecognisable. As Meg acknowledged in the days leading up to her son Joey's death,

---

[106] Meg Woodson, Turn It Into Glory, 1991, Hodder and Stoughton
[107] Meg Woodson, Following Joey Home, 1978, Zondervan Publishing House

the event would never be in the past. I also know with surety, Claire, I will never, ever forget your brave fight; never forget what you endured. How I went home and cried inconsolably that you were gone; that we would never share anything in this life again. That morning when the birds sang, when the warm hue of early summer was virulent in the air, and the sun shone brightly. . . .never would you experience the changing seasons again.

Val kindly cooked for me that evening and Bobby W., my pastor, and Peter H., our pastor of discipleship, came round too. The following day was one of reading emails, taking phone calls, doing your laundry from the hospital (how often one just goes through the motions). I went over to water your garden and check on your house; all I could think about was how the home you had so recently moved into would no longer be enjoyed by you.

Indeed, you never saw the spare bed I made up with such love and care, with your new duvet covers you had purchased from House of Fraser. You bought that lovely pale-pink throw for the small bedroom and the two pink cushions. (I gave these to Asha, and Rach was so moved and thankful, knowing that pink is Asha's favourite colour and that you had bought those with a view to your goddaughter coming to stay when she was older.)

It seemed such a waste, and indeed it was. Yet, even though you upsized in readiness for the lung transplant you never had, in your Father's house, where you now live, are many mansions with far more beautiful gardens, and you do not even need a ventilator or a lung transplant, and thus you no longer need your earthly home.

Still, you left so much behind and as George Bush said in his TV speech regarding those on board Flight 93 on 9/11:

"They left friends and family. . .promising careers, and a lifetime of dreams they will never fulfil. They left something else; a legacy of bravery and selflessness that will always inspire us."

Just like all those who perished in the events of 9/11, it is you, Claire, who has had to do the dying, not your family and friends, though our hearts have undoubtedly been broken in the process. So as we lay your body to rest in this Earth, we remember that God carries His lambs close to His heart (Isaiah 40:11). Being the great Shepherd He tends His flock, and in His arms He will gather his lambs and carry them in His bosom. Thus, He carried you on this Earth, and the wonder is that He now carries you in Heaven. So in our sadness, our memories will not only be about your struggle with a diseased body, but our gladness will resound of how you are now made perfect, so that this is not so much a mourning for your death, but a celebration of your life.

How utterly empty our lives would be if we believed that this life was all there is, but thanks be to God we know eternity awaits. You told me at one time, in those last days and in your mind's eye, you saw a picture of God dressed all in white. How I prayed that in that hospital room on your final morning on this Earth that God opened your eyes to see those angels coming at the time of your departure from this world. You had to see them, of course, once you left your body, so I know you were not only comforted, you were overjoyed.

I have told so many people, and my heart has broken countless, countless times at the suffering you had to endure; not just physically but mentally and emotionally in your last weeks. Nevertheless, I can only imagine the reality of that moment when God came for you, and took His lamb into His bosom, guiding you lovingly into His presence.

Beth Moore, in her book *The Patriarchs* says:

"God ties in our personal present with our future through an inner unrest Scripture calls 'longing.' I thank God that this world is not all there is. Our feet were meant to dance on another turf."[108]

You who loved dancing on earth, Claire, have found that alternate turf, and how can I not thank God that you are safe with Him?

---

[108] Beth Moore, The Patriarchs, 2005, Lifeway Press

Chapter Twenty-Six

The Eighth of June, 2012

Thus, my dearest Claire, as I dealt with the finality of your precious life drawing to a close, we held your funeral and cremation. It has been full indeed. It was a beautiful service, of which the reader can learn in the Appendix. As was your life, this day was full of love, full of gratitude, full of memories. . .and full of loss.

When I arrived home that evening, I was greeted by another stack of cards on my doormat. Equally, my inbox was aglow with emails, but instead of reading through them, I sat down and read your memory book until late into the night. So many of your loved ones have been so kind as to quote various Christian writers, who either wrote of or came to terms with grief. One such example is the following when Helmut Thielicke asks:

". . .Why is it just when life reaches its supreme moment we should suddenly be overtaken by the dread mortality and the fragility of life?"[109]

---

[109] How The World Began, trans. John W. Doberstein (Philadelphia: Muhlenburge Press 1961, p171) cited in Ron Dunn, (p71,When Heaven is Silent, 2002, Authentic Publishing, Milton Keynes)

I identify with this, Claire, because just about the time I had it all together (with you moving to a lovely new home in readiness for a lung transplant), everything fell apart. Dunn suggests again:

". . .As we grow older, our battles with God become more fierce, even more painful at times. The issues are more critical, the outcomes more profound."

He continues on page 61:

"When the hoped-for, prayed-for miracle doesn't come, when we are not delivered, when there is no miracle—this is the question that hounds us. . . .why?"

On page 100:

"Fair, that's all I ask God, but how can it be when my friend's children are graduating from college, starting careers, getting married, having children, while my child lies in a grave?"

I suppose, Claire, I will always have those lingering questions in the back of my mind. My discipline will come in waiting on the Lord for answers, perhaps only when we meet again in our eternal home. As I ponder these things, however, I realized once again that you are still teaching us; in your absence, you left behind memories and indeed, more than memories. Your attitude was never ,"Why is this happening to me?" but instead, "Look, I see my blessings in this."

That is why I consider the words of the great English poet, Alfred Lord Tennyson, who thought it was better to love someone (even if we subsequently lose that person) than to have never known love in the first place. You were given as a blessing to us for far shorter than we expected, but if we did not learn from you in thirty-six years, we probably were not going to.

Good thing you left us a few reminders.

Life is an Adventure – Dare It

A Silver Lining

Are there any benefits in having CF? In recent years I have been able to experience different parts of the world, which has been a real privilege. I caught the "travel bug" when I was in my late teens and I felt that I should get travelling in while I was sufficiently able to. My aim is to enjoy life as much as I can whilst I am able, and to see as many new places as I possibly can with the money and time I've got.

The year after I had my port-a-cath implanted, I felt reasonably well and a few of us from University went "inter-railing" around Europe. We visited eight countries in a period of three and half weeks and, although exhausted, we all enjoyed the experience. My family were quite concerned about me going, especially as I was unwell the day before I left! Similarly I realised it was a big responsibility for my friends, because if I was ill, it may well have jeopardised their holiday too. Trying to keep medication cool was a challenge. But I carried my portable nebuliser, together with my other travel gear in my back-pack all around Europe, with a little bit of help from my friends.

I have also been able to travel as part of my Christian service and such trips have included the Czech Republic with a group from my local church. We journeyed by road but this time medication went in a fridge in our pastor's motor caravan. The problem, however, was that the nebuliser wouldn't work but there were a couple of nurses on the trip who really looked out for me. A further privilege was taking food parcels and visiting refugees in the former Yugoslavia with a Christian organisation; this was an incredibly humbling experience.

Closer to home, I have undertaken a short spell of Christian service with the London City Mission and I have regularly helped with the youth work on the annual Caister week of the Fellowship of Independent Evangelical Churches. I continue to be engaged in co-leading a weekly youth group at my church. I love working with teenagers, partly because I think I am still such a teenager at heart. After my first degree, I took a year out and worked with the Christian Schools' Work Trust in Kingston-upon-Thames. It was a great experience. I enjoyed the work and benefitted so much from working with the team. I would love to work full time in Christian service one day. It was exciting for me to take the Christian gospel into schools and to show the teenagers that it is a relevant answer for their lives.

In many respects I'm very blessed having CF! I think that if I didn't have it, I would not have experienced half of the things that I have, and I have learnt so much through it. I don't think I would have chosen to have CF, but I know God has used me and blessed me more by having it. In recent years I have appreciated so much what it means to live with an illness like this. I didn't fully realise before but people do care about me. If I didn't have CF I would not have experienced half the things that I have done. Other people who are ill and yet who keep on fighting and don't give up are an encouragement to me. Some people keep me going just because they know what I am going through. Meanwhile life continues on the fast track and I will shortly complete a two year Master's course in Social Work. It has been my childhood ambition to be a social worker – though I am beginning to wonder why, as it seems to be one of the many stressful occupations!

Chapter Twenty-Seven

This Unnecessary Death

Dear Claire,

On the 2nd May, 2012 you were given such terrible news, and while it was so wrong for this information to be delivered without warning, we still were not told the entire truth. As awful as it was for me to hear, I am a nurse and healthy, while you were the patient and the one who was so ill; I cannot imagine what it did to your resolve.

Although I believe in the Christ-like tenet to forgive, as any mother would, I wanted the hospital to be aware of their misstep, so this tragedy could be avoided with other families. This is what I sought to accomplish regarding your final weeks in hospital, Claire. When I requested and read your medical notes, I was haunted by the "Do Not Attempt Resuscitation" (DNAR) form that was written on the 16th May stating you and I were both fully informed, yet we knew *nothing* about the order. Incidentally, as I understand it, it is now a legal violation of human rights to produce such a form without the patient or, if the patient does not have capacity, the next of kin being informed. As such, you can see the very real (and very difficult) action of forgiveness at work here.

I suppose, when I read the notes, it was not so much not knowing how you died but (odd as it may seem) the *process* of your dying, having been told so many falsehoods about it, went largely unnoticed by me. With those ever-lingering feelings of guilt, I only told a few select people about this and was so very grateful for their support.

I was explicit in my correspondence with the hospital leadership, and in my meetings with the involved staff and whilst very grateful for the medical care you received throughout your life time, I could not remain silent on the issue once I realised the huge gaps there were in what the team told us regarding your last illness versus what we had very specifically requested. A good summation of the drive to understand what had happened is quite eloquently summed up by Norman Maclean in *Young Men and Fire*:

"Unless we are willing to escape into sentimentality or fantasy, often the best we can do with the catastrophes, even our own, is to find out exactly what happened and restore the missing parts. Probably most catastrophes end this way without an ending, the dead not knowing how they died. . .those who loved them forever questioning 'this unnecessary death.'"[110]

Jean Vanier, in his foreword to Sheila Cassidy's book, *Sharing the Darkness: the Spirituality of Caring*,[111] echoes Maclean's thoughts, yet from a different perspective:

The dying. . .[and here the writer includes anyone with an incurable illness] are essentially people who are on a journey. They are an uprooted people, dispossessed, marginalised, travelling fearfully into the unknown. The condition and speed of the journey may vary – sometimes movement is barely perceptible, like the moving floors at Heathrow–but sometimes the

---

[110] Norman Maclean, Young Men and Fire, (University Of Chicago Press; Chicago, 1992)

[111] Jean Vanier, Forward to: Sheila Cassidy, Sharing the Darkness: the Spirituality of Caring' (2002, Darton Longman and Todd-Forward by Jean Vanier)

trucks hurtle through the night, throwing their bewildered occupants from side to side with all the terror of the line to Auschwitz. Above all they are dying alone and they are afraid. . . .what they want more than anything is that this thing should not be happening to them. . .but since this cannot be they want someone to comfort them, to hold their hand, to face the unknown with them.'

Ah, and yet, we dare to believe that God is good, Claire. I thought you were in the best hospital available, and we truly were from the physical aspect of your CF, but sadly the team failed with their dishonesty about your prognosis. That was what was so hard to bear, for you physically, but in a smaller context for me as I watched you struggle far more than you should have while the truth was evaded time and again.

After my meeting with the Chief Executive to get the hospital to finally acknowledge their lack of communication regarding your last admission, he sent me the following letter:

Dear Mrs. Salter

Thank you for coming to talk to Caroline S. and I about your beautiful daughter Claire. We were both moved by the way you spoke for Claire and others with Cystic Fibrosis and are so sorry for the missed opportunities for open discussion with Claire and you about the seriousness of her condition. Nothing we can say can undo what happened but as we told you, we met with the consultant prior to seeing you and I will talk again following.

In the notes you left us, you ask for my evaluation. Everything you raised in the meeting is there. In the meeting and from the written summary it is clear you did everything and more that a mother could for a much loved daughter and so am saddened that you should feel guilt and cannot forgive yourself for not being there for Claire. Our impression is that you were and that Claire knew. The responsibility is ours, for not listening to Claire's fears and your pain, for giving mixed messages and not addressing both your concerns honestly. I apologise and regret that this meant Claire died as you told us mentally and physically exhausted without having been given "permission" to stop fighting and leaving you feeling you were with her but not present and unable to spend the last weeks in the way you would both have chosen.

I appreciate your courage and sincerity in talking about your experiences and as I said at the meeting our door is open if you need to come back. I offer my sincere condolences for Claire's death.

Yours sincerely,

Chief Executive

It is worth noting that not only were my colleagues at the hospital where I worked extremely supportive, but one of the hospital staff where you were cared for, and who handled the complaint, said I had been patient, polite and honest in my approach. He recognised I was doing this for you; to try obtain some closure regarding why things went so wrong. After I met with the Chief Executive, I sent the following email to a handful of our friends that knew of my concerns:

Dear All,

I received the attached letter from the Chief Executive of the hospital where Claire was cared for, as a result of a meeting with him and the Director of Nursing a couple of weeks ago. Although I had prepared copious notes I managed to speak without them as of course, I have relived those last weeks of Claire's life so many times. On reflection, I should not have wasted time corresponding with the CF team but gone directly to the Chief Executive, as he was so understanding.

At the meeting last week I asked for the Chief Executive's evaluation, which he has now given me. I just wanted acknowledgement that things could have been so different. Claire suffered so much because of their dishonesty. . In case some of you wonder about his comment that I was "with Claire but not present," I explained to him that although I was in the room with Claire the morning she died, I was lying on the put-u-up bed after she had gone back to sleep and although awake, was unconscious of exactly when she died (the ventilator she was on was extremely noisy). Thank you again for your interest and support. Sincerely, Mave.

As a result of circulating the above letter, Claire, I received much support from our friends and loved ones. The following are just some of them:

Chris F. wrote:

"As you know, I first met Claire in hospital when we were both patients on the ward. I was struck by Claire's amazing ability to defy the ills of CF, which is best described as a terrible disease. Claire didn't cling to, rather she conquered life and I felt a soothing love of life radiated from her, like a mothering warmth. Such an amazing lady, I am proud to be called a friend."

Another Christian friend wrote:

"I am so pleased that you have actually found a respectful and understanding person, in the Chief Executive. I hope that his message to the medical staff regarding compassion, empathy and caring will teach the

entire team about honesty and truth, particularly when these are being requested."

From one of your nurse friends:

"Wow, that is an honest letter and words I believe you should have heard long before now. I know it will never be able to be undone or changed, but I really hope that they learn so much from their failures in the care of Claire and you. I have found it hard to accept that it had to end in such away so I can only imagine your heart ache. I admire your courage to find resolution. It cannot be easy for the doctors to admit their shortcomings and I can imagine your relief at the belated honesty. The tone of his letter is quite unprecedented and made my eyes fill with tears. I also feel really sad that you have had such extra heartbreak after Claire's death. Without doubt you would have been able to make choices if you had been better/ properly prepared and informed and it is something that I hope that the whole medical team learns from."

From Jackie R., at the Cystic Fibrosis Trust:

"Thank you for your email and the attached letter that you had received. I do so hope that this has gone some way to help you, especially after the most terrible time that you have gone through before and after losing your precious daughter. I really do appreciate you kindly emailing me and keeping me updated with any outcomes. Please do not hesitate if we can be of any further assistance in the future."

From Cynthia, a friend at church who also lost a daughter (in response that we were not told how ill you really were):

"Oh, Mave, it is so natural to 'want to know,' but for us as Christians, we have the edge! We can fill the void with the knowledge that it is all in His hands. This is such a fallen world and so many people these days lack credibility and conscience that it is often difficult to find truth when we need it most. Thank God He is truth and we have Him."

Lastly, Bernie wrote:

"I have been crying as I read this letter. I am one of Claire's friends who would have loved to say goodbye. I remember the last day I saw her and refused to really listen to her. I was not ready to even think about Claire dying but she knew. I remembered Claire calling me back as I was about to leave the room and said that she loved me. In hindsight, I think she knew that she would, more likely, not see me again. I wish I could have said more because I have so much to say to her."

I realize getting the hospital to admit what it did wrong will not bring you back, and that was, of course, never the goal. It is a mother's necessary right, however, to feel as though she did all she could to help other children and parents avoid the same suffering.

Regardless, you are with our Creator and I am here, and when I had accomplished what I intended, regarding an acknowledgement from the hospital, I suppose I had to face the cold truth that life had changed forever.

Months earlier I had gone through my diary cancelling all your appointments like port flushes, etc. Notes included dates to spring clean, buy you flowers when you returned from Jordan (except that you never went). . .I so wanted you to feel special and loved. Your friends, at my invitation, took mementos of you – clothes, shoes, jewellery. Rationally I know you would have approved, but when they took them, I wanted them back because deep down they are yours and I want you back. All this was a stark reminder that I now lived in a world of which you were no longer a part.

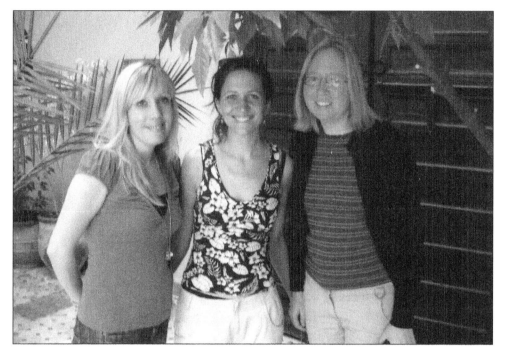

With Rach and Patricia in Morocco

After Words

A World of Which You Are no Longer a Part

It is odd, Claire, that some memoirs, now 30 years old and rather dog-eared to say the least, sat in the loft of our family home and then downsized with me to my new home in 2001, following your move to independence the previous year. I can remember you saying words to the effect of, "Oh, Mum, you keep them. Don't throw anything away –I'll know if you do!" and they had not been touched for all this time. Now you are gone and they, like all the memories I have of you, are so, so precious, and as I lovingly turn the pages of the scrapbooks you created I wanted to, yet again, know everything about every moment of your life.

I still have the rather tattered Christmas list that you kept from one year to the next. I cannot begin to thank you for all the beautiful cards and equally poignant words you wrote in all your cards to me, undeserved as they were. Each one special, each one treasured. Where did the years go, Claire?

Before I knew it, we were into May 2013, a year since you had died. On that mournful day, I looked back in utter sadness and disbelief that you were gone, but if I doubt God, Claire, I am denying His goodness.

I had emailed your Tiffin buddies:

"Going through Claire's boxes that were stored in the loft. I found Tiffin upper sixth yearbook –great photos/comments from/to each other and very nostalgic. I also found her school hymnbook (you had all swapped your hymn books between you and written in each others' the proverbial end of school messages such as farewell, but keep in touch. . So pleased Claire still kept hers.

Caroline T. emailed:

"It must be quite a journey for you to sort through Claire's correspondence. It is funny, but when we first went to Uni, email was just starting and I remember our first tentative emails to one another, Claire included. We always wanted to stay in touch with one another and the contact we had with each other was always so reassuring when everything else was new and a bit daunting. Ndullee brought her Tiffin hymn book to Book Group last time and showed where we had all written in it. It was a lovely reminder."

I also received an email from Rebecca M. to say:

"Us book club girls were at the Tiffin Girls' reunion ten days ago. We spent the day thinking of Claire, revisiting old haunts at school, digging up all the school photos (I know that Claire would have been very unimpressed at some of her and our hairstyles!) and celebrating all the friendships we made. We did miss Claire so very much that day, but in some ways it was like she was just sitting quietly with us, glass in hand and celebrating with us. We all thought of you too x."

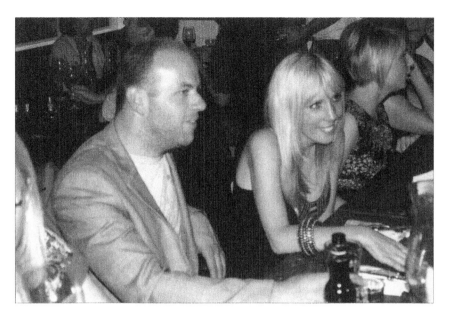

One of Claire's birthday meals, L-R Rhys, Claire, Emma

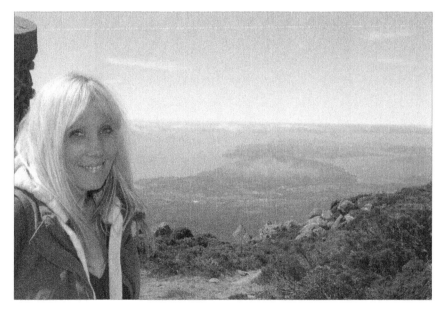

The last long-haul holiday with Emma

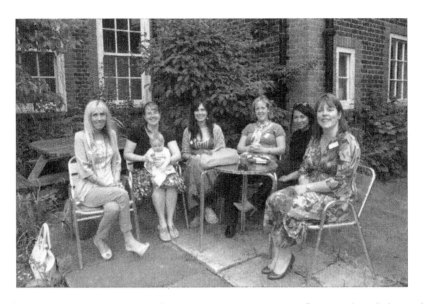

Tiffin Girls Reunion, May 2011, almost twenty years on from school days: 'friends forever!' L-R Claire, Caroline, Ndullee, Sarah, Naureen and Rebecca

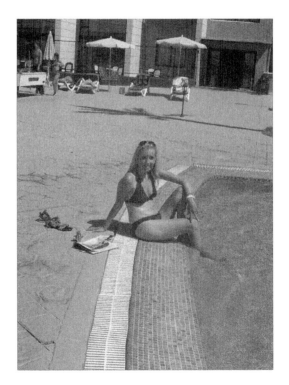

#29 October 2011, short break in Tenerife, prior to moving house, taken by travelling buddy, Jo R.

I found your calendars, Claire, from the years you were at Canterbury and have them displayed on my study wall. Your school books, uni and post qualifying social work course folders I have also kept since these are what helped define your life. I have retained the clothes that I could keep in the available storage I have, especially those most recent ones you bought, that defined you as the glamour queen you were; space at no. 43 has meant I had to be very selective, but many of the clothes you bought in the sales of Christmas 2011, as well as your jewellery and jewellery boxes, I have kept. I also have the full length gown you wore to the CF Ball in 2008 as well as the beautiful, sleeveless dress you wore to the Epsom Players evening at Epsom Downs Racecourse. This was to be the last formal dress you ever bought. I also have the swimsuit too, of course, unworn that you had purchased in readiness for your proposed holiday to Jordan.

I emailed many of your friends to say thank you for their help last year. It was based on a circular letter, so I only enclose a couple, but I also included Helen G., Jo S., Marianne T., Helen M. and many more.

2.5.2013 this to Jo R.:

"Hi Jo, a year ago today you kindly came up to the hospital to see Claire after she had been given bad news. She so appreciated your visit that day, as she did many of your visits. I also remember the last time you saw her on Saturday 19th May. She was so poorly but she appreciated seeing you."

5.5.2013:

"Hi Emma, a year ago today you so very kindly came up to the hospital to sit with Claire while I came home to do some laundry. (I was staying overnight for a week and both Claire and myself were running short of clean clothes.) That was one of many occasions when you stayed for me to

have a break and looking back I couldn't have done without you, so thank you so very much for all your help and friendship to Claire."

Claire, as I finally retired from my nursing post, I had time to send this letter to all your friends:

To all Claire's Friends and Work Colleagues, Family Members/Family Friends:

I could not let the first anniversary of Claire's sad death pass without saying thank you (especially to those I have been unable to contact until now) to all of you who played such an important part in Claire's life.

I enclose a "Footprints" book mark and the words from this famous poem by Margaret Fishback Powers.[112] The poem is meant to give people comfort when they are going through a hard time in their lives. This, together with a verse from Psalm 91 summed up God's care of Claire throughout her short life and especially, in the months leading up to Claire being admitted to hospital for the last time –I'm sure Claire knew how ill she was, but true to her character, she carried on working, socialising, helping out with the church youth group and loving her new home – however I believe she is now enjoying the best home she could ever have in Heaven.

Thank you again for all your prayers, texts, cards, gifts and support of Claire. I know she appreciated you all very much and indeed she expressed to so many, when she knew she was dying, her love and thanks. Thank you, too for those of you who were able to make it to her Funeral and Thanksgiving service.

---

[112] Footprints: The True Story Behind the Poem That Inspired Millions ©1964 by Margaret Fishback Powers. The Poem 〗Footprints〗 copyright © 1964 by Margaret Fishback Powers. Published by Harper Collins Publishers Ltd. All rights reserved.

I am writing about Claire's life in what I have called *Diary to My Daughter*. It is no literary genius, just an honest account of how she lived her life, "the embodiment of the values she believed in" (as Ndullee, a friend from Tiffin Girls' School said) and I will be using a lot of what you all said about her in your cards, texts, etc., but only referring to you all by first names. Although I was so privileged to be her mum, she was my teacher in so many ways and she gave me the "Time of My Life" (a phrase I used often when I wrote to Claire down the years). Equally she shared so much of her life with you all, because you were so important to her.

The Cystic Fibrosis Trust has a webpage in memory of all those who have lost their lives to CF (I am so grateful to one of Claire's friends who found this). Claire's star has been added (the photo is of Claire when she attended her last Charity Ball in September 2011, nine months before she died) and the details of accessing this are as follows:

http://www.cfstarsinthesky.org.uk

If you type the URL into a computer browser, then click on Appollo, then scroll down the page, you can turn the grid to "on" and Claire's star is grid reference B1, top middle.

"God made everything beautiful in its time." (Ecc. 3:11)

2015

Dear Claire,

As 2015 marches on and I write this final part of your diary for publication, it does not mean my fingers will cease to type, nor that my mind will no longer want to formulate words to continue to keep your memory alive. "I have a million hooks in my mind to hang the memories of you on,"[113] and there is so much more that

---

[113]   Unknown

I want to remember, so much more I want to say to you, in this year that would have been your fortieth birthday. What I have continually noticed during these three years is that whenever news items, for example, mention a date since 1975, my mind automatically remembers what age you were and where you would have been then; namely, school, university or work.

I have leafed through your birthdays book and discovered the dates that your closest friends turn forty this year also; those from school, university and church and bought a job-lot of cards for them. As Rach wrote:

"Oh Mave, it's such a tough time with all these birthdays. I know I so wanted Claire to be here to see many, many more. I look back to her last one, when we went to Kingston and it was one of the happiest meal times. Claire was on such good form and it was so much fun. And I can't quite believe it was her last."

Nostalgia (recalling sights and sounds of a Cotswold childhood) contained this line:

"...for it's the things that happened yesterday that have made us what we are today."[114]

Linda S.'s Mum wrote this poem, Claire, and how true it is.

Pat and I have been trying to think of ways to celebrate this special occasion. As I write, your church will open Claire's Conservatory in less than a month, and the aim is to invite many of your local friends. Paul, your pastor, said:

---

[114]   Jessie Margaret Hutson (nee Folkard) 1924-2010 (unpublished)

"We want the conservatory, Claire's Conservatory, to be bright, eye-catching and welcoming; just like Claire."

Victoria (your first prayer partner who also lived in Ranyard Close just up the road) and Ethan A. are coming from Canada for this. In addition, your beloved university, Kent at Canterbury, celebrates its fiftieth anniversary this year and one way they are marking the occasion is by way of the "Footsteps Project." Their website states:

As part of the University's 50th anniversary celebrations, students, staff, alumni and members of the wider University community can become part of the very fabric of Kent by having a short message or memory engraved on a brick, and set in a new celebratory pathway by the Templeman Library. The Crab and Winkle Path will commemorate the Canterbury and Whitstable Railway route (known locally as the Crab and Winkle Line), which ran directly below the University grounds. Set at the heart of the Canterbury campus, this new path will recognise those who have made the University what it is today[115].

Your inscription reads:

Claire Salter
Soc Psy 93-96
C.U member
RIP 2012 36 yrs
http://www.kent.ac.uk

---

[115] © University of Kent, Canterbury, Kent, CT2 7NZ

A few rows down is one that reads (and the initials are Ali's friends she met at uni):

Dear Ali, Memory keeps you in our hearts xx. C. G. H. K. M. S '97.

Kim told me that this is, indeed, Alison Browne, whom you wrote of in your *Horizons of Hope* chapter, and who died fifteen years before you, also from CF. How lovely that hers is so close to yours. I have been to Canterbury to view your special brick and take photos.

However, before I had the opportunity to go, our lovely friends, Trevor and Val A. were on the Campus for a Christian weekend recently and they found the bricks for you and Ale. Interestingly, they were staying in Park Wood accommodation, another tangible link with you. Val emailed on June 26, 2015:

"Feel so privileged to have seen a lasting monument to your precious Claire, but an even greater legacy is the memory of her life, as she loved and served her Saviour in this place."

Patricia A. and Sam O., who attended the 50th celebrations in September, also sent photos. I went down too, and spent a full morning photographing all your favourite haunts on campus, reliving your years there through my own eyes, snapping pictures of the Gulbenkian Café and the like.

Your fortieth birthday was remembered early this year by the annual CF Trust fund-raising sale at your old office base, Fairmount House on 15th July.

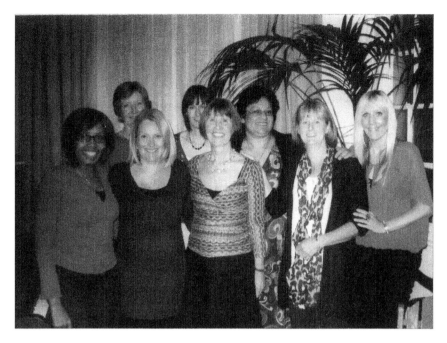

More than work colleagues, these are all fantastic friends, from L-R

Back row: Rosemary, Jo, Lata

Front row: Bernie, Heather, Marianne, Helen, Claire

Reception staff enlisted bakers in the building to supplement the cakes that your church friends, Carole, Lis, Nicola, Heather and Jean (as well as your cousin Kelly) made. The CF Fundraising group that you so faithfully remained part of in the last few years of life also contributed cakes.

The day following I wrote to all those who had kindly participated in this event:

I want to thank you so very much again for all your efforts towards the CF Cake Sale. The CF Trust banner we displayed said that Cystic Fibrosis is "no party" and that the Trust will not celebrate being 50 years old until all those with CF can. Sadly this didn't include Claire, nor thousands who have lost their lives to CF, but what you all did yesterday is testament to your respect for Claire and the CF cause. Claire joined the local fund-raising team a few years ago because, whilst she knew gene therapy wouldn't be in time for her, she wanted as many as possible to benefit from it in the future. One day gene therapy will be a reality so that lives may be saved, and *you, all of you*, would have helped contribute to that. Claire would have been so proud of you all.

Keleigh, Jemma and Jade remain so faithful coming all the way from Leicester for your birthday celebrations each year, joined by some of your local friends too, many of whom also met in Zizzi's for an evening meal.

On the family front, Jasmine Claire arrived in August, a daughter for Kelly and Chris and a sister for Tyler. How lovely that they chose her name with you in mind.

Slowly I accept your death into the narrative of my life though, like so many other bereaved, it is often difficult to do so, because you were so vibrant; so alive! I am a different person than who I was before you died. Of course circumstances change us, but I guess nothing more so than death. If someone were to accuse me of dwelling too much on losing you, however, of making a song and dance about your death, I would respond that I am as busy as ever and yet, not too busy to sweep aside the great loss your passing has meant.

It is important to give grief a voice; if God had not created us to love, then He would have made us differently. If we did not mourn, then heaven would be less longed for, so everything is relative. I cannot live in denial; I tried that during your growing-up years (as well you know; not regarding you but concerning another situation) and pushing down my true feelings only led to anger, despair and frustration. I know that to be emotionally healthy I need to confront life head-on. In the words of the song,[116] every time I had to say goodbye to you, especially on that last hospital admission, I did indeed die, but not just a little, by leaps and

---

[116]   Ella Fitzgerald, Every Time I Say Goodbye I Die A Little, lyrics and music by Cole Porter, published by Chappell & Company.

bounds, and that needs to be acknowledged too. However, God has promised that joy comes in the glorious new morning that awaits those that love Him.

The guilt, however, to which I have already alluded to in this diary, still raises its ugly head most days.

Earl A. Grollman suggests we chide ourselves that:

". . .too much has been left unsaid, unfinished, unfulfilled," and that unanswered "whys" are part of life. "You are especially enraged with yourself; why was I not more caring? You ask yourself again and again."[117]

Dunn suggests that:

Guilt is the inevitable consequence of grief and nothing is as irrational as guilt born of grief. Somehow in the sorrow-soaked thought process we see ourselves as partly or wholly to blame for whatever happened. We either caused it, contributed to it, or failed to prevent it. Guilt charges us with not loving enough, not doing enough, not being enough. Surely somehow we could have averted the danger and that eats at us. . . . .It is only "God's will" that absolves us.[118]

This theme is further supported in the book, *Death Be not Proud* by John Gunther, whose wife wrote concerning their son: "Missing him now I am haunted by my own shortcomings, how often I failed him. I think every parent must have a sense of failure. . . .after the death of a child. All the wonderful things in life are so simple that one is not aware of their wonder until they are beyond our touch.

---

[117]   Earl A. Grollman, Living When A Loved One Has Died, (Beacon Press, Boston, 1977)

[118]   Ron Dunn, When Heaven is Silent, p72 (2002, Authentic Media, Milton Keynes)

Never have I felt the wonder and beauty and joy of life so keenly as now in my grief that Johnny is not here to enjoy them."[119]

Readers of this Diary will know, Claire, that just as Meg wrote of major regrets regarding the parenting of Peggie, that like her, I wish I could do motherhood all over again. Similarly like Meg, keeping you alive and well meant never-ending activity (as Meg says: fixing nebulisers, physiotherapy and more) and that in an effort to keep her daughter alive, she actually pushed her away. She blamed herself for the "damage" she did to her beloved Peg and I identify wholeheartedly with her[120].

Whilst I am not making excuses for my behaviour, life was always so busy; there was always so much to do but my regrets haunt me. When you were a toddler you, as all toddlers do, asked many "why" questions. When I had tried to respond with patience and love, only to meet more questions from you, I would frustratingly say: "Because, just because." Now, Claire, I am the one to admit in a new way that not all questions have answers.

Despite my much frequented words that, "Life without you is too awful for words, that I don't want to do anything, go anywhere, see anyone," of course I do, because that is part of the fabric of life, whether we want to or not. I am, as usual, very busy. When I think of you, with your vibrancy for living, how dare I even think of butting out when you had so much living to do. As autumn approaches I am reminded of your growing up years, always mindful as you returned to school for another academic year and wondering how many you had left. Those feelings remain; I hate the evenings drawing in, I hate the dark days of winter and I hate remembering the circumstances in which you died. The words of a poignant song expressed these thoughts and feelings so clearly: *I Just don't Know What to Do with Myself*, written by Burt Bacharach and Hal David in 1962. The songwriters

---

[119] John Gunther, Death Be Not Proud: copyright ©1949 by John Gunther: A Word From Frances, p194, Harper Collins.

[120] Turn it into Glory, by Meg Woodson (1991 © Meg Woodson, Hodder and Stoughton)

speak of the pain of previously planning and doing everything for two people when only one is left. So my task is to recall happy memories and substitute those with the above.

Reader, if you want to help the bereaved, write, send cards, remind them how precious their loved one is to God; we love nothing more than to talk about the person we have lost. It does not matter if we cry; you are not upsetting us! Rest assured that when we have done battle with the world, socialised when we would rather remain at home, that we return there to weep anyway.

It is far easier to, in the words of the song by Jim Steinman, sung by Bonnie Tyler, "fall apart" (from the album *Faster Than the Speed of Night*) at home than in public, but please do not allow that deter you from talking to us about, I guess, the most important and utterly sad thing that has ever happened in our lives – the person we have loved above all others, and lost. In the busyness of life, we all forget, but if I may gently suggest, remember those for whom public holidays – especially poignant ones like Christmas and New Year – hold special pain. Even three Christmases on, I cannot go into shops displaying their seasonal wares, together with baubles and festive lights adorning the myriad of Christmas trees without choking up.

I know, however, I am not ready to forgive myself yet, Claire, because worst of all, I still cannot get those last few weeks out of my head. How you got through them feeling so ill and totally breathless. (When you were admitted your lung function was only 14% and it must have gone down so much further, but they never measured it again, thus we never knew.) How you coped with the panic of not being able to breathe, I cannot fathom.

My only conclusion, of course, is that despite all of this, you left a legacy few leave and now you are completely free. What I do know for certain, however, is I relate so profoundly to Kate, regarding Anna in *My Sister's Keeper*:

"I take her with me wherever I go. . . .there should be a law limiting grief. . . .a rule book that says it's all right to wake up crying, but only for a month. . . .that after forty-two days you no longer turn with your heart racing, certain that you have heard her call out your name,"[121] (p 405).

This grief rings true continually as seen in the poem below by Anna McKenzie, quoted in Sheila Cassidy's book, *Good Friday People.* Cassidy (a doctor in the Hospice movement but who was also imprisoned and tortured in Chile for treating an injured fugitive) says:

"The blank cheque written in solitary confinement has been cashed to the full and I know deep in my heart that His love is better than life itself."[122]

Claire, I could never pretend your suffering was equal to that of Cassidy, nor the times of heartbreak in your own life (and as you faced death, still with so much living to do, could be compared to many others). I do know, though, that suffering is personal to each one of us and those to whom this book is also dedicated, those who have lost children will, of course, have their own application. The poem "Good Friday People" is extremely contemplative:

And so we must begin to live again [How often you did this, Claire, when things went so wrong in your life; broken relationships, multiple hospital admissions; downright scary medical problems.]
We of the damaged bodies and assaulted minds
Starting from scratch with the rubble of our lives
And picking up the dust of dreams once dreamt.

---

[121] Jodi Picoult, My Sister's Keeper (reprinted with the permission of Atria Books, a Division of Simon and Schuster, Inc. MY SISTER'S KEEPER by Jodi Picoult. Copyright © 2004 Jodi Picoult.)

[122] Sheila Cassidy, Good Friday People (Darton, Longman and Todd 1991)

And we stand there, naked in our vulnerability,

Proud of starting over, fighting back

But full of weak humility at the awesomeness of the task.

We without a future that's safe, defined, delivered

Now salute you God,

Knowing that nothing is safe

Secure or inviolable here

Except you

And even that eludes our mind at times

And we hate you and we love you

And our anger is as strong as our pain

Our grief is deep as oceans

And our need as great as mountains.

So we take our first few steps forward

Into the abyss of the future

We would pray for

Courage to go places for the first time

And just be there

Courage to become what we have

Not been before

And accept it

And bravery to look deep within our souls to find new ways

We did not want it easy God,

But we did not contemplate

That it would be quite this hard

This long, this lonely.

So if we are to be turned inside out and upside down

With even our pockets shaken

Just to check what's rattling and left behind

We pray that you will keep faith with us

And we with you, holding our hands as we weep

Giving us strength to continue

And showing us beacons along the way to becoming new

We are not fighting you God,

Even if it feels like it

But we need your help and company

As we struggle on

Fighting back

And starting over.[123]

Writing this Diary is one of the saddest things I have had to do (the saddest, of course was saying goodbye to you, Claire) and I have to make myself consciously think of happier memories, even incredulous ones! You did the maddest things at times, like you and Jo R. driving all the way down to Swanage for Rich B.'s 30th birthday.

Or the time in your swine flu days when, once you were no longer infectious, I was permitted to take you out for a run in the car so that you could experience that expanse of space. Richmond was not too far away and we would go, wheelchair in tow, to the pizza restaurant for lunch, have a quick wander round the shops and then sit on Richmond Green to enjoy some sun. So whatever your death has taken away, it cannot erase memories.

In the book, *The Shack: Where tragedy confronts eternity* by Wm. Paul Young, set in Oregon (our favourite US state when you were sixteen years old and we holidayed there) tells the story of Mack's great sadness following the abduction, rape and murder of his young daughter, Missy. When Mack had conversations with God concerning Missy, he said:

---

[123] Anna McKenzie, Good Friday People by Sheila Cassidy (Darton, Longman and Todd 1991)

"I keep thinking of her so alone in that truck – terrified."

"Mack, she was never alone, I never left her, not for one instance."
Everything is as it should be. If God wanted us to know things, He would have told us. God did not purpose Missy's death, but that did not mean He could not use it for good."[124]

Wm. Paul Young quotes Frederick Buechner:

"You can kiss your family and friends goodbye and put miles between you, but at the same time you carry them with you in your heart, your mind, your stomach because you don't just live in a world, but a world lives in you."[125]

If, in this Christian novel, Mack could believe that Missy was never left alone, then I must believe the same for you, for God is good and we dare not doubt that. When my mind, as it inevitably does, reverts back to the sad times – the "Why, God?" times, especially about you not getting the transplant – I am reminded of this.

Post World War II, when my original family lived in the road adjacent to your church, money was very hard to come by, like it was for most people. I told you once that whenever, as children, we asked for certain items that were way beyond my parents' ability to provide, my mum would respond: "When my ship comes home." As a very young child I had a picture of a sailing ship bobbing about on the horizon, laden with treasure that belonged solely to my mum. I cannot even remember how old I was before I realised there never was such a ship! However, my memory reverts to those early days every time I reflect on this and yet the truth behind these words is eternal.

---

[124] Wm Paul Young, The Shack (p209, HarperOne, 2009)

[125] Telling the Truth: the Gospel as Tragedy, Comedy and Fairy Tale by Frederick Buechner (Harper Collins Publishers, New York) Copyright © 1993 by Frederick Buechner

I will not doubt, though all my ships at sea

Come drifting home with broken masts and sails

I shall believe the Hand that never fails

From seeming evil works good for me

And though I weep because those sails are battered

Still will I cry while my best hopes lie shattered

I trust in you.

I will not doubt though all my prayers return

Unanswered from the still, white Realm above

I shall believe in is an all-wise love

Which has refused those things for which I yearn

And though at times I cannot keep from grieving

Yet the pure ardour of my fixed believing

Undimmed shall burn.

I will not doubt though sorrows fall like rain

And troubles swarm like bees about a hive

I shall believe the heights for which I strive

Are only reached by anguish and by pain

And though I groan and tremble with my crosses

I yet shall see through my severest losses

The greater gain.

I will not doubt, well anchored in the faith

Like some staunch ship, my soul braves every gale

So strong its courage that it will not fail

To breast the mighty unknown sea of death

Oh may I cry when body parts with spirit

"I do not doubt," so listening worlds may hear it

With my last breath.[126]

In *The Velveteen Rabbit* by Margery Williams, the Skin Horse says to Rabbit:

Real isn't how you are made. It's a thing that happens to you. When a child loves you for a long, long time, not just to play with, but really loves you, then you become real. That's why it doesn't happen often to people who break easily, or have sharp edges, or who have to be carefully kept. Generally, by the time you are Real, most of your hair has been loved off, and your eyes drop out and you get loose in your joints and very shabby. But these things don't matter at all, because once you are Real you can't be ugly, except to people who don't understand.[127]

I agree wholeheartedly, Claire. It is people's suffering that makes them real, and real you were and still are, to the very core of your character.

While I want to cling to you, Claire, I realise I cannot, and the reason is best reflected in the poem, *Eternity* by William Blake (1757-1827):

He who binds to himself a joy

Does the winged life destroy

But he who kisses the joy as it flies

Lives in Eternity's sunrise.

---

[126] Ella Wheeler Wilcox. Streams in the Desert, December 9th, Chas E. Cowman, 1962 Cowman Publishing Company Inc. Los Angeles

[127] The Velveteen Rabbit, Margery Williams (copyrighted material. pg9, 1922, George H. Doran Company)

Adrian Barlow's blog suggests that Blake balances negatives against positives; the life-denying destructiveness of a selfish act versus the reward of a selfless gesture.[128]

In this same vein of thought, Elisabeth Kubler-Ross in *On Death and Dying* suggests:

Every hardship is an opportunity to grow. To grow is the sole purpose of existence on this planet Earth. You will not grow if you sit in a beautiful garden and somebody brings you gorgeous food on a silver plate. But you will grow if you are sick, if you are in pain, if you experience losses and if you do not put your head in the sand, but take the pain as a gift to you with a very, very specific purpose.[129]

Although I am challenged, Claire, to not become resentful, I refuse to taint your memories with any bitterness. When Paula D'Arcy lost her husband and daughter Sarah in a car accident she wrote: "One afternoon, my heart breaking, I began sorting through the clothes my Sarah would never wear. A dress lay across my lap. . .It evoked one more moment of bitter tears and confused disbelief. This was not the life I had chosen. It was not the life I expected. Life was not supposed to turn out this way.[130]"

Similarly this same author wrote: "Nothing else mattered then. Not my education, my training, my modest successes. They were a pitiful match for the hand flinging my world into a new mould. . . .Everything was expend-able. Life was the gift all along. . . . . .Who could believe the years would run out, young as we were? But they did run out. . .there was no next year. . .There had never been a guarantee."

---

128   http://adrianbarlowsblog.blogspot.co.uk/2012_04_01_archive.html

129   http://www.ekrfoundation.org/quotes/ Copyright © 2015 · All Rights Reserved · Elisabeth Kübler-Ross Foundation

130   Paula D'Arcy, Waking Up to This Day (p7, 2009, Orbis books)

In *Song for Sarah* this same author writes:

If we fuss. . .about our lives – if we make clothes and houses and work and events of great importance, then in the end we'll be fooled. In the end they are only temporary. There was to be something more but I missed it. I counted on tomorrow, and I counted on. . .you. I easily put off the question of what really matters, of what gives life meaning, of what is directing my life. Always so busy. He never guaranteed anything permanent except His love. I made all the other conclusions.

D'Arcy continues:

My eyes were lasers, keen hunters that found the homes where whole families lived-the ones with mothers, fathers and siblings-families that lived the way I thought life should be. . . .I didn't want the life being held out to me. That was the truth I was not speaking out loud. My secret thought was that there were two lives; the one I was supposed to have, and the crummy one I'd gotten. (p 50) [131]

Eareckson and Estes state:

His loved ones are very precious to Him and He does not lightly let them die.[132] (p 39)

---

[131] Paula D'Arcy, Song For Sarah

[132] Joni Eareckson Tada, Steven Estes. Steve Estes Foreword to the above book: (p39). Copyright © 1997 by Joni Eareckson Tada and Steve Estes. (Zandervon Publishing House, Grand Rapids, Michigan 1997.)

Have cruel or careless people broken your heart or stolen your dreams?

By the time their sin splashed onto your life, it was the will of God for you;

the God who loves you intensely and who will call them to account. (p88)

Yet, I know I had to forgive Claire, and focus on God, and your bright, happy memories. I had to trust Him, Claire. It is all I can do. Eareckson and Estes include this poem within the pages of their book (p88):

I didn't get to know her; there's something I need to say:

Please tell me your secret; I want to sit at your feet,

I need to know how you handle the pain that is your daily meat.

How do you keep on smiling when each day your health grows worse?

How do you keep depending on God when you're living under a curse?

Every time I see her; her smile comes from deep within

I know her fellowship with God isn't scarred by the circumstances she's in.

She admits her health is failing; she knows she's fading away

How can she remain so calm when I'd be running away?

My friend, can you tell me how you can trust the Lord

How can you stay so gentle and sweet when He seems to wield a sword?

You are to me a promise that even in the midst of pain

God is near and faithful if I will turn to Him again.[133]

In March and May of 2012, the sun shone warmly when you were in hospital. We ventured out with your wheelchair, oxygen cylinder strapped tightly to it, little realising that those journeys would come to an abrupt end in the middle of May.

---

[133]   Liz Hupp, p102, When God Weeps. Joni Eareckson Tada, Steven Estes. Steve Estes Foreword to the above book: (p39), (p88). Copyright © 1997 by Joni Eareckson Tada and Steve Estes. (Zandervon Publishing House, Grand Rapids, Michigan 1997)

For, as again in the words of Paula D'Arcy: "Roy and Sarah are badly hurt; Roy and Sarah are dying."[134]

You, too, Claire, were dying. How could this be when the summer stretched before us? When you had, only a few short weeks previously, moved into your new home that was meant to represent so much following your proposed lung transplant? Why did God create you so beautifully on the outside when your internal body was racked with disease? Perhaps an answer is found in Sheila Cassidy's *Audacity to Believe*:

. . .It somehow became clear to me that he wanted me to have faith in his plans for me, to be supple in his hands and happy to accept whatever he sent. I knew that this followed on from my decision I had made that day in the retreat house and on my mind and heart wrote out the cheque to God in which the price to be paid was left to the drawer. . .my cheque was so real that I could as good as see it. There were moments when the folly of my choice obsessed me, and I would snatch the cheque from the hands that held it so lightly and tear it up. Then slowly I took the pieces and sellotaped them together and once more offered my gift. Day after day I fought the battle until the crisp slip so boldly signed that day in March was crumpled and smeared with my tears and patched together, but it was still valid.[135]

On page 259:

That my life was to be of service to him I knew beyond any doubt but it had never occurred to me that that service might be undertaken somewhere very different from where I had chosen. . .I had written my blank cheque and invited him to do what he willed with me, yet now that the crunch had

---

[134]   Paula D'arcy, Song for Sarah, (p43, 2001, Shaw Books)
[135]   Sheila Cassidy, Audacity to Believe (p 258, 1977 Darton, Longman and Todd)

come I was afraid.' (p230). 'Could it really be that this is going to be the end of my life? Of course it could. But I thought I'd only just begun it. (p 231)

These were your sentiments, Claire, throughout your teen years, university and adult life. You wrote so often in your daily diary, "So much to do, and so little time to do it in." I guess this was your way of saying, even then, that you knew your life was going to be short and you wanted to cram as much in as you could. Cassidy continued (p 232): "I knew this was a time of testing and that I was at liberty to accept what he sent or to ask to be spared, and I knew that if my offering of myself had any meaning at all it must be unconditional and I must leave him free to use me as he wished."[136]

Like you, Claire, the world is full of amazing stories of the disadvantaged who learned to not only overcome but excel. As you know, I write this diary in memory of them and of those, too, who have supported them in their journey and quest. Of course it was your last illness and death that has had the largest impact on me, coupled with the mistakes I made throughout your life on Earth.

My Sister's Keeper[137] by Jodi Picoult may be a novel, but the research that went into it was amazing. It is a book you read for your book group, and that I read early in the mornings in your new home whilst you were in your last months of life, and needed as much rest as you could at weekends. I found the references to how a family coped with ill health and crises very akin to what life was like for you and I and so many, many who have to deal with illness and disability on a daily basis.

In it, Sarah remarks to Anna, her younger daughter: "I love you. I loved you before I ever saw you and I will love you long after I'm not here to say it. And I know that because I'm a parent, I'm supposed to have all the answers, but I don't. I wonder every single day if I'm doing the right thing," (p 388).

---

[136]   Sheila Cassidy, Audacity to Believe (p 258, 1977 Darton, Longman and Todd)

[137]   Jodi Picoult, My Sister's Keeper (reprinted with the permission of Atria Books, a Division of Simon and Schuster, Inc. MY SISTER'S KEEPER by Jodi Picoult. Copyright © 2004 Jodi Picoult.)

I echo those words, Claire; left frequently to cope alone, I really did not know what was right and what was wrong so often. Anna reflects regarding her mother: "She doesn't have much free time, since a calendar is something that can change drastically if my sister develops a bruise or a nose bleed," (p 10). Or, in your case, Claire, pneumonia, a port-a-cath infection, etc. Anna continues:

"Normal in our house is like a blanket too short for a bed – sometimes it covers you just fine and others it leaves you cold and shaking," (p 11).

There are really just too many parallels to list, but lastly, "a patient's body just gets worn down, from all the fighting. Little by little, pieces of them start to give up,[138] (p 41).

Yet, as I sit here pondering all of this, Claire, I am still ultimately comforted that God is good and we will be reunited again. On the back sleeve of his book *Shattered Dreams*, Crabb states: "God is always working to make His children aware of a dream that remains alive beneath the rubble of every shattered dream, a new dream that when realised will release a new song, sung with tears, till God wipes them away and we sing with nothing but joy in our hearts.[139]

This is now true of you, Claire; the shattered dream of not being healed, and yet God had a far better, more wonderful dream for you – eternity with Him. In *Streams in the Desert*, George Matheson asks: "Will I stand in God's house by night?. . .then I know at last that I desire not the gift but the Giver. When I can stand in His house by night I have accepted Him for Himself alone.[140]

---

[138] Jodi Picoult, My Sister's Keeper (reprinted with the permission of Atria Books, a Division of Simon and Schuster, Inc. MY SISTER'S KEEPER by Jodi Picoult. Copyright © 2004 Jodi Picoult.)

[139] Larry Crabb, 'Shattered Dreams' (2010, Waterbrook Press (division of Random House) Colorado Springs). Copyright ©2001 by Lawrence J Crabb Jnr, PhD

[140] George Matheson, Streams in the Desert, pg40 (1962, Cowman Publishing Company Inc. Los Angeles)

Your legacy lives on, right here on Earth, too. I am reminded daily, hourly, how you accepted so much, but it was not a passive acceptance, it was an active one. You chose acceptance – you elected it, you voted for it. However much you would have wanted to dash around and achieve a million things, your body would not permit that, so you decided to go with the flow and I am still, and will always be, in absolute awe of you. I have said so often that CF made you the person you became; that was so apparent from your childhood, teen and even more so your adult years. Despite not wanting to have CF, despite crying so often in the darkness of a hospital room, thinking that so few people understood, longing to be well enough to be home, disappointed when the doctors said you must stay even longer than first thought, it shaped you into the person that so many people know, that so many people admire. You allowed God to use your CF to His glory.

Whatever you would have wanted and longed to do with a long life, however much you would have been overjoyed with a successful lung transplant, however you wished to influence this world for good, you have been acceptant of God's plan for your life. Although we cried so often together, you may never know the count-less times that I cried alone for you, pleading with God, seeking Him earnestly in prayer that this guy that you love so much would be the one for you; would return your love. Yet with each unanswered prayer, and that last unanswered prayer for your life to be spared, I know that He is perfect and good. Seeing you overcome in all these heart-breaking situations strengthened my faith, not only in God, but in you, my beloved child, who overcame victoriously. My child, yet my teacher.

In the timeless words of the great Whitney Houston, "And I will always love you. . .[141]"

---

[141]   Whitney Houston, The Bodyguard, 1990, Grammy Award for record of the year

Conclusion

In her book *Waking Up to This Day*, Paula D'Arcy writes: "I think of a good friend who buried her young son. Years later someone asked her if she felt that he had been cheated of life because his years were few. Her response was striking. '. . . . .I got to participate for a while in the journey of that soul. For that I am unspeakably grateful.'"[142]

I cannot even begin to tell you, Claire, how I am also indescribably thankful that I got to share in your life.

Like thousands of others through the years, parents who have lost children "go on – not particularly because we want to, but because we have to, planting memories of our beautiful lost children, making sure they are remembered by remembering them, continuing to love them and I think, honouring them by getting on each day, one day at a time," (E. Kubler-Ross)[143]

You may have gone Claire, but my love for you has not diminished one iota. Indeed, it has grown, if ever that is possible. People have watched your life from afar; they have watched from near, and the message is the same – you were selfless in your pursuits. You evoked such love. You loved the perfume Allure and it has just crossed my mind that God used you to allure people to Him through your

142   Paula D'arcy, Waking Up This Day, p 80 (Orbis books, 2009)
143   Elisabeth Kubler Ross, by kind permission of the Elisabeth Kubler-Ross Foundation, www. ekrfoundation.org/

love. As Brian Edwards said at your cremation, the reason why so many attended was because of the person you were.

"Our function is not to live for ever, but to live this moment,"[144] You did that so, so well, Claire. Similarly, Beth Moore suggests that: "God ties in our personal present with our future through an inner unrest that Scripture calls 'longing'. I thank God that this world is not all there is. Our feet were meant to dance on another turf."[145]

Elisabeth Kubler Ross in her book *On Death and Dying* said: "The most beautiful people we have known are those who have known defeat, known suffering, known struggle, known loss, and have found their way out of the depths."

Even out of the depths of earth and into heaven, Claire.

She continues: "These persons have an appreciation, a sensitivity, and an understanding of life that fills them with compassion, gentleness, and a deep loving concern. Beautiful people do not just happen."[146]

I need constant reminders of your heavenly home because so often the pain of earth shadows this. Verse four of the hymn "Here is love, vast as the ocean" is one such prompt:

Millions since in earth and heaven

Drawing near the eternal throne

Called from every tribe and nation

One exulted Saviour own.

In that crowded congregation

I astounded find my place [Despite my broken heart, I am so grateful to God that you are safe there.]

[144] Joko Beck in: Paula D'Arcy, Waking Up to This Day, pg125 (Orbis books, 2009)

[145] Beth Moore, The Patriarchs, p239 (© 2005, Lifeway Press)

[146] Elisabeth Kubler Ross, by kind permission of the Elisabeth Kubler-Ross Foundation, www. ekrfoundation.org

Cleansed and clothed and by adoption

Made a child of God by grace. [147]

One glorious day I will not need all these Earthly *aide'memoirs* that deck my home and garden, and those that remain in your last home and garden, because I will be reunited with you in Heaven, with your and my God. How wonderful the grace of God is that He invited us into His family; indeed without that hope I could not have coped with losing you. In the book *A River Runs Through It* (we watched the film and I recall we both loved it; we went to Montana on one of our holidays and I feel an affinity with the book), Norman recounts the story of his family; the book finishes with thiIn the Arctic half-light of the canyon, all existence fades to a being with my soul and memories and the sounds of the Big Blackfoot River. . . . Eventually, all things merge into one, and a river runs through it. The river was cut by the world's great flood and runs over rocks from the basement of time. On some of those rocks are timeless raindrops. Under the rocks are the words, and some of the words are theirs.[148]

Similarly, Claire, I like to think that your words and your life will live on, as Norm wanted those that he loved to do also. Just as Paul, his deceased brother, is described by his father in the quote below, so you remain to me in my love and thoughts (older Norman narrating): "As time passed, my father struggled for more to hold on to, asking me again and again: had I told him everything. And finally I said to him, 'Maybe all I know about Paul is that he was a fine fisherman.'

'You know more than that,' my father said; 'he was beautiful.'"

---

[147] William Rees, circa 1870's, Baptist Book of Praise, 1900

[148] Norman McClean, A River Runs Through It (1989, University of Chicago Press)

Like Paul, Claire, you are beautiful, inside and out. Also like Paul, you were broken. We do not call brokenness this term for nothing; life is full of broken relationships, broken hearts and Jesus Christ's body was broken because of the world's largest broken relationship of all time.

C.S. Lewis describes the notion of the shadowlands as living between the sunrise and the sunset.[149] I know clearly you felt that shadow so acutely in your life and in your dying, as I do now in your death. While this world continues to separates us, I will always reach out heavenward to you, love you and honour you. I am not clever with words and have borrowed other folks' throughout this book, and why? Because grief is universal. Everyone has their own narrative and yet at the same time, we share something profound; that is why I have found it so comforting to read other people's accounts of their loss.

I also end with such too: Your human voice may well be silent but I will paraphrase the words of Blake Morrison[150] who said that although his father's voice had fallen silent, he continued to hear him. I pray that through the pages of this Diary others will hear you too Claire; that "being dead, you yet speak," (Hebrews 11:1-10).

Permission was granted too late to include the exact words from Roger Whittaker's song: "The Last Farewell"[151] within the pages of this Conclusion, but in paraphrasing them, I trust the meaning remains the same. He alluded to the fact that the person he loved and lost was indeed beautiful. . .that he had loved that person dearly and that no words could describe just how dear she was to him.

As your final words in the essay for *Horizons of Hope* reflect, Claire, the reason you were so beautiful was your heart for others. This undoubtedly bubbled up from your heart for God:

---

[149] C.S. Lewis cited in: Shadowlands: The True Story of C S Lewis and Joy Davidman, Brian Sibley, 2013, Hodder and Stoughton)

[150] Blake Morrison, And When Did You Last See Your Father? p231, (2007, Granta Books, London)

[151] The Last Farewell, by Roger Whittaker 1971 from the album: New World in the Morning

Life is an Adventure – Dare It

Endings

When the envelope flopped onto the doormat, the Cystic Fibrosis Trust symbol was clearly recognisable. To anyone unfamiliar with the logo it would probably just be seen as another advertising ploy, but this envelope was to introduce one of the best days of my life. I had been selected for a CF Achiever's Award in the "Services to the Community" category, and the envelope contained an invitation to the Hilton Hotel in Park Lane, London. I wasn't the overall winner, but I did come top in my category and benefitted from a healthy cheque!

So on December 10th, 1998, I arrived at the Hilton, went up in the lift and met with Terry Waite, who I later found out was to present my award. I met many other celebrities but my conversation with Terry Waite proved to be the best. Lots of CF winners of different categories were there and it was so great to meet them and hear their stories. We were all treated like royalty and enjoyed a fantastic lunch while we chatted and took endless photos. Terry Waite is one of my heroes because of his loving and caring attitude despite the years he was held hostage, most of which was spent in solitary confinement. It was during his captivity in the damp, dirty, underground cell that he developed chest problems and found it hard to breathe; that's why he can empathise with CF people so well. The whole experience of that memorable day will remain with me for a long time and this is one of the many examples of my privileges.

It is fitting that, having started with Ali, I should close with one of the poems she wrote. It was read at her funeral and it meant a lot to me and many others. Ali died in her early twenties and yet she was an inspiration to so many – a real fighter.

Ali's earthly race has come to an end but this poem speaks so strongly about her faith in God for her future.

"When I am strong

I will fight

And when I am weary of the fight, I will rest in you.

Knowing that you can carry me for a time.

In my fight

I will draw strength from your love

For your love cannot be beaten.

When I am alone, when I feel the icy touch of fear

I will take it in my hand and hold it out to you and in the heat of your love it will melt away.

When my heart feels isolated, when no one can comfort me and the crowd serves only to remind me of how alone I am

I will look within myself where you wait and I will remember to allow you to love me.

Then, when the joy is so strong that I cannot take life in quickly enough

I will remember to take a moment to sit with you and appreciate the beauty you created.

And when the night comes, I ask only that I be alive with peace and faith so that I may not fear the new day that lies beyond.[152]"

I echo Meg Woodson's words in her dedication to the book *If I Die at Thirty*[153] when she said of her daughter that all the best lines belonged to her Peg. In the

---

[152] Alison Browne, 1997 (Horizons of hope⬚ Edwards, B.H. © Day One Publications, 2000, ISBN 1903087 02-3.)

[153] Meg Woodson: If I Die At Thirty pg 95 (1975, Zondervan Publishing House)

same way, Claire, this Diary is yours and thus you must have the last word and what better than the text you shared with your friends on that Wednesday in May of 2012:

"My lovely friends. . . .You have made my life so wonderful, special, exciting and fun; let's pray there are more times to come. I love you all and wanted the opportunity to say how amazing you are, each and every one of you, and the love and support you have shown me over the years has meant more than words can ever say. . . . . Now let's get praying and down to business. Xxxxxxxxxxxxxx."

Appendix One

Correspondence Received
On/After the 25th May

I t did not take long for the news of your death (or should I say your entrance to eternal life) to reach everyone connected with you. There were letters, texts, emails and cards that flowed in from people who knew you from various circles expressing their feelings for you, including one from the G. family. Kate was so faithful in visiting you in hospital over the years. Emails also came from the hospital where you died. These are such early days, but they are coming in thick and fast. The cards are too numerous to list; however I hope you are both humbled and also proud of the love shown to you.

They represent family, school, university (both Kent at Canterbury and Reading) and church friends, various friendship groups you belonged to as well as from colleagues, past and present. (Your cousin Kelly, as well as Jo and the Hedge family, kindly provided print outs from your Facebook posts). Room prevents me including everyone's. Space also prohibits inclusion of all the sentiments expressed by so many, thus I have had to edit them.

From School Friends*:*

I recognised so many names from Tiffin Girls' School (TGS) and it was comforting to read these Facebook posts, as well as a few who were not familiar to me, including Ruth Jones, (whom I believe you last saw at the TGS reunion in 2011) and Lynne Frost (but maybe I just do not identify with their names if they are now married!).

Ndullee S.:

Dear Claire, . . .I'm not sure that any words can do justice. Even as a child you showed enormous emotional maturity and were always the first to extend a hand of kindness. I feel so lucky to have had you as a friend. You've always been there for me. You lived life to the full and made every day count. It's some small consolation to me to know that you experienced more in your short life than many do in twice as long. You lived your life according to the principles you held so dear and touched many people with your love and kindness. These are a few of the things I'll remember: your smile; the eleven year old girl I met at school; looking absolutely fabulous in thigh-high boots; dragging an oxygen bottle around in killer heels for Becca's baby shower; coming to my hen weekend despite being so poorly you could hardly walk; coffees at Fortune's; dinners at Carluccios; the roast you once cooked for book group; and a lovely dinner at your new house just after you'd moved in. I can't believe you're gone. Love you xxx.

Catherine D.

Heaven has a new angel now – Claire was a beautiful person in every way and will never be forgotten by those who knew her, but will always be missed.

(Catherine included the lovely poem "Weep Not For Me" by Constance Jenkins.)

Rebecca Mac:

Claire had the biggest group of friends of anyone I know. I don't think anyone was a bridesmaid as many times as our Claire; each time a different outfit; each time looking fabulous. Claire's social diary was notorious; you had to book yourself in with her weeks in advance. She had time for everybody, made everyone feel special and never burdened anyone with her troubles. I met Claire aged 11 at our first day at Tiffin Girls'. Throughout university and all the junctions of our life and our friend's lives Claire was there. Claire got me into medical school. Asked, "Tell me something about a patient or a disease that you have encountered," at interview, I told Claire's story. In my medical finals I was asked, by chance, to describe the ion channel disruption in cystic fibrosis. Claire was with me again. It was in our monthly book group with Sarah, Ndullee and Caroline that I will remember Claire most. It never mattered if Claire hadn't read the book, she had usually been jetting off on an exotic holiday, driving all weekend to get to a friend's party, wedding or baptism. Or she had been working really hard and just needed some sleep. Boy, could that girl sleep! We knew in our hearts that we would lose you at some point, Claire. I just wish that day hadn't come. Sleep well, my beautiful friend, you'll wake in heaven.

Sarah M.:

Dear Mave,

Those of us from book group met up last week, and although it was sad in that it brought home to us that Claire really was gone, we shared some great memories of her.

I loved her independence and assertiveness which came on so much from her early days at Tiffin to her working days as a social worker. I admired so much her determination to work and live a normal life despite her illness. All the times she felt bad but hid it and cared so much about all our relatively minor issues. I do not know anyone who had as many friends as Claire.

Caroline T.:

Claire has been a presence in my life for many years. I first met her at Tiffin Girls' School and couldn't understand why she was interested in me! Later I realised that she wasn't nosey, she just cared. I got to know Claire better through Christian Union and her prayer and thoughtful answers to questions helped me to know Jesus as my Lord. She has remained a shining example of how to express God's love to the world.

Us book group girls will miss her so much. Claire was the common thread that ran through all our lives and I have often thought that she has been the glue that kept us all together over the years. That glue will never dissolve now, even though she is not with us anymore. That is just one of her many legacies. Claire played a key part in my being saved. If she hadn't patiently prayed for me and shown me what being a Christian was like, I don't think I would be a Christian now. I truly owe her my life.

Melanie G.:

Simply put, Claire was one of my oldest and best friends. . . I remember her support during some of my more difficult moments; she was one of the few people I truly trusted and felt able to talk to during these periods. She was passionate about things that really mattered to her: family, friends, church, her career, fashion, travel and maxing the moment, living life in the fast lane, gathering experiences. When I think of her achievements, I am amazed at all she crammed in such a short space of time and used to wait with baited breath for the next instalment. (Mave, whilst a good degree of this gumption comes down to her tenacious personality, a good deal is also a result of the way she was raised and the values you instilled in her. I also have great respect for you as a mother for allowing her to live her life as she wanted to even when you were concerned about choices she made and pressure she put herself under making so few exceptions for her illness.)

Claire was never defined by her CF; that was just an incidental by the way. So I was shocked on hearing of her death, always believing she'd fight off another infection and that there would always be one more tea and cake session. . . . Love you, Claire xxx.

Claire E.:

From standing freezing cold at the bus stop on the way to school to trips away to the caravan, I have happy memories of a very special person. You will never be forgotten and this sadly puts life into perspective. . . .I have been in contact with some of the other girls from school too and they all send their thoughts and love, as does my mum.

Lynne F.:

"He shall wipe every tear from their eyes. There will be no more death or mourning or crying or pain," Rev. 21v4. A far better place. One of the loveliest girls in the school. Thinking of her friends and family.

Helen R.:

Unexpected and sad news today. Thinking of Claire Salter and how she used to power round the track to do the 1500m (even representing our form at sport's day). Hope you are in a better place now. Xxx.

Faye W.:

I am very grateful for my friendship with Claire. I loved her greatly as so many people did.

Zoe W.:

Though I haven't seen you for many years you are always dear to my heart and often in my thoughts; a gentle, caring, determined and passionate soul on this earth, who touched everyone's life that you met. So inspiring, never complaining of any burden that you had to bear, I feel blessed to have had you as a friend. You will always be in my heart. Love you, Claire xx.

Ruth J.:

Claire, what an amazing woman – an inspiration to all those who knew her or ever met her. Her capacity for friendship was unending – always there for people no matter what. You will be so missed.

Beth L.:

I am truly sad to hear about Claire. She was absolutely unique and one of the kindest people that I have ever met. She will be missed by so many people, myself included. Thanks for sharing the details for tomorrow with all the old Tiffin Girls. We will be there for her.

From University:

Ruth H.:

This world has not seen a more beautiful person than Claire. I thank God for her life, love, courage and her constant determination. What a precious gem, a beautiful expression of God's creation, a much loved and deeply missed dear friend. I will always hold you close to my heart and thank the Lord for the joy, love and laughter you brought to my life. She enriched my life so much xx.

Isla M.:

I feel so blessed to have been able to see so much of her in the years since we met at uni and house-shared during our second year. She was such an encouragement to me last year and really understood what it was like to be away from home and in hospital. Claire blessed so many people. Her warmth, compassion and perseverance were a testimony of God's grace in her life.

Ele F. (Her nickname for Claire was "Mozzie," after mosquito due to Claire's slight size, from having CF):

I am so sad. Claire was a beautiful, funny, stubborn and vain Mozzie and we loved her that way. I think she would have found it unbearable to say goodbye and we have found it even more unbearable to let her go. The good thing is that Claire knew she was an angel passing through, so she lived her life to the fullest. She did all she wanted to do that her body allowed her to do. I am so lucky I got to spend some time with her.

Caroline S.:

So good to visit you in hospital, Claire, but so utterly sad that now you are gone. Xx.

Simon and Lynn W.:

Despite knowing that this day would come, it has still been a shock that Claire has been called home, but at the same time we rejoice she is safe in her Father's arms. Claire played a big part in our lives, from early friendship at university, as Lynn's housemate and of course, bridesmaid at our wedding. We will miss you, housemate, bridesmaid and super friend; so full of life with the most amazing smile. A real testimony to God's love. All our love.

Keleigh, Jemma and Jade:

Keleigh first met Claire at the University when attending the Christian union. Claire stood out from the crowd for Keleigh as she would always make an extra effort to speak to her and notice when she hadn't been to a meeting for a few weeks. . . .We never realised the full extent of living with CF until Claire joined us on a trip to Spring Harvest. Her morning medication routine was very time time-consuming but she never allowed CF to stop her from doing things. We would often talk to Claire about finding a man; our husbands couldn't understand why she hadn't been snapped up years ago, but there were few men who were able to meet her high standards with equally strong Christian values and morals. Claire was an independent young woman and determined to do as much as possible for herself. Love always to our dear friend Claire, xxx.

Patricia A.:

I first met Claire at university, when she took me under her wing; I was a foreign student and feeling a bit lost. . .this was the start of a very special friendship, enjoying, among other things, evenings out in Wimbledon Village and Kingston, travelling to Morocco together, organising a hen party and being bridesmaids. My favourite memory is when she came to Cape Town to visit me and going horse-riding on Noordhoek beach. I remember how impressed I was with her courage. Claire, you hold a special place in my heart and always will. You are such a beautiful example of compassion, determination and being true to yourself. You didn't let anything stop you from getting the most out of life, and you'll be an inspiration to me forever. I love you and miss you.

Geraldine L.:

Dear Claire, how I long to meet you for a long lunch in Covent Garden and sit opposite your gorgeous smile.

Sally and Dave, Karen and Guy (It was Karen, who lived in one of the five rooms on Claire's floor in Darwin College who wrote that first Christmas you were all at uni: "Hope you have a wonderful Christmas with your family, Claire. Thank you for being so nice.")

Sally:

Karen and I both knew Claire from University and she was a kind, supportive person who made us feel really welcome and included. She was also sensitive and intelligent. In typical Claire fashion, she suffered in silence, unwilling to be a burden on anyone, didn't make a fuss during her times of illness and did her utmost to make the most of her time here on this planet. We had really good times together and our lives have been enriched by her being in them. For such a short time on earth, she made a massive difference to all our lives. Draw strength from how much she has influenced the lives of others, helped so many people and left so many with loving memories. I know she certainly made a difference to my life. I have never met such a beautiful person, both inside and out.

Kim P.:

Claire's life was certainly not an indifferent one. She has always been brave, although, the way she lived her life we never realised how brave she actually was. . . . To endure years of such a tough illness and having to fight so hard for every breath. She made it look a lot less difficult than it must have been. I re-read Claire's chapter in the book and realised how much we had taken Claire's illness and her bouncing back so often for granted. Our little group from Kent Uni will miss her when we meet up; she was so lovely and genuine. She's left so many people with so much more than they would have had if it wasn't for Claire's friendship.

Anna J.:

Claire, you were my fresher's friend and we met on my first day at uni; a beautiful girl with a beautiful heart.

Becky and Simon D.:

Claire, where would I be without your wisdom, prayers, hugs and smiles at uni? You kept me walking in the knowledge of God and sane! Love you more than you will ever know.

Emma N.:

"And though your heart already knows, sometimes I like to say, you've made the world more beautiful – I'm glad you came my way," (source unknown).

Samantha O.:

Claire was such a wonderful and selfless person and I will miss her. She touched my life profoundly when I was going through a difficult time and she radiated God's love in action with her love for others and she was always so kind and generous. Thinking of your beautiful smile.

Matt D. (an inter-railing buddy):

Claire was a dear friend of mine and a truly fantastic person. At uni, It didn't take Claire long to get stuck in to the Christian Union, and she soon joined the weekly prayer and bible study (Flip) group. I was always amazed at the resilience and courage Claire showed through her illness. Claire was a real credit to you and I will miss her so much.

Sarah S.:

Claire was my prayer partner at UKC and introduced me to Barton Road Church. Through both we became good friends and Claire's support and love kept me in touch with God even when I wanted to run away! Claire's spiritual maturity, outlook on life and acceptance of her illness were a great inspiration.

JPH:

Claire was the year above me at UKC and I was always struck by one thing, her smile. In the midst of her obvious suffering (always coughing, etc.) I can remember she would always look at people and smile. Claire was a courageous, bright and humble person. She was a true soldier of Christ, who through thick and thin, just kept going with such grace and compassion. She always seemed more concerned with others' welfare rather than her own. What a woman of God. Claire, you were loved by all who knew you.

Lorna D.:

To a truly inspiring and beautiful woman of faith. So devastated to hear the news. You lived life on earth in all its fullness and we know that you are now shining bright for all eternity. But we will miss you Claire.

Work Colleagues:

Emma S-K (Royal Borough of Kingston Social Work team):

Claire, so shocked, so sad, it's ten years since I saw you but it's enough to say you were an unforgettable friend. You were so brave, so funny, so beautiful, so principled, so fresh. You lit up our lives around you. Rest in the arms of your Father.

Sue W. (One of Claire's previous managers):

I am writing on behalf of everyone at this Area office in Reigate to let you know how deeply felt is Claire's loss to this group of colleagues, and particularly her friends from Mole Valley and St. Faith's with whom she worked before. She was a well-respected and much loved colleague and friend.

Claire's success in life is such a credit to you both; she was an amazing person to contribute so much to life, achieving many different things in a very grounded way, always helping others. It was always a joy to see Claire; she was the kind of person everyone stopped to talk with at Fairmount. Please accept our deepest sympathy as we share in your sadness at this time.

Janet F.:

I wanted to write to express my sadness at Claire's death, but also to tell you what a wonderful social worker and manager Claire was. She was an inspiration to her colleagues for her positive attitude and respected for her knowledge and skills.

I was Claire's senior manager for many years and I personally liked and admired her. Claire worked at 100% at all times and was very dedicated. She never let her health hold her back and always pushed herself to achieve her goals. Claire was a very able manager who gave thoughtful and reflective supervision to her staff. She was very supportive and encouraged others to emulate her high standards of practice. She also had a high level of personal and professional integrity which remained her touchstone through more difficult times in Surrey. Claire never wavered in her ability to grasp each situation she found herself in, whether as a social worker or a manager. With my sincere condolences.

Your team members (Sandra, Julie C, Carole, Scarlett, Ntombie, Trish, Oliver, Annemie and Kulu, the latter two also talked about the same faith they shared with you):

Dear Claire, missing the fashion show each day. We have so many golden memories. To a very special, beautiful lady – I am amazed at what you achieved and how you pushed yourself on all levels.

Claire, always available to help, a true person who would never not listen when asked a question. Greatly missed, you have been such a loss to our team. Your absence has been felt by everyone. You will live on in the hearts of those who had the good fortune to know and love you.

You gave so much to so many. We are all so lucky and blessed to have known you.

Oliver Fernandes:

Claire was a beautiful, intelligent, kind and fun person, who was inspirational to me both personally and professionally. I will never forget Claire's incredible strength in dealing with her work despite her failing health. She was often reluctant in telling her colleagues about her CF; instead she was clear she wanted to be assessed on her qualities as a social worker.

Another read:

I have such fond memories of our time at St. Faith's Family Centre. I looked up to you so much when I first started with Surrey in 2004, so impressed with your dedication, professionalism and calm manner (that we needed later in 2009-again you came up trumps). It was a pleasure to have known you.

Helen G.:

I will miss Claire more than words can express – such a dear, wonderful person and friend to me.

Jo S.:

Dear Claire, my colleague but much more my very special and loved friend. I treasure your friendship; so many happy memories that make me smile. We were so lucky to have had you in our lives. With love and wish there could have been many more great times. Xxx.

Marianne T.:

Claire and I just seemed to fit together in the team. Claire put the needs of her team and the children, whose well-being meant so much to her, before her own. She worked tirelessly for Surrey Children's Services, always playing her own health needs down. In fact, many never knew how unwell she was at times, but that is how Claire wanted it. Claire and I have laughed a lot over the years and that's how I shall remember her, head thrown back, beautiful fair hair streaming over her shoulders and both of us almost helpless with laughter. Of this I am sure, Claire is now at peace and her suffering is over.

Lex and Mike T.:

Beautiful inside and out. Dreams come in big sizes so you can grow into them. You certainly grew into yours. I'm a better person for knowing you. Sleep tight, beautiful lady. Xxx.

Barbara K.:

Claire, your cheeky smile, gutsy determination and sense of fun and humour plus your sensitivity and courage are an inspiration for us all!

Ann Curtis:

I loved knowing you, Claire. God bless.

Heather H.:

So sorry to get this very sad news yesterday. You are going to be missed by more than you could have ever known. Sleep well, Hunny [sic]. Xx.

Susan L.:

Claire was a lovely colleague to work with, always supportive and dedicated to her work. But more than that she was a great person to be around – such personal integrity and a deep faith, as well as a great sense of fun. Hers was a life lived with purpose.

Angela T.:

I first met your beautiful daughter about eight years ago, during the early stages of my social work degree, when Claire became my Supervisor. She gave good, stern direction and incredible support. She really cared for the children, our clients. She taught me to have more courage on the job. Once she told me I needed zero-tolerance towards a mother who had compromised her parenting. Claire was not afraid to tell it like it is.

Fiona W.:

Hello Mave. I worked with Claire at St. Faith's Family Centre some years ago when my brother died suddenly and I found the lead up to Christmas in 2006 very difficult. Claire recognised this and gave me a beautiful Poinsettia plant, realising that it would be a difficult time for me. Claire's kindness at that time has stayed with me over the years.

Janice:

Dear Claire, . . .Some people just pass through our lives and others, as they pass through, influence us in a special way –thus you have influenced me. You will be so missed. Xx.

Elaine H, WECP Team:

I heard the sad news through my work, and we (my department) were so shocked. Claire was so loved and respected by everyone she worked with, she will be much missed. Claire, your smile, your laugh will always be remembered. Xx.

Hanna W.:

Dear Mrs. Salter, It was my good fortune and privilege to work with Claire some years ago. I always admired her integrity and professionalism in all that she did. She was one of the most conscientious Assistant Team Managers I ever knew. She rarely spoke of her disability and never expected anyone to make allowances for her. I will always remember her for being a sincere and lovely young person.

Sandra S.:

Claire never made a fuss and thought of others before herself. I think only her inner group really had an idea of how poorly she was. She had shared with me just after Christmas how serious her health was. However, Claire did not let on to others how ill she was. Each day she arrived in some other gorgeous outfit and those crazy high shoes she insisted in wearing, often working later than she should. Her wish was to be allowed to do her job, a job she continued to be very good at right up until her last day. Claire was determined to carry on her great passion of work, but was also scared she would be "put out to pasture, not that there was ever a suggestion of this by management who continued to value her contribution to our team, however, I know Claire hid how ill she was for that reason. Leaving work would not have suited her at all! She had incredible mental and physical strength. Xx.

Various Friendship Groups

Jo R.:

To my best friend. Since knowing Claire from childhood, I was lucky enough to become a life -long friend. Claire and I shared many fond memories through the years and got through our good and bad times together. She was a loyal friend who inspired many, many people. She will never, ever be forgotten. A huge gap has been left; your memory lives on as I continue to remember and cherish the years I knew you. I love you and miss you so much. Life will never be the same. My VIP xx.

Leah, Kate and Zoe wrote:

Dear Claire, there are no goodbyes. Wherever you are, you will always be in my heart.

Claire, you will be the brightest star in the sky and there will always be one star that shines more brightly.

Rach M.:

Claire was never one to sit back and enjoy the ride; she lived serving others and so clearly showed that as she struggled to work in the midst of an infection, she never stopped giving, even if she had had to slow down for a transplant. I don't understand why she died; I have so many questions but I have to believe that one day in eternity what we see now only in part we will see fully and I guess that's where faith kicks in. For me, knowing her has changed me. She had such an enhanced emotional intelligence, was extraordinary in how she did life, how much she cared, how much she loved life, and how strong, and so very much fun she was.

Mave, the last time I saw her in hospital she related how you had told her how impressed you were at how much she had achieved – being a qualified social worker in a management position, all the qualifications and training she did, being able to hold down a full-time job, living her life to the full and by herself and doing all the travelling. Claire really valued that conversation. She treasured what you said and was so pleased that she had surpassed your expectations.

Bernie P.:

I remember the last day I saw her in hospital; I was not ready to even think about Claire dying, but she knew. I remembered Claire calling me back as I was about to leave the room and said that she loved me. In hindsight, I think she knew that she would, more likely, not see me again. I wish I could have said more because I have so much to say to her.

Emma Jane T.:

You were "here to be my light, bringing out the God colours in the world," Matthew 14, the Message. Something you did effortlessly. I wouldn't have missed my friendship with Claire for the world.

Helen M.:

My beautiful friend, I'm so glad we went to lunch together after a training morning in October 2000. . . .Then there were the tennis seasons. I have wonderful memories of our talks about Wimbledon. . . .I loved us dressing up and meeting in Wimbledon Village in a bid to celeb spot a tennis player. We'd laugh over a pasta dish and you always made me smile. . . .It was lovely staying with you in your new home this year. I loved talking to you about your interior design ideas. . . .You have been a truly amazing friend, an inspirational friend and a beautiful friend. The wonderful times we shared I will always treasure. I love you Claire; my family did too.

Mummy has a photo of Aunty Claire in our dining room and tells us about her. We think she is very pretty! Love Sebastian and Rafferty.

Rob M.:

Claire, you gave me determination and inspiration to run two marathons and several half marathons in aid of CF. I am a pretty good judge of character and to me you were one of the kindest, friendliest, most resilient and honest people I could ever meet. It has been a pleasure to have known you.

Betty M.:

Words cannot express how saddened I was to read of Claire's passing. When we met in Zambia approximately 3 years ago, one would not know that Claire had a serious illness, a remarkable young woman who did not allow her illness to dominate her life. Her warm, welcoming personality, courage, determination and love of life will be missed by all who knew her.

Rhys:

My friend Claire, you are the very best of people. You showed me what it truly meant to be a friend. I will miss you very much. You have all my love always. X.

Yasmine and Bruce M.:

I met Claire in 2000, when we worked for the same Children and Families' team as Social Workers. I will miss Claire so much and am so privileged that she was such a great friend to me. Her love, interest and concern for others were exceptional, always putting her own difficulties aside. Claire was the most amazing and incredible person I know. I feel very honoured that I was her friend. She was and will always be an inspiration to us all.

Jo C.: (from Reading University)

When I last visited Claire, I couldn't get over the amount of medication she was on. I kept saying to her that if this was what was needed to get her to transplant, then just go with it, as afterwards she would have been so well. However, there was part of me that felt it was too much to ask her to keep going when her lungs were so badly damaged and I can't imagine half of what she went through.

Ruth W.:

So glad that Robbie got to have cuddles with his Auntie Claire, will miss our catch ups; you were an amazing woman and a credit to the Social Work profession.

Charlie:

The memory most in my mind is of the last time I saw her, when we met up for a meal with Jo and Ruth last autumn. She was then clearly more ill than I'd ever seen her but still full of laughter, gossip, determination and zest for life.

Jennifer W., your piano teacher:

Claire was such a caring and loving girl, always ready to help someone else Looking back I see she came to me for piano lessons from 1982-93 (the year she went off to university) – she was always a pleasure to teach, I will never forget her.

Tara S. (one of your CF friends):

I was thinking of Claire today and went onto her Facebook page. As you know, I met Claire in hospital during a stay there and we kept in touch, but when I heard the news of Claire passing I really wanted to say how sorry and sad I was. Claire always seems to me to be such a positive person and she always left me feeling as though, through her inspiration, I could take on the world! Reading about Claire's faith has given me a renewed enthusiasm for living life as a Christian. I will always remember her.

Sarah and Nigel C.:

I will never forget the fun we had in Yugoslavia, loved sharing a room with you and washing in "green water"!! Love you loads.

Elisabeth N.:

Oh, how I will miss her, but will never forget her. She was an inspiration; her love of life, all the places she managed to see, the things she did, the joy she spread. A true Angel was Claire, one more in God's heaven. I truly believe God broke the mould when He gave Claire such a loving and caring heart.

Church Friends:

Debby S.:

I am saddened, so saddened to learn about Claire's departure and can only begin to imagine the welter of emotions you will be experiencing on top of being drained and exhausted emotionally and physically from these past weeks during her rollercoaster stay in hospital. As your beloved only child, Claire has been the axis of your daily life. . .May He give you His peace and reassure you that not only was His (and your) beautiful Claire not alone, but that what transpired at that point was the most wonderful thing which had yet happened to her.

Dave M. wrote:

Claire, I know you won't get this; you don't need messages of encouragement anymore, because God took our lovely little sis in Christ to be with Him. I know you are beyond pain now but I still feel pain. . . I am crying like a baby. But my incredibly lovely little sister, I end up smiling because you're now with your Saviour. He saw how lovely you are and wanted you home with him. So I guess I'll have to join the queue of those who want to see you again in glory.

Rachel J.:

Claire was the bravest person I have known and she was the best friend I have had. As we grew up together we shared so many happy times; camps, clubs, laughter, tears, joy and sadness – all the things that made our friendship so strong. I was so grateful I was able to come and see Claire one last time when she was in hospital. I will be thinking of my precious friend Claire as I will be unable to attend her funeral.

Claire N.:

Thank you, Claire, for being the most wonderful example of godly womanhood to me. Your life and outlook inspired me from the very first time I met you. I've never known anyone else like you.

Ali S.:

My son Nathan remembers taking Claire to the wildlife park when she visited in 2010, where we saw kangaroos and Tassie devils . He has got into a habit of ending his prayers, "Thank you God that Claire is with you in heaven for ever and we shall see her again." I've realised my children have never seen Graham and I was so tearful and so sad until the time we were told about her passing. The one thing I will always remember about Claire is that she always had time for people.

Helen and Stuart C.:

Claire was such an incredibly wonderful, precious friend and special person and I will miss her so much. I will so miss her courage and extreme thoughtfulness. Even in the worst episodes of her illness, she always thought of others. She will leave a huge hole in our lives. I am incredibly grateful to God that she was in my life for 20 years and for the blessing she was to me and all who knew her. A wonderful example of Christian womanhood. 'Til we see her again, 'til heaven.

Mark and Hannah W.:

Claire, you were a truly caring friend to me and Hannah and so many others. Your attitude towards making the most of your life has always shaped ours and will continue to do so. Our lives are all the poorer for your absence but all the richer for the example you left. Wait for us.

Dear Mave and Pat, We are lost for words at the passing of Claire, but please know this:
many, many people are mourning with you both
many have been touched by the life Claire lived
many have been inspired by her character
many will keep alive the example she set to others.

Natalie H-G.:

Yesterday I and many others lost a wonderful friend, one who put the interests of others first, even until her final days. You are the most courageous, beautiful, amazing woman. . . . "Dancing Queen," xx.

Dave W.:

Claire, you were the best friend anyone could ever ask for, always concerned for others even though you were suffering so much yourself. You will be deeply missed. Xx.

Nicola W.:

Memories of Claire: Leading youth work with her was great fun; she was always up for a laugh. Claire was great at getting alongside the young people and she never let CF stop her from doing what she wanted to do. We (Natalie, Maz, Claire and myself) met as a prayer group —they were great evenings. She loved life and her God; she was a great friend who will be greatly missed by all our family. I asked Becky what Claire loved: "Shoes" was the reply.

From some older church members:

During your last hospital stay, three couples who had prayed for you regularly throughout your life wrote the following.

Ivan and Dorothy W.:

Every time we see Pat we hope to hear that you are back in your lovely new home, but alas, not yet. We know how you feel about being in hospital so just want to say again that you are so much on our hearts and in our prayers.

From Jim and Audrey W.:

What you are facing today, never for one moment think you can't cope. When you've run out of strength, and can't fight on, God will send reinforcements – start looking for them. Just trust Him, Claire; He loves you so much and He knows what He's doing.

David and Betty Simm:

We are upholding you, Claire, before the Throne of Grace and entrusting you to our loving Lord. We love you so much.

Also, Margaret E., who knows from personal experience what it is to care, and to look on helplessly in the chronic illness of her own daughter, Karen, said:

My mum passed the baton of prayer to us the day she died. She used to pray for you every day and now we do.

Emma and Matt S.:

My beautiful friend, you will be sorely missed. Your outlook on life is one that will influence me forever. It was a privilege to have had you in my life. We had such fun and I have so many wonderful memories. What I will remember most is the time you always gave me and that you were always more interested in how I was than in yourself. What a wonderful, wonderful lady you were and I know you are safe with your Father in heaven now. Love always.

Lesley Ann B.:

I felt her warmth today. I miss you so much, honey. Thank you for always being there. You still have such an Impact on my life, even when you're not here. All my love and gratitude, Lesley. x.

Pippa M. (n response to photo put on Face book):

Wow, stunning photo of Claire. . . Been thinking about you, wish you were here. X.

Daniel O.:

Thank you, Claire that you have been so influential in people's lives. The few weeks you spent at Impact was great. You were always a person to talk to about most things and that is all down to your loving and caring character.

Victoria A.:

My beautiful friend Claire. I have so many wonderful memories of our times together in Ranyard Close and beyond. I am so privileged to have you as my friend. I will miss you terribly but have the peace of knowing that I will see you in eternity. I love you, my sister in Christ. From Claire's sense of humour, I have learned how to laugh at myself, from her unwavering faith in God, I am challenged to desire a deeper relationship with God myself. From her thoughtfulness, I am learning to show more consideration to other people. Thank you, Claire, for your precious gift of friendship. I will never forget you. Lots of love.

Kat S.:

I might not have known you as well as my family but they were extremely fond of you and from them I knew you were a beautiful person. A brave fighter with a huge heart and determination. A true treasure gone but never forgotten.

Rebecca W.:

My dear, dear auntie and close friend! You will be missed by everyone you have met and touched with your kind and caring heart. You were so incredibly strong and fought for many years. You will be missed on Christmas Eve.

Steve D.:

You seemed to always be my youth leader from Spectrum, to Impact and beyond. You were often the butt of our jokes but always took it well. You were always loving, you were there for us, and never scared to ask the difficult questions. Above all you modelled to us the selfless love of Christ and always sought to point to Him in all that you did.

Suzanne T.:

I'm running the Lululemon half marathon in Vancouver in memory of Claire Salter, an inspirational, selfless and beautiful friend who gave much of her time to supporting the charity.

Michelle S.:

Oh Claire, the bravest, most beautiful person I have ever known. . . .It has been over fifteen years since we last saw each other but to me it only seems like yesterday. . .you touched my life with your smile, your love and faith in God. We shall meet again in heaven. Rest well, Angel.

Simon and Lynn F.:

I remember very vividly, several years ago now, Claire standing on the platform at the Kings Centre, talking about her role as a "'year outer" in the Schools' Work. I thought then what a plucky, determined Christian girl she must be not to allow CF to stop her doing what she wanted to do for God.

Sarah P.:

I've never known anyone like Claire in my life. I doubt I will ever meet anyone like her again, without question the nicest person I have ever met. Truly selfless, beautiful, positive, kind, funny. Her genuine interest in everyone around her and her zest for life will always be a shining example to all who had the privilege of knowing her. I always admired her determination to live life to the max. I wish I could be even half the person Claire was.

Celia and Andy C.:

Claire was a unique person, her witness and testimony in the face of such a serious health condition was incredible. The Lord truly blessed and used her and we thank God for having the honour of knowing her.

Millie C.:

Claire, you fought for so long, you're safe now; God has you. We all love you. RIP.

Written the day of your Funeral and Thanksgiving Service (Memory Book and Facebook Entries)

8th June

Ellen C.:

Today is the Thanksgiving service for a wonderful, beautiful person, both inside and out. Claire, you are already missed and will continue to be until we see you one day in heaven.

From Family:

Uncle Keith:

My Dear Claire,

I remember clearly sharing so many good times in your life. One of the best was you and your friends coming down to Devon on the coach to stay with me enjoying the views of the River Dart. Then we would all watch the Regatta Tennis Tournament, which I like to think gave you your love of tennis, that we would go to see so often at Roehampton and Wimbledon. I realise how many, many friends you had who all loved you so much. I loved you too and I always, always will.

Cousin Kelly, Chris and Tyler:

To Claire, we will miss you so much and will never forget you. You were so kind and thoughtful. . .I loved how you thought about everyone else and their problems. I love how you worked so very hard and still made time to have a catch up with me. Love you always.

Cousin Lee:

Just wanted to say that you are missed by many. You touched so many people with your ability to always remain happy no matter how unwell you were at the time. One lasting memory I will always have was of one Christmas time when you had just got out of hospital and still rather unwell but you still looked great even with the breathing apparatus you had to use. You were constantly smiling and laughing.

Cousin Kev:

The ladies that spoke, you were wonderful in your words and self-control. It was a magnificent turn out to celebrate her life and to say goodbye to a great member of our family and a great friend to so many. Bye Claire. X.

From your friends and work colleagues:

Abigail A.:

Claire's funeral was such a moving testimony both to her sparkling character, as well as to her precious Saviour. Am praying that as He sustained you to care for Claire and to pay tribute to her today, so may He continue to uphold you all.

Sue Cunningham (Aussie Sue):

A beautiful service for a beautiful girl. Enjoyed all our fun when at St. Faith's together. You are sadly missed.

Phil and Louise W.:

It is with utter sadness that we heard of the passing of Claire. I can remember quite clearly telling her at our wedding that she was the nicest person I had ever met. Such a wonderful thanksgiving service today, which really shows how much she is loved and thought of by touching so many people's lives. She was always such fun to be around, always smiling, always interested in us, always listening, such good humour – laughing so very often. I remember more serious times too, at house-parties away with the youth work and when sharing concerns for the young people in our group. She really is a credit to you, Mave. It was a real, loving and beautiful tribute to Claire and you conducted yourself in a way that Claire would be so proud. May you know wholeheartedly how much she is loved and how much she will be missed, until we meet her again.

The following was written regarding you in Surrey County Council's North East Newsletter in June 2012:

"It was a very sad day in the NE Area due to the death of Claire, however I think she would have been happy with the amount of people that came to her funeral to show how much she was loved and will be missed. One thing we can do in memory of Claire is to keep up the good work we do with the children and families and make her proud. Alex K. (Editor)."

In the same newsletter, from your colleague, Susan G.:

In Loving Memory of Claire. This month we sadly said goodbye to one of the most inspirational people that many of us will ever have the honour of knowing. Claire Salter, after a long battle against Cystic Fibrosis took her rightful place alongside the other angels in heaven. Claire never showed or burdened others with her on-going health needs, if anything she showed those around her in almost 37 astonishingly packed years what you can achieve in your life, if you have the determination and ambition that she had.

Claire was such fun to have around and was so completely dedicated to her job. She was a great colleague to have in the management team and took a real pride in her work. . .well, in everything she did. It is difficult to comprehend sometimes just how much Claire did achieve given her significant illness! Those that were there heard from family and friends about her love for shopping, which was evident in the way that she dressed so amazingly every day, her love for chocolate, which was evident in her locker and her love for life. Claire was a member of her local church and also a valuable member of a book group. It was here that she would share her most recent dating disasters and have the others in the group roar with laughter. I will remember Claire with such fondness.

Kevin R.:

What uplifting services! I was amazed at the numbers at both and it was great to catch up with some people we haven't seen for years.

Helen and Cliff H.:

Mave, your tribute to Claire was so beautiful. Such strength! Such love! Claire, we all loved that smile and your gentle ways. As Pastor Paul said, your beauty was breath-taking here so, wow! to your heavenly body. Thank you for all the memories

Naureen S.:

It was a really touching, moving and also uplifting funeral. It almost felt as though she might be milling around her guests, looking fabulous and flashing that winning smile. I will miss her and feel privileged to have known her. What an inspiration to us all. Vivacious, kind, beautiful, glam-orous, cheeky, brave and determined. I was also impressed by you, your composure, your spirit and your amazing ability to speak so eloquently to so many people on what must have been one of the most difficult days of your life. Claire showed immense courage, but so did you.

Julie and Nevin H.:

What a wonderful farewell; how beautiful, gifted, anointed and popular Claire was. The tributes painted such a fantastic picture of an abundant life –so rich, so outward facing and so full.

Maria and Ray J.:

We have just been saying how amazing the services were. The tributes from Claire's friends were beautiful. Everyone who was present heard the gospel; everyone heard how a Christian is to live and die. Claire suffered much more than we will ever know but she was loved more than we will ever know too, especially by our Lord.

Val dropped a card through my letter box that evening. It read:

My Dear Mave,

I can't let this day pass without thanking you and Claire for arranging such an amazing Thanksgiving day for the life of one amazing lady. Both the services were incredible and the way you spoke so movingly at them was just absolutely wonderful and must have touched the hearts of everybody there.

We want to pledge to continue to pray. . .for every person who heard the wonderful hope of the gospel, having seen it modelled by both you and Claire, and maybe read it in her book. But we also want to assure you and Pat particularly that we will be upholding you in these next few days and weeks as the reality of your dreadful loss becomes more obvious. We pray that the one whose name you honoured today will strengthen and renew your sad hearts. Thank you for giving us such an example and testimony of trust in your Heavenly Father even in the midst of your darkest hour.

. . .Claire would have so enjoyed seeing the crowd that assembled in her honour. She would have loved it!

I found this text from Patricia on your phone in the early hours of 9th June: *Good night, sweet Claire. I'm not ready to say goodbye yet, so sleep well. Thank you for touching my life so deeply.*

Later Correspondence

Rach M. (you were bridesmaid to her in 2008):

11.10.12: Thinking of Claire today and how she felt so ill at the wedding but you would never know, she looked stunning as usual. Claire brought me and so, so many others such love and sparkle to our lives. She was set apart, anointed, blessed, extraordinary. And despite the CF and what it made her go through, it also somehow made her so special, or perhaps it wasn't the illness that did but the way she handled it. . .brought out the very best in her. Fighting the illness made her such a strong person, such a rock to so many others too.

Your colleague, Brian B., Senior Building Maintenance Officer, who kindly parked your car/carried your brief case in to the office so often when you were just too unwell to do it yourself, wrote:

Hi Mave, just a quick line to say I have the pleasure of letting you know I have fitted Claire's bench in the office grounds and it looks fantastic.

1ST Anniversary and beyond:

These are a few of the many cards, emails and Facebook posts I received on the first anniversary of your death.

From Darrell and Barb B., who lost their daughter, Carrie in a road traffic accident (you and Carrie share the same anniversary date):

We are keeping you in prayer especially as you approach this one year anniversary of Claire's passing. I found the first anniversary a day of conflicting emotions; amazed that I had made it through the year and then knowing there was yet another year and years in front of me. Darrell and I both felt a little like what was expressed in the "Footprints" poem –God had indeed carried us through those many months.

Rich B.:

Tomorrow a year will have passed since you left and I'm still struggling to verbalise the sadness I have at losing a unique friendship, along with my gratefulness for knowing such a positive and inspirational person. I miss you. X.

Jo R.:

A year ago today we lost the most special friend in our lives; you meant so much to so many of us. Words can't really describe how I have missed you this year and still think of you every day. I will never forget your love of life and adventure. We were so fortunate to have had you in our lives. You are truly missed. Xx.

Rebecca M.:

Wearing trendy shoes today in her memory.

Chris F.:

As you know, I first met Claire in hospital when we were both patients on the ward. I was struck by Claire's amazing ability to defy the ills of CF, which is best described as a terrible disease. Claire didn't cling, rather she conquered life and I felt a soothing love of life radiated from her, like a mothering warmth. Such an amazing lady, I am proud to be called a friend. X.

In 2014, with such dedication Keleigh, Jemma and Jade drove all the way down from Leicestershire for the third year in a row to celebrate your birthday in Richmond Park, along with Rach. They wrote afterwards:

The weather was perfect and it was just so lovely watching the balloons soar into the sky. We still can't believe our beautiful friend is no longer with us and we miss her dearly.

Sue Chambers:

It was a privilege to be able to remember Claire at work today. The cake sale was amazing. The raffle raised £265.00. Mave put up some lovely photos. xx.

Jo R. Photo of the red roses and white gypsum placed in Hook Evangelical church for your anniversary caption read:

In memory of the most glamorous and amazing friend anyone could wish for. Remembering my amazing friend today, two years on, who touched so many people's lives. Miss you x.

Helen G. wrote on the occasion of your second anniversary:

Thank you for making it possible for us to meet and what a lovely time in Richmond Park, to let the balloons and butterflies go just made the day. So relaxed and Claire would have loved us all to do just what we did. Reflect on the lovely day we had and the roses you have put in places/ given to people, so meaningful. It is so clear how much Claire was adored and how she will never be forgotten.

Paul, your pastor, emailed:

My daughter, Bethany, was interviewed in the service this evening about going to York University to study social work. She was asked why she wanted to do this and Bethany related how Claire used to take her out for coffee when she was 13 and how she became a role model for Bethany; how much she inspired her, and so now wants to do social work herself. Claire's legacy of love and inspiration lives on; as she does in glory, perfect glory.

Appendix Two

Excerpts from Claire's Funeral
and Thanksgiving Services, June 8th, 2012

To ensure as many of those that knew you were aware of the arrangements for the above, we wrote a letter and posted it on Facebook. Your church notices recorded the sadness and shock that everyone felt following your death, as did my church. Peter H. (on behalf of the ministry team) wrote:

Dear Friends, I am writing to inform you with deep sadness that we heard this morning of the death of Claire Salter in hospital. She has finally lost her long battle with cystic fibrosis, a battle she fought so positively and courageously. But she has now entered into the presence of the Lord who loves her and whom she loved; what a comfort it is to know that this is a place where there is no more illness.

Committal Service –Rev Brian Edwards

Brian (your pastor in your growing up years) preached at the Crematorium on John 11:1–6, "Lord, the one you love is ill."

I expect you have never heard a funeral message on that verse! It's not very positive or hopeful – anyway, it's a bit late to remind Jesus of that now.

Ah, but there are a few very good reasons why I have chosen that verse. I have known Claire all her life. I married her parents and dedicated her as a little baby. And I cannot recall a time when Claire was not sick. Time without number over almost thirty-seven years Hook Evangelical Church have prayed earnestly for Claire: "Lord, the one you love is sick." A wonderful encouragement in that verse and a strange mystery.

"The one you love."

Claire was one whom the Lord loved. Not because she was sick or because she was a beautiful person, but because He loved her – that is what Christians call the undeserved grace of God. None of us deserve God to love us, but that love God had for Claire did not begin when she became a Christian. The best part is that God loved her before even the creation of the world. The Bible is full of reminders that God's love is eternal. And God showed that love by sending his Son, Jesus Christ, to live here a perfect life and to die an unjust death in order that Christ could take upon Himself the guilt and sin of all who are genuinely sorry for disobeying his laws and living to please themselves rather than to please God.

And Claire was genuinely sorry that she was not what she knew God wanted her to be, or how he wanted her to live. When asked what is the greatest commandment, Jesus replied: "Love the Lord your God with all your heart and with all your soul and with all your mind, and your neighbour as yourself," (Matthew chapter 22, v34-36). And Claire knew that she, like all of us, had failed on both those counts.

I well recall Claire coming to me at the close of kids' camp and saying, "Pastor, I want to become a Christian." And she never looked back.

She would say to me now, "Tell them about the Saviour who loved me." And that is exactly what I am doing right now.

But the other half of our verse reads: "Lord, the one you love *is sick*." Why? There is the paradox. If Jesus loved Claire, why was she so sick? Why did He not heal her?

Well, look how the Bible story continues, v. 6, "When he heard that Lazarus was sick, he stayed where he was two more days." Lazarus got worse and died.

Now you all know what a beautiful woman Claire Salter was. Oh she was not perfect – ask her mum and Auntie Pat – but we all know her attractive personality, her bright, winning smile. You can see it now. Claire always made you feel that *you* mattered. Ask after her welfare and she would quickly brush it aside with, "And how are you?" We all know her courage and determination. In her own story in *Horizons of Hope* she headed it, "Life is an Adventure – Dare It." Oh she dared it, all right. Check out her itinerary: Eight countries across Europe, Czech Republic, Yugoslavia, South Africa, Egypt, Israel, USA – and more. "Have medication, will travel" was her motto – the only qualification was a cool box or fridge in which to store that bundle of medication.

But Claire was a beautiful person because Jesus Christ was her Lord and Saviour. He made her the person she was. If you do not see that, then you have sadly missed the open secret of Claire's life. She never doubted God or His love, or that He is good and has a plan in all things. I don't mean she understood all things. Beneath the outside, Claire admitted that she was scared of pain and her medical future. Tearful of course, but trusting through tears.

Why was the one whom Jesus loved sick and why did she die?

Come back to our story. Jesus said, "It is for God's glory," (v 4).

Often Claire struggled to find a meaning in it all. And you may say, "How was all this suffering for God's glory?" Let me give you just one answer.

Look around this crematorium. How many here? Why? Because you have been greatly influenced by her life. That is to the glory of God. Claire humbled us all. Claire unintentionally rebuked us for our petty grumbling. Claire shone a light into all our lives. Claire showed us what caring for people really means – genuinely caring, not just doing a job. Claire revealed a Christian faith and love for her Saviour Jesus Christ that was a challenge to the fit and healthy. In short, Claire's life of sickness brought honour to God.

But why did He let her die? She was only thirty-six. But no Christian ever dies too soon. So, come to the close of our little Bible account.

Jesus said to Martha, "Your brother will rise again."

"Oh I know that," said Martha. "At the resurrection at the end of time."

Then Jesus told her something very wonderful: "He who believes in me will live, even though he dies; and whoever lives and believes in me will never die."

Claire lived and died, but because she believed in Jesus and trusted Him, she is not dead now, only her body. She is alive with Christ. The Christian believes firmly in the future resurrection, but for now, death is not the end. Claire is not dead now. She is with Christ and all her pain and suffering are gone and forgotten. No more needles, no more coughing, no more physio, no more medication, no more weakness, no more struggling to live. She is alive with Christ in all the fullness of life.

But I must close as we take our final leave of Claire's frail, weak, earthly body. Do you have the same confident assurance that Claire had? One day, this will be you. Will your friends and family have the same certain peace and joy for you that we have for Claire?

It starts at the cross where Jesus died and where Claire asked for forgiveness and for a new life – and that she has now abundantly.

Let Claire have the last word from her own story in *Horizons of Hope.* Listen to her voice:

"There are times when I get tremendously excited about the thought of heaven. . . . . However, I know God wants to use me while I am here and I hope that, despite myself I can somehow reach in to other people's hearts and touch their pain. God has been so faithful and loving throughout my life that I know I can and must trust Him for what lies ahead."

Words of Thanks (from Claire's Mum)

This service has largely been planned by Claire. At certain times over the past few years when she hit a bad patch, she added her reflections. Her family really appreciate each one of you coming today and for the amazing support you gave to Claire through the years, especially during the final weeks of her illness. Claire, when she knew she was dying, specifically asked me to add my thanks to that of hers.

In thanking Claire's general practitioner (GP) practice, I expect that she must have been their most expensive patient, but all the medication and care she needed, they provided. I had such lovely cards from the two GPs, and when I went to see the one who was assigned to Claire, she wept and said that she would never, ever forget her courage and her acceptance of such an awful illness. Dr. Carole B. wrote: "It was so sad to hear that our brave, beautiful Claire has died. Her courage, unfailing positive attitude in the face of that awful illness were truly an inspiration and I will never forget her."

Her partner in the GP practice, Dr. Jane D. wrote: "Claire was so brave, strong; a lovely girl and so unfair to have such a short life. I know several of her friends, Beth, Catherine, etc. who thought the world of her. We shall miss her."

Although we know Claire hated hospitals, I want to thank the whole CF team who cared for her throughout her life. This is just one of the comments made by hospital staff: "Claire was a special, amazing person – a true inspiration with masses of determination, who lived her life to the full. It was a privilege to witness first hand her enormous strength and courage. We admire her tremendously."

Then I want to thanks Claire's church – Hook Evangelical – for their support to Claire in every way and throughout her years of illness, so many of you here today, also my church in Chessington. It's humbling to know the amount of people in churches and groups around the country that have been praying for her.

Claire kept in touch with lots of school friends from Tiffin Girls', and some of these formed a book group a few years ago, which Claire also attended. Their tributes, together with other friends from school, have been included in *Diary to my Daughter* that I have started to write. This will also contain eulogies from both Kent and Reading University friends, as well as various friendship groups Claire belonged to, and also her church.

I would like to read a couple of the letters from managers within Surrey Social Services. This was penned by Claire's last manager:

"I am writing to say how sad I was to hear of Claire's death last week. Although we were all very aware that Claire had a life-threatening condition, she bore it with such resilience and courage that we felt that she would be with us for a long time to come.

"I first met Claire in April 2010 when I took over the management of the Looked After Team, where Claire was an assistant manager. I liked her immediately; she was young, committed and extremely hard working. Claire, at that time, was concerned as she had been involved (to a small degree) with a review into a case which was held by one of her social workers. She was understandably concerned about the implications and outcomes of this review. As it turned out Claire had nothing to worry about as it was clear that her actions in the case were exemplary, but it was typical of her sense of responsibility and devotion to the job that she loved to do. Claire was an excellent social worker and manager; she was very in tune with the needs of children and their families. She could take on the most difficult of

parents and achieve a resolution through her empathy, understanding and skill. Most of all, though, I remember her courage. She would never back down from a difficult task or conversation; she was able to be calm and yet firm and she would never leave the office without ensuring that all her work was in order.

"Claire was loved by everyone in the office; she always had a multitude of friends who dropped over for a chat. She was young, attractive, charming and great fun to be with. I personally found her an enormous support. She was always sensitive to how I was; she was very kind and made time for others. I absolutely believe that she loved her work and that she was very happy with us at Fairmount House. We are all so sad she is no longer with us. She is greatly missed both now and will be in the years to come.

"I know that you must be so proud of everything that Claire achieved in her life, she was such a remarkable young woman and you must miss her so much.

"With kindest regards,

Penny Mac.

A letter from the Deputy Director-Children, School and Families read:

"As I would have expected, Claire's passing has touched many. I have had messages from a number of people outside of Children's Services who have worked with her over the years. The strong characteristics of her love of life, desire to seize every moment and her resolute good nature have carried through each job she has undertaken or team that she has been part of.

"Some of my dearest memories of Claire reflect her dedication: Walking the floor at Fairmount of an evening and suggesting that maybe, 'It's time to pack up and go home," Of course the expected response was, 'I'm just

finishing off.' Yesterday I spent some time with Claire's team. They spoke warmly and with affection of a much loved and respected professional colleague and friend. The room was full of personal treasured anecdotes of a woman of great faith and emotional strength as well as a highly respected professional colleague, supporter and dedicated children's manager.

I do so wish Claire could have read these letters; she was always concerned that she was not performing well because of her daily battle with her illness, but she received verbal and written commendations from senior managers, which is confirmed in the above.

I just want to tell you a little of Claire's last fight to get well over these past few months and the latter weeks when she was in hospital, to show you what an important part you all played. In January of this year, despite already being very ill, Claire continued to work long hours in her job. She also helped with her church youth group, but by February it was clear she was losing ground rapidly. Following one of her hospital out-patient appointments she texted a friend:

"Feeling rough, but going home on intravenous antibiotics again as they don't have a bed; otherwise I'd be in. Have been on three weeks of IVABs and signed off for rest of week. The consultant asked Mum to continue to stay at my home as am struggling to breathe. Decisions to make regarding my health and work; things quite difficult."

One of Claire's school friends came to stay for a weekend in March, and ever concerned with other people Claire texted me:

"You okay, Mum? Off to church with Faye. Shall I take IVABs out of fridge before I go?"

Claire texted Chris, another patient with CF:

"Love my new house, it's great but haven't been doing well since New Year, so now infection is really bad; am sure will be better soon."

However, Claire went into hospital in March and texted friends:

"Morning, just to let you know am being admitted to hospital today as am not responding to these IVABs (5th week now) please could you pray that I get better on new treatment and have a stronger appetite? (I don't want to even eat chocolate!) Thanks, Claire. She came home from hospital for a few days at Easter, although very unwell. Such was her dedication to her Social Work job that she insisted in going to work for a couple hours for three days but then was taken from work by ambulance back to hospital and never returned home.

A couple of weeks into her hospital stay, Claire was told she was seriously ill. For the rest of her time in hospital she fought to get better and I'm bound to say this as her mum, I know, but in all my years in nursing I have never seen someone fight so hard. But Claire also knew the stakes were high. At the same time, however, despite requesting complete honesty regarding Claire's prognosis, sadly the hospital staff were not transparent and led us to believe she was on the road to recovery. Of course there were many text exchanges but I mention just a few here to help plot the course of those last weeks and demonstrate Claire's dependence on God.

To one of her friends, Maz, who was also in hospital, Claire wrote:

"Just so scared as still not responding to treatment. Just can't get these thoughts out of my head. Prayer is the only thing to get me through. Infection levels in blood are rising still – 178 but were only 20 when I was

admitted. Now on non-invasive ventilation mask to give my clapped out lungs a break. Love you a lot and praying for you too, Maz."

Sample text exchange from Rosemary B. read:

"We really missed your leadership at Horizons last week, so get better fast 'cause we need you! 'I find rest, O my soul in God alone. My hope comes from Him.' Claire, I send these Bible verses to be helpful but if you would rather I stopped I understand."

To which Claire replied:

"No, I love them, please keep them coming. That's what I'm focusing on – know God is in control, whatever the outcome. Please pray for heart rate to go down, for me to keep eating, un-wellness to stop –such strong, over-whelming feeling of illness going through my body – not had it before, very scary. I'm getting soooooooo exhausted now. Thanks and love to you all. Xx."

One of Claire's best friends from childhood, Jo R., arranged for a TV personality to visit her. That evening Claire texted:

"Thank you for arranging a magnificent day, Jo. Wasn't it fantastic? Thank you for being such a special friend to me."

That same day Claire texted another good friend, Helen G.:

"Drew picture of my garden at the weekend and incorporated the sweet peas. Xx."

Claire also texted me later that evening, as part of her lovely, caring nature to ensure I arrived home okay:

"Have googled carbon monoxide – it's very interesting. Will show you tomorrow. Love you lots."

To which I replied:

"Do you mean carbon dioxide?"

Of course her response was:

"Oh yes I do! Love you so much, Mum, thank you for being you."

Claire's friend, Sarah C. texted:

"Great news about infection levels being down a bit. We all prayed at house group last night." However, Claire replied:

"Thanks, Sarah, still not turned the corner; quite unwell today. Treatment not working."

On 16th May Claire texted some friends:

"Please pray, as I feel my infection has returned overnight as feeling very ill again. Pray I will have confidence in God and if my infection levels are up I have strength to keep fighting – thanks."

On 18th May, one week before Claire died she texted her Auntie Pat:

"Awful evening; oxygen levels suddenly went down by 10% then started coughing up mouthfuls of blood in corridor – medical team spent all evening stabilising me and another IV line put in –so scary. Asked Mum to stay but she stayed till 9:30pm. [I can't tell those gathered here today, how distraught and wretched I felt reading this now.] *Despite this, blood infection levels (CRP) down again from 44 to 31; such an answer to prayer, let's pray it continues. Xx."*

Keleigh texted on behalf of Jemma and Jade too:

"So great to get a text back from you. I'm in tears. Hang on in there mate, we all love you so, so much."

To which Claire responded:

"Don't be sad; I will keep fighting as much as I possibly can. Just need a little miracle to get these drugs to work now as there are no other options. Love you lots. Very up and down, but managing a shower with help from Mum and walked a few steps today. Will keep in touch if I can but tending not to use phone if I'm feeling very unwell."

Then on 22nd May (the day I asked one of the doctors for a frank and honest appraisal of Claire's condition):

"Please bring a marguerite pizza from Pizza Hut. Can't speak and Mum stressed. Please get people praying I push on through this. I feel so low,

so exhausted and that all the hard work I've put in to getting better has reaped little reward. Pray for hope renewed and strength and quick results now to keep me going. I'm desperate."

Whilst to her friend Bernie, (who had texted: *"Keep the faith."*):

"I'm just so scared, Bernie; they changed the IVs last night and I feel very unwell this a.m. I'm concerned if this doesn't work, where will I be left? God has everything in control but it just feels my health is so out of control."

Then to Jo R.:

"Taken a big dip, Jo, but looking forward to seeing you today, although you should be prepared for my changed appearance, all thanks to IV hydrocortisone and have ventilator mask strapped to my face/head."

Rosemary B. texted again: *"Keep me as the apple of your eye, hide me in the shadow of your wings. Remember, prayer is happening everywhere for u and prayer is strong."*

One of the last texts Claire received (apart from those that Dave M. and Chris F. sent after her death) was from Xenia, a friend of Saj and Rach which read:

"You are so precious, such a jewel. Claire you may be exhausted and feel you have nothing left, but we are doing battle for you in prayer."

Throughout this time, the Bible promises remained written on the white board in Claire's room and "prayer was made" (Acts 12) for her up and down the UK and abroad, as Andrew S. wrote:

"Hi Claire, I gather you are having a really *tough time and needing a lung transplant. I've been praying for you and getting my friends to pray too. Big hugs, xx."*

Claire received many, many cards, texts, gifts and visits and this kept her fighting spirit active. Yet at the same time, the paradox was that Claire talked of how she felt God was preparing for her to die and we were able to have lots of chats of her Christian hope of heaven. Those were very special times. Claire loved sunshine. She continued to believe in it even when the clouds hid it; it would be silly not to. So with God, she knew He was there even if He appeared silent as far as improvement in her health was concerned.

Niccolo Paganini came out before his audience one day and discovered that his violin had been stolen and another left in its place. "Ladies and Gentlemen, I will show you that the music is not in the instrument but in the soul." And he played as he had never played before; and out of that second-hand instrument, the music poured forth until the audience was enraptured with enthusiasm and the applause almost lifted the ceiling of the building.

The entry for September 28th continued: "It is your mission. . .to walk out on the stage of this world and reveal to all earth and heaven that the music is not in conditions, not in things, not in externals but the music of life is in your own soul."[154] Claire learned that staying alive was not what mattered most, but her ultimate trust in God. She also knew that "the woe and the waste and the tears of life belong to the interval and not the finale."

To use another thought from *Streams in the Desert* for June 13: "Rest is not a hallowed feeling that comes over us in church; it is the repose of a heart set deep in God." And among all the fears that Claire battled with, I believe she knew

---

[154] Chas E Cowman, Streams in the Desert, September 28th (1962, Cowman Publishing Company Inc., Los Angeles)

that God was in control.To begin with, Claire had loads of visitors and she really appreciated this. My sister, who shared her care with me together with you, her family and friends, buoyed her up. Of course, the last week of her life was the hardest. Claire was on a ventilator and could not breathe without it. Gradually she withdrew from social contact, stopped visitors, didn't use her phone and each day she would say, "This is it." But through it all, the messages and cards kept coming and she was aware of this.

On 25th May, when Claire lost her battle with CF, a friend sent me this quote:

"God is not caught unaware. He wrote the biography of Claire's life long before she was born and thus was fully mindful of the time of her departure."[155]

When Claire was eventually discharged on the third occasion from the High Dependency Unit in 2003, I started organising a folder of special quotes and readings I had collected through the years into what I called a "Gems" folder. Among many quotations, it contained the following:

J.C. Ryle wrote: "God never removes his people from the world till they are ripe and ready. He never takes them away till their work is done. They never die at the wrong time, however mysterious their deaths appear sometimes to man. . .The Great Husbandman never cuts his corn till it is ripe. Let us. . .take comfort about the death of every believer. Let us rest satisfied that there is no chance, no accident, no mistake about the decease of any of God's children. . .God knows best when they are ready for the

---

[155] *Source unknown*

harvest."[156] What's more important is to remember how Claire lived, not how she died.

I received this personal letter from a social work friend of hers who knew Claire well:

"Claire is beautiful, bubbly and talented. Her social life and holidays are what she enjoyed most. Her managers and colleagues alike in Social Work told her often she would go far. That is, until CF held her back in many aspects of life. She would look longingly at cyclists as they made their way through Richmond Park, while her mode of transport was by car. Her gruelling treatment programme is aimed at keeping the effects of CF at bay. Her countless hospital admissions, the pain of many investigations and feeling ill, however, never deterred her. Her courage and determination, like so many others with CF, is exemplary."

Personally I would add that Claire was not resentful; many times she put me to shame with her outlook on life when most of her friends married and had families, excelled in sport and their jobs because they had no illness to deter them, when my reaction was often one of bitterness. But her wisdom to me was amazing: "Don't go down that road, Mum. It isn't worth it."

In the last *X Factor* programme one of the competitors sang the Beatle's song, "She's got a Ticket to Ride," (1965). Claire got her ticket to heaven ahead of us. We make choices whether to be involved in other people's lives or not. You chose to be involved in Claire's, and she in yours and I am so grateful for the richness she experienced by knowing you all and I believe it was these friendships that in part

---

[156] J.C. Ryle, Holiness 1956 James Clarke and Co, London

kept her going. Thank you all so much for your cards, letters, emails. Claire would be so proud to have known of your support.

At the end of this service we'll exit to Westlife's "Flying Without Wings," (1999). This was one of Claire's favourites and reminded her that her hope of heaven was very real, that she would be free from the shackles of CF and truly have breath enough to fly. So thank you so much for the truly valued contribution you brought to Claire's life and know that she appreciated you all. As no doubt she enriched your lives, you equally did hers. Remember, "Memories are the best gift of all."

Thanksgiving Service

"Embrace Life and Expect Glory"
Rev. Paul Pease (Claire's Pastor in her adult years)

This is a thanksgiving service for Claire, a wonderful young woman who so many people loved. In fact, I don't think I've ever come across someone so young who is loved and cherished by so many people. So many people speak so highly about her and we pray that what we do here will help us in our grief, will renew our hearts to make the most of our life as Claire did of hers, and will prepare us for eternity, as Claire was prepared for that great adventure.

Claire was a believer in the Lord Jesus Christ and all we do now reflects that great fact and certainty, and ensures that though we grieve, yet we do not grieve without hope. 1 Corinthians 15 v58, "Always give yourself fully to the work of the Lord because you know your labour in the Lord is not in vain." Claire's life counted –this scripture assures us that all we do in this life matters. Claire embraced life as much as she could and did as much as she could, and did so many things for so many people and it all counted.

Claire loved life – she loved being alive. There were some of the things that Claire loved about life.

1. Loved (interested in) so many people – visited you although you were hundreds of miles away or even halfway round the world. Mileage was no barrier for Claire; she stayed in touch with people because she cared. She was generous to so many people, always had time for people. She was a real people person.

2. Loved having fun and enjoying herself; loved to laugh about many things and even laugh at herself. New Year, Christmas and birthdays were always so special to Claire. Her birthdays were always celebrated as if they were her last and she always wanted as many people as possible to share them with her.

3. Loved to look good – she could turn heads. She loved to dress nicely and look pretty.

4. Loved her work because it helped people, often struggling to get into work even though at times she felt so ill. A sense of responsibility and commitment to her team and those she cared for.

5. Loved children and young people. Had a great concern for them and took a special interest in them; their well-being, their future, what they would do with their lives. Claire worked in just about every youth ministry we had at Hook, in just about every team and age over the years. "She always seemed to be my youth leader from Spectrum to Impact," wrote one of our members. Leading youth work with her was fun, but rightly serious about the big issues in life. She was ever ready to meet with the young people for coffee, a chat about life, the universe and everything.

She really wanted to live life to the full, overcoming so much in order to do so:

- Fighting her CF
- Overcoming infections and illnesses regularly
- Trying to get out of hospital as quickly as possible.

Such an inspiration to us all, so determined; refusing to give in to her CF. And she made the absolute most of the years God gave her. So in honour of Claire, I would encourage you to make the most of life whilst you have it.

The most amazing thing about Claire was that she loved God and had a really strong, unwavering faith in Him.

But one life is not enough. You get one shot but I want another life –a next one, a life after this one has ceased. So did Claire – Claire expected glory.

The Christian hope is really amazing. It's for the resurrection of our body, reunited with our sinless souls and living in the presence of God forever and ever.

What happened to Jesus will happen to those who love him

As He has a resurrection body, so we will have the same. Claire will have a resurrection body – this was her firm hope.

A body that shines with splendour. If Claire looked so good this side of heaven, what will she be like in heaven? And now Claire is in the presence of God.

This resurrection body will be given to Claire freely, but she knew the immense cost to the one who will give it. Jesus Christ accomplished this by His death on the cross. He took our sin away but at such a cost to Him – pain, shame, agony – but He did it because he loved Claire and us and now Claire and all who love Him are guaranteed another life, in a new world with a brand new body. She will be presented to God as the gorgeous bride of Christ, without spot, stain wrinkle or any other blemish.

Claire attended many weddings on earth. She would be at them all, entering into the joy of the happy couple, but secretly longing that one day it would be her turn. Well, now she is with the Man who loved her so much He died to save her – The God-man, Jesus. And she is extremely happy with Him and will live with Him in glory, not like some fairy tale of happily ever after, but in reality, world without end. Having dared the adventure of this life, Claire is now in paradise with Christ.

Finally, we give thanks to God for Claire's life and we will go on missing her. Her work was therefore not in vain, for it was in the Lord, hence her smile, bravery, inspiration counts because it counted to Him. To know Claire was to be touched by someone who suffered so much, but who always reached out to others. Caring for others overflowed naturally into her everyday life.

But hear her whisper as she looks you full in the face, with her encouraging smile and that sparkle in her eyes saying, "Life is an adventure-dare it. Embrace life; expect glory."

Claire, as an aside, and in response to Paul's reference to you wanting to be married, Rach wrote on the evening of 8th June:

CF never made her resentful or bitter. I can remember in the last year we talked about the frustrations of seeing others have it all and she was telling me that it was pointless letting resentment build up, or to go down the route of, "It's not fair." Claire was the person who really rejoiced when good things happened to others, even when fearing that it would not happen to her. She could really identify with the pain people felt when there was loss or a time of waiting. I prayed so much for Claire to be married, Mave. She was not short of offers during and after uni, but Claire had so much get up and go and needed someone of equal character. She said she tried to rejoice with them as it's their moment. Gosh, such grace – I don't know how she did it as I knew it hurt, but Claire could really rejoice with them. Incredible, really I think about that often now. . .She was so much fun. Claire changed (and still does change) people; we have a different perspective in our life because of her.

Tribute by Jo R.

I feel so privileged to have this opportunity to pay tribute to my best friend, Claire. Claire and I were close friends since childhood from growing up in the same church. My lasting memory of Claire as a child was when I had arranged to play at her house. I turned up to find Claire standing on the pavement carrying a blue bucket. I peered inside to see a white rabbit peering up at me. How Claire loved that little rabbit.

I always knew Claire was a special person; she loved and cared for her friends and family deeply and was always so concerned for their well-being before her own. She was always so glamorous and beautiful. How we laughed together that there was never seemed to be a mirror or shop window she wouldn't look at her reflection in! Having said that, if I looked like Claire I would want to keep looking at myself, too!

Claire and I loved our clothes shopping trips together; she knew exactly how to dress for every occasion. We would spend many hours wandering round the shops, stopping to sit down for a coffee break if she got overtired. I did often suggest to her that these little breaks were also to rest her feet due to the six inch heels she insisted on wearing!

I have many treasured memories of holidays abroad with Claire as she loved the sun and exploring new places. How we laughed on these holidays about the time she would take to get ready to go out, spending what seemed like hours in the bathroom, often flooding the bathroom floor each time she had a shower!

During her last stay in hospital Claire spoke fondly of a TV personality she had seen from the programme *Made in Chelsea*. After much deliberation about this and to cut a long story short, he came to the hospital to visit her. Just before he was due to arrive I walked into her room and saw her sitting there with hair and make-up perfect. How I admired her strength and determination despite being so ill.

A few minutes before he was due to arrive she asked me to check her breath, to see if she needed to clean her teeth again. I asked her how close she was planning to get to him! Although she was so grateful to me for arranging the visit of this celebrity, it was really Claire who was the star and I think he realised that too after meeting her.

The last time I saw Claire we held hands and told each other how much we loved the other. Little did I know it would be the last time I would see her, but I thank God for that final hour I spent with her.

Lastly to Mave, Claire achieved so much in her life and I know you are so proud of the person she was.

Tribute by Rachael M.

I will never forget when I first met Claire at University. It was Freshers' Week and we were at a Christian Union event. She was sitting on my right with her long blond hair and a big smile and was surrounded by almost half of her corridor mates who she had invited along. Two things struck me then about Claire, she was both glamorous and popular.

We used to joke with Claire that we never saw her "dress down" or wear flat shoes; even when we went to visit a farm last year with my daughter, Asha. . .Claire's artistic streak was apparent in her dress sense and her love of interior design. She said if she wasn't a social worker she would love to be a personal shopper. . .

I don't have to say how very popular Claire was, nor the fact that she was bridesmaid eleven times and also a godmother. She had both wide and deep friendships. As I got to know Claire at University, the most striking facet of her personality was how much she cared. She really looked out for and reached out to people, taking them under her wing. Claire truly reflected the kindness of God. She was the most dependable of friends. . .Claire was such a loving person, so supportive and trustworthy. She was the keeper of many secrets, I think partly because she allowed you to be vulnerable with her, to share your heart.

Nothing would hold Claire back at University; she immersed herself in student life and activities. Despite getting breathless whenever "It's Raining Men", (Paul Jabara and Paul Shaffer, 1979)

or "I Will Survive" (Dino Ferkans and Freddie Perren 1978) was played at a party, Claire was first on the dance floor. She lived life to the full and as I re-read the chapter she wrote in *Horizons of Hope*, I realised that over three times she talks about how determined she is to "live life to the full." Claire was certainly not a passive observer of life, but an active participant.

Claire was incredibly caring, but she was also amazingly courageous and strong. Beneath her calm spirit was a fighting heart; she fought on a daily basis, even to do the most mundane things. She would occasionally say that getting ready in the mornings with all her medication, physio and strength it took was sometimes such hard work, yet alone holding down a most demanding and responsible job and then maintaining her super-packed social life. In her chapter Claire writes: "When I take time off I feel that Cystic Fibrosis is winning and I don't like to be defeated."

Daily life could be such a struggle, a battle, yet I can't remember her moaning about this; Claire just got on and did it, never complaining about what she couldn't do, instead doing everything that she could. It made me smile when I read in her chapter about her volunteering at school for the 1500 metres, knowing she would come last but she still went for it, determined to do it. It was when I went on holiday with her that I was reminded of how much Claire had to go through with all her medication and the limitations of her health, as when I saw her she looked so well and rarely shared the daily struggles she went through.

One of our first of many holidays together was our European Inter-railing trip in our second year of University, when with Will and Matt we visited eight countries in three and half weeks. Claire's determination enabled her to carry a heavy rucksack for most of the trip despite surviving on Milka chocolate and McDonald's chips! The trip gave her a real desire to travel and explore and with her mantra of living life to the full, she crammed in every opportunity to do this. A few years ago, when the list was a bit shorter, she said she wanted to tell everyone at her funeral all the countries, etc. she had visited.

I don't want to be standing here reading a tribute to Claire. I wasn't ready to let her go. I so wanted her to experience what it's like to go running up and down stairs, to get up in the mornings and not think about taking medication and doing physio, and to dance without being breathless. And despite the mountains of prayers, especially over the last few months, Claire is now not with us. But as Claire wrote: "When I view life in the light of eternity I remember that God has a reason for everything. Although I don't understand it fully now, one day I know I will."

I, we, have to trust in God. Claire, in her last few weeks took comfort in God's Word and she said to me in our last conversation that she knows that God is a loving God and that she can only depend on Him. Claire loved life, despite its challenges for her, and we loved her so much; our lives have suffered a great loss. The comfort I have is that now when I think of Claire in eternity I see her running, the sun is shining on her long blond hair and she is happy and so, so free.

Tribute: Helen G.

My dear friend Claire,

So many thoughts come in to my head when I think about dear Claire and I was honoured to be asked to put a tribute together.

When I think of Claire I can smile and think of chocolate, glitter, high heeled shoes, holidays, jewellery and the wonderful chats we had. I can then cry and think why she isn't still alive as she loved life so much. It was admirable how much fight Claire had in her to live an adventurous and exciting life and how she lived life to the full.

I have known Claire for over nine years, first as a colleague then as a friend. Our friendship grew over the years and it became very special. I valued our working relationship and treasured our friendship for many reasons.

Claire was so dedicated to her work and would always put every child she worked with first and would fight for their rights. She helped children achieve their goals. Talking about goals, I remember a nine year old boy we were taking into care and while we were telling him what was going to happen, he asked if we could play football with him. Well, I don't think Walton Recreation ground had seen anything like it! Claire used her shoes as a goal post at one end and her smart handbag at the other and there she was, kicking a football with this young boy –could turn her hand to anything, our Claire!

Another memory I have is of Claire and I in Horley at nine o'clock one evening, trying to return a thirteen year old to her foster placement. We were in the car and this young person was on foot. We would spot her and follow her going one way and she would change direction when she saw us, until such time we both gave up and met back at the foster carer's home after she was picked up by the police.

I think I have said this to many people and now I can say this from the bottom of my heart; Claire, I was very lucky to know you and I feel privileged you came into my life. Thank you.

I know that all my work colleagues and all Claire's friends would join me in this tribute to Claire as each and every one of us has a memory of such a wonderful person. I will always hold a very special place for you in my heart. God bless you, rest in peace, I will miss you so much.

Tribute by Bernie P.

Words are so inadequate to express how much Claire meant to me and talk about the everlasting impact she has made in people's lives - she was one of a kind. . .I met Claire approximately thirteen years ago when she was a newly qualified social worker in front line child protection. As a bright, motivated and conscientious person, she was eager to make a difference in people's lives and a success of her career, irrespective of her health difficulties.

It was very evident from the outset that Claire cared deeply for people, which made it so easy to connect with her. Throughout her career, she remained committed, dedicated and motivated and continued to work full time. And she developed into a successful and excellent assistant team manager. She has achieved great success in her career, receiving compliments from so many: parents, managers, barristers and a judge and Claire was quite chuffed about that!

For her excellent work that she produced, she always remained very modest. Unfortunately some of her hard work was not acknowledged, but it did not hold her back to try and achieve the best outcomes for those she served and for her team. Most of the time Claire would be one of the last, if not the last person in the office and as an assistant team manager she would be one of the few managers who would work late, ensuring that her staff were supported as they dealt with crisis situations. She made colleagues feel supported and valued, always willing to listen and lend a hand but would also challenge when required in a gentle, but firm way.

During this time Claire became a close and trusted friend. We shared many joyful and sad moments and little adventures, too. These memories have been my comfort during this time. One of the things of many I admired about Claire was her ability not to allow anything to hold her back and to live life to the full. Her love permeated through all she did; she was such a gentle, caring, loving, generous and encouraging person and friend. Even during her challenging moments she remained selfless, wanting to support others and putting her own needs last. I was always inspired by her character, her love and fighting spirit and she would never give up, always remaining faithful.

I will never forget our final moments together as I left her hospital room for the last time shortly before she died. Although she wanted to live she was also ready to surrender to God. Even during her last days on this earth, she made me and others feel loved and valued and continued to inspire me by her faith. Although I am comforted by the fact that she is at peace, our loss is indescribable, so painful.

I'd like to read a short poem that is so applicable. The author remains anonymous:

When God saw you getting tired and a cure was not to be,
He put his arms around you and whispered, "Come to me."
He didn't like what you went through and He gave you rest.
His garden must be beautiful, He only takes the best.
And when we saw you sleeping so peaceful and free from pain,
we wouldn't wish you back to suffer that again.

Today we say goodbye and as you take your final rest,

that garden must be beautiful because you are one of the best.

Today I stand here to say goodbye to my beautiful and precious friend and say thank you to God for putting such a jewel in my life.

Family Tribute to Claire by her Mum

On Claire's behalf, thank you all so much for coming today, for your messages of condolence and many tributes to Claire.

I've had the time of my life being Claire's mum and the great paradox is longing for her to stay, but knowing she had to go, to do the hard part of dying. As we laid Claire to rest earlier this afternoon we know that God carries His lambs close to His heart. Thus he carried her on this earth, despite his rod falling on her so many times (and another paradox is that it is His rod that comforts us) but as Margaret Fishback Powers[157] wrote, when only one pair of footprints were seen, they were His. Therefore in our sadness our memories will not only be about her diseased body, but how she is now made perfect, so that this is not so much a mourning of her death, but a celebration of her life.

This is my personal, earthly farewell to my all and best. We know, Claire, that you were torn with a longing to stay; too soon to die, too soon to say goodbye, [158]and yet paradoxically we know that God took you when your earthly work was done. You will not grow old, as those who are left grow old, age shall not weary you, nor the years further condemn.[159]

---

[157] Margaret Fishback Powers *Footprints : The True Story Behind the Poem That Inspired Millions* ©by Margaret Fishback Powers. The poem "Footprints" copyright © 1964 by Margaret Fishback Powers. Published by Harper Collins Publishers Ltd. All rights reserved.

[158] Art Buchwald Too Soon to Say Goodbye 2007, Marcia Rosten publishers

[159] Paraphrase from: Ode of Remembrance taken from Laurence Binyon's poem 'For the fallen' The Times, September 1914

Claire was born on a Wednesday on one of the warmest days in July of 1975. I could tell you about, "Wednesday's child, full of woe," (from the nursery rhyme "Monday's Child") but I want to tell you about God's child. Despite lots of chest infections as a child, Claire was very active and, being an only child, always had lots of friends round to play. She loved spending time with her Auntie Pat; Pat and Pete used to take her out regularly, as well as enjoying great holidays at our family caravan.

Claire was a pupil at St. Mary's infant and junior schools in Long Ditton and still kept in touch with one of her teachers. Margaret S. wrote, following news of Claire's death:

"During a lifetime of teaching and being in contact with so many children, there are inevitably some who, for many and various reasons, remain clear in one's mind and memory; Claire was one of those. She was such a courageous little girl – always a pleasure to have in class. It has been a privilege to see her grow up into such a delightful young woman, and to have had her so faithfully keep in touch with me.

"Whilst Claire was in my class my husband was quite ill. One afternoon he decided to walk down the hill to meet me from school. He soon realised he had overdone it and stopped against a garden wall. Claire, who knew him quite well, was on her way home from school when she saw him. She sat on the garden wall talking to him until I appeared on my bike. To me that incident sums Claire up; at eight or nine years of age she had the understanding and compassion to stay as a support and comfort, having realised his need. I will never forget her."

At eleven she went to Tiffin Girls' school. Although Claire found the transition from a small (mixed sex) junior to a large (single sex) senior school very hard to begin with, she made strong and lasting friendships (many of which continued until her death) and reading through her school reports, they speak of her being a kind, supportive member of each class she was in. She also became a prefect in the sixth form and co-led the school Christian Union.

Having completed her A levels, Claire went to the University of Kent to read Social Psychology. She loved her university experiences and joined the Christian Union (also co-leading a group) where, again, she met many friends. She led an active student life, and linked in with her fair share of voluntary organisations, for example, Amnesty International, Niteline (a listening service for students) , a mentor for an Eating Disorders' group, as well as attaching herself to helping the homeless in Canterbury and the weekly Soup Run. Like most students, Claire worked in her vacations, although she did go Inter-railing around Europe, too.

One friend (Sally S.) said of her:

"Claire was an inspiration to so many, touched so many hearts and lives and will be sadly missed by all. She made me feel so welcome and feel so special in her company. I don't think I could have asked for more support than I received from Claire at University when I lost a member of my family, she always knew the right words to say."

Another wrote:

"There are certain people who touch our lives in a certain way and having known them, we will never be the same again."

After uni, Claire took a gap year and worked with the local Christian Schools' Work Team. This cemented her desire to be a children's social worker and she went to Reading University to do her Master's in Social Work course. One friend, Jo C. said:

"It was our first day on the course and come lunch time I was standing alone, knowing no one. Claire came up and asked if we could lunch together. Since then we have been the closest of friends."

Claire returned to work and live in Chessington, first with the Royal Borough of Kingston, then with Surrey Children's Services. A colleague wrote:

"Claire had a gift; she loved people and people loved her. My life has been better because she has been in it. She was an amazing young lady, whom we admired immensely."

I have included a couple of high points of Claire's career, although there were many. As Claire gained promotion and moved teams her manager, Sue W., wrote (Spring 2009):

"Scary stuff losing you to Fairmount – you have been an inspiration in the team, such a lovely colleague and worth your weight in gold. Thank you for your huge commitment. So jealous of your new team – they are very lucky to have you."

In a personal card from this same manager, 9.4.09:

"Dear Claire, thank you for being such a skilful assistant team manager and a lovely person to have as part of the team. I have hugely valued your calm and intelligent approach to all our challenges over the past months. All

your hard work and dedication to the cases and to staff has really helped us stay afloat. I will miss you hugely, but the best of luck in your future career. Please stay in touch. Love, Sue."

Feedback from Claire's tutor for her Post Qualifying (PQ) Child Care Award (2005) read:

"This is a strong portfolio where the candidate has clearly met all the practice requirements in her reflective commentary. She makes some interesting comments about balancing the needs of children and young people, whilst working with parents to promote change. The opportunity to undertake group work in today's current social work climate is rare and by all counts this candidate enjoyed this piece of direct work. A clear pass."

With Claire's increasing need for medical equipment at home (plus her collection of shoes and handbags!), she upsized and moved house last November to a lovely new estate a mile away in Hinchley Wood. Although Claire only enjoyed her new home for a matter of weeks, she loved planning it and living there. She had designs to spend lots of time in her new garden this summer, but sadly that did not come to fruition.

As a society we want to emulate the dead, put them on a pedestal, and to some degree we should, but Claire was honest enough for it to be told, "warts and all." Those of you that knew her well would recognise this saying: "I'm in a mood!" She could be really stubborn at times and nothing and no one could get her to change her mind – she certainly didn't listen to me!

Claire failed as we all do and it would be wrong to paint her as a perfect person for, until we reach heaven, we are all flawed. She knew what it was to be sorrowful over her sin, to want to turn the clock back, to have regrets about how she lived parts of her life. We all lose our way to some degree at times, and Claire was no exception.

Claire had not only a physical, life-threatening illness to cope with, but all the other hurts and heartbreaks in life that we experience; some more than others. Of course she shared her most intimate thoughts with her trusted friends but she also shared some things with me and I know that despite her outward appearance and zest for life, she could also be really sad at times; she was a broken person, like we all are. Loss is part of life's journey that I am sure we can relate to.

Claire was fiercely independent; she was very much her own person and made her own decisions. She certainly didn't want me living with her but I was allowed to stay at various times in her adult years when she needed extra help! It was with God's help and her sheer willpower that she wanted to live as normal a life as possible. Claire was a giving person. . .it's said that we make a living by what we receive in the form of a salary, but that we actually make a life by what we give (attributed to Sir Winston Churchill 1874-1965).

Claire loved life; of that we are certain and her pastor, Paul, has already alluded to this. She loved people, holidays, the proms, Wimbledon tennis (this love she got from my brother, who was an avid amateur tennis player), Hampton Court flower show, ballet (her favourite was *Spartacus*) all kinds of pop concerts, the cinema.

She also had a deep faith in God. I'm told that her faith, love and compassion were evident in all she did. And as a parent, I can only add that I believe her independent nature, indomitable spirit and sheer determination, together with God's help, was what made her, against all odds, live so well and so long in terms of her CF. Claire didn't choose to have CF, but she certainly chose how to live with it. Trevor A., both a former pastor at the church I attend and the then chairperson of the Schools' Work Trust (now known as Insight) once wrote that Claire was "a shining beacon of loveliness and grace."

All parents know that the hardest thing to do is to stand by helpless at your child's disappointed hopes, yet God, following the feeding of the five thousand in John chapter 6 v12 asked the disciples to "gather up the fragments [the broken bits]. . .let nothing be wasted." And in God's plan nothing is wasted, not even death. Many of you have either written or spoken of your sadness at Claire's passing and have been so kind as to encourage me to keep going in the face of grief. *Streams in the Desert* (March 11) says: "Sorrow came to you yesterday and emptied your home. Your first impulse is to give up and sit down in despair amid the wrecks of your hopes. But you dare not do it. . .other lives would be harmed by your pausing; holy interests would suffer. Weeping inconsolably beside a grave can never give back love's banished treasure. . .sorrow makes deep scars; it writes its record ineffaceably on the heart which suffers. We really never get over our great griefs; we are never altogether the same after," (J. R. Miller).

Claire never let CF get in the way of life. She may have had CF, but until recently, CF did not have her. She chased her dreams and fulfilled a good number in her short life; however, naturally some remained unfulfilled. Claire always knew her days were numbered, though she did hope she would make it to lung transplant. She had loads of holidays and packed so much into her life. These holidays were not always indulgent. She loved to see other cultures and one of her favourite trips was to Vietnam. Another was to visit a friend working with street children in Belem, Brazil.

However, as already alluded to earlier today, Claire was far more ill than any of us really knew; myself included. She survived swine flu three years ago, but she was living on borrowed time. One of the hospital consultants wrote that they didn't know of another CF patient who was still working full time on such a low lung function as Claire had. She certainly had her fair share of difficulties from a multitude of complications of her illness and her fair share of disappointments and heartbreaks in life.

In the past few years and in her spare time, Claire worked tirelessly for the CF Trust, because although she knew gene therapy would not be in time for her, she desperately wanted those younger than her to benefit. She was deeply touched by the introduction in the book *The Private Worlds of Dying Children* when the author stated: "I have failed unless this study contributes to the memory of these children. . .who still must suffer."[160] Thankfully the prognosis of people born with CF has increased year on year, but still lots can be done to improve their quality of life. Rosie Barnes, at a charity ball in 2008 as one of the past Chief Executives of the CF Trust, spoke of research into gene therapy arguing, "In total this research will cost us X million pounds, but we hope it will save priceless young lives."

Claire ensured she saved enough money to enable her to give up work following her lung transplant. As we know, sadly that hope did not become a reality. When I think of Claire and all she endured, my heart leaps with pride but it also breaks. Claire, who found it so hard to breathe, will know what it is like when I say she "Take(s) my breath away" (1979, Rex Smith).

I may not have entirely agreed with the way Claire chose to live her life, but she was her own person; she refused to let CF get in her way of living a full life. Her philosophy, as we know from this Order of Service, was as Mother Teresa wrote: "Life is an Adventure –Dare It" and, as in the film *Steel Magnolias*: "I would rather have thirty minutes of wonderful than a life-time of nothing special."

When considering Claire's death, I love the words used by Annelle to Shelby's mum after Shelby dies: "Miss M'Lynn, I don't mean to upset you but I hope it will be a comfort to you that Shelby is with her King. . .when something like this happens, I pray very hard to make heads or tails of it. I think in Shelby's case she wanted to take care. . .of everybody she knew. . .and her poor body was just worn out. It wouldn't let her do everything she wanted to do. So she went to a place

---

[160] Myra Bluebond-Langner, The Private Worlds of Dying Children (Princeton University Press; First Edition 1978)

where. . .she will always be young. She will always be beautiful."[161] Claire's and Shelby's fragility of life was so apparent and yet the depth of strength was palpable. That's the paradox of her life; body frail but mind strong.

There is much, had I had the power, that I would have liked to have changed about Claire's life, but nothing regarding her eternal destiny. I have accused God so often; asked Him why she suffered, but have I stopped to thank Him for the goodness and joy she found in life, that she gave to me and that people found in her?

At the Fellowship of Independent Evangelical Churches (FIEC), in the 1990s, John MacArthur spoke on 2 Corinthians 2:14, "But thanks be to God who always leads us as captives in Christ," or in the author's words, in "triumphal procession." MacArthur said that: "It's enough to march in the parade, to wear the uniform, to advance behind the General." As Christians we see the triumph. . .it's enough to be a clay pot.

A friend emailed this to me just this morning and I felt it appropriate to include it here. Jean Vanier states in his forward to Sheila Cassidy's book *Sharing The Darkness*, "It is about people who are very earthy and very vulnerable; people who no longer wear masks because they do not even have the energy to maintain them. It is also about the people who truly care about those who have become vulnerable and who are dying. These. . .are experiencing their own deepest fears.'[162]

My thoughts have remained full of Claire's last hospital admission, but is that nightmare all that there is? What of hope? We have certainly heard a lot of that today and another email I received quoted C.S. Lewis. "They say of some temporal suffering, 'No future bliss can make up for it,' not knowing that Heaven, once attained, will work backwards and turn even that agony into a glory."[163]

[161] Robert Harling, Steel Magnolias page 66, 1988, Dramatists Play Service Inc.

[162] Sharing The Darkness: the Spirituality of Caring, 1988, Darton, Longman and Todd

[163] C.S. Lewis, The Great Divorce, *1946, Harper Collins.*

Despite her illness, I didn't know that having Claire as a daughter could have made me so happy; she slowed me down, the roles have been reversed and she has been my teacher.

In Isaiah's vision (chapter 6) he saw the Lord high and exalted, seated on a throne. Above Him were seraphim, each with six wings. With two they covered their faces, with two they covered their feet and with two they were flying. For the latter years of Claire's life, CF had a profound effect on her, but now, as we have previously heard, she is free. So Claire, fly high, and hear the words of Christ: "Well done, good and faithful servant, enter into the joy of the Lord," (Matthew 25v23).

But my concluding words must be to you who stood by her, supported her. For years a picture hung in a London hospital, depicting a race. Underneath the caption read, "The race is not always to the swift, but to those who have the courage to keep on running." This is linked to the verse in Ecclesiastes 9:11a: "I have seen something else under the sun: The race is not to the swift." Reference has been made to Claire's track sports where she was determined to run, even if it meant coming last. No, Claire was not a good athlete in the sense that we use that word, but in the race against CF, in the race of life, she was so encouraged by all of you to keep going. Each one of you stood on the side lines, cheering her on. Thank you.

References

Prologue

1   Norman Maclean, A River Runs Through It (University of Chicago Press, 1976; reprint, 2001)

2   Harold S. Kushner, When Bad Things Happen to Good People, (Penguin Random House 2002)

3   Sheila Cassidy, Audacity to Believe, (Darton, Longman and Todd, 1977)

4   W. E Sangster, Let Me Commend, Paperback (Wyvern Books, 1961)

5   Margaret Fishback Powers *Footprints : The True Story Behind the Poem That Inspired Millions* © by Margaret Fishback Powers. The poem "Footprints" copyright © 1964 by Margaret Fishback Powers. Published by Harper Collins Publishers Ltd. All rights reserved

6   http://www.wholesomewords.org/missions/biopaton7.html (also see:) John G. Paton, D.D. Missionary to the New Hebrides, An Autobiography, edited by the Rev James Paton, B.A. (Elibron Classics © 2005, Adamant Media Corporation)

7   Beth Moore, The Patriarchs: Encountering the God of Abraham, Isaac, and Jacob (Lifeway Christian Resources, 2005)

8   Beth Moore, The Patriarchs: Encountering the God of Abraham, Isaac, and Jacob (Lifeway Christian Resources, 2005)

Chapter One

9   Tears In Heaven, Written by Eric Clapton and Will Jennings, from the album Rush, Warner Bros. Records, January 1992

10   Source unknown

11   O Sacred Head Now Wounded, composed by Hans L. Hassler 1601

12   Thank You Mum For Everything, Helen Exley (Helen Exley Giftbooks, 2007)

13   Sheila Cassidy, Audacity to Believe (Darton, Longman, Todd, 1977)

14   David Rhodes Faith in Dark Places, (Triangle, SPCK 1996)

15   David Rhodes Faith in Dark Places, (Triangle, SPCK, 1996)

16   Myra Bluebond-Langner, The Private Worlds of Dying Children (Princeton University Press; First Edition 1978)

17   Bruce B. Wilmer, Feelings, 1987 Wilmer Graphics

Chapter Two

18   Roberta Flack, The First Time Ever I Saw Your Face, From the album First Take (Atlantic 2864, March 7, 1972, Written by Ewan MacColl)

19   Chas E. Cowman, Bird In A Winter Storm (Cowman Publishing Company Inc., 1962)

20   Reprinted with the permission of Atria Books, a Division of Simon and Schuster, Inc. MY SISTER'S KEEPER by Jodi Picoult. Copyright©2004 Jodi Picoult

21   Meg Woodson, Turn It Into Glory, (Hodder and Stoughton, 1991)

22   B.H Edwards, Horizons of hope (Day One Publications, 2000)

23   B.H Edwards, Horizons of hope (Day One Publications, 2000)

24   Cat's In The Cradle. Words and music by HARRY CHAPIN and SANDY CHAPIN ©1974 (Renewed) STORY SONGS LTD. All Rights Administered by WB MUSIC CORP. All Rights Reserved .Used By Permission of ALFRED MUSIC

Chapter Four

25 Slipping Through My Fingers, SONGWRITERS: ANDERSSON, BENNY/ULVAEUS, BJORN by permission of Bocu Music Ltd. Photocopying is illegal without the consent of the Publisher.

Chapter Five

26 Record each treasured moment, (Source unknown)

27 The Way We Were Words and Music by Alan Bergman, Marilyn Bergman & M Jarvin Hamlisch © 18th May 2015, Reproduced by permission of EMI MUSIC PUBLISHING LIMITED, London W1F 9LD

Chapter Six

28 PS I Love You, Compiled by H. Jackson Brown, Jr. 1990 Rutledge Hill Press, Nashville

29 William Sangster, 'He is able' (Wyvern Books, Epworth Press 1962)

Chapter Eight

30 Graham Kendrick © 1988 Make Way Music. www.grahamkendrick.co.uk.

Chapter Nine

31 Author unknown

32 Author unknown

33 Joni Eareckson Tada, Glorious Intruder: God's Presence in Life's Chaos, pg 209 (Multnomah Books, 1989)

34 Joni Eareckson Tada, Glorious Intruder: God's Presence in Life's Chaos, pg 211 (Multnomah Books, 1989)

35 Love Is A Many-Splendored Thing (Twentieth Century Fox Film Corporation, 1955)

36 'I Will Survive' performed by Gloria Gaynor, released in October 1978, written by Freddie Perren and Dino Fekaris. From the album: Love Tracks.

37 R.E.M. , Everybody Hurts, Automatic For The People (Warner Bros, 1992)

38 Source unknown

39 Source unknown

Chapter Eleven

40 Written by Charlie Chaplin in 1966 and performed by Petula Clark

41 R.E.M., Everybody Hurts, Automatic for the People (Warner Bros, 1992)

42 Steel Magnolias, 1988, Robert Harling, Dramatists Play Service Inc.

Chapter Twelve

43 Source unknown

44 Written by Bryn & Sally Haworth. Performed by Sarah Lacy (© *1983 Kingsway Thankyou Music)*

Chapter Thirteen

45 Lori Gottlieb, How to Land Your Kid in Therapy, The Atlantic, June 7 2011

46 You Are Always On My Mind, Songwriters: Johnny Christopher, Wayne Carson, Mark James, , published by Lyrics © EMI Music Publishing

47 Wendy Mogel, Ph.D, The Blessing of a Skinned Knee: Using Jewish Teachings To Raise Self-Reliant Children 2001, Scribner

48 Meg Woodson, Turn It Into Glory, 1991 Hodder and Stoughton

49 John White, Parents in Pain, p36 (Downers Grove: Intervarsity Press, 1979)

50 Ron Dunn, When Heaven is Silent, p171 (Thomas Nelson Inc, Nashville, 1994)

Chapter Fourteen

51 Anonymous, quoted in 1000 Places To See Before You Die, by Patricia Schultz. (2010, Workman Publishing 2010)

Chapter Fifteen

52 www.cwr.org.uk
53 Author unknown

Chapter Sixteen

54 John Lennon, "Beautiful Boy," in *Double Fantasy (*Geffen, 1980)

Chapter Seventeen

55 Horizons of hope' Edwards, B.H. (Day One Publications, 2000, ISBN 1903087 02-3)

Chapter Eighteen

56   Origin uncertain

57   Brennan Manning, Abba's Child (NavPress, Colorado, 2011)

58   Brennan Manning, Abba's Child (NavPress, Colorado, 2011)

59   Michael Kearney, Mortally Wounded: Stories of Soul Pain, Death and Healing, (Touchstone Books, an imprint of Simon and Schuster 1997)

Chapter Nineteen

60   Marion Stroud, The Gift of Friends (Lion Hudson Plc, 1995)

61   Crystal Lewis, Beauty for Ashes, on Beauty for Ashes (CD released by Metro One Inc, September 23, 1996)

62   Amy Carmichael, Gold Cord: The Story of a Fellowship, (© 1932 by the Dohnavur Fellowship. Used by permission of CLC Publications) May not be further produced. All rights reserved

63   Timothy Dudley-Smith, Above the Voices of the World, (1987)

Chapter Twenty

64   Author unknown

Chapter Twenty-One

65   Chimamanda Ngozi Adichie, Half of a Yellow Sun (2007, Random House, LLC)

66   Say What You Want by Texas, Album: White on Blonde, 1997 ,Songwriters: McElphone, John, Spiteri, Sharleen, Smith, Clifford. © EMI Music Publishing,

Sony/ATV Music Publishing LLC, Warner/Chappell Music, Inc., Universal Music Publishing Group, BMG RIGHTS MANAGEMENT US, LLC

Chapter Twenty-Two

67 Author unknown

68 Anonymous

69 Slipping Through My Fingers, SONGWRITERS: ANDERSSON, BENNY/ULVAEUS, BJORN by permission of Bocu Music Ltd. Photocopying is illegal without the consent of the Publisher.

70 Author unknown

71 Nicholas Wolterstorf Lament for a Son, Wm. B Eerdmans Publishing Co, 1987

72 B.H.Edwards, Horizons of hope, 2000, Day One Publications

73 Frederick Buechner, Wishful Thinking, 1993, Harper Collins, used by permission of the Frederick Buechner Literary Assets, LLC

Chapter Twenty-Four

74 Walter J. Burghardt, 1980 (in: Horizons of Hope):'Tell the next generation', New York Paulist Press, p315

75 Manning, B. 1994 Abba's Child. Navpress, Colorado, p148-150

76 Shout to the Lord, by Darlene Zschech, (Integrity's Hosanna! Music)

77 Turn it into Glory, by Meg Woodson (1991 © Meg Woodson, Hodder and Stoughton)

78 Following Joey Home, by Meg Woodson (© 1978, Zondervan Publishing House)

79 Turn it into Glory, by Meg Woodson (1991 © Meg Woodson, Hodder and Stoughton)

80 Meg Woodson, Following Joey Home, 1978 Zondervan Publishing House

81   Meg Woodson, Turn It Into Glory, (Hodder and Stoughton, 1991)

82   Sheila Hancock, (cited in: Sue Mayfield) Living with Bereavement, 2008, Lion Hudson Plc

83   Sue Mayfield, Living with Bereavement, 2008, Lion Hudson Plc

84   C.S Lewis, A Grief Observed (Faber and Faber, 1961)

85   Meg Woodson, Following Joey Home (1978, Zondervan Publishing)

86   Chas. E. Cowman, Streams in the Desert May 30, (1961 Cowman Publishing Company, L.A. Copyright by Mrs Chas E Cowman 1925)

87   Jesus Will Walk With Me, Haldor Lillenas,

Chapter Twenty-Five

88   Brennan Manning, Abba's Child (NavPress, Colorado, 2011)

89   Following Joey Home, by Meg Woodson (© 1978, Zondervan Publishing House)

90   Robert Frost 1969, Stopping by Woods on a Snowy Evening. From The Poetry of Robert Frost, edited by Edward Connery Lathem. (Copyright 1923, © 1969 by Henry Holt and Company, Inc., renewed 1951, by Robert Frost.) Also: Johnathan Cape. Reproduced by permission of the Random House Group, Ltd.

91   Ruth Picardi, Before I Say Goodbye (Penguin, 1998)

92   C. Austin Miles (1868-1946)

93   Meg Woodson, Turn it into Glory, 1991 © Meg Woodson, Hodder and Stoughton

94   Sheila Cassidy, Good Friday People (Darton, Longman and Todd 1991)

95   George Matheson, 1842-1906 (November 7th 1962, Cowman Publishing Company Inc. Los Angeles)

96   Graham Kendrick, Here in this holy place (Copyright © 1983, Thankyou Music)

97   Following Joey Home, by Meg Woodson (© 1978, Zondervan Publishing House)

98   p223 Sheila Cassidy, Audacity to Believe1977, Darton, Longman and Todd Ltd.

99 Time of My Life, Composed by Franke Previte, John DeNicola, and Donald Markowitz. Recorded by Bill Medley and Jennifer Warnes (RCA Records Label, September 24, 1987)

100 Anne R. Cousin, in The Christian Treasury.

101 Extract taken from the song 'I Will Glory In My Redeemer' by Steve and Vikki Cook Copyright © 2001 Sovereign Grace Praise *Adm. by Capitol CMG Publishing worldwide excl. UK, admin by Integrity Music, part of the David C Cook family, songs@integritymusic.com

102 Phyllis McCormack, Crabbit Old Woman (Nursing Mirror, December 1972)

103 SEASONS IN THE SUN, Adaptation anglaise de Rod KcKuen S/les motifs de l'oevre orginale <<LE MORIBOND>> Paroles et Musique de Jacques Brel © Warner Chappell Music France et Editions Jacques Brel. Music and original French lyric by Jacques Brel -English lyric by Rod McKuen © 1961 by INTERSONG PARIS, S.A.-Edward B Marks Music Co: Sole Licensing and Selling Agent for USA, Commonwealth of Nations, including Canada and Australia and New Zealand and Eire - All Rights Reserved -CARLIN MUSIC CORP. London NW1 8B

104 Source Unknown

105 Streams in the Desert, Chas E. Cowman (1962, Cowman Publishing Company Inc., Los Angeles)

106 Meg Woodson, Turn It Into Glory, 1991, Hodder and Stoughton

107 Meg Woodson, Following Joey Home, 1978 , Zondervan Publishing House

108 Beth Moore, The Patriarchs, 2005, Lifeway Press

Chapter Twenty-Six

109 How The World Began, trans. John W. Doberstein (Philadelphia: Muhlenburge Press 1961, p171) cited in Ron Dunn, (p71,When Heaven is Silent, 2002, Authentic Publishing, Milton Keynes)

Chapter Twenty-Seven

110 Norman Maclean, Young Men and Fire, (University Of Chicago Press; Chicago, 1992)

111 Jean Vanier, Forward to: Sheila Cassidy, Sharing the Darkness: the Spirituality of Caring' (2002, Darton Longman and Todd)

After Words: A World You Are No Longer Part Of

112 Footprints: The True Story Behind the Poem That Inspired Millions ©1964 by Margaret Fishback Powers. The Poem 'Footprints' copyright © 1964 by Margaret Fishback Powers. Published by Harper Collins Publishers Ltd. All rights reserved.

113 Unknown

114 Jessie Margaret Hutson (nee Folkard) 1924-2010 (unpublished)

115 © University of Kent, Canterbury, Kent, CT2 7NZ

116 Ella Fitzgerald, Every Time I Say Goodbye I Die A Little, lyrics and music by Cole Porter, published by Chappell & Company.

117 Earl A. Grollman, Living When A Loved One Has Died, (Beacon Press, Boston, 1977)

118 Ron Dunn, When Heaven is Silent, p72 (2002, Authentic Media, Milton Keynes)

119 John Gunther, Death Be Not Proud: copyright ©1949 by John Gunther: A Word From Frances, p194, Harper Collins.

120 Turn it into Glory, by Meg Woodson (1991 © Meg Woodson, Hodder and Stoughton)

121 Jodi Picoult, My Sister's Keeper (reprinted with the permission of Atria Books, a Division of Simon and Schuster, Inc. MY SISTER'S KEEPER by Jodi Picoult. Copyright © 2004 Jodi Picoult.)

122 Anna McKenzie, cited in: Good Friday People by Sheila Cassidy (Darton, Longman and Todd 1991)

123 Anna McKenzie, Good Friday People by Sheila Cassidy (Darton, Longman and Todd 1991)

124 Wm Paul Young, The Shack (p209, HarperOne, 2009)

125 Telling the Truth: The Gospel as Tragedy, Comedy, and Fairy Tale by Frederick Buechner (Harper Collins Publishers, New York) Copyright © 1993 by Frederick Buechner

126 Ella Wheeler Wilcox. Streams in the Desert, December 9th, Chas E. Cowman, 1962 Cowman Publishing Company Inc. Los Angeles

127 The Velveteen Rabbit, Margery Williams (copyrighted material. pg9, 1922, George H. Doran Company)

128 http://adrianbarlowsblog.blogspot.co.uk/2012_04_01_archive.html

129 http://www.ekrfoundation.org/quotes/ Copyright © 2015 · All Rights Reserved · Elisabeth Kübler-Ross Foundation

130 Paula D'Arcy, Waking Up to This Day (p7, 2009, Orbis books)

131 Paula D'Arcy, Song For Sarah 2001, Shaw Books

132 Joni Eareckson Tada, Steven Estes. Steve Estes Foreword to the above book: (p39). Copyright © 1997 by Joni Eareckson Tada and Steve Estes. (Zandervon Publishing House, Grand Rapids, Michigan 1997.)

133 Liz Hupp, p102, When God Weeps. Joni Eareckson Tada, Steven Estes. Steve Estes Foreword to the above book: (p39), (p88). Copyright © 1997 by Joni Eareckson Tada and Steve Estes. (Zandervon Publishing House, Grand Rapids, Michigan 1997)

134 Paula D'Arcy, Song for Sarah, (p43, 2001, Shaw Books)

135 Sheila Cassidy, Audacity to Believe (p 258, 1977 Darton, Longman and Todd)

136 Sheila Cassidy, Audacity to Believe (p 258, 1977 Darton, Longman and Todd)

137 Jodi Picoult, My Sister's Keeper (reprinted with the permission of Atria Books, a Division of Simon and Schuster, Inc. MY SISTER'S KEEPER by Jodi Picoult. Copyright © 2004 Jodi Picoult.)

138 Jodi Picoult, My Sister's Keeper (reprinted with the permission of Atria Books, a Division of Simon and Schuster, Inc. MY SISTER'S KEEPER by Jodi Picoult. Copyright © 2004 Jodi Picoult.)

139 Larry Crabb, 'Shattered Dreams' (2010, Waterbrook Press (division of Random House) Colorado Springs). Copyright ©2001 by Lawrence J Crabb Jnr, PhD,

140 George Matheson, Streams in the Desert, pg40 (1962, Cowman Publishing Company Inc. Los Angeles)

141 Whitney Houston, The Bodyguard, 1990, Grammy Award for record of the year

Conclusion

142 Paula D'arcy, Waking Up This Day, p 80 (Orbis books, 2009)

143 Elisabeth Kubler Ross, by kind permission of the Elisabeth Kubler-Ross Foundation, www.ekrfoundation.org

144 Joko Beck in: Paula D'Arcy, Waking Up to This Day, pg125 (Orbis books, 2009)

145 Beth Moore, The Patriarchs, p239 (© 2005, Lifeway Press)

146 Elisabeth Kubler Ross, by kind permission of the Elisabeth Kubler-Ross Foundation, www.ekrfoundation.org/

147 William Rees, circa 1870's, Baptist Book of Praise, 1900

148 Norman McClean, A River Runs Through It (1989, University of Chicago Press)

149 C.S. Lewis cited in: Shadowlands: The True Story of C S Lewis and Joy Davidman, Brian Sibley, 2013, Hodder and Stoughton)

150 Blake Morrison, And When Did You Last See Your Father? p231, (2007, Granta Books, London)

151 The Last Farewell, by Roger Whittaker 1971 from the album: New World in the Morning

152 Alison Browne, 1997 (Horizons of hope' Edwards, B.H. © Day One Publications, 2000, ISBN 1903087 02-3.)

153 Meg Woodson: If I Die At Thirty p 95 (1975, Zondervan Publishing House)

Appendix Two

154 Chas E Cowman, Streams in the Desert, September 28th (1962, Cowman Publishing Company Inc., Los Angeles)

155 *Source unknown*

156 J.C. Ryle, Holiness 1956 James Clarke and Co, London

157 Margaret Fishback Powers *Footprints : The True Story Behind the Poem That Inspired Millions* ©by Margaret Fishback Powers. The poem "Footprints" copyright © 1964 by Margaret Fishback Powers. Published by Harper Collins Publishers Ltd. All rights reserved.

158 Art Buchwald Too Soon to Say Goodbye 2007, Marcia Rosten publishers

159 Paraphrase from: Ode of Remembrance taken from Laurence Binyon's poem 'For the fallen' The Times, September 1914

160 Myra Bluebond-Langner, The Private Worlds of Dying Children (Princeton University Press; First Edition 1978)

161 Robert Harling, Steel Magnolias page 66, 1988, Dramatists Play Service Inc.

162 Sharing The Darkness: the Spirituality of Caring, 1988, Darton, Longman and Todd

163 C.S. Lewis, The Great Divorce, *1946, Harper Collins.*

Lightning Source UK Ltd.
Milton Keynes UK
UKOW05f2308140116

266326UK00004B/6/P

AUDACIOUS
JOURNALISM

AUDACIOUS JOURNALISM

The Arts, Style & Depth

ANIETIE USEN

origami

Parrésia Publishers Ltd.
82, Allen Avenue, Ikeja, Lagos, Nigeria.
+2348154582178, +2348062392145
origami@parresia.com.ng
www.parresia.com.ng

ISBN: 978-978-55874-2-5

Printed in Nigeria by Parrésia Press

TO ALL OF YOU

ESPECIALLY

Dele Giwa, Ray Ekpu, Dan Agbese, Yakubu Mohammed, Soji Akin-rinade, Nyaknno Osso, Kayode Soyinka, Dele Olojede, Dele Omo-tunde, Ayogu Eze, Etim Anim, Soji Omotunde, Nosa Igiebor, On-ome Osifo-Whiskey, Dare Babarinsa, May Ellen Ezekiel, Eyo Nsa, Chuks Iloegbunam, Louisa Aguiyi-Ironsi, Lawson Omokhodion, Richard Ikiebe, Mike Akpan, Bala Dan Abu, Ben Edokpayi, Kola Ilori, Wale Oladepo, Austen Oghuma, Rolake Omunubi, Peter Ishaka, Ely Obasi, Janet Mba, Abdulrazak Magaji, Emenike Oko-rie, Sola Lufadeju, Mercy Ette, Nats Agbo, Sylvester Olumehense, Ibrahim Moddibo, Joyce Osakwe, Soni Ehi Asuelimen, Sam Omat-seye, Ben Nwanne, Okagbue Aduba, Chuzzy Udenwa, Ajan Agbor, Abiola Oloke, Bola Ojo, Utibe Ukim, Olu Ojewale, Bose Lasaki, Steve Agwudagwu, Tony Eluemunor, John Ebri, Jossy Nkwocha, Clarice Azuatulam, Armstrong Abangson, James Uloko, Dotun Oladipo, Matthias Igbarumah, Chris Uroh, Joseph Ode, Wale Akin Aina, Obong Akpaekong, Tunde Asaju, Sam-Loco Smith Bryson, Veronica Edafioka, Esta Ezekiel, Josh Arinze, Chris Uroh, Emeng Udosen, Chris Ekam, Israel Wilson, Joseph Inokotong, Dozie Arinze, Lucy Ekopimoh, Sly Edaghese, Ose Omijeh, Chris Ajaero, Stella Ochoga, Tobs Agbaegbu, Henrietta Okeke, Dollor Ogowe-wo, Akpa Edem, Obiora Ifoh, Marshall Okop, Wale Ajao, Felicia

Anidu, Dan Akpovwa, Ine Fetepigi, Levi Ogundina, Obi Azuru, Mary-Anne Aipoh-Ikoku, Uzo Nzegwu, Emmanuel Bodemeh, Paul Adams, Chuks Onwudinjo, Taiwo&Kehinde Shultz, Afolabi Adesanya, Conrad Akwu, Emmanuel Ebong, Angela Aboderin-Emuwa, Aniekan Umana, Clement Okitikpi, Jerry Ekwere, Emman Effiong, Iyah Onuk, Eki Adzufeh, James Onwuegbe, Letty Diai, Dili Ezughah, Muyiwa Akintunde, Ibim-Toby Semenitari.

AND TO

Nduka Obiagbena, Waziri Adio, Simon Kolawole, Segun Adeniyi, Eniola Bello, Kayode Komolafe, Davidson Iriekpen, Eddy Odivwiri, Krees Imodibe, Tayo Awotosin, Frank Nwabueze, Akpo Esajere, Chris Mammah, Lekan Otufodunrin, Segun Fatuase, Des Wilson, Parchi Umoh, Obiota Ekanem, Ekaette Ekpo, Ikpong Essien-Udom, Ekikere Umoh, Josephine Edikan Umoren, Sam Akpe, Udeme Nnana, Anietie Iyoho, Etim Etim, Oba Obadare, Ernest Essien, Comfort Essien, UduakAbasi Udofia, Ekom Udofia, James Essien, IDJ Essien, Idorenyin James, Udy James, Rev. Dr. Uma Ukpai, Pastor Mrs Philomena Uma Ukpai, Anietie Ebong, Favour Ebong, Edet Akpan, Glory Akpan, Udeme Udofia, Victoria Udofia, Onyema Ugochukwu, Godwin Omene, Emmanuel Aguariavwodo, Timi Alaibe, Chibuzo Ugwoha, Chris Oboh, Christy Atako, Bassey Dan-Abia, Victor Ndoma-Egba, HE Nsima Ekere, HE Akpan Isemin, HE Victor Attah, John James Akpanudoedeghe, Umana O. Umana, HE Etim Okpoyo, HE Yakubu Bako, Nuhu Bamali, Samuel Adjogbe, Asikpo Essien-Ibok, Lucky Awobasivwe, Windy Isong, Ben Udobia, Sunday Ekpo, Okon Nseabasi, King James, Kokoette George Umoren, Felix Afe-Johnson, Timothy Zachaeus, Kunle Omotosho, Godwin James, Felix Onwiodukit, Victor Adeyanju, Tunde Kupolati, Imoh Ukpong, Mbuk Mboho, Chris Ekpenyong, Patrick Usanga, Ahunna Imoni, Ndidiamaka Ezugu, Chijioke Amu-nnadi, Charles Akpan, John Araka, Pius Ughakpoteni, Napoleon Ekperi, Solomon Edebiri, Davies Okarevu, Toye Abosede, Okejoto Gochua, Mary Funke Bello, Queen Mensah, Mercy Udoro, Lucky Ogbuji, Theresa Arokwe, Anderson Ukeh, Azafi Omoluabi-Ogosi, Olukayode Qosim Olowu, Oluwafemi Ayodele, Celestina Briggs, Bamijoko Agbomedarho, Chinwoke Okeuhie, Nnamdi Okoroji, Dan Ajunwa, Dein Fyneface.

AND MORE ESPECIALLY TO

Etim Duff, Jessie-Philip Usen, Stella Usen, Edima Udobia, Johnson Udobia, Ekemek Usen, Ukeme Usen, Dara Udobia, Mfreke Esu, Esu Esu, Bernice-Grace Esu, Imaobong Essien, Abasifreke Essien, Miracle Essien, Kuyik Usen, Mary Utin-Nkanu, Otuekong ON Obot, Victor Ekpo, Lucy Udoh, Emmanuel Udoh, Joseph Udoh, Tony Udoh, Cletus Udoh, Itoro Uko, Emma Uko, Idongesit Udoh.

AND ABOVE ALL TO

My Father, The Almighty God; My Lord and Friend, Christ Jesus; and My guide, My Comforter-and-Helper-in-Chief, The Holy Spirit.

To all of you listed above, wherever you are, I have just three things to say:
1. THANK YOU
2. THANK YOU VERY MUCH
3. THANK YOU VERY VERY MUCH.

CONTENTS

AFRICA

AMERICA

WORLD

INTERVIEWS

SPORTS

FOREWORD

Audacious Journalism is the audacious book on the art and science of journalism, from the perspectives of a field artist, who lived his life for almost thirty years – from the crunchy and crusty space of the sparsely furnished operating room of rookie reporters, to the uncertain jungle of scary wars where no conventions are observed and the compensatory comfort of the boardroom in his later years.

Audacious! That is perhaps the best descriptive word for the courage with which journalists carry out their often unappreciated tasks. Anietie Usen, the author of this book describes the news hounds at the legendary Newswatch magazine, as reporters who were "brought up to be audacious". Audacious Journalism is therefore an encyclopedic escapades and collection of thrilling stories,opinion articles, sports, political and other feature stories which he wrote over his long period of tutelage with some of the best editors and printed media at the time.

In all, there are over a hundred stories reflecting both his eclectic interests and the body of assigned duties. In its full title the book seeks to serve as a source of information, entertainment, education as well as play the role of a how-to text. While it does not set out clearly to play a direct pedagogical role, any good student can glean from its content , the arts, style and depth of news writing, feature writing and providing entertainment even when the subject matter is a serious one. The author shows great skill in caption writing - some of his captions or story titles are drawn from literature, politics and sports. One cannot avoid such titles as **The House That Quacks Built, His Excellency The Farmer, University of Criminals, The Despot and The Pope, Hello! Is Mobutu Still There?** and many such captivating titles.

Mr Usen shows a high degree of creativity in his writing style, such that if he wished, he could also double as a thriller writer. He is at home with political imageries as much as he relishes deep clerical issues. When the reader goes through this collection he cannot afford not to view the author as one who throws up some serious matter up for discussion but then reclines in a corner of the room watching you get worked up with the travails of a nation, Africa and a world, where "**a tyrant bites the dust**", where "**rebels are on the move**" and where "**the pen battles the gun**" and comes out triumphant.

I see this work as a collector's item which would be found useful both in the classroom and newsroom. It is joining such works as Dan Agbese's book on Feature writing and other how-to books, which have become invaluable in the teaching and training of journalists in Nigeria and elsewhere around the world. It is a meeting point between theory and practice and of town, gown and crown.

Des Wilson
Professor of Mass Communications

TO START WITH...

The first story I wrote for *Newswatch* was torn into pieces and flung into the dust bin by Dele Giwa, my editor-in-chief. As I stood there before him, completely frozen by the force of his fury, he stormed out of his office into the deputy editor-in-chief's office next door, shouting, "Ray, Ray, Ray, look at this boy. I sent him to do a story and he turned up here with a PR stuff. He says he thought the man was my friend. Who cares whether anybody is my friend or not. Warn him o."

My baptism of fire began three days earlier. Barely two hours after I assumed duties as Reporter/Researcher in March 1985, I was summoned to see the editor-in-chief. He had sent his messenger to fetch him any reporter in sight and I had the misfortune of being picked from the five pioneer reporters in the newsroom. As I walked into his office nervously, a tall and suave gentleman was in his company and they were chatting, laughing and screaming like school boys over a pot of hot coffee. They were obviously very good friends, perhaps school mates, and as I later found out, from his part of the country in then Bendel State.

The boss simply turned a bit impetuously in my direction and said rather inattentively: "My friend, you go now and get some tour advance and proceed to Benin for this assignment. This gentleman is behind the exhibition. Okay!" As I took the invitation from his hands reverentially and motioned to step out, he called me back. "My friend, I hope you know production is on Wednesday and that's 48 hours from now."

I had never travelled by air for an official assignment, although I had worked briefly for a major national daily before I was recruited (or should I say conscripted) by *Newswatch*. So, all the way to Benin and back in Okada Airline, the best private airline in the country at that time, I was smiling coyly and poised to impress my boss with a lavish praise of his friend. That became my undoing. The story was unsalvageable. This is the painful saga of how I missed a byline in the maiden edition of the phenomenal magazine.

My pain, however, became my gain just a few months down the line. I learnt the lesson of professional detachment the hard way, but via the fast lane. In four months I became the first *Newswatch* staff to be promoted. This was two months ahead of the prospective confirmation of my appointment. The boss suddenly became my friend and first nicknamed me R&D and later the Whiz Kid.

In 18 months, I was already on the editorial board of *Newswatch,* rubbing shoulders with celebrity editors like Ray Ekpu, Dan Agbese, Yakubu Mohammed, Soji Akirinade, Nosa Igiebor, Dele Olojede, Dare Babarinsa, Onome Osifo-whiskey, Chuks Ilogbulam, May Ellen Ezekiel, Dele Omotunde, to mention a few. In six or so years of professional escapades, I won virtually every local and national award in sight; and became part of the incredible editorial crew that held Nigeria and the international readers spell-bound for years. We were treated like folk heroes everywhere we arrived to investigate and write stories. Kings and queens sought our attention, sometimes in vain. *Newswatch* was read like a Bible across the nation. Like the Holy Bible in China, some editions of the magazine were scarce commodities, often photocopied and circulated underground in many parts of Nigeria.

My arrival at *Newswatch* as a reporter/researcher was probably as dramatic as the saga of my first script. I had stopped over at the 62 Oregun Road, Lagos, office of the new outfit, just to see a good friend, Nyaknno Osso, the celebrated newspaper librarian, who had moved from *Nigerian Chronicle* in Calabar, South-South Nigeria, to join the fledgling news magazine. At that time, only the preview edition of *Newswatch* had been published. Osso was seeing me off from his second-floor office when he suddenly said, "Oh! Ani, why don't you say hello to Ray before you go?" I had never met Ray Ekpu face-to-face before that time. But I felt sufficiently familiar with him through his inimitable and must-read columns in the *Nigerian Chronicle* and later *Sunday Times* and *Sunday Concord*. A towering editor and respected national figure, he was a source of inspiration to youngsters in the profession and beyond. So, I quickly jumped at the offer by Osso. But on getting to his first-floor office, Ekpu's secretary told us he was conducting an interview for new staff, in company of Giwa. Osso then suggested I dropped a note for the big man. The secretary readily provided a note pad on which I wrote something like: "Dear Ray, I stopped over to see and congratulate you on your latest venture. I would have loved to wait and meet you in person, but I have to hurry back to meet my deadline. See you another day. Anietie Usen, *The Punch*."

Osso and I were on the ground floor moving towards the taxi that brought me; when someone ran downstairs to say Mr. Ekpu wanted to see me. Back to his office, a robust, fine-looking man stood halfway between the secretary's office and the inner office, with the door half opened. "Are you Anietie?" he asked irritably with a hoarse voice that sounded like the bellows of rolling waters. Before I could say yes, he flew into a fit of anger with a flurry of questions: "Am I your mate? How old are you? Who told you that you can call me Ray? Don't I look old enough in your eyes to be addressed as Dear Sir or Dear Mr.Ekpu?" I was choking for words, and still struggling to say something, when someone obviously important inside the inner office said, "Ray, who is that?" "One small boy at *The Punch* that we talked about this morning," Mr. Ekpu replied. "Let me see his face," the man in the inner office said in a commanding tone.

Lo and behold, it was Dele Giwa, the editor-in-chief, whose face I had only ever seen in the newspapers. Four or five well-dressed and sober job seekers, in my age bracket, sat in front of the famous journalist. They were obviously being interviewed for employment in the new publication. One of them, I can recollect, was Angela Aboderin, the scion of the famous Aboderin dynasty, who later rose to the apex of the advert department of *Newswatch*. Giwa turned his attention away from them and directed a battery of questions at me about the story I had done for *The Punch* in that day›s edition. It was on the serial demise of gerontocratic Soviet leaders, and I had accurately predicted the emergence of Michael Gorbachev as the successor to Konstantin Chernenko. "How did you know he will be the next leader? Did you study in Russia? Do you write only on international issues?"

The big man was obviously thrilled by my answers and analysis of Soviet politics. While still answering one of his questions, he stopped me halfway and said sharply: "Come for your letter on Monday." I thought he meant a letter of interview. But when I arrived that Monday, what I got was a letter of appointment as reporter/researcher on a salary of N4,500 per annum. The snag, however, was that I was on N4, 800 per annum at *The Punch*. But I decided to take the plunge as a small fish, in where I anticipated, would be a big river.

Newsroom was simple, Spartan and almost bare. Small wooden tables coupled with stilted and stiff chairs, a typewriter and a transistor radio were all that sat in a small austere hall on the first floor directly opposite the office of the editor-in-chief and his deputy. Only Akirinade, the general editor; Igiebor, the associate editor and perhaps Omotunde, also an associate editor, had what could perhaps be regarded as a table of their own. In those days, television was a luxury. Not even the Editor-in-Chief could indulge in such gadgets. In any case, the NTA, the major television station in Nigeria then, was only televised for perhaps six or so hours a day, mostly in the evenings. Even before 12 midnight, a national anthem was all you needed to know that the station was gone, till hopefully, the next evening. Telephone? Perish the thought. Later, however, we had one ebony black receiver initially in the editor-in-chief's office. A parallel line was later connected to the newsroom. But the amount of time and energy it took to wind that black box to life would sometimes leave your index finger sore with pains.

What was lacking in luxury in the newsroom was well compensated for by the incredible enthusiasm and gusto of highly skilled reporters, who were trained and spurred to squeeze water out of stones. The newsroom comes alive every evening once newshounds, who had spent the day filtering their ways into secrets deals of government and company officials, begin to drift back to base. The yelling and celebrations that greeted scoops were tonics for more scoops. Heaven help reporters who came back from their beats so often with excuses. You would be told in many ways, that "in *Newswatch* we do not publish excuses but stories." Deadlines were nightmares. My friend and colleague Louisa Aguiyi-Ironsi captured the terror of deadlines with a sticker on the newsroom wall that said: DEADLINE AMUSES ME.

My initial beat was Aviation with additional oversight on research institutions. To start with, I got permission to fly with the Nigerian Airways to all 16 airports in Nigeria at that time. This was part of my orientation in that beat; *Newswatch* would not bargain for less. I remember when we did our first cover story on the mismanaged Nigerian Airways in September 1986. Nosa Igiebor, who anchored the story and Conrad Akwu, the staff photographer had to fly with the FLYING ELEPHANT, as the Nigerian Airways was called, to London to observe first-hand the operation of the airline from the international end. I flew the local routes, including a day in the cockpit of an Airbus A310 with Captain Philip Machaunga and co-pilot Johnson Omodiagbe. We foretold Nigerians in that story that the Nigerian Airways was becoming Nigerian *Air-Waste* and *Err-ways*; if urgent steps were not taken to sanitize the place, the overweight and sluggish FLYING ELEPHANT would simply drop dead. And, it came to pass.

Aviation was a sensitive beat, but not anyway as sensitive as the Dodan Barracks, the seat of Military Government in Nigeria. Tommy Edamina (not real name), a rugged and fast-talking professional, was our Dodan Barracks Correspondent. One after-noon, Tommy and I just returned to base, a few minutes before 4 o'clock; he from Ikoyi and I from Ikeja. The Newsroom was bus-tling as usual at about this time. Then the big man, Giwa, emerged from his office and joined us in the Newsroom. "How was your day,"he began to chat with some of us. Then he got to Tommy. "How was Dodan Barracks today, Tommy?" "No problem sir. Ev-erywhere is calm," Tommy answered with a smile. Just then, the prime time, 4 o'clock news on Radio Nigeria began. The first item on the news was a shock. The newsroom was brought to a pin-drop silence. "The chief of general staff, Nigeria's No.2 man, Com-modore Ebitu Ukiwe, has been sacked, with immediate effect. In his place, the Chief of Naval Staff, Rear-Admiral Augustus Aik-homu, has been sworn in..." The newscaster had barely switched to the next news item, when the boss turned, furiously, at Tommy and said: "Tommy Edamina, you are fired." That was it.

For the next few minutes, the newsroom was motionless, even after the furious editor-in-chief, had walked the short dis-tance back into his office. Three or so minutes later, amidst the palpable tension that engulfed the newsroom, a messenger from Giwa's office stepped into the newsroom and all eyes were on the usually unnoticeable fellow. Walking straight to where I stood, he said: "Anietie, *Oga* wants to see you." I was scared to my marrows. My heart was literarily in my hands, when I walked into Giwa›s office. "Anietie, you are the new Dodan Barracks Correspondent from today. Get a letter for Duro (Onabule), the chief press Secretary to the president, tomorrow, before you go," he said, still looking unhappy with the breaking news that caught us completely unawares.

If there was anything I knew about my new beat, it was simply the fact that it was, in *Newswatch*, a do or die assignment; the waterloo for any ill-equipped reporter. For a *Newswatch* magazine reporter, the task was tricky and laden with booby-traps. The radio and the television reporters would be first with the breaking news. The newspapers would follow early the next morning. The news magazine that would be published sometimes one week later would have to be both ingenious and resourceful to still find something new and news-worthy for the reader on the same subject. My first assignment was to find out why the nation's No.2 man was unceremoniously removed from office. Who were the dramatis personae in this saga of military politics? How was the power play played out? How did the military cabal arrive at the new No.2 man? Will the falcons hear the falconer and will things soon fall apart, if the falcons cannot hear the falconer?

It was no secret that *Newswatch* and Dodan Barracks, were not the best of friends. The *Newswatch* correspondent in the seat of power must, of necessity, walk a tight rope everyday. For me, the atmosphere was simultaneously hostile and unwelcoming, especially as I showed too much independence for the comfort of the State House. My kind of assignment had little or no respect for press releases. In fact, I held press releases in contempt and relied more on irregular but reliable sources, which often unsettled and ruffled a number of feathers in the seat of power. For the first one month, I had a running battle with a particular aide of the president who threatened virtually every Monday to withdraw my accreditation. Whenever I reported this back to the Editor-in-Chief, he would say in his usually dismissive way: "Anietie, don't worry yourself. The trouble with (name withheld) is that he didn't go to school. Ignore him." You couldn't work with Giwa and failed to feel important. He wouldn't hear that a government official invited you for an "empty lunch." "Look, Anietie," he would say, "you are the one who should invite that man for lunch, and not the other way round."

I remember when Ekpu, the deputy editor-in-chief, wrote one of his masterpieces titled A HOLLOW RITUAL. It was a chart-buster. It got us, of course, into trouble, as usual. We were summoned to appear before the Justice Uwaifo Tribunal set up by the military government at the defunct National Assembly Complex in Tafawa Balewa Square, Lagos. The entire hall was jampacked with journalists and members of the public who came to show solidarity for *Newswatch*. Gani Fawehenmi was our lawyer; I was picked to cover the trial. I had never met Fawenhinmi in action. In an incredible display of legal erudition and oration, he held the tribunal spellbound as he punctured holes in the case against Ekpu and *Newswatch*. As he marshaled his arguments masterful-ly, I jumped up in the sky and screamed, clapping. I didn't know it was an offence to do that in a tribunal. Then, a soldier with the rank of a major walked up to me and tapped on my shoulders in an attempt to take me out of the hall. Unfortunately for him, my boss, Dele Giwa was sitting right behind me. The moment the soldier touched me, Giwa sprang to his feet and almost wrestled the man in khaki to the floor. There was pandemonium in the place. "Who the hell do you think you guys are in this country," he shouted. "Look, the way they are promoting you, if I were in the army I would be a General by now," he said, his eyes bulg-ing. Apparently to avoid undue attention and distraction, Justice Uwaifo managed to bring some order to the place, but not with-out a scathing criticism of the column that brought us to his tri-bunal. We all walked out virtually free from the place, jubilating.

A go-getter, Giwa's style as a newsman and manager of newsmen was many-sided, albeit directed at making his dream magazine a runaway success. His blueprint for me as State House correspondent was simple and subtle: while it was important to cultivate the company and relationship of the high and mighty in the State House, it was sinful to neglect a bond with the low and minor. Soon, I discovered that the boys who were staff officers, protocol assistants, confidential secretaries, typists, clerks and messengers sometimes knew in black and white and first hand, what some top ranks scarcely got to know. I hardly missed their weddings, birthday parties or that of their wives and children. I learnt to play squash and golf because some of my sources were addicted to the two sports. I was a scrabble buff and there was a staff officer of the rank of major who would drive all the way from Ikoyi to my house in the Ikeja suburb of Ogba most weekends just to play scrabble with me; sometimes till day break.

As far as the State House was concerned, I took my briefing only from the executive editors, principally the editor-in-chief. We had regular briefing and debriefing sessions, formally and informally. Whatever tip or lead I picked up would be relayed immediately to the boss. Delay is dangerous, he would say. Often he had more leads and would want me to crosscheck some and report back. Besides the office, I was sometimes invited to his Talabi Street residence, mostly on Sundays for briefing and debriefing.

Then came the big bang. On Friday October 17, 1986, Giwa invited me to see him at home on Sunday afternoon to "compare notes." Dressed in my new cream shorts and T-shirt, and trekking leisurely from my Ogba, Ikeja residence to his house, just 20 minutes or so away, I was already at the entrance of Talabi Street, with the twin duplex he shared with Ray Ekpu within my sight, when I heard the infamous explosion from a letter bomb that terminated his life. Horror-struck and unable to stand the gory site of his mutilated and burnt flesh, I was at once torn between escaping for safety and staying put to do a blow-by-blow account of the tragic Sunday.

There was no doubt in my mind that I had just walked into the epicentre of a momentous event, and that as the State House Correspondent I had a very unpleasant job on my hands. To begin with, the envelope that masked the letter bomb carried the official address and logo of my beat. When the messenger of death handed over the killer envelope to Billy, Giwa's young son, who innocently passed it to his father, in his study, in the presence of Kayode Soyinka, our visiting London Bureau Chief, the remark my boss made just before he opened the envelop was "oh, it must be from the president." The press statement we issued immediately after Giwa gave up the ghost pulled no punches but directly accused the presidency of murdering the legendary editor. The next morning, duty demanded that I go to work in the very office we had accused of killing my boss.

Of course, I was the cynosure of attention as I walked angrily into the place. State House was engulfed with tension. A pall of confusion and bewilderment hanged ominously over every office. Nigerians had never heard; talk less of witnessing a gruesome atrocity of that magnitude. As I walked into the press centre, two minutes walk to the president's home and office, all eyes were on me. I was probably the most unwelcome Nigerian in the State House today. Reporters from other media houses across the country hovered around me to hear first-hand snippets of the dreadful event. While mystified junior State House staff huddled in small groups to grieve over the strange incident, equally baffled top civilian officials and military brass locked themselves behind closed doors to ponder on an appropriate response to the pointed accusations by *Newswatch*, which were already making headlines across the world.

Amidst the tension, a funny incidence that signposted the mood of the nation took place right in the premises that hosted both the office and residence of the military president. Out of the blues, a deafening explosion seized the air. There was nobody left standing, including uniformed men. Everyone ran for cover. Few minutes later, we all emerged from hiding and peeped through the windows to discover it was not a military coup, which was in vogue those days, but a worn out car tyre of one of the reporters that gave up at last.

The first effort by the State House to wash its hands off the assassination of Giwa was panicky, hesitant and timid. The president did not want to speak directly to reporters. The idea of a press statement by the presidential spokesman was also jettisoned. Reporters waited for more than twelve hours after Giwa had been bombed before they were told that Rear-Admiral Aikhomu, the No.2 man would address a press conference. When eventually the press conference was confirmed, reporters were surprisingly taken away from the seat of power, the usual venue of press conferences, to the State House Annex, on Marina Road, Lagos, some 30 minutes drive away.

Security at the venue was on red alert. Gloom was written visibly on every face. With Aikhomu were two other top military brass, who curiously were in contact with Giwa in the last days and hours before the bomb. We in *Newswatch* had linked them, and in fact, identified the two officers as arrowheads in the horrific saga. Aikhomu said he had nothing to say to Nigerians but to present the allged culprits to speak for themselves about their involvements with Giwa just before his demise. Tunde Togun, a top officer of the intelligence corps managed to brave some complicated explanation. But Colonel Halilu Akhilu, the director of military intelligence, was a nervous wreck, blustering his way through a confusing tale of woes. I had never seen a soldier so lily-livered and faint-hearted. He was sobbing at a point. Aikhomu had to order all tapes and camera shot down. Fierce-looking security operatives stamped their authority in the hall to ensure compliance.

I simply removed my own tape recorder from the banquet table and placed it on my laps under the table, sufficiently concealed by the table cloth. I am not sure *Newswatch* was able to publish everything about Akhilu›s contradictory denials. Barely 24 hours before the letter bomb that killed the famous editor, Akhilu had phoned Giwa to inquire about his house address. One of the questions that caught the military intelligence chief off-guard was why he made the curious inquiry. He said almost sobbing, that he was on his way to the airport and wanted to stop over and see Giwa at home because in his Hausa culture if you have a friend and do not visit him at home, you are not regarded as a true friend. When someone followed up with a question on whether he did visit Giwa afterall after he got the address, he got stuck, gazing at the ceiling endlessly without an answer. Aikhomu brought the drama suddenly to an end. The attempt by government to exonerate itself fell flat on its face and raised more questions than answers.

Thereafter, Dodan Barracks became for me a veritable warfront. Reporting the Machiavellian operations of the military government, with the uncanny accuracy of an insider became more or less my forte and the exclusive preserve of *Newswatch*. Some government blunders which often went unnoticed were dug out and placed in the public glare, all in an effort to make them sit up or ship out. In one incident, State House had announced a rash of political appointments to constitute a Constitutional Review Committee. Overnight they put together an elaborate swearing-in ceremony in Abuja. Unknown to government and virtually all Nigerians watching the ceremony, one of the so-called 'wise men' sworn in with fanfare was a local teacher with identical names with the actual appointee. In the course of chatting with some of the appointees in their five-star hotel rooms, I stumbled into the blunder and quietly launched an investigation that took me to the villages, homes and offices of the two namesakes in far away southern tip of Nigeria. Under a week, the incredible story was on the desk of Dan Agbese, now my deputy editor-in-chief. The moment he glanced through the story, he literarily jumped at it, with the caption "Right Name, Wrong Person." The newsroom was agog with laughter. Public reaction was amazing. Six newspapers culled the story from *Newswatch* the next morning. Many editorials on the subject were to follow.

As I bathed in the glow of the scoop, *Newswatch* decorated me with the Editor-in-Chief Prize for Professional Enterprise. In the citation, the editor-in-chief said: "It is a story that depicts in a rather poignant manner the festering sore in the Nigerian public administration system. It is a story that underlines our absent-mindedness as a nation and I am happy that you were sufficiently alert to notice it. The story is well told, with a little tinge of unintended humour, and we would have loved to laugh, if it were not such an unlaughable affair." Guess what my prize money for the "magnificent" story was: N500 (about $3). That was good money in 1988 and big motivation for years to come. Staff motivation played a key part in the runaway success *Newswatch* enjoyed for years. Good reporters such as Dele Olojede, May Ellen Ezekiel, Ajogu Eze, Ben Edokpayi, Nosa Igiebor and Dare Babarinsa were celebrated in-house and made to feel like superstars out there.

Yakubu Mohammed, the managing editor, almost blew my mind one day when he told the world in his *Editorial Suite* that I was the Irving Wallace of *Newswatch*, "a writer of thrillers, a risk taker, an adventurer, the right stuff." As he put it: "If there is a difficult assignment, he (Anietie) will not hesitate to volunteer. He is a very calculating fellow, who is often lured by the sense of adventure and the desire to achieve. You may say he is of the right stuff."

So many professional awards were to follow my stories, one of which came with an overseas scholarship and won me the fellowship of the Thompson Journalism Foundation in the UK. While I grew famous in the media with the nickname of "Whiz kid," I became a marked man and very infamous in the State House. Soon, Duro Onabule, the presidential spokesman, announced my expulsion and ban from the State House. It wasn't the ridiculing of the absent-mindedness of the military regime that made me a persona non grata in the State House. It was a serious matter that shook Nigeria to its foundations.

I was in Benin, Midwest Nigeria one Sunday morning, when some young officers guarding the State House, suddenly turned the nozzles of their armored tanks at the bedroom of President Babangida, and reduced the place into rubble. Major Gideon Orka, the mastermind of the coup, was a familiar face in Dodan Barracks and the young lieutenants who manned those armoured tanks were boys, I and other State House Correspondents met nearly everyday and sometimes interacted with. Once I heard the marshal music and the coup speech by Orka announcing the overthrow of Babangida, I knew I would be 'overthrown' instantly if I were not in the State House immediately. With my new Peugeot 505, I took on the usually four-hour Benin-Lagos Express road in less than three hours. I parked my car at the Federal Ministry of Information on Awolowo Road, Ikoyi and found my way through shortcuts and side gates into Dodan Barracks.

The place was a ghost town. The main gate I had avoided was ajar. The walls of the first floor apartment hosting the living room and bedrooms of the first family were ripped open. Water from burst pipes was flowing and splashing freely everywhere. Some wall decorations and smashed picture frames were hanging precariously on their way down. A heap of debris covered the chairs, settees, and tables. Scared stiff that I might have walked into a firing squad, I ran back and hid myself in the toilet of the press centre, peeping constantly and nervously through the window overlooking the inner premises, not sure exactly what had become of the coup. About an hour later, I heard the movement of vehicles. It turned out to be that of Yussuf Mamman, the influential press secretary to the vice-president. In his company was the NTA crew of two. The terrified landlord was to surface soon. Looking dazed, with unkempt hair and dusty uniform, he spoke only with the NTA, confirming that the rebellion has been crushed. Thanks to Sani Abacha, the chief of army staff and close friend of the president, who mobilized loyal troops to crush the uprising. All I did for *Newswatch* was capture the atmosphere of mayhem, painted a picture of bedlam and granted readers nationwide a graphic insight into the day of infamy. A fine gentleman and aide-de-camp of the President, Lt.Colonel U.K. Bello was killed in the coup. My bosom friend, Major Nuhu Bamali, who was a staff officer in the president's office, was promoted to Lt.Colonel and appointed the new ADC. But that was not sufficient to spare and keep me one day longer in the State House.

My ban from the State House made news and was played up by some media houses. It was high time I ventured elsewhere. As head, Foreign Affairs Desk, my first assignment was to cover the Soviet withdrawal of troops from Afghanistan. The trip from the onset was fraught with danger. I flew via Swiss Air from Zurich, Switzerland, into Karachi, Pakistan. Within minutes of touch down in Karachi, I was arrested and quarantined. It took the efforts and intervention of American Embassy officials to secure my freedom two long days later.

Now freed, I headed to Peshawar, the highly inflammable boarder town between Afghanistan and Pakistan, aboard the Pakistani International Airline, PIA. The entire Peshawar was a minefield. You couldn't step out anywhere on your own in a tempestuous city besieged by terror. The first day I stepped out on a guided mission to interview a Mujahideen commander, I returned to find a wing of my hotel in rubbles, courtesy of a bomb left in the saloon of the hotel. On my second night, I was smuggled into Afghanistan by some pro-American intelligence and diplomatic personnel, who were at that time the main backers of anti-Soviet Islamic fighters, now known as Taliban.

Meeting with these unsmiling medieval figures in their caves at night, presented for me an extreme dimension of professional hazard. I wished I was still quarantined in Karachi, rather than find myself in dark ominous caves. It was the first coming of Benizar Bhutto as prime minister of Pakistan. I was to return to Karachi and Islamabad to file stories of Bhutto's battle against

Islamic fundamentalists, which of course she lost, two decades later - along with her life.

It was however the civil war in Liberia that translated into a veritable nightmare for me and three other Nigerian reporters; with two of my colleagues killed in cold blood. I was just returning from Cotonou, capital of Benin Republic, to cover the country's presidential elections when Ekpu, now my editor-in-chief, called me into his office and said: "Anietie, I think you have to proceed to Liberia immediately." I had thought on my way back from Benin Republic that I would take a few days off to see my wife, Stella, and baby daughter, Edima, in my home State in far away Akwa Ibom, but the urgency in Ekpu's voice showed this was not a mere suggestion but an order.

With me in Benin Republic to cover the presidential elections was my bosom friend Krees Imodibe, the political editor of *The Guardian*. Together, Krees and I were the first journalists to interview the victorious Nicephore Soglo, in his house, after he defeated Matthieu Kerekou to end nineteen years of military rule in the small West African country. Krees was doing for Guardian what I was doing for Newswatch and our paths crossed ever so often at various assignments. Besides, we shared a common humble background of grass-to-grace. We were both orphans and houseboys at a point in time, and we both managed to acquire university education via the help of kind-hearted people. We both gate-crashed into journalism, having initially studied courses not directly connected with the media. In the case of Krees, he was heading for a career in teaching and actually went first to a teachers training college famously known in Nigeria as College of Education. We both used to drive all the way from Lagos to Agenebode, his village in Edo State to eat bush meat and return to Benin to while away time in his sister's restaurant.

Predictably, just as *Newswatch* ordered me to proceed to Liberia, *The Guardian* also dispatched Krees for the same assignment. Along with Krees and me was Tayo Awotosin of the *Daily Champion*, and Frank Nwabueze of *National Concord.* The four of us were the first Nigerian reporters to cover the Liberian civil war from the onset, unprotected by any peacekeeping force, which was in any case not in existence at that time. I had known Frank casually in one or two assignments, but I had never met Tayo until that assignment in Liberia. He was a tall, lanky and gentle fellow, the direct opposite of my friend Krees who was short, robust and swift. While the three of them were lucky to fly directly into Monrovia, I got stuck in Conakry, the capital of Guinea, as Air Guinea, the only Airline that was still braving the Liberian route, was no longer willing to risk the trip.

The only option left for me was to go to Freetown, capital of Sierra Leone by road and find my way to Monrovia via Kenema, the Sierra Leonean boarder town with Liberia. This was a 700-kilometers journey through tortuous and treacherous Nigerian-like roads, but I was determined to be in Liberia. My unscheduled trip to Sierra-Leone became a blessing. I turned up in Freetown about the same time peace talks between the Liberian warring factions were being hurriedly put together. I made contacts with both factions to the peace talks, checked into the same hotel with them and interviewed key delegates, including Samuel Doe's minister of information and filed my reports back to Nigeria.

When the peace talks collapsed under 48 hours, I saw horror written on the faces of most delegates. They told me it was not safe for me to travel to Monrovia when virtually anyone who had the means was hurrying out of the country. But I was desperate to be in Monrovia. *Newswatch* must report this war from the theatre of war itself, I kept telling myself. I found my way by taxis and buses to Kenema by night, and spent the night in a rebel-infested dingy hotel. Here, I began for the first time to feel and smell the danger lurking ahead. I couldn't sleep at all that night because of rampant gunshots in the area and violent squabbles by the marijuana-smoking and drunken rebels. The thought of returning to Nigeria flooded my heart all night, but in the morning, I met a Liberian Muslim leader who was at the peace talks. He was desperate to go to Monrovia to evacuate his family and nothing would deter him. I was desperate to go into Monrovia for my professional family and nothing would deter me. With his driver and me in the front seat of a new car, we took off on one of the most dangerous journeys that I have ever undertaken.

The custom post between Sierra Leone and Liberia was deserted. The smooth 100-kilometer road between Kenema and Monrovia, tarred by the Nigerian government, had no other vehicle except our Peugeot 406. He opted for bush tracks rather than the main road for the better part of the Liberian end. Even on the bush tracks, we drove at breakneck speed unmindful of tree stumps and ditches. Broken down vehicles, household items and sick aged people dumped by fleeing refugees littered the bush tracks and foretold the perilous terrain ahead of us. It was a race against time but no one could deter this man, for a second, from getting his wives and children out of harm's way.

Monrovia itself was a ghost town. Everybody was hiding either from marauding warriors or from flying bullets fired by the two sworn enemies. To worsen matters, it was on a day all the professionals in Monrovia (doctors, engineers, architects, journalists) had the temerity to take a peaceful protest to the Presidential Mansion, to beg their president to simply walk a few steps down the seaside and board an American luxury ship stationed behind the mansion to sail him to exile. President Doe's response was a torrent of teargas and bullets.

The frantic man who brought me from Sierra Leone dropped me suddenly as we approached the city center and pointed hurriedly at a certain direction where I could possibly find a hotel, as he turned right obviously in the direction of his neighborhood. In the middle of nowhere I choked for divine help. Within minutes two soldiers emerged from their trenches and seized me. They were troops loyal to President Doe. One yanked my bag off me immediately while the other pushed and kicked me as he barked orders for me to move in the direction of a nearby storey building. A senior officer in mufti who sat partially hidden by the half-wall took over from his untamed boys and grilled me. Confirming that I was a Nigerian journalist just arriving from Sierra Leone, he kept me for safety and later detailed two other untamed soldiers to help me locate the nearest available hotel. The first two hotels we went refused to open their gates. At the third hotel, they shot into the air in anger, forced their way in. I was handed over to the panicking hotel manager, with a warning to ensure my safety, if he loved his life.

The next day when a bit of life returned slowly to some parts of the dying city, I ventured out to the ministry of information, where I met and reunited with Krees, Frank, Tayo and other foreign journalists, including Elizabeth Blunt of the BBC. That evening, I moved over to the small hotel where Krees, Frank and Tayo were staying right in the heart of Monrovia. The owners and workers in the hotel had virtually deserted the place. Electricity had since stopped. Water was in very short supply. Toilets were unsightly. Marijuana-puffing ruffians and other suspicious faces made up the bulk of the remaining guests. We hardly spent time in the hotel, until nightfall when we returned from the embassies, government and aid agencies to ferret and confirm information we pick from some sources including deserting soldiers.

After a fierce gun fight broke out on a Saturday night around our hotel, we became restless and decided that we should find our way home the next morning. I barely slept that night. It was clear the warfront was shifting dangerously nearer and a street by street fight to control Monrovia would have begun. By six in the morning, I was banging on the doors of my Nigerian colleagues to dress up and flee with me to Sierra Leone. My first port of call was Krees' room. He was already up, too, but surprisingly said he wanted to wait for a few more days. As I entered his room, he was writing a letter, hurriedly, which he said I should help deliver to his managing director, Mr. Lade Bonuale. I dashed to Franks' room and he came out with me to Krees' room where we argued again about the exact situation on ground and the right time to escape. I left Frank with Krees and rushed to Tayo's room. He was brushing his teeth. We spoke hastily with the tooth brush in his mouth. He, too, said he would want to wait a bit more. That was the last time I saw him. Krees and Frank escorted me in a somewhat jolly mood to the nearby waterfront that Sunday morning, where I boarded a Sierra-Leone bound bus laden with refugees. They stood back and waved at me as the clumsy old vehicle struggled to make its way to the main road. That was the last time I saw my bosom friend Krees. When I got to my Paramount Hotel room in Freetown that Sunday night and tuned to the BBC, I was shocked to hear that the road I had just passed had been captured and taken over by rebels, cutting off Monrovia from the rest of the world.

(Perhaps, this is the first time the following information would be made public). With Monrovia cut off and the city center besieged and bombarded by rebel forces, Krees, Tayo and Frank decided to find their way to the Nigerian embassy outside the city centre. The only trouble according to my investigations and interview with several refugees was that Frank was suddenly struck down with severe diarrhea and could not move one inch out of the hotel. Out of sympathy for Frank, Krees and Tayo could not flee the city centre in time in spite of the bombardments. Krees and Tayo did everything they could to help Frank take flight with them, but Frank was virtually dying in their hands. At a point, Krees and Tayo decided to carry Frank on their shoulders, with one of Frank's hands hanged on Krees shoulder and the other hand on Tayo's shoulder. It was an impossible task for the sick man more so because Krees was nearly half the height of Tayo. At a point, Frank himself, certain that he would die, encouraged Krees and Tayo to abandon him for their safety. That was the last time the dying Frank saw his ill-fated colleagues.

Frank was later picked up on the road by some Burkinabe soldiers, who fought on the sides of Charles Taylor. His saving grace was his fluency in French language. Besides, Frank had only just returned from Burkina Faso to cover some events, before he was assigned to Liberia. When the Burkinabe soldiers verified he was a sick Nigerian journalist who had only recently visited their country, they had pity on him. Medical help soon came. He was later put in a refugee ship which brought him in the company of other refugees to Freetown.

But Krees and Tayo were not so lucky. They were seized directly by Charles Taylor's invading troops, who were angry with the Nigerian government for backing the Samuel Doe army. Taylor, in retaliation, had handed down orders to his troops to deal ruthlessly with Nigerian refugees caught in the conflict. A British journalist working with the London *Sunday Observer* later told me in Paramount Hotel, Freetown, how my friends Krees and Tayo were killed along with many other Nigerian refugees, whom Taylor alleged were spies. "They were executed in front of reporters...The two Nigerian journalists were shot as spies." I played down the story and perhaps made scant reverence to it in my reports at that time because I could not imagine it and did not for once think Taylor could so brutally execute some journalists, given his background as an American-trained man.

Why can't I go and talk to the President, I said to myself, as I walked past a white, simple roadside storey building that was introduced as the Office of the President of Sierra Leone. I was not assigned to interview the famous man when I left Lagos but I knew for sure my editors would jump for joy, if I went the extra mile and sat down with a foreign head of state. Getting an exclusive interview with an African head of state is not a day's job; it requires elaborate protocol. But *Newswatch* reporters were brought up to be audacious. I confess that at some point, some of us, *Newswatch* reporters became overconfident and were seen as cocky even by colleagues from other media houses.

My overconfidence was in display that afternoon in Freetown as I walked in to see the Press Secretary to the President. "My name is Anietie Usen. I am the Associate Editor of *Newswatch*, Nigeria's No.1 news magazine. I want to speak to Mr. President, possibly today." The gamble paid off. Within an hour, I was driven in a black State House car up a winding, hilly road into a cul-de-sac that hosted the residence of President Joseph Momoh. For another hour and a half, right inside the study of the president, next to his disheveled bedroom, I squared off with a man whose face was familiar across the continent and beyond. I converted his press secretary into my photographer. *Newswatch* made it a cover story. One thing that struck me about the Sierrra Leonean President's home was the number of President Babangida's portraits in his house, right down to his study. There were more portraits of the Nigerian leader on display than President Momoh. I couldn't help but ask President Momoh why it was so. "Nigeria is our big brother. President Babaginda is my personal friend," he said. It was one escapade that proved not just Nigeria's influence in the West African sub-region, but the respect *Newswatch* enjoyed internationally.

Covering the political crises in Sierra Leone and Liberia, as well as in Pakistan and Afghanistan was the first audacious assignment I undertook in a profession I literally gate-crashed. The rest is contained in the book in your hands now. Enjoy!

NIGERIA

THE COVETED CROWN

At the zero hour, tension mounted and engulfed the banquet hall of the Abuja Sheraton Hotel, where thousands had crowded to hear the result of the hotly contested post of chairman of the National Republican Convention, NRC. It was 10 o'clock in the night and now, after 10 hours of balloting and counting of votes, the moment of truth had finally come.

Ibrahim Mantu, a charismatic candidate and one of the favourites for the top job, who sat defiantly in the front row of the hall, began to look nervous. He dipped his hand into the breast pocket of his white caftan, brought out pieces of kola-nut and began to chew them rapidly. He was just three metres from the table where the votes were being counted and the heap of votes for Tom Ikimi, his leading opponent, had convinced him he was heading for a defeat. His eyes turned blood-shot and without knowing, he began to tap his right foot against the floor impatiently. His close friend and political associate, Renshammah Kiya Rimi, who sat by his side, leaned towards him and whispered into his ears, apparently telling him to keep his cool. His other close aides flanking him consulted quickly among themselves and asked him to go, like other candidates, and await the election result in his tenth-floor Sheraton executive suite. But Mantu, determined to brave it to the end, refused.

Outside the hall, plain-clothes security men took strategic positions, keeping an eye on large groups of sharply divided supporters, who monitored proceedings on 16 close-circuit television sets. Ibrahim Alfa, retired air vice-marshal and chairman of the Transition of Civil Rule Committee, sitting on a raised platform all day with Humphrey Nwosu, National Electoral Commission, NEC, chairman, and Jerry Gana, chairman of MAMSER, shifted in their seats and braced up for the election result, the climax of the NRC convention.

The hall rumbled with a murmur. "S-i-l-e-n-c-e! May I have your attention please," Stephen Agodo, national administrative secretary of the NRC, stiff as a ramrod and holding the statement of result in his hands, screamed into the microphone. The hall froze into dead silence. "I, Stepen Agodo, national administrative secretary of the National Republican Convention, hereby certify, that I conducted the election of the national chairman of the National Republican Convention on the 22nd day of July, 1990; that the election was contested; that the candidates received the following votes: (1) Portwright Akaighe: four votes; (2) Bassey Etim Akpan: 66 votes; (3) Austin Izagbo: 76 votes; (4) Ibrahim Mantu: 878 votes; and (5) Tom Ikimi: 1,757 votes. I hereby certify Tom Ikimi duly elected." Ovation.

An hour before the result, Ikimi's aides monitoring the counting had sent words to him, in his Noga Hilton executive suite, breaking the good news and requesting him to hurry down to the Sheraton banquet hall, some five kilometres away. As Mantu stood, shook his head and walked away, his head unbowed, the jubilating crowd of Ikimi supporters made efforts to put the man high up on their shoulders, but Ikimi resisted the idea. He did not show any visible sign of joy or excitement over his victory. He did not hug anybody. He did not stand up with a clenched fist raised in the air. He did not even say a word into the many microphones shot into his face by reporters. As Alfa and his team took their leave, Ikimi, looking very scared and panicky, stood up and virtually raced out of the hall, confounding his supporters and reporters who had waited to capture his mood. The faces surrounding him and the voice urging him to slow down appeared too strange for his comfort. The fire of celebration went off quickly as his numerous supporters found no real motivation to celebrate. In his moment of glory, Ikimi looked less than a kingpin.

Outside, a tranquil crowd dispersed slowly, drifting away into their thoughts. Nobody cheered. A journalist and former university teacher, who preferred not to be quoted, made an effort at explaining the melancholy. I think his (Ikimi's) victory is not his victory and many people here are worried about the implication of his victory for the NRC, the bespectacled radical writer said. May be right. May be wrong. Whatever the case, Ikimi's victory July 22 completes a clean and resounding victory of the northern caucus faction of the party over the southern faction. Like Ikimi, all the 13 other candidates, on their powerful ticket, floored their opponents in landslide victories. Mantu's 878 votes were, in fact, the highest any opponent of the northern caucus could muster.

Stephen Lawani, a Benue indigene and candidate for the post of deputy chairman, polled 2,027 votes, while his best opponent, E. Dimike of Imo State, had 314 votes. Usman Alhaji, a 29-year-old indigene of Kano State, recorded 1,990 votes to win the key post of national secretary, while his main rival, Oruamba Anjuba of Rivers State, got 358 votes. Abba Dabo, former chairman of Liberal Convention, LC, who was considered a heavy weight for the job, came a distant third with 216 votes. For the post of national financial secretary, Abubakar Galadima of Borno State defeated Mohammed Jiddah, also from Borno State, by 1,848 votes to 232 votes. Chris Adighije from Imo State registered 1, 648 votes to outscore Iyanam Iyanam of Akwa Ibom State for the post of national treasurer. Doyin Okupe, a medical doctor and an indigene of Ogun State, defeated Sulia Adedeji of Oyo State by 1,073 votes to 653 votes for the post of publicity secretary. Olufemi Fani-Kayode, son of Remi Fani Kayode, adopted earlier as the northern caucus candidate, came a distant third with 493 votes. Aliyu Jibrin Yelwa of Sokoto State was returned unopposed for the post of national auditor, while Rufus Olagunju Ariyo of Ondo State floored F. O. Offia by 1,858 votes to 353 votes to become the national legal adviser. Kabir Abdullahi, Abdulkadir Mijinyawa, Audu Yakwo, Tijani Ramallan, Onikepo Oshodi and Ojo Afolabi defeated 14 other candidates for the job of ex-officio members, to complete a 100 percent win for the northern caucus.

Back in the safety and comfort of his campaign headquarters at Nicon Noga Hilton Hotel, Ikimi was calm, reassured and relaxed as he read his acceptance speech to a crowded press conference. "This is the dawn of a new awakening. We have a challenge to rise above division and seek the betterment of all Nigerians. I accept (this) verdict with humility and from this moment, I rededicate myself to the service of our party for the progress of our country," Ikimi said in a sonorous voice. He quickly extended his "hand of brotherhood and fellowship" to his defeated opponents and pledged to be a chairman for all the interests within the party. As he put it: "We remain members of the same family because the NRC is one vast Nigerian family. I welcome you to participate in the new politics of dialogue, (because) I shall listen to and speak with all the constituents of our party without fear or favour."

Ikimi, an architect, touched peripherally on the political programme of the NRC and gave some clue to what kind of government the party would run, if it wins the big political race. Said the new chairman: "Our party will (be) a beacon of efficient and responsible administration, not only in Nigeria but Africa. I believe in accountability to the electorate. This will be the hallmark of our tenure of office. We will work not just to manage wealth but use our abundant resources to create employment and prosperity for all. We shall ensure that Nigeria achieves its true destiny and greatness. We invite all Nigerians to join in this movement."

In the question and answer session that followed, Ikimi was voluble or, as someone put it, "too eloquent for an architect." Said Ikimi on the issue of presidential candidate for the party: "Look, when the time comes for nominating the presidential candidate, we shall sort it out amicably; we shall go through primaries, a process that is well known and admired in other parts of the world, and we shall make a success of it. So, it is still possible that a southerner can make it. But if it is not a southerner, whoever will be the nominee will gain our support because he would have gone through the mill."

The controversy over the NRC presidential candidate remained the Achilles' heel of the party in the race towards 1992. It haunted the party all the way to the just concluded convention. It created wounds that may take time to heal. And it almost threw spanners in the works of the Transition to Civil Rule Committee.

On July 19, less than 48 hours before the convention kicked off, the temporary secretariat of the NRC and SDP at Abuja Sheraton sat down around 10.00pm to finalize arrangements for the convention, work out the election procedures and screen nominees for the election. Present at the meeting, which was presided over by Agodo, were Adamu Fika, SDP national administrative secretary; Nwosu, Gana and the 44 state administrative secretaries. The meeting had barely gone half way when it ran into a knotty problem. All the 78 nominees for 14 party positions had either been petitioned against or found to be "invalidly nominated." There were "glaring and inexcusable" cases of double, multiple and outright wrong nominations. Most nomination forms even carried forged signatures. A closer investigation seemed to convince the committee that those irregularities were carried out by political opponents in an effort to get their opponents disqualified. But there was no way of knowing whether nominees themselves had not tried to short-circuit the process. After some arguments, Gana, according to an insider, suggested the idea of mass disqualification of all nominees. Agodo, *Newswatch* learnt, objected "because of the cost and the fact that the convention was already at hand." But most officials at the meeting went with Gana's suggestion. The matter was quickly referred to Augustus Aikhomu, vice-admiral and Chief of General Staff, CGS, Nigeria's No.2 man, who had just arrived Abuja that evening and the man authorized the mass cancellation and extension of deadline to 6.00pm. Friday, July 20.

When the shocking news was broken the next morning, panic and confusion gripped thousands of delegates and candidate trooping into the federal capital territory. At first, leading NRC chieftains contemplated a boycott of the convention. Said Dabo in his seventh floor Hilton executive suite: "Have you seen any-body fill any new forms? We may boycott it. It is a blow to the political class." By deadline the same evening, only 10 candidates had submitted their forms. The deadline had to be pushed for-ward again to 4.00 pm, the next day, July 21, when the conven-tion started. At the end, 63 candidates scaled the hurdle. It was a very difficult hurdle. For a candidate to be duly nominated, he required 44 signatures, two from each state and Abuja.

Delegates and their signatures suddenly became hot com-modities, purchased only by the highest bidder. With the po-larization and fractionalization of delegates between north and south, east and west, middle belt, minorities, etc., over the pres-idency issue, even the highest bidder could not get a signature. A campaign staff to one of the candidates for the chairmanship told *Newswatch* that the backers of his boss had to charter three aircraft to different parts of the country to quickly purchase sig-natures from party members who had not been caught up by the presidency fever. One candidate told *Newswatch* he paid as much as N4,000 for two signatures inside the Hilton Hotel, July 20. "You can't believe it, but I am determined not to chicken out of this election," the candidate, a public relations consultant, said.

That Friday night, July 20, was a night of long knives. Tension, distrust and political intrigues had combined to erect huge walls between different parts of the country. It had been speculated all day that all southern delegates arrived Abuja determined to vote for Mantu, considered a northerner, even though peripherally so. Northern delegates were also believed to reserve their vote for southern chairmanship candidates, in a similar ploy to pock-et the presidency. There were at least two well-known southern candidates at that time, Akpan and Ikimi, and it was still hazy which one among them would have been endorsed by the northern caucus.

Would the masters of the game split their votes between the two southerners, paving the way for Mantu? Several secret meetings between delegates from the same states and other states lasted throughout the night. Inside Hilton's eighth floor suite, a meeting of Akwa Ibom State delegates, summoned by Akpan, ended inconclusively barely an hour after it started at 10.00pm. It was a bad omen. Akpan had called the meeting to solicit "total support" in his bid to be the chairman. He told delegates present that he had the blessing of the northern caucus and that Mantu had pledged to step down for him. He was wrong on both counts. Mantu, stumping between Sheraton and Hilton hotels, where most delegates camped, had not contemplated such a decision. In fact, his enthusiastic troops of campaigners were singing around the lobby of the hotel at that time. His campaign had by then become the most well-organized.

Akpan also told the group that he was, not blocking the chances of the south to produce the next president as alleged by some delegates. He said he had plans to resign midway into his tenure, if that would guarantee the south the ultimate political prize. The crowd murmured in disbelief and began to step out one after the other. Later that night, when Akpan sent his nomination forms to Cross River State delegates for signature, the group, led by Anthony Ani, an accountant, gave him a thumbs down. Even among Akwa Ibom State delegates, his state delegates, Akpan had only the support of a tiny fraction of delegates led by Etukudo Ekproh, a young gubernatorial aspirant whose camp had performed badly in the state party elections. Majority of delegates from the State, led by Lambert Udo, the State NRC chairman, and Akpan

Isemin, a governorship aspirant, preferred Mantu, in solidarity with the limping southern caucus.

Later that same night, a joint meeting of the northern caucus with some "elders" of the west began in the Hilton's executive suite of Ibrahim Gusau, former minister in the Shagari administration. Present at the meeting, in addition to Gusau, were Adamu Ciroma, Maitama Sule, Remi Fani-Kayoda, Ahmed Kusamotu, Olagunju Adesakin, Oyo State NRC chairman, Segun Oribote, Ogun State NRC chairman, and Bosede Oshinowo of the Lagos State NRC, among others. After several hours of hard bargaining, the meeting came up with a ticket. Akpan, hitherto a favourite of the northern caucus, was out-manoeuvred, out-manipulated and dumped. Endorsed were Ikimi and the team that later made a clean sweep for the caucus. Kasamotu, said to be eyeing the vice-presidential ticket, boasted last week that he sponsored Ikimi's candidature: "Yes, I ensured his victory. I made it happen."

But Okupe's candidacy for the publicity secretary job against Femi Fani-Kayode became a sour spot in the alliance. The elder Fani-kayode, *Newswatch* learnt, was livid that the northern caucus had turned their back on his son's candidacy at the last minute. Fani Power, as Fani-Kayode is fondly called in political circles, had a week earlier, in Lagos, made his son's candidacy on the powerful ticket possible, amidst the crisis over a zoning formula. He had then, according to *Newswatch* sources, "compromised the southern solidarity" and agreed to support the northern caucus on the issue, provided his 30-year-old son was given an express ticket to the party's key publicity job. The deal was struck. But a few hours to the close of nomination, the caucus had been swayed. Adesakin, supported by Oribote and Oshinowo, as well as Kusamotu, opted for Sulia Adedeji from Oyo State, the same State with Fani-Kayode. Adedeji's candidature, *Newswatch* learnt, was actually Kusamotus' strategy to split Fani-Kayode's vote and pave the way for Okupe. He succeeded. Adedeji polled 653 votes, 160 votes more than Fani-Kayode's 493, clearing the way for Okupe who carried the day with 1,073.

The Yoruba delegates, as a result of internal friction among their leaders, became a fragmented force. Four meetings to reconcile their differences and make them fight as one team did not quite succeed. The third such meeting July 21, in the banquet hall of the Sheraton Hotel, which was also to be addressed by Mantu, collapsed when more than half of the delegates said they would not listen to Mantu.

The meeting of the Igbo delegates from Anambra and Imo states called by Emmanuel Iwuanyanwu in his Hilton Hotel suite that same night, did not fare much better. Majority of delegates from Anambra State, controlled by Hyde Onuaguluchi, the controversial Sabbath priest, did not even bother to attend the meeting. The Imo delegates, who formed the bulk of attendants at the meeting, decided their votes would be better cast for Mantu.

Chucks Muoma, renowned lawyer and NRC chairman of Aba local government area, told *Newswatch* the decision to vote for Mantu derived from the long-standing agreement within the party that the national chairman of the party would be elected from the north, while the president would be elected from the south. "We have to keep faith with that gentleman's agreement. We believe that this is the only way we can dislodge the misconception that the NRC is a northern moslem party. Any political manoeuvre that deviates and disallows the southerner, no matter his State of origin, to run for the presidency, will lend credence to recent coup plotters' allegation that there is a plot by a section of the country to dominate the government in perpetuity," Muoma said.

With the leaders of the western and eastern states going their separate ways in factions and fractions, the political goal desired by Muoma was bound to fail. And with the perennial mutual suspicion among the south taking over at Abuja, the entire southern delegation was like a flock of sheep without a shepherd. Yemi Ademefun, engineer and NRC member who wants to be the governor of Ogun State, could not hide his concern over the situation. Said Ademefun: "I must confess we have a big problem in The South. We are not united. We cannot speak with one voice and The North will always exploit us unless there is some measure of understanding, cohesion and discipline amongst us."

The Cross River State NRC delegates, numbering 58, the smallest outside Abuja, appeared, for a while, the most disciplined of the southern delegates. Led by Anthony Ani, delegates in the group would not sign nomination forms or negotiate with candidates outside the knowledge of Ani. Guides, some of them former Constituent Assembly, CA, members, were brought in, all the way from their home states to monitor the State delegates. But soon, cracks began to appear on their walls of defence. Joseph Wayas, former senate president, *Newswatch* learnt, was the trouble. He wanted the State delegation signed, sealed and delivered to a particular candidate disapproved by leaders of the delegation. He was rebuffed, but he won some converts. Discipline broke down. From then on, it was every man to his tent.

The breakdown of tight control over delegates by their leaders spread quickly like wildfire throughout other States. Money became the solvent that melted the hearts and iron-clad defences of many delegates. In attempts to win over some States' delegation enbloc, *Newswatch* gathered, sponsors of one chairmanship candidate paid huge sums of money, ranging from N200,000 to N250,000, to leaders of some State delegations. Following the mass cancellation of nominations, desperate candidates were paying as high as N2,000 per signature. That shattered almost completely the guards put up by delegates, some of whom are unemployed. Said one angry delegate to his leader: "Chief, chief, don't harass me again o! Is it zoning I will chop?"

Aikhomu knew about the havoc money was creating at the convention and when he stepped out on July 21 to address delegates at the convention, he had some unpalatable words for those he called "money-bags." Said Aikhomu: "It is shameful that certain Nigerians who had had access to money are constituting themselves into a political nuisance. We have records of such individuals. We condemn their role and we warn them to desist from their current practices." Turning attention to ordinary individual members of political parties, Aikhomu said they should "learn to be self-sufficient and to price their individual integrity above money." He urged them not to mortgage themselves or succumb to corruption or influence of "persons who have no ideas to offer but money." As he put it: "The negative impact of money in the political process can marginalize competent Nigerians with vision and leadership credentials. It can create a class of mediocre rulers who will succumb to corruption and undemocratic practices. You and your party must check this tendency, because your party and the entire political system will be the greatest losers if you allow yourselves to be infested by moneybags."

On the issue of zoning, Aikhomu said though the government was conscious of the need to reflect "federal character" in the political parties, the practice should not be reduced to an immutable law. "The zoning of offices should not be the overriding principle. The search must be for clear and credible candidates for leadership at all levels of our political system. This administration does not and will not subscribe to zoning for elective political offices because it restricts the choice of credible candidates and can enthrone mediocrity," Aikhomu said. It was the same speech that Aikhomu returned to Abuja to read three days later when the Social Democratic Party, SDP, convention kicked off July 24.

The SDP convention was a sharp contrast to the NRC convention. It began in the manner of a rural carnival. Virtually each State delegation arrived the federal capital territory with traditional dance troupes. Rural faces, most of them on their first visit to Abuja, roamed the vast hotel premises, visibly excited by the sheer beauty of the five-star edifice. Frenzied drummers, acrobatics and maiden dancers attracted large crowds inside and outside the gates of Abuja Sheraton Hotel. Most States came dressed in uniforms and special attires that distinguished them from other delegates. Lagos State delegates looked resplendent in the green *aga* hats. You would not recognize Garba Hamza, multimillionaire philanthropist and Lagos delegate, in his beautiful *aga* hat. "I am enjoying every bit of it," he told *Newswatch* in the midst of friends who crowded around him outside the hotel.

The opulence and flamboyance that characterized the NRC convention had taken a back seat. Instead of Mercedes Benz, BMW and other flashy cars, a large number of delegates arrived in lorries and buses, most of them hired from state transport corporations. Instead of Hilton and Sheraton hotels, where most delegates of the NRC were camped, the SDP delegates stayed in cheap, seedy hotels in far-away Suleja, Keffi and majority in Kaduna, a grueling three-hour drive to Abuja, and ate outside in roadside restaurants. A female delegate from Bendel State arrived with her husband and a food flask July 24 at the Sheraton Hotel. "I brought my own food because I know that all this Sheraton food is very expensive." She was right. Adinner of *eba, tuwo or amala* at Abuja Sheraton goes for N104.50

In spite of the poverty and fanfare that accompanied the SDP to Abuja, delegates arrive ready to do political battle. *"Sai* Arzika, *sai* Arzika" (Unless Arzika, unless Arzika), a large crowd of supporters of Mohammed Arzika, a chairmanship candidate, shouted as they drummed and ran around the venue of the convention with banners and posters. *"Sai Baba, sai Baba"* (Unless Baba, unless Baba), a separate crowd of supporters of Babagana Kingibe, the only opponent of Arzika, responded with a deafening chorus. Weeks before the convention, it was clear the SDP convention would feature a straight fight between the Arzika camp and the Kingibe camp. A camp of "progressives," the Arzika faction, made up of members of defunct People's Solidarity Party, PSP, was heavily backed by at least 10 former governors of the Progressive Peoples Alliance, PPA, while Kingibe's conservative faction received the support of Shehu Yar'Adua, former Nigerian No. 2 citizen; Arthur Nzeribe, billionaire businessman; Olusola Saraki, former senator and millionaire king of Kwara State politics; Paul Unongo, former minister and rising star of Middle Belt politics; Femi Adekanye, former PSP national coordinator and rising star of Yoruba politics, to mention a few.

Early Monday morning, July 23, just as the NRC delegates departed, Arzika stormed the venue of the convention with his team and published posters, pictures and names of 14 candidates, including himself, running on the PSP ticket. The candidates, including Yemi Farounbi, deputy chairman; Alexis Anielo, secretary; Frank Kokori, financial secretary; David Iornem, publicity secretary; J.J. Fwa, treasurer; Ado Indabo, auditor; Ogana Lukpata, legal adviser; as well as six ex-officio candidates. It was one mistake that could have been avoided. It foreclosed any last minute deals with the PFN faction and portrayed the PSP faction as rigid and uncompromising.

Far away in Kaduna, where the PFN faction camped most of its delegates to avoid a close look at the list, top leaders began to plan their counter-moves. John Ekong, former CA member who was supposed to be on the PFN ticket as the secretary candidate, was dropped. In his place, the PFN caucus endorsed Ebere Osieke, a professor and choice of Nzeribe. It was a move that was aimed at countering the weight of Anielo, a former CA member sponsored by former governor Jim Nwobodo. The PFN, which had also penciled down Iornem for publicity secretary, sent for the management consultant. Iornem was already campaigning under the PSP ticket, his station-wagon Peugeot campaign vehicle bedecked with Arzika's pictures side by side with his own. He was asked to choose between the two camps. Iornem chose both. He was asked to remove Arzika's pictures from his campaign vehicle. Iornem refused. The PFN quickly dropped him from its ticket and brought in Markos Shamma, a reverend gentleman, at the last minute. Also recruited at the last minute by the PFN was Ademola Babalola from Oyo State to fill the post of deputy chairman. The PFN had reserved the position for Farounbi but the veteran broadcaster had preferred the Arzika camp. Though the two camps, on their own, supported Kokori and Lukpata, attempts by some members of the party on the eve of the convention to sit the two camps down and reduce areas of conflicts failed as each side was already poised for a show-down.

The first opportunity for the two sides to clash in the public came 10.00am, July 24, inside the capacity packed venue of the convention. Arzika and Kingibe were given three minutes each to speak to 2,938 delegates. Present were Aikhomu, Alfa, Nwosu, Gana, Agodo, Fika and some 1,000 supporters watching proceedings on close-circuit television sets. When the NRC chairmanship candidates were put to the same test three days earlier, Ikimi and Mantu performed well and this boosted their chances. Now, the idea, a brain-wave of Gana, had become a star attraction of the convention. Arzika was invited first to the podium. A loud ovation accompanied him all the way. He was calm, collected and mature in his approach as he began his speech *extempore.* He briefly went through highlights of his career in government, business and politics. He turned to the party and spoke of the rivalry as being "healthy." Then he struck his best line: "My fellow compatriots," he began on a deliberately slow pace, "there will be winners in this election, but there will be no losers." It was a line that was roundly applauded. It earned Arzika a gread deal of respect and cut for him the image of a father of the party.

Kingibe was exuberant and flowing with confidence. His carriage, diction and style gave him out as a good soapbox material. He gave Arzika a pat with one hand and then a blow with the other hand. Said Kingibe: "Yes, I agree Arzika was in the civil service, but I was not just there, I rose to the top of that service. I agree he was in the Foreign Service, but I climbed to the apex of the Foreign Service. Yes, I agree he worked in the State House as a private secretary, but I was also there as a principal secretary." Then Kingibe turned combative, this time in the direction of the government and the NRC. He took up Aikhomu on his speech on "moneybags." Said Kingibe: "Your reference to money-bags, Chief of General Staff, sir, is appropriate, but the issue should be more appropriately directed at the NRC because we don't have money-bags in the SDP." That earned him the vital across the board ovation.

Majority of delegates and reporters packed in the hall declared Kingible the winner of the debate. But Arzika could not be called a loser. He may have come across as soft and too sober. But opinion began to form among delegates about the need for a strong and competent leader that can build a solid foundation for the SDP. Majority of the delegates also began to express concern over Arzika's home-base in Sokoto and said that could make him vulnerable to political pot-shots by Sokoto power brokers, who are believed to be core NRC. Said Jibrin Jiddah, a delegate: "That is a weak link. Once the chairman is neutralized, the entire party would find itself in limbo."

But Arzika had other weak points to contend with in the race. His close association and virtual dependence on former PPA governors, especially Abubakar Rimi and Lateef Jakande, became a political albatross. In the north, he was regarded as a "surrogate of banned Yoruba politicians." In the west, the disdain against the pervasive tentacles of former PPA governors had sparked off something like a mini-rebellion, which was later to affect Arzika's chances in the election.

After Tokunbo Dosumu, daughter of late legend Obafemi Awolowo, was frustrated and harassed out of politics by banned followers of her late father, other young and promising politicians began to put their foot down in defiance of the old war lords. Femi Adekanye, businessman and former university teacher was one of the rebels. He broke ranks with the Yoruba PSP "elders" and with other young men and women, joined forces with the PFN faction of the SDP in an action that was considered a political suicide. By convention time, however, the young man had mustered sufficient political forces to deal a blow on Arzika'ss ambition.

At the convention, the west was no longer a monolithic political entity with a bloc vote. From Ondo State, where Adekanye started his crusade, the anger of maltreated newbreed had spread to Oyo, Ogun, Lagos and Bendel states. In Ogun State, Titi Ajanaku, former chairman of Abeokuta LGA, and Dayo Abatan, former student union leader, had led the campaigns for Kingibe. In Oyo State, Ganju Adesakin, the State SDP chairman, who had earlier defeated former governor Bola Ige-sponsored candidates in the State election, kept a distance from the PSP faction, in favour of Kingibe. From Lagos State, Femi Bamgboye, chairman of SDP in Ikeja LGA, led his supporters to vote for Kingibe in defiance of former governor, Jakande. In Bendel State, Abel Ubeku, a presidential aspirant who sources say "could no longer tolerate the attitude" of the banned former governors, led a Bendel State delegation that voted largely for Kingibe. Screamed an elated Adekanye inside the Sheraton venue of the convention after Kingibe had been declared winner. "This is a newbreed result. The point that has been made today is that we are tired of being rubber stamps of banned politicians."

In the result, Kingibe floored Arzika by 1,651 votes to 1,191 votes. Ademola Babalola, hurriedly drafted by the PFN into the race, recorded a shocking victory over Farounbi by 1,457 votes to 1,355 votes. Ebere Osieke, and other PFN candidate, won the key secretary post by 1,383 to 1,131 votes against Anielo, said to be sponsored by PPA's former governor, Jim Nwobodo. The Kingibe ticket also won the post of treasurer for Hammani Bazza, who polled 1,440 votes to beat Jorman Fawaz of the PSP camp. Mohammed Sambo Koko, who contested for the post of auditor on the platform of PFN also defeated PSP's Ado Indabo. Unlike the NRC election, the SDP's was not a one-sided victory by a faction. The PSP's Iornem narrowly defeated Shammah by 1,723 to 1,666 votes to secure the post of publicity secretary. The two camps also won three ex-officio members each, while Kokori and Lukpata, endorsed by both sides, had no difficulties winning their posts. Said an excited Kingibe in a short victory speech: "Let's go back to our (SDP) house. There shall be no factions again."

That pledge may be hard to fulfill in both parties, as the big race for President Ibrahim Babangida's seat kicked off in earnest last week, just as the convention rounded off. As delegates and observers trooped out of Abuja last week full of praises for the efficient conduct of the elections, it appeared, however, that the most urgent task facing the new party leadership is how to manage their victories. Said a senior western diplomat, who witnessed the historic party conventions: "It has been a very orderly exercise, but it remains to be seen whether the new party leaders have the generosity of heart to accommodate their defeated opponents and facilitate a smooth transition to civil rule."

A FIVE STAR CONFUSION

Dodan Barracks, Nigeria's seat of power, may not have bargained for such a mess. But this hot February afternoon, the day Eme Awa, Professor of Political Science, was sacked as chairman of the National Electoral Commission, NEC, witnessed a proportion of confusion that left the government reeling in embarrassment.

The usual Monday National Security Council meeting had extended to Tuesday. It was a marathon meeting and State House correspondents were banking on a list of new cabinet promised by the president. Except for Sani Abacha, Chief of Army Staff, who had been dispatched to Saudi Arabia the previous night at the head of government's delegation to the finals of the Under-21 World Cup tournament, all other service chiefs as well as the chairman, Joint Chiefs of Staff and the Chief of General Staff, CGS, were present.

At about 1.00 pm, Yussuf Mamman, press secretary to Augustus Aikhomu, was summoned to Aikhomu's office. Soon, Mamman returned to his office with breaking news. "The federal military government has decided to effect some changes in the membership of the NEC," he said with an air of importance. Minutes later, a two-page press release announcing the "change" signed by Mamman and stamped "No Embargo" (meaning it should be published immediately) was given out to the correspondents. The press release announced the appointment of a nine-member electoral commission headed by Olakunle Orojo, retired chief judge of Ondo State.

Other members of the commission, according to the press release, were Al Gazili, Adele Jinadu, Festus Emeghara, Ahmed Kiyawa, Gabriel Ijewere, Aliyu Haidara, Eno Irokwu, Dagogo Jack and Aliyu Umar as secretary. The release also announced the deployment and swapping of positions by the NEC's resident electoral commissioners in the 21 states and Abuja. In a brief chat with correspondents, Mamman volunteered the reason for Awa's removal and the necessity for a new commission. "The shake-up has been carried out in order to invigorate the NEC and inculcate some dynamism so that the body can face the challenges of organizing the next election. This change is with immediate effect," Mamman said.

As some correspondents whose media houses are based outside Lagos rushed for the telephone, their Lagos-based colleagues jumped into their standby cars for a quick drive to their offices. Their reports filed, some reporters left for home but the unexpected was yet to happen. At exactly 3.55pm. Mamman dashed back to the press centre. The place was empty.

"Please there is a change." He said nervously to a handful of correspondents who had waited to see the end of the Security Council meeting and watch the live telecast of the World Cup encounter between Nigeria and USA. To replace Orojo, the just appointed chairman of NEC. Mamman said, was Humphrey Nwosu, Professor of sociology and one-time commissioner for local government in Anambra State.

"Why? The question flew at Mamman relentlessly, but he had no answer. His concern was how to get the new name across to the media houses quickly. The correspondent of the Federal Radio Corporation of Nigeria , FRCN, had just rushed back (from his office just one kilometer away) and prime time news at this station was just five minutes away. The change was immediately effected through the radio but most correspondents who heard the 4.00pm national news from their offices thought the radio man had made a mistake and refused to change their stories. They showed their editors the press release to prove that Orojo was the new NEC chairman.

But even in the State House, that was not the end of the confusion. Soon after 4.00pm, Mamman was summoned again. Two more names had surfaced as members of the NEC, Yunusa Oyeyemi, a NEC member who had been dropped, was given back the job, and Patrick Odo, a new face was named into the commission. Mamman was still unable to explain the confusion and the piece-meal manner the names were coming in. To further complicate matters, the prime time NTA news, regarded as the official voice of the military government, that evening announced a "nine-member" commission but showed 12 names including that of Orojo, as members of the commission. The confusion in the newspapers the next morning was worse. Asked the *Nigerian Tribune* in a banner headline: "Who is new NEC chairman."

That morning, March 1, Mamman had to "put the record straight" with another press release listing the correct chairman and members of the commission. But somehow the puzzle was compounded. The names of Festus Emerghara, who was appointed a member in the first press release and that of Patrick Odo, who was appointed after the first press release, had now disappeared entirely from the list. The "final list" also showed that apart from Awa, four other members of the commission were removed. They were Adamu Fika, Garba Gumi, Christopher Akande and Umaru Sanda Ahmadu, who was the secretary of the commission. To take over Ahmadu's job was Aliyu Umar, (a one-time secretary to the government of Niger State, who was later appointed a federal permanent secretary by the Shagari administration.

The bungled reconstitution of the NEC continued last week to raise questions. Why was Awa removed? Why was Orojo appointed and dropped suddenly? Or, in fact, why did the government have to reconstitute and reorganize the NEC midstream? Duro Onabule, President Ibrahim Babangida's chief spokesman told *Newswatch* that changes and appointments in government were normal and the same applied to NEC. Said Onabule: "There is nothing sacrosanct about changes or appointment of any person into public office. Anybody could be appointed or dropped at anytime."

However, other inside sources in the State House told *Newswatch* that Awa was perceived by government to be unnecessarily rigid, weak, and unable to shoulder the huge responsibilities in implementing the political transition programme. "The whole place was untidy," the source said. "That's not to suggest corruption. No. But he was clearly unable to take charge of the place." According to the sources, there was also a personality clash between Awa and the commission's secretary, Ahmadu. Said the source: "This running battle between him (Awa) and the secretary had been going on for sometime now and government had thought he could put his feet down and sort things out but he couldn't. The decree that established NEC says he (the chairman) is the chief executive but he wasn't asserting himself."

Though government sources attributed Awa's removal to lack of dynamism, other well-informed sources last week traced his problems to his uncompromising stance on certain contract awards. One such contract, our source said, was for the supply of communications equipment to NEC for the conduct of the forth coming elections. A top government official was said to have taken interest in the contract and wanted the contract awarded at the cost of about N80 million. But Awa, *Newswatch* learnt, insisted that the contract was overpriced and said the equipment could be purchased elsewhere at less than half the quoted price. "From then on,"*Newswatch* was told, "Awa was seen as a threat to the economic and political interests of some officials." Still some sources said that Awa had appeared "too radical and politically at variance with the known outlook of the government."

The issue, it appears, may remain contentious for some time to come, but the sudden dropping of Orojo, which added a credibility problem to government was a clear case of government undoing itself. Orojo, according to reliable State House sources, was not consulted before he was appointed to the sensitive job. When he was later contacted at the last minute, "the man simply declined the appointment." Most State House correspondents who found this out last week were taken aback. Only a week earlier, on February 20, the president had pledged after an AFRC meeting that the practice of "appointment and dismissal by radio," adopted by most military regimes in the country, was on its way out.

The political implications of the haphazard handling of the

NEC appointments were, however, what bothered political analysts the more, last week. Oyibo Chukwu, a member of the Constituent Assembly, CA, told *The Guardian* last week that the changes were "curious," especially against the background that no "serious" reason was given as to why NEC was reconstituted. Nse Umoren, another CA member, saw the change as a result of the belief that the Awa-led group could not have conducted a free and fair election. Said Umoren: "If the change is politically motivated, it leaves much to be desired." Yet another CA member, Michael Umonta, interpreted the dissolution of the NEC as an indication that government does not want to hand over power to "just anybody."

In Lagos, the development generated the same feelings of forbearance and uncertainty. Gani Fawehinmi, a Lagos lawyer and well-known government critic, said the reorganization typified "a breach of faith on the transition programme." Fawehinmi's colleague and friend, Olu Onagoruwa, added that the shake-up at NEC was an "ominous sign that the transition programme was not going very well. That the NEC is not stable... and that our (political) future is very bleak." Onagoruwa said government should have investigated Awa better before his appointment. "If they have now found a better man, then they were guilty of misjudgment in the first place," he said.

For Awa himself, his removal was a big load off his neck. As he put it in his last day in office: "The chairmanship of the National Electoral Commission is a very hot seat. I have tried to do this job very honestly to ensure a free and fair election, but perhaps, somewhere along the line, there has been a clash with the normal trend in Nigerians politics. (However), I will like to be remembered as someone who tried to do his job honestly."

RIGHT NAME, WRONG PERSON

The charming and confident middle aged man had savoured what he thought was the greatest moment of his life. Before the full glare of television light, he had been sworn in as a member of the Constitution Review Committee, CRC, by President Ibrahim Babangida. The ceremony, he recalls, was very elaborate. Elite ceremonial guards had turned the scene at the palatial NICON Noga Hilton Hotel, Abuja, into something of a Buckingham Palace. Floral decorations, dangling chandeliers as well as glossy green-white-green flags danced gently inside the exquisite conference hall. Seated already with him and chatting in whispers were fellow CRC members, their relations, top officers of state and a large crowd of pressmen.

He remembers the brisk and colourful arrival of the President, escorted by a cavalry of ceremonial guards. "Ladies and gentlemen" a dashing protocol officer had announced, "The President of the Federal Republic of Nigeria." A standing welcome. The national anthem. Everyone was back to his seat.

He remembers himself standing before the president, sober

and happy, with a Bible in his right hand and the text of the oath in the other hand. He can still hear his strong sonorous voice ringing through the microphone: "I, Asuquo Sam Inyang, do hereby swear... So help me God." The applause that followed and the signature he scribbled on the register are still very fresh in his mind. Most of all, he remembers the president pumping his hand in congratulation and the private discussion he and other CRC members had with the president soon after the ceremony. Pensive, he also remembers the horde of reporters and photographers seeking interviews and struggling to take his picture. He sighs, pulls himself together and tries to sleep off. He can't.

His mind wanders further. He remembers the joy that descended on his family when he returned from the swearing-in ceremony. His mind flashes back to the celebrations and congratulatory letters he received from his friends, colleagues and relations. In agony, he turns once more on his bed and tries to figure out how his wife, children and family can quickly handle and overcome the embarrassing situation. No solution. He sighs again, and tries to sleep. Again he can't. Daybreak.

For Inyang, 47, the headmaster of the Army Children School, Rainbow Town, Port Harcourt, trouble started on the night of September 2. He was watching the network news with his family, when the names of those appointed to serve on the CRC were announced. One of the manes was A. S. Inyang. "They were my full initials and surname, and many people who saw it started coming around to congratulate me," Inyang said. Somehow, Inyang managed to maintain his calm, asking those who wanted the appointment to be celebrated to wait till he could confirm it.

The next day, the same names appeared in most newspapers. Greeted by a barrage of congratulations everywhere he went,

Inyang headed for the federal ministry of information's office at Port Harcourt to find out whether he was, indeed, the appointee. The ministry did not know. Inyang was advised to try the governor's office. The governor's office did not have the list either.

A rather cautious person, he decided to wait for his letter of appointment. But his friends told him that appointees were notified via television, radio and newspapers, to report at the NICON Noga Hilton Hotel, Abuja, September 6, for the swearing-in September 7. On his persistent argument that he knew nobody who would have recommended him, many people reminded him that he is a teacher of pupils, some of whose parents are ranking army officers in the government. They may have wanted to compensate his 14 years as a teacher of their children, the argument went.

On September 6, Inyang left for Abuja. On presenting himself and his identity card at the hotel, he was checked in along with other appointees. A decorated elevator lifted the man to his exquisite fifth floor suite. "It was at that point that I thought if I was not the right person I would have been so told," Inyang recalled.

At the swearing-in ceremony the following morning, the man took time to pronounce his names in full. "I, Asuquo Sam Inyang..." There was no sign something was wrong or out of order. In an interview with *Newswatch* in his tastefully furnished suite that evening, Inyang did not hide his appreciation for the unknown person who recommended him. "I am still surprised," he said. "I feel deeply honoured to serve my country at this level. Another member of the CRC, Awwalu Yadudu, a lecturer at Bayero University, Kano, spoke in the same vein: "I am quite surprised. I was very reluctant to come here. There are so many Awwalu Yadudu and I may not have been the one appointed."

Yadudu was right. There was another A. S. Inyang, too. One

month after Inyang was sworn in, the other Inyang surfaced. As it happened, he was the right Inyang.

After the CRC's inaugural session the committee took a four-week break to enable the public send in memoranda. On resumption October 4, Inyang returned to Abuja. He was accorded all the protocol due all CRC members and was checked into the Agura Hotel with his colleagues. Thirty minutes later, he heard a tap on his door. Trouble was knocking. Thinking it was probably one of his CRC colleagues, he put aside the constitutional documents he was reading and opened the door. A stern-looking man, who said he was an officer of the CRC, walked into the room. "There is a mix-up somewhere, Sir. You have to check out of the hotel now. You were wrongly sworn in. The right person in Anyang Sylvester Inyang."

Inyang, for once, wished it was all a dream. It wasn't. He paced round the hotel room, shocked and consumed by distress. "I became restless. I tried to say something but was so confused. Then I managed to tell the man, they should have written to me at Port Harcourt during the break since they had my address. Then I tried to phone some of the CRC members. It was the height of embarrassment in my life."

On October 10, Inyang, still restless, wrote to L. M. Okunnu, the cabinet office permanent secretary in charge of the CRC. He got no reply. Five days later, the headmaster telephoned Okunnu, again to ask for an official explanation of his predicament. The woman told him not to "bother" her, but wait for the letter. On November 19, more than two months after Inyang had been sworn in, the letter finally arrived Port Harcourt. It said Inyang's swearing-in was an "error."

"Look at the situation this way," Inyang told *Newswatch*, "I took six months leave of absence. A colleague was appointed to take my position as headmaster, on acting basis. Then, suddenly, everything crashed. How do I explain that? I feel ashamed. I need something to take me out of the scene for a while. Really, I need the break, if you know how I feel."

The case of the headmaster is not unique. It has only attempted to bring into focus the unfortunate system of making key government appointments via television and radio, without the slightest consultation with those appointed. A few years ago, a prominent community leader in Kwara State was hospitalized after an experience similar to the headmaster's. His name was announced on the television and radio as one of the newly appointed commissioners. That night, the entire community and his friends as far as Ilorin, the state capital, descended on his house.

There was a big party, which lasted throughout the night. The next day, the man, accompanied by his family and a large crowd, went for the swearing-in ceremony. Shockingly enough, he was not the one appointed and virtually had to be dragged out of the venue of the ceremony by the security men. Late Obafemi Awolowo, the respected Nigerian statesman, rejected an "appointment by radio" in 1976 to serve in the constitution drafting committee, because he was not consulted. As one observer argues: "This is a very disrespectful way of making key appointments. This is certainly not a serious way to run a government."

THE CRASH OF FLIGHT 086

Time was 5.03pm, on November 7, 1996. A routine flight from oil-rich Southern Nigerian city of Port Harcourt disappeared from the control tower radar screen as it was getting ready to land in Lagos. Frantic efforts to spot the aircraft in the hazy evening skies yielded no result. Moments later, Flight 086 plunged head-long into the bottomless lagoon of Ejirin, near Lagos.

The Boeing 727 went down with 143 souls. Internationally-backed massive rescue operations came up with a piece of wing, the size of a reading table and an orange-coloured box curiously called the Black Box. That was all rescuers could salvage from the wreckage of Nigeria's worst air disaster.

Tears flowed. Sorrow and horror gripped the nation. General Sani Abacha, Head of State, made a four-minute nationwide broadcast that graphically expressed the grief of the nation. He described the tragedy as one of the saddest events in the history of Nigeria.

True. So many factors combined to make that horrible November evening a sad day for Nigeria. On board Flight 086 were some of the best brains in Nigeria, trusted hands in the oil industry, irreplaceable fathers and bread winners, newly-wedded couples who were flying off for a blissful honeymoon and children. There were also 29 foreigners on board.

Besides, Flight 086 was manned by one of the best fliers the country has ever had. Dafe Sama, the captain and folk hero of his people, was not just the trainer of many Nigerian pilots, he was the national president of Nigeria's Association of Aircraft Pilots and Engineers, NAAPE. What's more, here was Nigeria's favourite airline, Aviation Development Company, ADC, reputedly safe, efficient and reliable. It was the only airline in the country quoted on the stock exchange.

What actually happened to Flight 086? Was ADC sabotaged? Did Flight 086 develop an engine problem? Was it airworthy in the first place? Or was the airplane blown into pieces by bombs as some suggested? Did the crash have something to do with the Ogoni crisis as some intelligence theories speculated? Did secret agents of government, hot on the heels of its critics, plant explosives in the airplane to settle scores with one or two of them on board?

For 14 montns the search for answers kept the nation in suspense. For the investigation panel set up by government, mum was the word. The closest government volunteered to date on the tragedy was given by Ita Udo-Imeh, Air Commodore and Aviation Minister. He said the crash of Flight 086 was caused by "human factors."

Last November, Jerry Agbeyegbe, pilot and new president of NAAPE, demanded for the report of investigations into the crash. After months of investigation, *Newswatch* has, at last, unraveled the puzzles of "human factors" that caused the air disaster. The

Black Box of Flight 086 which consists of the Cockpit Voice Recorder, CVR, and the Flight Data Recorder, FDR, is in *Newswatch* possetion and has thrown sufficient light on why the ADC flight crashed.

The FDR was taken to the American National Transport Safety Board, NTSB, for transcription. NTSB passed no judgment on the crash but transcribed every conversation and noise in the Black Box. The Black Box, *Newswatch* can reveal, recorded everything properly. The recordings reveal that nothing was wrong with the ADC aircraft and that the status of the engine was perfect.

The flight ran fully the three phases of emergency, suggesting that there was no pre-flight impairment in the aircraft condition. There was also no sign of trouble at all before the crash on the outskirts of Lagos. The transcripts of CVR and the FDR pointedly confirmed that the cause of the crash was a "traffic conflict situation." Indeed, *Newswatch* can now reveal that Flight 086 was barely 30 seconds away from colliding with another Boeing 727, called Flight 185 which was wrongly released into the air by air traffic controllers.

Flight 185 belonged to Triax Airline. It was heading for Enugu. Nigeria would have recorded a double tragedy that Thursday evening but for the fact that ADC Flight 086 was equipped with a traffic collision avoidance system, TCAS. With TCAS in Flight 086, the pilot saw Flight 185 flying directly at him. In a sudden manoeuver to avoid collision with Flight 185, the pilot of the ADC aircraft lost control and the plane plunged into the Lagoon.

Said a senior airport official: "Well, I can tell you that somebody fumbled. That evening, we would have lost two Boeing 727s and maybe double the number of casualties but for the TCAS in Flight 086. This is why ADC deserves some commendation."*Newswatch* investigations show that the journey for Flight 086 from Port Harcourt began on a beautiful note. Flight 086 called the approach controller, APC, at Lagos Control Tower at 1547.27 hours:

ADK 086: Lagos approach eh good afternoon, (This is) ADK 086

APC : ADK 086, good evening. Go ahead

ADK 086: A Boeing 727, eh Port Harcourt to Lagos. Flight level 240 degrees on board 144. Crew of 01 eh correction 10 included, endurance take off 0220

APC: Say again, total crew?

ADK 086: 10 Crew included

APC: ADK 086 is cleared no delay for VOR approach, runway in use 19L.

The summary of that coded conversation was that the captain of Flight 086 informed Lagos Approach Controller of his movement and received clearance and confirmation to proceed accordingly. Six minutes later, Flight 086 called APC again to inform him he was right on course. The reply from APC was "Go ahead." Then Flight 086 said "next call descent" meaning, "I will call you again when I am ready to descend."

Flight 086 kept the promise. At 1556.42 hours, about three minutes later, Flight 086 called APC notifying him of his position and requesting for descent. At this point APC was busy with another flight called Flight 645. A few seconds later, he returned to Flight 086 and sought confirmation that it wanted to descend. Flight 086 answered in the affirmative, giving all necessary data. By now, Flight 086 was at 69 nautical miles to Lagos. No tension. No anxiety whatsoever in their conversation. Meanwhile, APC was making efforts to speak with Flight 645 but Flight 645 requested Flight 086 to help. Flight 086 came in and helped APC relay the message:

ADK 086: "QNK 645, Lagos is calling you"
Flight 645: "Ok, Sir, if you can relay (to Lagos I am flying at) eh 56, level 220

The flight continued normally only with banters between the crew that sometimes drew hearty laughters. Again at 50 miles to Lagos, flight 086 notified APC of its descent and its position. The reply from the tower was: "Roger, ADK 086 descend to 160 (meaning O.K. ADC Flight 086, descend to 16000 feet above mean sea level").

At this point the NTSB – transcribed tape indicates that the radar controller in the control tower took over from the approach controller, as messages moved to the radar frequency. About the same time, Flight 185 to Enugu had been cleared to take off from Lagos opposite Flight 086 which was already descending into Lagos. Tragedy was about to strike. But Flight 185 was completely unaware and uninformed about Flight 086 because, like most aircraft in Nigeria, it was not equipped with TCAS. All the same, a hearty conversation began between the radar controllers and the pilot of Flight 185, at 1553.10 hours.

Flight 185: Radar, good evening. Flight 185 with you on the right turn
Radar: Flight 185, good evening. Radar identified (you) on departure. Verify you are passing 1400.
Flight 185: Charlie, Charlie (Yes, yes)

Radar: You want a left or right turn?

Flight 185: O. K. we'd like a right turn

Radar: No problem, you turn right, heading 330 degrees. I read you continue turning, heading 330.

How wrong! There was a problem. That was certainly a fatal instruction. The ascending Flight 185 was heading directly into the descending Flight 086. Apparently uncomfortable, Flight 185 pilot sought again from the radar controller to confirm the instruction given him.

Flight 185: Radar, eh, Flight 185, eh, again, can we turn further right, sir?

Radar: Flight 185, turn right, heading 360, 360.

Flight 185: Roger (meaning O.K) right 360

Radar: (second later) Flight 185, (you are) 6 miles North West of the field. Turn right; resume (your) own navigation.

That was a big mistake, aviation experts told *Newswatch* in the course of investigations. It was too early for the radar controller to allow Flight 185 to resume flying on its own, experts agree. The radar controller however put a seal to that at 1558.15 hours.

Radar: "Flight 185 (you are) 10 miles east of the field. Radar service terminated, maintain squawk.

Flight 185: Good night, Sir

As it turned out, it wasn't going to be a particularly good night. Not for radar controllers, not for the entire nation. And just then,

the pilot of the ADC Flight alerted the radar controller of his position. That was at 1600.14 hours!

Flight 086: Lagos approach, eh ADK 086, eh coming out of 210
for 160 44 miles (meaning: Lagos approach controller, eh,
this is ADC Flight 086. We are at 21000 feet above mean sea
level. We are descending to 16,000 feet above means sea level. We are 44 nautical miles to Lagos)

Radar: ADK 086, squawk ident (meaning ADC Flight 086, Identify yourself)

Flight086: Ident (meaning: I am doing so or I am identifying myself).

Radar: (about a minute later) ADK 086, radar identified at 41
miles south east of the field, fly heading (hesitating) fly heading eh, 320, vector round traffic, descend maintain FL50
(meaning ADC Flight 086. I have identified you on radar at 41
nautical miles, south east of the field. Fly heading, fly heading, eh, 320 degrees, Descend and maintain 5000 feet above
mean sea level).

Flight086: Down to 50, heading 320 (meaning: I understand. I
have been cleared to descend to 5000 feet above mean sea
level and to fly heading 320 degrees).

At this point, it was just 30 seconds to disaster. Then confusion
started. The tower controller began to betray anxiety.

Radar (1602.41 hours): ADK 086, what is your actual heading
now?

Flight086: (1602.46 hours): We are heading eh 3 .15, turning
320.

Radar (1602.51): Maintain heading 300, maintain heading 300
Flight 086 (1602.56): Ah, we..

Then the TCAS in Flight 086, came alive.

TCAS 91602.57 hours) Traffic, traffic (meaning hey, you have another aircraft approaching you and may collide with you)

Flight086 (1602.58 hours noticing Flight 185) I have it OK, we have the...

Radar (1603.01 hours): Say again?
Flight086 (1603.03 hours): I have the traffic and I continue my heading to 330, to avoid him.

Radar (1603.08 approving Flight 086 plans) That's better.

It was not better. Three seconds later, TCAS in Flight 086 changed from what was initially a traffic information alert to what is called Resolution Advisory: an emergency warning on how to quickly avoid collision with Flight 185 which was now imminent.

TCAS (1603.11): Reduce (descent), reduce, reduce, climb, climb, climb (meaning, you've got a serious problem. Reduce descent to avoid collision. Climb up climb up, climb up).

What was heard next in the black box tapes was a sound similar to a high speed clacker. That was nine seconds after the TCAS warning. Five seconds later the sound of a horn followed along with sustained screams, that apparently came from horrified crew members and passengers. Then a rapid knocking sound followed, similar to the sound of a knocking car engine. The screams continued. A voice believed by experts to be that of Sama was shouting orders: "Power! Power!! Power!!!"

Experts interpret this to mean emergency commands to the pilot flying to "throttle, throttle, throttle" to gain the needed climb. One retired captain said this indicated that Sama was "still conscious and battling to recover that aeroplane until impact."

Back at the control tower, Flight 086 had disappeared from the radar. But the controller did not think at first it was anything serious. After his last message ("That's better) to the ill-fated aircraft, he had switched attention to guide Flight 645. Returning to Flight 086, 30 seconds later, he called five minutes without any reply. Then an unidentified aeroplane within the vicinity joined to call Flight 086. "ADC 086, Lagos wants you," the unidentified aircraft said. No answer.

Now panic began to descend on the control tower with repeated calls to the crashed aircraft. "ADK 086 Lagos, ADK 086, Lagos, how do you read? ADK, ADK ADK." Then a helping hand came from another aircraft called Flight 615 which was also coming into Lagos.

Flight615, Lagos (radar), what is his destination, we will try and raise him for you. Soon Flight 645 was also brought in to help. "Could you help raise ADK 086?" the radar controller requested. "ADK , ADK, ADK. No response. Worried, Flight 645 asked the radar controller:" Lagos, is he in-bound or out-bound?" The radar controller had no time for interviews." ADK..ADK..ADK 086 Lagos?" he went on.

With the calls becoming more frantic, other incoming flights began to suggest where ADK 086 could possibly by located: radar scope? radial? Tower frequency? Every frequency? On the tarmac? No dice. One in-bound flight was requested to hold on for 15 minutes as the run-way was being cleared for a long possible emergency landing.

Flight615 (to Radar): OK, Lagos, what was the last level you gave him?

Radar: FL 50, sir,

Flight615: And did he respond?

Radar: Ah, he responded and he was even a traffic to (Flight 185) when they crossed I called him. I couldn't see him again.

Like the radar controller, nobody has seen ADK 086 and 143 souls it flew ever since. It seems now the energies of government and aviation authorities are focused on averting a recurrence of the Ejirin experience.

In a paper presented November last year to the Vision 2010 sub-committee on aviation, K.K. Sagoe, the nation's head of aviation accident investigation bureau, classified the ADC Flight 086 crash among "accidents caused by contributions from the Air Traffic Control."

Said Sagoe: "Recently, negative contributions by the air traffic controller services are surfacing in the accident scenario in Nigeria. The accident of Boeing 727, registered 5N-BBG near Ejinrin village on 7th of November, 1996, comes to mind. A Boeing 727, (Flight 185) was departing from Lagos to Enugu, while a Boeing 727, that was operated by ADC Airline was about to commence its approach to Lagos on a flight from Port Harcourt. At 16,000 feet above means sea level, both aircraft found themselves on a collision course. The ADC aircraft was equipped with traffic collision avoidance system and hence was alerted to the danger. In an anti-collision avoidance manoeuvre, the aircraft plunged into the waters of the lagoon at a speed in excess of 500 knots. The investigators traced the origin of the accident to the fact that the air traffic controller released Flight 185 to fly under its own navigation far too early before the two aircraft were certain to have been positively and vertically separated."

As a result, aviation authorities have made acquisition of TCAS a priority for all airlines in Nigeria. *Newswatch* learnt from reliable sources that government has already given all airlines in Nigeria up to the year 2003 to equip their aircraft with TCAS. That decision was conveyed to them last December. Although, they initially resisted the idea, thinking that it was government's way of avoiding the repairs and efficiency of traffic equipment, it later agreed to comply with it in the interest of safety.

Said a senior staff of the air worthiness division of FAAN: "The question of installing TCAS is non-negotiable. In fact, government wanted TCAS installed immediately, because of the sad event of Flight 086 but we had to strike a compromise when some airlines demanded for a time frame of five years."

Accordingly, training of pilots and air traffic controllers on operation of TCAS is in the offing. In addition, both aviation authorities and AON have resolved to put pressure on government to provide functional radar coverage to the whole country. AON appears also to have convinced government to train air traffic controllers properly because of apparent difficulties they encounter daily in working with them. Government and AON appear also to have agreed to enforce existing regulations concerning compulsory use of transponders. Transponder is a radio device which transmits its own signal on receiving it. Operators may have agreed that the serviceability of their transponders is suspect. Aviation regulations require that all aircraft must not only be equipped with transponders, they should be switched on before takeoff. Monitoring and enforcing this regulation have been lax in the past. Indications are that aircraft without service-able transponders may not be given clearance to take off in the near future.

Newswatch investigations further show that "human factors" have been blamed for 90 percent of plane crashes in Nigeria. Ac-cording to records by aviation accident investigators, apart from two accidents namely, the Nigeria Airways Boeing 707 crash of December 1994 and the crash of Falcon 20 operated by Aero Contractors in September 1995, all the other accidents could have been avoided if the human element of the operation has been performed accurately.

For instance, the accident of the Gulfstream aircraft that crashed into a telecommunication mast in Jos in June 1996, kill-ing Mohammed Wase, a colonel and military administrator of Kano State, was traced by investigators to human factor. Investi-gations show that "the clearance of the aircraft by the air traffic controller was to a navigational aid that was known to be unser-viceable with radial error of more than 10 degrees."

Similarly, the Fokker F-28 aircraft from Lagos to Enugu which crashed November 1983, three miles to run way, killing 53 per-sons, was caused by human factor. *Newswatch* learnt that the pi-lot of that aircraft may have suffered from "spatial disorientation or dizziness." The pilot, who did not die in the crash, later died in a road accident, when the car he was driving suddenly veered off the road killing him and his children.

While the tragedy of Flight 086 appears to be keeping avi-ation authorities on their toes for more than a year now, avia-tion officials may not have taken visible and adequate steps yet to cater for the well-being and sagging morale of staff charged with the sensitive responsibilities of manning multi-million dollar equipment and guiding hundreds of aircraft a day to safety.

Sagoe identified poor salaries and economic status of air traffic controllers vis-à-vis pilots as one reason for accidents and lack of confidence by air traffic controllers. Said Sagoe: "This lack of confidence of the controllers was clearly evidenced in the ADC accident."

FLYING BLIND IN NIGERIA

Hans Werner, a captain of the Lufthansa Airline, left the Koeln Airport, Bonn, West Germany, for Nigeria on August 2, 1986. The 10-page pre-flight information bulletin he got at the Koeln Airport sufficiently warned him of the situation at the Murtala Muhammed International Airport, Lagos and the Aminu Kano International Airport, Kano.

The bulletin said several navigational, approach and landing aids that would help Werner to pilot his big bird safely in Nigeria were either unserviceable or unavailable. In Kano, the Distant Measuring Equipment, DME, the Non-Directional Beacon, NDB, the Instrument Landing System, ILS and the runway lights, were all said to be unserviceable. Werner was even warned of the possibility of stray animals on the Kano apron. A similar situation is said to exist at the Lagos airport.

What all these meant for Werner was that, he was to rely more on what, in aviation terms, is called Visual Flight Rules, VFR, which means using one's naked eyes for a hi-tech job. An experienced pilot with tens of thousands of flying hours, Werner consoled himself and took off. But the German pilot was to have the fright of his life. As he was embarking on the final descent, just a few minutes before touch down at the Murtala Muhammed International Airport, the lights at the airport went off, Werner found himself screaming, unconsciously. But he recollected himself just in time to get the aircraft up again on what is called a holding pattern, flying around the airport for about seven minutes before power was restored. He was lucky that he had enough fuel.

For many pilots in Nigeria, what happened to Werner is almost a daily experience. So many things are wrong with Nigeria's airports all at the same time. On August 12, Nigeria Airways operated a flight with the Airbus A-310 flown by Captain Philip Machunga and co-pilot Johnson Omodiagbe. It was a frustrating experience for them. "Oh, it's blind flying we are doing here," Machunga said to *Newswatch*'s Anietie Usen, who was flying with official permission in the cockpit. The two young pilots had been calm all the way but they became frustrated at a point when their contact with Kano could not give them the accurate information they needed to land. "Most of the time, we are not friendly with these air traffic controllers. Most of them are not well trained. They keep feeding you with very inaccurate information," Omodiagbe said as he shouted messages across to the air traffic controllers at Kano.

Machunga said the DME, the NDB and most of the other navigational, approach and landing aids are unserviceable. "That gives us extra work and it's risky," the pilot said. Whether in Kano, Lagos, Port Harcourt or any other international airport in Nigeria, the problem of navigational aids is the same.

On land, the situation is equally frustrating. The Kano airport has virtually nothing apart from the immigration and customs checking counters. Communication equipments are dead. There are no conveyor-belts and high loaders to carry loads to and from aircraft. Said Richard Ebodaghe, Nigeria Airways' acting district manager in Kano: "We virtually have to carry loads on our heads here." What is worse, Kano Airport is probably the dirtiest international airport in the world. The airport building constructed in the 1940s is a shadow of its former self. The paint has peeled off the cracking walls. Doors and windows are broken and without locks. The toilets are unkempt. Said Garba Ahmed, Acting Editor of *Triumph,* a Kano-based newspaper: "This so-called international airport in Kano is a disgrace to this country."

Sokoto, Maiduguri, Ilorin and Kaduna airports are tagged international airports because they serve as exit points for pilgrims. They lack navigational and ground facilities just like Kano. Similarly, the N4 million Calabar "international" airport which used to serve as transit station for Nairobi, Yaounde and Brazaille passengers, does not have something as basic as telephone facilities.

In 1985, the N250 million Murtala Muhammed International Airport was voted "the worst in Africa" in a survey conducted by a London-based international magazine, *Hotels and Business Travels.* Also, the International Aviation Transport Association, IATA, said three months ago that security measures in the foremost international airports, Lagos, Kano and Port Harcourt were "very inadequate." That earned Nigeria an instant rebuke by the International Civil Aviation Organization, ICAO, which a year earlier, had described Nigeria's air space as a "red zone."

The annoyance of IATA and ICAO may have stemmed from rampant raids on aircraft at the Lagos tarmac. Ethiopian, Ghanaian and Spanish aircraft as well as a Nigeria Airways' plane and two private aircraft had been raided and robbed by bandits at the airport.

At their inception, most of these airports, especially Lagos and Port Harcourt were in good shape. It did not take long before things started to fall out at the joints. Abubakar Sule Natiti, the air commodore who is in charge of aviation department said that the necessary aviation facilities at the airports were unserviceable because of lack of spare parts, but said that government has approved N3.5 million for the purchase of navigational and landing aids. How soon the aviation aids will be put back in shape remains a matter of conjecture.

DEATH OF THE ICONIC PRINCE

His last days were sad, painful and humiliating. They contrasted rather sharply with his days of pomp, power and pageantry.

For Shehu Musa Yar'Adua, 54, retired major-general and icon of Nigerian political class, his final journey, Monday December 8, 1997, bore a cruel mark of fate. He died uncared for, in a remote prison yard at the guinea-worm infested town of Abakiliki, Ebonyi State.

The news of the death of Nigeria's one time chief of staff (vice president), who was serving a 25-year prison term for alleged complicity in a coup plot, sent shock waves, anger and uncertainty across the political landscape of Nigeria. His death quickly eclipsed the news of the House of Assembly elections in the national media; except on the Nigerian Television Authority, NTA, which did not even mention the calamity, but preferred to announce the death of a mother-in-law of a naval officer.

The outpouring of grief for Yar'Adua was spontaneous and profuse. "When I heard this news I did not believe it. I don't believe that we have missed that young, sound, organized, tactful and good Nigerian. He was a firm believer in democracy, an astute manager of crisis, full of useful thoughts and calculation and always interested in uniting people," Olusola Saraki, a prominent Nigerian politician and a kingpin of the Congress for National Concensus, CNC, said.

Kwairanga Mohammed Joda, millionaire businessman and UNCP governorship aspirant in Adamawa State was close to tears when he spoke with *Newswatch*. "It is such a difficult issue for me to discuss please," he said, his voice shaking. "This is the first national leader to die in this circumstance. "I regret this day," Tanko Yakassai, a famous Kano politician said. Sule Lamido, the former secretary-general of Social Democratic Party, SDP, described Yar-Adua's death as "a great tragedy."

The same feelings were shared in other parts of Nigeria. Lamidi Adedibu, the coordinator of the Democratic Party of Nigeria, DPN, in South-Western Nigeria, said Yar'Adua was "a formidable Nigerian politician who never allowed tribalism to influence his judgment."

Lateef Adegbite, Secretary-General, Nigerian Supreme Council for Islamic Affairs, NSCIA, said Yar'Adua's death was a "great blow and embarrassment to Nigeria and could have been averted."

Many prominent Nigerians in their reactions called for a thorough investigation into the death. "Nobody will believe that government did not have anything to do with his death. It is important that government explains the circumstance of his death" Yomi Ademofun, a presidential aspirant of the National Republican Convention, NRC, in the 1993 elections said.

Onalapo Soleye, former minister of finance spoke in the same vein. "People who were holding him would have to account for his health and death. They must tell us something about him," he said angrily.

Gani Fawehinmi, a leading Nigerian lawyer said: "We want a high powered inquiry to be conducted by the United Nations into the circumstance of Yar'Adua's death."

The first reaction from a non-Nigerian body came from the United States Embassy. In a two-paragraph statement, Wednesday, December 10, the embassy expressed profound sadness at the untimely passing on of Yar'Adua. Describing him as an "exceptional public figure and an outstanding son of Nigeria," the statement called on the Nigerian government to release detainees and political prisoners as promised by the head of state, General SaniAbacha in his November 17 anniversary speech.

Perhaps if immediate action had been taken on the promised freedom, the embarrassment of Yar'Adua's death in prison could have been averted. This is what human rights and opposition groups harped on most of last week. They felt the death of Yar'Adua had proved them right. They seized the opportunity to point accusing fingers at government. Civil Liberties Organization, CLO, in a statement signed by Ayo Obe, its president said "the Nigerian military dictatorship has finally achieved what it set out to do on March 1995, when it arrested Yar'Adua." The CLO demanded to know how many more (Nigerians) held in prisons for political reasons and trumped-up charges must die in chains before the government do the right thing."

The National Democratic Coalition, NADECO, the leading opposition group said they have been loud about human rights abuses by the government with little support from politicians. "Now that Yar'Adua is dead, they will come to their senses because we don't know what government will do with other detainees, many of whom we know are sick and deserve urgent medical attention," Abraham Adesanya, veteran lawyer and acting leader of NADECO said.

UbaSanni, coordinator of Campaign for Democracy CD, in northern Nigeria told *Newswatch* that he had recently formed a Free Musa Yar'Adua Committee and that he was horrified by the news of his death. "The people of the North can never forgive this administration for allowing Yar'Adua to die in such a degrading way," Sanni said.

Ever so often, the public surprises the establishment by a great display of public grief. This was the case in Katsina, the home town of the late politician, when his body arrived for burial Tuesday morning. The tragedy had been announced since 5am during prayers in all mosques in the city. When the body touched down in an Air-force plane at 9.45am, it was difficult to suppress tears and public outrage. Many cried openly like babies and the large crowd that lined the street chanted *Allah Sai Sharia,* meaning God will judge.

At the Katsina Stadium where more than 20,000 people came to pay their last respect to their own prince, the mood was at once that of repressed anger and frustration. The late general's younger brother Umar, often broke down. He and Yussuf, another brother, recited the Koran and cursed loudly in Hausa. "He who kills with sword will himself be killed by the same sword when the time comes," Yusuf cried apparently quoting the Koran.

Binta, the widow, was in Kaduna, 300 kilometres away, when she heard the news apparently on Radio Kaduna which received a faxed release by the Katsina Emirate Council around 7 o'clock that morning. She phoned to request that the remains should not be buried until she arrived. The ceremony was consequently delayed. On arrival, she looked at once inside the Muslim traditional coffin, *Makara,* and began to weep uncontrollably. The crowd wept with her.

Wrapped in white linen, Yar'Adua was buried at 1.30pm at the Dalmarina cemetery, amidst wailings of people who insisted he was framed up with charges of coup plot which led to his death.

"Let everybody know today in the presence of Nigerian leaders here present that we don't believe that Yar'Adua committed the offence for which he has paid for with his life" an aggrieved man in the crowd shouted to the hearing of some key Nigerian leaders who descended on the serene northern city on hearing the sad news. As tension mounted, Suleiman Chamah, a colonel and military governor of Katsina State, who had rushed back from Abuja, appealed to the people of the State to remain calm.

Given the short notice of the burial, the caliber of dignitaries present was impressive. It was a gathering of who's who in Nigeria. Ibrahim Coomassie, police inspector general; Tukur Mani, permanent secretary, Federal Ministry of commerce both from Katsina, Mohammed KabirUsman, Emir of Katsina, Mohammadu Bashir, Emir of Daura; Babagana Kingibe, former Minister of Internal Affairs and running mate of MKO Abiola, Kola Abiola, son of MKO Abiola, the detained politician; Atiku Abubakar, presidential aspirant of SDP in the 1993 elections, Adamu Ciroma as well as a host of former ministers and governors. As at press time, top political leaders from all parts of the country, were still trooping to Yar'Adua's family home to condole with the widow, and the 76-year old mother of the former Nigerian leader. But there was no formal federal government presence at the funeral. The government never issued a formal statement on the death either.

A different kind of crowd headed for Abakiliki, the dusty, ancient town where Yar'Adua died. Prominent in this crowd were reporters who needed to piece together the last days of the Katsina prince. To call Abakiliki a town is charitable. The main road has just been graded. Almost everything including the white fence of the government house is brownish with dust. Most of the houses are built with mud. Named the capital of the newly created Ebonyi State a little over a year ago, Abakiliki made international news in 1995 when FIFA cited outbreak of guinea worm and cholera as part of the reasons it refused Nigeria permission to host the under-20 World cup competition.

Last week, Abakiliki was making a different kind of news. Men and women and even school children clustered around the street to talk in whispers about Yar'Adua. The rusty prison where Yar'Adua spent his last agonizing days stood some 300 meters away from the Government House. It stinks. It overflows with inmates and septic waste. It was built several decades ago for 70 inmates. But last week, when Yar'Adua died, there were more than 150 prisoners, more than double its colonial capacity. The toilet and bathrooms are unsightly. Passerbys hold their noses tight when they come near the prison. Waste water from the prison toilets and bathrooms flows onto the main road. Portable water is in short supply, in spite of a borehole dug recently. Electricity is luxury, and very often out of the question. Here was the last abode of Nigeria's former No. 2 citizen.

He had a bare corridor-size room to himself. But often the heat kept him on the veranda, his chin cupped in his palms. "He was always smoking," one prison official told *Newswatch.* In conversation with warders and other inmates, "he often expressed sadness that he was framed up but thankful to God for sparing his life," another prison staff said.

Bouts of depression were said to be his constant partner. "Sometimes he would just sit alone for endless hours staring into a blank space without a word," the prison official said. *Newswatch* learnt that his health started deteriorating drastically when he was transferred from Enugu prisons to Abakaliki. Prison officials finally raised alarm late last month on his health. Investigations in Abakaliki, Enugu and Abuja show that it wasn't until Monday night December 8, when Yar'Adua collapsed that serious effort was made to take him to the hospital. He arrived the University of Nigeria Teaching Hospital, UNTH, a dead man, according to hospital sources. "He was brought in here dead," a doctor who said Yar'Adua had earlier in the year been treated for high blood pressure told *Newswatch* at UNTH. UNTH is 150 kilometres from Abakaliki.

For angry Nigerians who were demanding to know what or who killed Yar'Adua, the two suspects have names that begin with letters ABA. The first suspect could well be Abakaliki and the second suspect is Abacha. For five weeks according to *Newswatch* investigations, messages consistently poured into the presidency in Abuja, asking for approval to transfer Yar'Adua to a hospital for proper diagnosis of his ailment. He was said to be complaining of weakness and difficulty in breathing among other things.

Newswatch sources in Abuja said the first few letters on the matter were received by Kingibe, who was still the minister of internal affairs. Kingibe took the letters personally to the presidency. He was said to have met with cold shoulders of Abacha everytime he got there. On one occasion, *Newswatch* heard Kingibe was pointedly instructed by Abacha to "stick to other pressing matters." Kingibe was obviously concerned because of his relationship with Yar'Adua, considered as his political mentor. The presidency, according to *Newswatch* sources, saw nothing critical in Yar'Adua's case to warrant Kingibe's special attention.

However, the matter reached a critical point in the first week of December when dispatches from Abakaliki were said to have been coming on a daily basis. That was when approval was given for his hospitalization!

Abacha was again informed shortly before midnight Monday, December 8 that Yar'Adua was critically ill. A few hours later he was confirmed dead. Aso Rock immediately got in touch with the Katsina emirate council of which Yar'Adua was a member. He was *Tafidan Katsina*. The council broke the news to the late general's family.

Government released the corpse to the emirate council and provided a plane to fly it to Katsina. After that, security in Abuja and most parts of the north was put on red alert to forestall any breakdown of law and order. Government ordered the police, the state security service, SSS, and the directorate of military intelligence, DMI, to recall all staff on leave for essential duties until further notice.

In Abuja, there was an increase in surveillance by plainclothes security men. Some of them drove in taxis and commercial buses, monitoring the trend of discussion on Yar'Adua. Junior and middle level workers at government offices were seen discussing in hushed tones.

At the top, discomfort and dismay was palpable. This was more so because government was said to have recently initiated discussions with Yar'Adua and other political prisoners through the National Reconciliation Committee, NARECOM, headed by Alex Akinyele.

In one of the meetings with Yar'Adua several weeks ago, government officials, according to our sources, discussed with him the possibility of a conditional release. But Yar'Adua, *Newswatch* was told, argued for an unconditional freedom, insisting that he was not guilty of the offence for which he was jailed. He was said to be in high spirits after the meeting, just before the bout of sickness that gave him the final knock-out.

What killed him? There is no official confirmation but speculations are rife. Some reports have attributed his death variously to cardiac arrest, lung cancer, inflamed liver as well as constant stooling and vomiting. Offiong Bassey, Chief cardiovascular technologist at the Lagos University Teaching Hospital, LUTH, tried to establish a link between the three ailments. He said cardiac arrest is "the sudden stopping of the functioning of the heart, when a person is being confronted with bad news, a frightening situation or severe stress." According to him cardiac malfunction could arise from disease of the heart and it could also be a result of untreated hypertension. Some of the symptoms of cardiac arrest, he said, include frequent stooling. "As someone becomes stressful, he has a general bad feeling, notices an increase in heartbeat and visits the toilet regularly. He could even be tempted to think that he has diaorrhea," Bassey said.

Depression, says psychologists, can also spell fatality. For men who have lived the better part of their lives in comfort, finding themselves alone in the squalid confines of a prison could make the difference between life and death. Derin Olorunshoba, psychologist and lecturer at LUTH told *Newswatch*: "It can be very traumatic and even fatal for a person who had enjoyed freedom and comfort at the highest possible level to be incarcerated. He could say "No this can't be me. They will come and remove me." But when the expectation is cut off, he would become unnecessarily tense, go to toilet more frequently than normal, lose his appetite, develop sleeplessness and other sickness you cannot really place your finger on and before you know it, his life is in danger zone."

Concern was widespread last week on the fate of other political prisoners and the implication of Yar'Adua's death for the already battered image of Nigeria abroad. "Whose turn next"? was the big question NADECO asked last week. Said Mike Ozekhome, a constitutional lawyer: "This is an eye opener. Government should immediately release Abiola, Olusegun Obasanjo, former Nigerian Head of State, imprisoned along with Yar'Adua, and all other political prisoners before it is too late."

Sunday Ovba, a former SDP stalwart and associate of Yar'Adua said when Nigerians talk about Nelson Mandela's 27 years in prison, they don't really have an idea of the prison conditions in Nigeria. "Our prisons are actually next door to hell. It is intolerable. There is no Mandela that can survive in Nigerian prisons," Ovba said.

Whatever were his failures, Yar'Adua's courageous contributions to democracy in and out of uniform, put him in a class of his own. In his press conference, February 17, 1995, barely 24 hours after his release from a five-day detention, he equated his experience in detention to "bearing the cross of democracy in Nigeria." He had emerged as a visible and vocal critic of the Abacha administration, constantly demanding an exit date and brief tenure for the administration. He sued government after his release. Although he later withdrew the suit at the intervention of peace-makers, the battle line had been drawn. He was perceived by government and political observers as the unseen hand behind the constitutional conference vote in December 1994, which set January 1996 as the terminal date for Abacha. At a press conference in Lagos, he said pointedly that Nigerians had lost faith in the military. As he put it: "It is indeed regrettable that the military annulled the June 12 election. Annulled with that election is the confidence of Nigerians in the military and the military organized form of democracy." (He was arrested again on March 8. Most people concluded he was picked up again, for his insistence that the Abacha government was an extension of the Babangida administration, which annulled the June 12 election. Nobody thought Yar'Adua and Olusegun Obasanjo former head of state could wind up in a tribunal for trying coup plotters.

Even military authorities said that their arrest had nothing to do with the coup plot, because they were arrested by the police and not the army. Fred Chijuka, Brigadier General and Army Spokesman at the time, said on several occasions that the army had nothing to do with the arrest of Yar'Adua.

At the time of Yar'Adua's arrest, Obasanjo was in Copenhagen, Denmark, attending a United Nations conference on the elimination of poverty. Although Walter Carrington, then the United States ambassador to Nigeria, warned him not to return to the country on the strength of security information at his disposal, Obasanjo returned, saying he had nothing to fear.

A day later, he was arrested. Six weeks later, the two men among others appeared before a military tribunal trying coup plotters. It was a drama that shocked the nation and the international community.

Many thought both men were persecuted for their political beliefs. There had been bad blood between Abacha and the two men since November 1993, when Abacha came to power. Yar'Adua and Obasanjo, *Newswatch* learnt, told Abacha at separate meetings that their support for the government would depend on his announcement of a transition programme, which should also state his hand-over date.

The charge of coup plot against them became quite a curious coincidence which eventually discredited the guilty verdict on the two former Nigerian leaders. Aware that Nigerians received the guilty verdict with a pinch of salt, government decided to televise video clips of proceedings at the tribunal. Screened by NTA on a Sunday evening, October 1995, and watched by millions of Nigerians in stone silence, the entire nation was shown a frightened Yar'Adua being implicated by R.S Bello Fadile, a colonel who allegedly spearheaded the plot.

An anonymous narrator said Yar'Adua's involvement in the coup plot started, when Sambo Dasuki, a lieutenant colonel, and former aide-de-camp to former President Ibrahim Babangida, and son of the dethroned Sultan of Sokoto, Ibrahim Dasuki, was prematurely retired from the army. Yar'Adua was said to have used the retirement to instigate Dasuki to join efforts to change the government.

In his own confession, Bello-Fadile claimed he met Yar'Adua twice and introduced himself as coming from Dasuki. He alleged that Yar'Adua promised to support the coup fully. Yar'Adua was enraged and almost jumped out of his seat in reaction. But even in his angry response, what he said either in confession or in defence was not audible to viewers. The only phrase that was audible was when he spoke about the retirement of Dasuki. Even then viewers could not hear the beginning of the sentence. Nor could anyone say when the sentence ended.

A weaker link in the televised tribunal proceedings was that there was no evidence of any cross-examination of Bello-Fadile by either Yar'Adua or Obasanjo. Lawyers who reacted to the confession said such cross examination would have shown the date of the alleged meeting, how the meeting was secured and who was instrumental or participating. "We take note of the absurdity of Bello-Fadile's confession. By the statement of government, Colonel Bello-Fadile (had) pleaded not guilty of coup plotting," Lateef Kareem, a lawyer had said in a press release.

Other critics of the video confession said the suspects may have made their confessions, under duress. They cited the case of Akinloye Akinyemi, a former army major who said the agony he went through before implicating M. A. Ajayi, a retired lieutenant colonel, was unbearable. Said Akinyemi, while apologizing to Ajayi, in the video clip: "Sir I am sorry. I struggled but I went through a lot of pain and it reached a point where no one could believe my story and I tell them. I am sorry I betrayed you. The pain was so much."

In the process, the televised confession wound up with more questions than answers. One of such questions followed the retired general even last week to eternity: did he actually participate in the coup as Bello-Fadile said, even in the face of his avowed campaign for a return to democracy?

It is impossible to say how the Yar'Adua saga would have ended if he did not die in prison., Whether he would have emerged a hero or a villain. But on Tuesday morning last week when Nigerians awoke to the devastating news of his death, there was little doubt that whatever were his iniquities in the past, he would be remembered with sympathy, as the first Nigerian leader who died in prison.

ABACHA'S LAST HOURS

Sani Abacha, Nigeria's ruthless military ruler, betrayed no sign of illness at his last public appearance, just hours before he died. Swaggering alongside the departing Palestinian leader Yasser Arafat at the Nnamdi Azikiwe International Airport in Abuja and dressed in a trendy purple caftan, he was strikingly ebullient and confident in his gait.

A few hours later, he was back at the airport, this time a dead man, wrapped in a white bed sheet, inside an open traditional casket. Shocked relations and State House officials who carried his body to the airport hurriedly thrust the corpse into the luggage compartment of the aircraft. Then, on second thoughts, they brought it out into the main cabin, with the body rolling uncontrollably in the open casket and almost falling off the gangway.

There were no formalities, no ceremonies, no red carpet, no salutes. Even the traditional 21-gun salute and military parade that are part of the funeral rites of a national leader were absent, as the presidential jet shot into the gloomy evening skies, bound for his home town of Kano. It was the same aircraft on which

Abacha was supposed to fly the next day to Burkina Faso, for the Organisation of Africa Unity (OAU) heads of state summit, where he would have received pats on the back for doing a great job of restoring peace and democracy to Liberia and Sierra Leone. Now he was heading in an unwanted direction: to the grave.

His sudden death was attributed to cardiac arrest, more commonly known as heart attack. He was known to have suffered from cirrhosis of the liver for at least 11 years. This was further complicated by kidney impairments. But he was receiving good medical attention from some of the best doctors in the world, who flew into Nigeria from Israel or Saudi Arabia. His doctors were said to have agreed at one stage that he needed to spend at least a month in a specialist hospital overseas but he rejected the idea, fearing that subordinates would exploit his absence to push him out of power.

Journalists who broke the news of his declining health were arrested and detained. He later admitted publicly that he was recovering from sickness. In the past six months he seemed to be enjoying good health, even putting on some weight in the process. But the extra weight, *AfricaToday* learnt after his death, was actually caused by steroids in the medication given him.

Even though his poor health was public knowledge, Nigerians are still not sure whether their ruthless strongman died a natural death. Some newspapers even reported he was poisoned, while other media outlets indicated the dreaded general was in the amorous company of a beautiful foreigner. *AfricaToday* could not confirm that but investigations by *AfricaToday* reveal that the general suffered a heart attack in one of his guest houses in Aso Rock, Abuja, where he had gone to perhaps, "to relax a bit." He was said to have gone to the guest house unaccompanied by tight security after he returned from bidding Arafat farewell. General Jeremiah Useni, the minister for the Federal Capital Territory and his close friend, was said to be with him at the guest house that night and would have been one of the last to see him alive. One of those present noticed the big man suddenly gasping for breath and foaming in his mouth. The guest raised the alarm and contacted senior security aides at Aso Rock. Doctors summoned to revive the reclusive ruler, who ruled Nigeria with iron fist, battled for more than two hours before they gave up hope. At least two people, including the "guest", were helping security personnel, as *AfricaToday* went to press, to put together a clearer picture of the last few minutes of Abacha›s life.

The news of Abacha's death shocked the world and evoked sympathy from many African leaders, who had known and respected him for his fierce Pan-African policies. In Nigeria, however, the death of their strongman sent millions of people into wild jubilation. His five-year reign was considered too cruel and repressive and his quest to transform himself into a civilian president had brought the country to the nadir of war. Said a radio talk show host on the air: "This man took over power in crisis, ruled in crisis and died in crisis. What an era."

In most parts of the oil-rich but poverty-ridden country, the celebration took the form of a carnival staged before television cameras and reminiscent of post-coup jubilation in Africa during the 70s and 80s. In Kwara state, in The North, students and taxi drivers defied heavy downpour and took to the streets with a mock coffin, singing anti-Abacha songs. They seized the condolence registers opened by the government and tore them into pieces. In Katsina, home town of Shehu Yar'Adua, the former deputy head of state who died in prison six months ago, the sentiments were similar. Groups of youths gathered at Yar'Adua's residence to pray and celebrate.

Abacha's death "is a blessing. It is God's answer to the national prayer for peace and stability recently organised by the federal government. It is the divine way by which the Almighty wants to intervene in the ongoing political crisis... to avert bloodshed, anarchy and the possible break-up of the country," Alhaji Yagub Isha Bataganawa said.

The Guardian, a liberal Nigerian newspaper reported that many residents of Uyo, Akwa Ibom state, and Oweri, Imo state, trooped to the beer parlours to make merry on hearing Abacha's death confirmed. Students destroyed billboards and posters displayed by groups that supported Abacha's presidential bid. Said a former governor of Anambra state, Dr Chukwuemeka Ezeife: "Abacha's legacy is a bumper harvest of lessons for all of us that are alive. He performed his demolition job with ruthless efficiency. Today we stand at the brink of disaster. But dry bones shall rise again."

The jubilation became so embarrassing that former head of state General Yakubu Gowon and religious leaders were forced to publicly condemn and discourage it. Said the usually outspoken Anglican Bishop of Akure, Reverend Emmanuel Bolanle Gbonigi: "This sense of jubilation at someone's death is sad. It should not be so." But one member of his church countered by saying "when God drowned Pharaoh in the Red Sea, Moses and the children of Israel rejoiced with songs."

Some of those who knew Abacha defended his record, despite the imprisonment and killings of opposition leaders and activists that took place during his five years in office. "I do not think many people understood him well. You needed to get closer to him. He loved this country and the entirety of its people. He was a good man," Abacha's special adviser Wada Nas told the BBC. A senior military officer who spoke to *AfricaToday* said "though Abacha's style and approach to governance gave soldiers and the military a bad name, he exhibited great courage and admirable firmness that endeared him to some of us. Except for his vulnerability to psychophants who eventually destroyed him and dragged him into this unfortunate issue of self-succession, he was an authentic Nigerian hero."

Abdulsalam Abubakar, a general and now the new head of state, together with the other Provisional a Ruling Council, PRC, members woke on June 8, to discover that their good friend and tough boss had died suddenly, without naming a successor. His number two man, General Oladipo Diya, is on death row, accused by Abacha and summarily convicted of plotting to overthrow Abacha.

When the PRC met that afternoon, members pretended to be more concerned with grief and the burial than who takes over from the late head of state. Africa Today's sources say it was the Inspector General of Police, Ibrahim Coomasie, who introduced the question of appointing a new head of state to fill the vacuum Abacha had left. "He was better placed to introduce the subject others were skating because he is the law and order man and he was not in contention for the post," says our source.

Once the issue was tabled, tension quickly replaced grief. Below Abacha were three lieutenant-generals: Useni, the convicted Diya and Mohammed Haladu, the former industry minister. Diya was clearly out of the picture and Haladu had been hospitalized abroad for some months. This left the PRC with Useni, the most senior general on the PRC. He was a classmate of Abacha in the command and staff college and had remained a close friend till the last moments. Naturally some eyes turned to him.

At that point the PRC adjourned for the burial. When it reconvened at 11 o'clock that night. Rear Admiral Mike Akhigbe, chief of naval staff, braved the odds and nominated Abubakar, the chief of defence staff, instead. Akhigbe was quickly supported by Air Vice Marshall Nsikak Eduok, the chief of air staff. Our source said only one officer mildly disagreed with Abubakar's nomination. The consensus was that Abubakar was No.3 in the military hierarchy, while Useni was performing a purely administrative responsibility as a minister in the government. Useni was later given the chance to speak and the PRC agreed that Abubakar be promoted instantly to the rank of a full general. "Politically, Abubakar was the number three man behind Diya. Useni is a minister and politically comes far behind the service chiefs, although a lieutenant-general. Apartfrom that, Abubakar inspires confidence because he is strictly a professional soldier with no known links to politicians," says our source.

Abubakar does not come across as a power-hungry man. He is known to be a credible and resolute officer who takes genuine interest in the integrity of the military as well as broader issues like stability, justice and fair play, which have eluded Nigeria for years. But does the Nigerian military have the conscience and the will to move the country forward after 30 difficult years in power? The next few months will tell. As Abacha himself said in an address to media executives in 1994: "The past becomes an albatross only if we fail to learn from it and heed its lessons. It is now time to seek a sober understanding of what went wrong."

EYES ON THE ROCK

A green Lexus car pulls out of the Murtala Muhammed International Airport, north-west of Lagos. The car turns left and edges towards the main road, chased frantically by a convoy of more than 50 cars. The striking Lexus is suddenly swamped at a T-junction that empties commuters into the rest of Lagos. Dozens of anxious heads squeeze out of the windows. Screams of "Ekwueme, Ekwueme, Ekwueme" fill the warm night air.

Alex Ekwueme, the silver-haired architect, Nigeria's vice-president from 1979-83, who is widely respected and regarded as a strong contender for the presidency, waves from the back seat, his wife, Beatrice, by his side, a permanent smile on his lips, clearly overwhelmed by the sheer outpouring of enthusiasm for his candidature in the February 1999 elections.

Ekwueme, 66, one of the founders of People's Democratic Party (PDP) arrived on a British Airways flight at 6.30pm from a two-week overseas trip, to receive a tumultuous reception from thousands of drumming and dancing supporters. It took another three hours to squeeze him out of the airport. "I had never seen a thing like that. I was just wondering what I had done to deserve such a show of love," the multi-millionaire politician told *Africa-Today*.

Enugu, Ekwueme's home-base in South-East Nigeria may be a long way from Lagos, but Ekwueme is pulling quite a crowd here these days. In Kano, up north, the next day, and in Zaria and Abuja the following day; and then in Benin and Enugu that weekend, the story was the same. And for good reason. The unpretentious Nigerian politician, who has spent the past five years stone-walling the despotism of General Sani Abacha, is counted among the few politicians in the country still left with some of the credibility and integrity needed to salvage Nigeria. Not only that, it is the first time since the end of the Nigerian civil war 28 years ago, that a politician from what was Biafra has seemed to attract trans-ethnic support for the top job.

Just a few days before Ekwueme declared his presidential ambitions, Chief Emeka Odumegwu Ojukwu, the former Biafran head of state, had told *AfricaToday*, in his Independence Layout residence in Enugu, that "there is a grand design to keep Igbos out of power and make them perpetual "hewers of wood and drawers of water." This, he claimed, is why his party was not registered. This has combined with routine factors of Nigerian politics, to bring into sharp focus the place of the Igbo people in Nigeria. Are the Igbos, the cream of whose leadership largely lubricated the Abacha self-succession machine, well-placed to take over the leadership of Nigeria? Or have the Igbos, who waged a three-year war of secession, been fully reconciled and reintegrated into Nigeria?

Coincidentally, just hours before Ekwueme touched down at Lagos from his American and European tour, General Olusegun

Obasanjo, former Nigerian head of state, who as brigadier and commander of the Third Marine Commando brought the civil war to an end in 1970, also declared his intention to contest the presidency on the same PDP platform. Though Obasanjo's candidacy is receiving a widespread thumbs-down, especially in his home base in the south-west, the respect and support he enjoys elsewhere, especially outside Nigeria, has singled him out as possibly the only man who can thwart the ambitions of Ekwueme and Igbos to confirm their Nigerian-ness.

That is not to play down the presidential bid by another Igbo man, Emmanuel Inwuanyanwu, the multi-millionaire publisher, who like the late M.K.0 Abiola also owns an airline and a football club. Inwuanyanwu was a close friend of General Abacha until the last days of the dictator and was often regarded as the ordained vice-president in Abacha's ill-fated civilian incarnation. Now, he is a leading figure in the All Peoples' Party (APP), which Nigerians have sarcastically christened "Abacha's Peoples' Party." That is quite a cross to carry. Though Nigerians are a forgiving lot, they don't seem to be in a hurry to forget the Abacha era- the darkest part of their chequered history. And that makes Inwuanyanwu's chances pretty slim.

Inwuanyawu told *AfricaToday* in his luxurious residence in Victoria Island, Lagos, that General Abacha was a good man who was spoiled by his advisers. "He is a good example of what bad advisers can do to a leader," he said. But that flies in the face of the confessions by many Abacha aides that they were simply executing the orders and wishes of their master. And in a week the Nigerian government announced it had already recovered N65 billion (about $753 million) from Abacha's wife and children, the APP, analysts say, must gear up for a rugged road to power.

Strikingly, the presidential race remains an all-southerners affair, an indication that Nigerians may have settled for Section 299 of the draft constitution, which recommends a rotational presidency, even as government curiously pushed out the draft for a further six-week public debate. Accordingly, those eyeing the seat of power — known as Aso Rock — include southerners such as Don Etiebet, former petroleum minister (PDP); Philip Asiodu, another former petroleum minister (PDP); Samuel Ogbemudia, former labour minister and governor of Bendel State (PDP); Anthony Ani, former finance minister (APP); Gamaliel Onosode, renowned technocrat (APP); Bola Ige, former governor of Oyo state and a leader of Alliance for Democracy (AD); Olu Falae, former finance minister (AD); Richard Akinjide, former justice minister (PDP), and Tunji Braithwaite, leader of the Democratic Advance Movement (DAM)

While south-westerners insist on taking the shot because they were recently deprived of the job after their son Chief Abiola won the election, south-southerners maintain that they are the producers of Nigeria's oil wealth yet have nothing to show for it. But the complaint of marginalisation in the affairs of the country seems to be loudest of late in Nigeria's south-east.

Says Stanley Macebuh, a leading Nigerian journalist: "The Igbos are marginalised to the extent that their access to the decision-making process in this country is very, very limited. It has its practical effects when you are making decisions about what roads to construct or repair or what road not to bother with. Quite often, if you look at the people sitting there to make decisions, you'll probably find that there is no Igbo man there. The decision-making process is [therefore] so warped and so much against the interest of the Igbos."

It is a line of thought most Igbos subscribe to. Says Ojukwu: "We are marginalised in every way. Is it only now that we realise that we are the biggest minority tribe in Nigeria? Look at our roads, you will see clearly the evidence of marginalisation. I find marginalisation in education and in political appointments. You see certain departments of government people from the east are never allowed to have access to. Ojukwu has now joined the APP.

But this feeling cuts across party lines. Ifeanyi Nwosu, former general manager of SCOA and a PDP member, says it is difficult to point to any federal presence by way of industries 'and infrastructure. "Just think about it. Can you point to any important project or industry sited by the federal government in the southeast? In Owerri, we had to levy ourselves and raise money to build an airport. Have you seen such a self-help project elsewhere in Nigeria?" he said in an interview with *AfricaToday*.

Last August, a group of Igbo people known as Movement for the Survival of Igbo Race (MOSIR), took a full page advertisement in a Sunday newspaper to state their case for the attention of the new Nigerian government. "When thinking of government presence in Igboland, the establishment that comes readily to mind include the National Museum of Colonial History, Aba, and the National War Museum, Umuahia, two relics of a past marked by the spoliation of Igbo wealth and ruthless wastage of blood of Igbo youths." Some other Igbos have pointed to a situation where, of 25 top government departments and corporations, ranging from oil, communications and banking to the military and para-military establishments, none is headed by an Igbo man. On top of that, others have drawn attention to the fact that "inconsequential portfolios are often assigned to ministers of Igbo origin." Accusing fingers go in more than one direction. "For the past 38 years, Nigeria is governed by the north for the appeasement of the west and total neglect of the east. The Igbo is not in the sharing equation," Arthur Nzeribe, APP member and maverick politician, who connived with the military to scuttle the victory of Chief Abiola in the 1993 presidential elections, said in an article published in a pro-Igbo magazine.

Macebuh sees the problem from another perspective: the military. "Logically, you cannot talk about the neglect or marginalisation of one of the three major groups in the country but in practical terms. It is the case and the reason is that we have had for too long a central government run by the military: the military that is top heavy with northern echelons and personnel." Macebuh continues: "During Shagari's tenure, and I believe in any civilian set-up, things would be fairer because a political party needs support from every part of the country and if you have to have that support, you must pay attention to everybody. So it is the military marginalisation, rather than marginalisation per se."

Ekwueme tried to explain this at the fifth annual conference of the World Igbo Congress held in London last October: "As a result of the civil war, the Nigerian armed forces became denuded of Igbo officers and men. The Igbos were not available for recruitment into the Nigerian Defence Academy (NDA) during the traumatic years of 1967-70. The consequence of this has been weighty. Given the total military dominance of Nigeria's politics it is easy to appreciate the full extent to which Igbo absence in the higher echelons of the Nigerian armed forces during the period has contributed to Igbo emasculation." According to Ekwueme, "it is important for the Igbos to know where the rain started to beat them because our elders say that he who does not know where the rain started to beat him would not recognise where and when it stopped."

Perhaps the rain will stop when Ekwueme becomes president. But he does not see himself or his mission in terms of Igbo nationalism. "In fact, all Nigerians are marginalised. It depends on what aspect of our existence you are talking about. There are Nigerians who are marginalised politically. They are kept out of the position of authority in government. There are Nigerians who are marginalised economically. They are kept out of the commanding heights of the economy by those who control it. There are Nigerians who are kept at the margin of the bureaucracy. There are those who feel that they are left out of the armed forces... So every Nigerian suffers from one form of marginalisation or the other. My mission as president, if I become one, is to ensure that all these areas are properly addressed [because] everybody in this country is marginalised," Ekwueme told *AfricaToday*.

For the Igbo, the question of citizenship is as important. Because of their passion for trade and commerce, there is virtually no community in Nigeria where Igbos are not found trading, settling and erecting business empires. Perhaps they own more houses outside their states than any other set of people in Nigeria. This, coupled with their civil war experience, often makes them very reluctant to breach the peace. Yet, they often find that when the chips are down, as it is wont to be in Nigeria, they are not considered as part of the community where they live and their investments are the first at risk. Says Macebuh: "One of the basic grievances when Igbos talk about marginalisation is actually the fact that an Igbo man who has lived in Kano all his life (was born there and today is probably 45) still cannot claim Kano as his home. That is a very serious constraint."

These are some of the issues that would naturally be expected to take the front burner in the coming elections. But it is not likely that they will. In Igbo land as in other parts of Nigeria, the December 5 council elections —the first since Abacha died and the first in a series of elections that will culminate in a civilian government on May 29, 1999 —will revolve around attachment to individuals, including, of course, Abacha. In a way, the coming elections could as well turn out to be a battle between pro-Abacha or anti-Abacha Nigerians, and nowhere else will that battle be fiercer than in the six Igbo states.

Though the PDP is rated ahead of the other eight political parties, the APP with its enormous financial muscle remains a real threat. It is most likely that the Abacha factor would later determine the shape of alignment of the smaller parties. And what shape Nigeria takes thereafter and indeed in the approaching century will be easy to discern after the referendum.

That indeed is a big enough issue, even in Igbo land.

THE PRISON IN HELL

The man died just before lunch. A plate of beans pottage kept at the foot of his hospital bed was covered with flies. His sore mouth and sunken eyes were barely closed. The rusty leg-iron that fettered him to the bed had left his right ankle badly bruised and swollen. From a distance, one could count the number of his ribs. His collar-bones stuck out, giving him the ugly look of a drought victim. The doctor's report simply said Muazu Mohammed, Prisoner No. 1519/86 of Kano Central Prison, died of "acute malnutrition." Life in a Nigerian prison is hard, inhuman and cruel.

Mohammed was not sentenced to death. He was just one of the 46 prison inmates in Kano State who died last year as a result of the horrifying condition of prisoners in the State. Rabiu Bello, Mohammed's prison mate, died of pneumonia. Abdullahi Dahiru, also of Kano Central Prison, died of sclerosis of the liver; Sumaila Bala, a detainee in the same prison, was killed by tuberculosis. Haruna Juli, of Gumel prison, lost his life to gastroenteritis; Mesa Tsoho died of meningitis; Abdulmumuni Salisu, of Goro Dutse prison, died of dehydration; while Audu Abubakar of Birnin Kudu prison and Umaru Ali of Kazaure prison died of heart failure and what doctors called "hypodermic shock" respectively.

Karimu Lawal, a 32-years-old detainee in Ilorin, Kwara State had thought he could survive the brutal and horrible conditions of the prison. He did not. Four hours before his death, a judge on tour of the prison had taken pity on the sorry state of his health and ordered that his case be taken to court the next day. But Lawal, who had survived three years in detention without trial, could not survive another day to prove his innocence. When an Ilorin magistrate court called his case the next morning, Jimoh Ishola, a warder, stood up instead. "My Lord," he said, "Lawal died last night and his body has been taken to the mortuary."

Paul Ogba, 30, died on his way home, a few hours after his release from Umuahia prison. He was one of those "lucky prisoners" released on amnesty by the Imo State government to mark a recent independence anniversary. Before the good news came, Ogba had been receiving treatment for "severe malnutrition" at the Queen Elizabeth Specialist Hospital, Umuahia. Then a warder came to the hospital and said, according to hospital's records, that Ogba had been given amnesty and "should be allowed to go immediately," despite the condition of his health. Dizzy and tottering on his steps, the home-bound ex-detainee took a taxi heading for his village. One hour later, he arrived home, a corpse.

From Aba to Zaria and from Shagamu to Sokoto, *Newswatch* investigations show that Nigerian prisons have become a national disgrace, something akin to a hell hole. Like the Hobbesian State, life there is brutish, nasty and short. Convicts who survive the ordeal of the prison come out usually worse, mentally and physically wrecked. The death toll is heavy. In the first three months of this year, 42 inmates died in Ikoyi prison, Lagos. The same prison recorded more than 300 deaths between January and November 1988. Worse affected were those awaiting trial. They made up more than 200 of the dead, while regular prisoners accounted for 97 deaths. At the Kirikiri Maximum Security Prison in Lagos, the number of dead prisoners for this year could not be ascertained. But *Newswatch* found that in June and July 1988, some 37 detainees awaiting trial died; none of them had been charged to court.

The federal prison at Ilesa, Oyo State, probably has one of the worst records of deaths in Nigeria. In April alone, five prisoners died there following an outbreak of yellow fever. In just three months (June, July and August) last year, 67 died, 37 of them in two weeks. In September, October and November, another 70 died. Sources at the Wesley Guild Hospital, Ilesa, where most the prisoners died, told *Newswatch* that the chief killers of the prisoners in Ilesa were none other than kwashiorkor, tuberculosis and scabies. According to officials of the Ilesa local government council, who allocated land for the burial of the prisoners, 15 of those who died from kwashiorkor last year were "given mass burial in a shallow grave, most of them naked." Sad. Heartbreaking.

Embarrassed by the constant outbreak of diseases in the prison, prominent indigenes of the area have protested to the federal government to quickly remove the "death chamber" from their town. Oluwadamilare Awe, chairman of the LGA, making a strong case for the relocation of the prison, told Adedeji Oresanya, a colonel and governor of the State, that the multi-purpose maximum prison had "become a graveyard for inmates." Adekunle Aromolaran, author and Oba of Ilesa, added a weighty voice to Awe's protest. As the only federal institution in the area, Aromolaran said the prison "has not served any useful purpose." He, therefore, suggested that the "graveyard" should be done away with so that the community could use the land occupied by the prison "for farming and other beneficial projects" relevant to the economic survival of the town.

The Auchi prison in Bendel State has a similar tale of woe. In the first three months of this year, 22 prisoners were killed by scabies and other infectious diseases. The figure portends an ill omen for the small prison which recorded a total of "only 30 deaths" throughout last year. In Benin City, an up-to-date figure obtained by *Newswatch* shows that 15 prisoners have so far died this year. The breakdown shows further that six died in January and three each in February, March, and April. In Enugu, there is an unconfirmed report that the death toll averages two in a day. Even in Eket, Akwa Ibom State, a small prison meant for minor offenders serving short term sentences, the mortality rate is high. The situation was so bad in November and December last year that there were at least three deaths every week.

At the root of the problem are poor medical services, deplorable sanitation, acute overcrowding, starvation and severe hardships which inmates undergo in the prison and police cells. Nkadi Okocha-Ejeko, medical director of Ejeks Clinic, Benin, recently initiated a free-medical-service-for-prisoners project in Benin in response to the poor state of medical services in Nigerian prisons, which he said is "non-existent." He is right. There is only one doctor and a nurse attached to Ikoyi and Kirikiri (medium and maximum) prisons (two of the biggest prisons in Nigeria) during working hours between 7.30am and 3.00pm. Official records in Kano show that uptill last February not a single kobo of the year's financial allocation to the prison service had been released for purchase of drugs.

Fola Kuteyi, a chief magistrate in Akure, halted proceedings in her court recently to donate money for the purchase of food and drugs for Adam Frank, an accused. She said that she took the decision as a fellow humanbeing and "because of lack of proper care in prison custody." Frank, a Ghanaian, was standing trial for "assaulting" his former master, a policeman. He appeared in court yawning, emaciated, pale and ravaged by skin diseases. He was scratching his body from head to toe. Kuteyi could not bear the sight for long. "The nature of my job is to serve humanity," Kuteyi said. "I don't like the ghost of a person I am seeing here."

Convicts who survived death in Nigerian prisons are but walking skeletons, a ghost of their former selves. Food is a major problem. Tunde Thompson, a journalist jailed during Buhari/Idiagbon regime, said in his book, *The Fractured Jail Sentence,* that the quality of food served, especially to those awaiting trial, is so nauseating that to talk about quality would be to do extreme violence to language. "You couldn't call it food really," Chris Nderibe, a philosophy graduate of the University of Nigeria, Nsukka, said. Nderibe was arrested following a students' demonstration and detained for several months. He narrated a graphic story of the food situation in the prison. "You wouldn't give that food to your dog. That's the truth. At one stage, we (detained students) went on hunger strike. What they did was mix a little paste of what passed for gari and give you some bitter liquid which is supposed to be soup."

Nderibe, at an interview with *New Africa* magazine last September, recollected a particular incident which illustrated how truly horrible the food situation in the prisons is. "This particular day, rice was served. Not that it looked like anything you expect a human being to eat. We were still on hunger strike, so we rejected our share. It was then I witnessed the most pitiable experience of my life. The non-student inmates jumped at the rejected food. A fierce struggle ensued and in the process, the plates fell down, over-turning their content on the filthy, smelly floor. Then the famished inmates scooped the food ferociously straight from the floor into their mouths in the manner of wild dogs."

As more journalists, students and Second Republic politicians returned from prisons to tell stories of malnutrition, kwashiorkor and death, government last January raised the daily feeding allowance per prisoner from N2.50 to N4.50. But the price of food went up too, some by more than 500 percent, wiping out whatever improvement the increase could have made to the prison diet. Prisoners remain famished and malnourished. To make matters worse, prison officials are known to pilfer the food meant for prisoners.

Moje Bare, a jurist, headed a panel that probed the prison riot last year in Benin City. Goodwill Osunde, a controller of prisons at Abuja and former head of Benin prison, told the panel that the riot, which claimed 24 lives, was partly caused by the theft of food by warders. "I am aware that the diversion of prisoners' food by some prison workers was one of the reasons for the crisis," Osunde told the probe panel. As a result of the findings of the panel, the ministry of internal affairs directed prison controllers throughout the country to ensure strict monitoring of warders handling prisoners' food. The problem, however, appears to defy solution for now. When *Newswatch* visited the Benin prison, prisoners were head shouting *"cargo don go-o."* "Cargo" is the prisoners' slang for food. Prisoners usually raise such an outcry when they see their keepers stealing their food.

Nigerian prisons have been variously described as horror

chambers, medieval dungeons and torture camps. Perhaps, the worst problem is overcrowding. Festus Iyayi, a former university lecturer, was held in a Benin police cell for one night in July 1988. Here is his story: "In that seven metres of corridor, there were 51 of us. In each of the cages meant for inmates, there were at least 12 inmates. There is no water in the cell. There was no toilet. The urinary and the toilet are the three basins on each of the cages and on of the bare floor, three feet away from me, on the corridor."

John Shagaya, a colonel and minister of internal affairs, said that about 58,000 prisoners in the country were being housed in prisons meant for 28,000 inmates. This represents 30,000 or 51.7 percent more than the available space. Take Ikoyi prison. It was built in 1961 to accommodate 800 inmates. It is currently housing 2,500 convicts and suspects. The Benin prison, built in 1906 for 220 inmates, is now stuffed with 797 inmates. *Newswatch* found that the place is so choked-up that both prisoners and those awaiting trial sleep in shifts on the bare floor. Some stand for so many hours before it is their turn to sleep for just one hour. It sounds stranger than fiction but there is just one water tap for 797 inmates in Benin prison.

In Maiduguri, the congestion in both the new and the old prisons has reached a stage where inmates squat all night to sleep. Mohammed Ibrahim, a student of the Ramat Polytechnic, Maiduguri, was locked up in the prison for five days after a motor accident in which he knocked down a kid. "It is terrible in there," he told *Newswatch*, "both the sick, the living and the dead are dumped together in one room. There is virtually no ventilation. The weather now is very hot. The room is stuffy. There is just no space to stretch your legs. A cell meant for 30 people is swelling with 120 prisoners and detainees. People squat all night to sleep." The old Maiduguri prison, built to accommodate about 300 prisoners, now has 856 inmates, while new prison, with a capacity for 400, actually houses 1,211.

The situation in Kano is even worse. A small cell meant for 20 inmates now accommodates 200, while 3,000 convicts and suspects are packed into a place built for just 1,500 people. Sule Adamu, 31, who said he spent two years in the state central prison, had a chilling story to tell. "For more than a year, I had nothing to wear. My uniform had torn into rags. I converted my jumper into something like a pair of shorts by putting my legs through the hands and finding some way to wrap it around my waist, just to cover my genitals," Adamu said.

According to the ex-convict, "a man in the Nigerian prison must demean himself by doing what he should do in the private in the full glare of more than a hundred other people. We were all sick. We spent all day scratching our bodies, writhing in pains and coughing. Every day, someone next to you died and you knew it could be your turn the next moment. You are allowed outside the cell one hour a day or, if you are waiting trial, one hour a week. One day, we went to fetch water and I saw a reflection of myself on a glass door. I was something like a bag of bones. I was so unnerved; I didn't know when I started weeping. Only a few people can recover from the trauma of where I found myself. I do not know when I can completely put it behind me."

Josiah Oki was acting chief judge of Bendel State when he visited Auchi prison. What he saw was so repulsive that he told prison officials a piece of his mind. He said the prison was unfit even for cattle. "Even the cattle will refuse to be kept in this kind of cell," Oki said.

Nnamdi Aduba, a criminologist and lecturer at the University of Maiduguri, has conducted extensive studies and research into the condition of Nigerian prisons. He told *Newswatch* in Maiduguri that one of the most unfortunate things about Nigerians prisons is that 60 percent of those in jail are suspects. As a result of the trauma, those awaiting trial have mental problems. Said a prison welfare official: "The investigations of their cases are endless and they do not have any idea when they will leave the prison. Their relatives desert them. Psychological torture sets in and the inmate simply goes mad. He can't even remember his name or where he comes from. Now, how do you obtain a relevant information from a mad man or associate with him? At the end of the day, you find out that we are running a psychiatric home."

Perhaps, the most unfortunate and ironic dimension to this national malaise is that majority of those who undergo this devastating physical and mental torture are either young persons, poor individuals, first or minor offenders who can be legally sanctioned in many other ways outside the jail house. Statistics nationwide show that more than 55 percent of the prisoners are first offenders. About 80 percent are serving short-term imprisonment (under two years). More than 60 percent are awaiting trial, while 33 percent of the convicts are serving terms for stealing without violence.

Ibrahim Antar, Attorney-General and Commissioner for Justice, Borno State, early in the year decided to go round and take a look at some of the prisons in the State. At Potiskum prison, about 140 kilometres east of Maiduguri, he found a sick, pitiable woman who was suffering from mental depression. She was serving a five-year jail term. The Attorney-General inquired about what brought her to the overcrowded prison. The assistant superintendent of the prison, Abubakar Adams, told him: "The woman was jailed five years for stealing one naira." Antar was shocked. To be sure, theft is a criminal offence; but not a few thought, like Antar, that her jail term was a bizarre travesty of justice.

Majority of the 2,000 people awaiting trial at the Ikoyi prison have spent, believe it, nine years in custody for minor offences which, on conviction, would have carried not more than two years jail term. Rough estimates available to *Newswatch* show that more than 50 percent of Ikoyi prison inmates are there for such offences as wandering, affray, conduct likely to cause a breach of peace, all of which are bailable offences under Nigerian law.

Worse still, these minor offenders, young and old, are dumped together in the same cells with hardened criminals and mentally deranged convicts. Eniola Fadayomi, Lagos State Attorney-General and commissioner for justice, visited the Ikoyi prison with some reporters some weeks ago. The reporters were not quite allowed to have a close look at the prison and its inmates. "All press men should go out. You are not wanted here," S.T. Dakwat, the assistant director of prisons ordered. The reporters resorted to wait outside for Fadayomi to brief them later. When she came out, she just shook her head and volunteered: "I can tell you the situation is deplorable." "Is it true that under-aged people are being kept with hardened criminals?" one reporter asked. "I cannot disclose that. It is too sensitive to allow the public to know," the Attorney-General said.

The public has been told by the Civil Liberty Organization, CLO, a human rights group, that under-aged and minor offenders are locked-up together in the same cells. Said the 1988 annual report of the group: "Different categories of prisoners are kept in the same cells without taking into account their ages, offences and criminal record. The mentally insane are kept in the same cells as the sane."

An international expert in police and prison matters came to Nigeria early last year to investigate the conditions of police cells and jails which he intended to publish in the authoritative *Criminal justice International* Journal. Peter Nwankwo, himself a Nigerian but based in the US, was given some access to most of the country's prison. In March last year, he granted an interview to the London-based *New Africa* magazine. "I didn't witness anyone being tortured, but do you know something? They clamp suspects still awaiting trial and hardened criminals together. This is both legally, socially and morally indefensible," he said.

Mohammed Lawan Gwadabe, a lieutenant colonel and governor of Niger State, said of the conditions of prisons in the State: "A situation whereby hard and condemned criminals or sick prisoners are made to share cells with those awaiting trials, including in some cases juveniles, cannot be said to be normal or acceptable." Godwin Abbe, his Akwa Ibom counterpart, used the word "shocking" to describe what he saw in Eket prison. "These kids should definitely not be here," Abbe said, visibly annoyed. The governor saw cases which the *Pioneer,* a government-owned newspaper, described as "hardly comprehensible with children below the age of 15 (rotting away) in overflowing cells lacking even in the slightest suggestion of comfort."

The prison authorities do not accept the blame for over-crowding. They say that they have no option but to incarcerate whoever is sent to them. They pass the buck to the police and the courts. The police, on their part, pass the buck to the courts, arguing that they are compelled to detain suspects whose cases are not promptly disposed off in courts. Judges say that the judiciary is understaffed and the courts overcrowded. Yahaya Mahmud, a chief magistrate in Kaduna, gave a vivid picture of the situation in the Kaduna judiciary. "We have six judges in the State, three of them on part time (because they are heads of some special military tribunals), but there are over 2,500 pending cases in the courts," he said in a seminar paper titled "Administration of justice in an Ideal Society."

Oki, chief judge of Bendel State, put the problem in perspective in an interview with *Newswatch*: "There are many factors responsible for the overcrowded prisons. The police may still be carrying out investigations on the matter. Sometimes, the police may have finished investigations and sent the file to the ministry of justice and because the director of public prosecution's office is flooded with many cases, they are unable to attend to all the case on time. The accused person's lawyer may not show up in the court and the case has to be adjourned. The police have no vehicle to bring accused persons from prison to court. I had an experience in Ughelli. Lawyers were seated. I was there but the police didn't bring the accused persons, so the court couldn't sit."

So where does the blame lie? The prison service, without doubt, is beset with a myriad of problems, including acute shortage of facilities to do their work. Duty vehicles, ambulances, telephones and other communication equipment are hard to come by in virtually every prison in Nigeria. *Newswatch* investigations show that the entire Kano prison service has no "single vehicle it could call its own." It is common in Kano City to see a prisoner carrying a fellow prisoner on his back to the hospital, escorted by a warder.

Olawuwo Oyesola is a warder with the Nigeria prison in Ibadan. Last December, he wrote a letter to The Editor of the *Daily Sketch,* the Ibadan-based government-owned tabloid. He sought to explain to the editor why the situation in Ibadan prison was so horrible and why the press should not nail warders for the problem. He wrote: "The Oyo State command of the prisons service has not got a single vehicle. Warders assigned to take prisoners to the hospital have to pay for public transport from their own pockets. There are occasions when warders are detailed to take prisoners to other towns to attend court. The warders also must make the transport arrangement. They are asked to make claims at the end of the month which are never honoured. The prisons department has formed the habit of going to the customs office in Ibadan to beg for vehicles. Are we not under the same ministry of internal affairs?"

The question of discrimination in the treatment of prison officials by the internal affairs ministry was at the root of a threat last March by warders in Lagos to go on strike. They complained of delays in payment of salaries, leave allowances, as well as shifting allowances approved by government since 1988. They are also demoralized because of poor conditions of service and "discriminatory treatment." They say their salaries are inferior compared to those of immigration and customs officials, all of whom belong to the same ministry. Such discrimination, one superintendent told the *Daily Champion* last February, "does not give the warder a sense of commitment or job satisfaction." Another point of grievance is the slow pace of promotion in the service. Said one warder: "If you go on training, you will be promised promotion but, ten years after that training, you will remain stagnant." He asked: "How can government be doing that to us in spite of the very sensitive job we are doing?"

Most Nigerian prisons were established during the colonial period by the 1916 Ordinance. But experts and commentators on prison affairs are not amused that 75 years later and 29 years after independence, when the British who introduced the prison system to Nigeria are carrying out massive reforms, the state of the Nigerian prison remains pathetically inhuman. The sheer mental and physical torture, as well as the alarming mortality rate in the prisons, have combined to provoke the conscience of many Nigerians. Are our prisons geared to correct and rehabilitate inmates and make them better citizens or are they slaughter houses or concentration camps or, still, a breeding ground for better trained criminals?

On paper, the role of the Nigerian prisons service is tripartite. First, they are responsible for "safe custody of persons legally interned." Second, they "treat" them and third, they are supposed to rehabilitate them. Ideally, the Nigerian prisons service also believes that the treatment and the rehabilitation of offenders could be achieved through carefully designed and well-articulated administrative, reformative and rehabilitative programmes aimed at inculcating discipline, respect for law and order and the dignity of honest labour in convicts. In reality, however, it is a different ballgame altogether. Rehabilitation and correction are made impossible because of the acute shortage of facilities such as vocational workshops and libraries in the prisons. For instance, the Calabar prison has only a carpentary workshop. The workshop trains only three prisoners because of acute shortage of tools. Libraries, where inmates can study and prepare for examinations and advance their careers while in prison, are virtually non-existent. In Maiduguri, for instance, *Newswatch* found only two books in the prison library: a Bible and a Koran. In the absence of these facilities, Nigerian prisons are in the words of Edem Koofreh, chief judge of Cross River State, "colleges for criminals."

A prison, as one official told *Newswatch*, is not a holiday resort. But the conditions in our prisons could certainly be better. Penal systems in Europe today thrive on how best prisoners could be utilized for their own and the benefit of the society. In most parts of Europe, prisoners even engage in wage labour. Minor offenders serve their sentences in factories chosen by correction departments. This ensures that the convict is not radically distanced from his family and the society. Interested convicts even undergo training and earn diplomas and degrees, which they use for employment upon discharge from prison.

To come nearer home, the Zimbabwe prisons services strives to impart productive skills on its inmates to aid their reintegration on release into the society. There is a strong involvement of prisoners in agriculture and many prisons aim at self-sufficiency in food production. This involvement, according to reports, saves the government an estimated 350,000 Zimbabwean dollars annually. The government also benefits from the prisoners through the supply of meat, milk and vegetables from the prison farms. There is also what is called prisoners building brigade, PBB. They are involved in building of houses. Since 1980, the PBB is said to have constructed more than 300 houses for prison staff at prison locations in Harare, Chipige, Nkayi and Gokwe among other places. Prisoners at Chikumbi, the formidable maximum prison outside Harare, have also built a modern milking-parlour, a pig breeding unit and an abattoir.

In Nigeria, the situation appears to be the reverse. Prisoners are wasted away at a great lose to themselves, their families and the society. Lack of rehabilitation programmes has made it possible that the only thing an ex-convict can ever hope to look forward to in Nigeria is a successful crime career. Plans over the years to carry out long overdue reforms remain what they have always been: plans. Government, as *The Observer* said in an editorial recently, remains "rather tall on promises and very short in concrete actions." The result is that prisoners' conditions throughout the country continue to degenerate from bad to worse.

The plight of Nigerian prisoners and the penal system have, in the past few months, occupied the attention of human rights groups, philanthropic organizations, churches and individuals. The Prison Fellowship of Nigeria, PFN, a voluntary organization concerned with prisoners' welfare, last month dispatched an SOS to the government, pleading that the "brutality, dehumanization, wickedness and the degrading congestion of dunghills we call prisons" be urgently looked into and checked. "The way we are managing criminal behaviour in this country is a sad commentary on our humanity," Odunaike, president of the organization, said. Ghana-born Apianda Arthur, regional director of Prison Fellowship International, PFI, who was in Nigeria last month, urged top government officials to strive and upgrade prison standards even in their own interest, because every Nigerian is a "potential prisoner or could find himself in the prison any-day."

Arthur, a former top government official in the deposed Hilla Liman administration in Ghana, was jailed by Jerry Rawlings. Speaking to the FPN in Lagos last April, he said it was his habit, as interior secretary, to divert fund meant for prisons to other departments but "when I landed eventually in Ghana prisons, I was faced with a squalid situation that heightened my belief for a total overhaul of prison conditions throughout Africa." Jim Sharkey, a Catholic priest who has been at the vanguard of improving the conditions of prisons at Eket, says some of the ways to overhaul prison conditions in Nigeria are to introduce "paroles or suspended sentences for minors, as well as counseling to stem anti-social behaviours." Sharkey, an Irish who has spent 30 years in Nigeria and works in conjunction with the local prisoners' welfare committee to donate food to prisoners at Eket, say the conditions of inmates, especially those awaiting trial, are deplorable.

The Nigeria Association of Prisoners' Welfare, NAPW, says the first step to improve the condition of prisoners is to set up a special tribunal to decongest the prisons while more prisons should be built to take care of the increasing number of suspects and convicts. But Emmanuel Olowu, a criminologist, says building more prisons or what he calls "custodial expansions" is "irrelevant, inefficacious, inappropriate and violates contemporary criminological and penalogical wisdom." According to him, the building of more prisons usually leads to a tendency by law officers to throw more people into jail, in the vain belief that there is adequate space to keep them. Besides, the building of more prisons, he said, results in increase of operational cost such as feeding, clothing, beddings, transportation of inmates and provision of medical, educational and other facilities. On top of that, he said, the present prison staff of 18,000 would have to be increased with the building of more prisons and that would add to the strain on the prisons budget, probably beyond the financial capabilities of the government. He suggests a "holistic and multidirectional" approach. As he put it: "It must aim at reducing the country's high rate of unemployment, reducing the crime level by formulating and implementing relevant socio-economic policies, as well as improving our unscientific criminal justice system. That, put together, will reduce to a manageable size the population of prison-bound criminals."

A PRISON TO DESIRE

The high brick walls are hardly noticeable. On all sides, they are dwarfed by sky-scrapers that embrace the skyline and make up the bulk of the high-class offices and shops in this bustling city centre of Cardiff, capital of Wales, in the United Kingdom. A smooth narrow road ends abruptly at the foot of the brick wall.

This sunny afternoon, the huge remote-controlled glass door slid open effortlessly to admit *Newswatch* to Her Majesty's Prison, Cardiff. Hardly any black man is in sight except *Newswatch* audacious reporter, Anietie Usen. Even the English spoken here is strange, a mouthful of accented intonation, akin only to what the evangelicals call speaking in tongues. This afternoon, there are 486 inmates locked up in three blocks of three storeys built in 1884. In the visitors' hall, about 50 of them sat opposite their relations across a row of five long tables, trying to say as much as they could within the 30 minutes permitted each prisoner.

More than 200 were in the workshops busy with their handicraft. Another 100 were sitting or lying on the lush lawns enjoying their one-hour break, sun-bathing. Inside the three-by-five metre rooms, two or three prisoners sat on their beds, smoking. The walls were covered with pornographic pictures.

"What magazine's that you are reading?" Alan Rawson, governor of the prison, asked as he knocked and stepped into the room with *Newswatch*. "Oh, what else?" the inmate replied, laughing as he displayed the centre-spread of the nude women magazine for the governor to see.

There were two eight-spring beds a small table and a locker squeezed into the room, leaving a narrow passage between the two convicts. The room was designed for one convict. But now some of them even accommodate three convicts, on six spring double-bunk beds. In mathematics, that is 200 percent overcrowding.

The prison governor was ready with an explanation. "A degree of overcrowding is expected in a prison like this because we keep short-term prisoners not exceeding 12 months. Virtually all British prisons of this kind are overcrowded," he said.

Of the 486 inmates, 152 were non convicts awaiting trial. Non-convicts in Cardiff, however, do not await trial for nine years as in Nigeria's Ikoyi Prison. They are taken to court every seven days until their cases are disposed of.

Rawson told *Newswatch* that Cardiff prison alone services 26 magistrate and three crown courts. At the end of the middle block is the prison kitchen. Bill Hendry, the officer in charge of the kitchen, supervised 20 healthy inmates as they prepared dinner. Five large containers were filled with creamed potato chips ready to be served. Rice was being cooked on several electric pots. Apart from rice and chips, the menu for dinner pinned on the kitchen notice board also included chicken curry, stuffed mar-row and macaroni. The menu register placed on Hendry's table showed the next breakfast: bread rolls, cheese, sausages, bacon, fried and boiled eggs, tea, coffee and chocolate. "They (inmates) seldom complain about meals. When they do, it's probably about poor appetite, in which case they may request for sweet or tea only," Hendry said.

A part of the main block of the prison houses a well-equipped hospital. The hospital has three doctors and 13 nurses. All kinds of treatment except major surgery are undertaken here. Unlike some Nigerian prisons, deaths of inmates are rare in Cardiff. Said Rawson: "The last time anybody died here was about five years ago when an inmate committed suicide."

To keep prisoners busy and useful to themselves and the community, Cardiff prison runs evening GCE classes and 10 trade workshops. Prisoners learn such trades as painting, plumbing, plastering, television and radio repairs, etc. But perhaps one of the largest rehabilitation centres in the prison is the tailoring workshop.

David Tyler, the head of the workshop, said that his men sew at least 43,000 trousers a year. A pair of jeans is supplied to the prison store headquarters in London at the price of £6.40. Said Tyler: "We in Cardiff sew the bulk of jeans worn by prisoners in the country. As you can see, they are as good as the ones you would buy at Marks and Spencer."

Part of the tailoring workshop houses the laundry which is equipped with modern washing machines. Prisoners' clothes and beddings are changed once a week and prisoners are assigned to wash, dry and iron the dirty ones. For their jobs in the workshop, prisoners are paid four pounds a week. "This is actually pocket money meant for their cigarettes and sweet," Rawson said.

During weekends, one of the large workshops, the metal recovery workshop, is converted into a cinema hall. Inmates are also allowed to watch television in groups of 50 in the night. Thereafter, they are locked inside their rooms and a chamber pot is kept in the room for toilet conveniences,. In the morning, the pots are "slopped out," if you know what that means.

Chamber pots and "slopping out" remain a major criticism against Cardiff prison. "It is a very dirty practice and something just has to be done about it," a female staff of the National Association for the Care and Rehabilitation of Offenders, NACRO, said, although she told *Newswatch*, she had no authority to speak to the press. Rawson said "slopping out" will be eliminated when the building of the new prison with private toilet facilities is completed.

The prison governor works with some 290 staff, 206 of whom are uniformed men. The least paid warder earns £13,500 per year. That, as at now (1989) is well over N150,000. "I believe the staff are well paid and motivated. That is why they perform their duties very well," Rawson said. That duty is explained by a poster on the wall of his office. "Her Majesty's Prison serves the public by keeping in custody those committed by the court. Our duty is to look after them with humanity and to help them lead law-abiding and useful lives in custody and after release."

THE HOUSE THAT QUACKS BUILT

Blood soaked clothes. Crushed pieces of furniture. Twisted iron rods. Broken pots, plates and rubble. These are all that remain of House No. 26, Idusagbe Lane, Idumota, Lagos. Like a pack of cards, House No. 26 came down almost leisurely in a slow motion and brought down with it two other adjoining bungalows. Eleven people were crushed to death. The horror of the tragedy still hovers like a ghost above the debris.

The killer building was just a bungalow until 1977, when Sanusi Hassan, the landlord, brought some bricklayers who did what they thought was the reinforcement of the foundation. Thereafter, Hassan would come around as he pleased to add a few rows of blocks on top of the bungalow. Soon, he became a proud owner of a one-story building. Then, he added another floor to it. Everything was still fine until work started on the third floor. Then the house came down in a heap of rubble.

Barely two weeks after the Idumota disaster, another house collapsed at Ikorodu, Lagos, killing four children. Several other children were severely injured. The house was used as a coaching class for about 60 children. On the fateful day, some pupils were still arriving in batches, while early comers were busy playing and waiting for their teachers when the bungalow caved in.

Ten days later, yet another house collapsed in Calabar, Cross River State, shortly after a heavy rainfall, killing three women and leaving many others with plastered legs and bandaged heads.

The incidence of collapsed buildings is not confined to Idumota, Ikorodu and Calabar. Similar tragedy has become a recurring decimal in several parts of Nigeria. This situation has raised much concern and anxiety about the safety of lives and property. Lagos has recorded an alarming proportion of this tragedy. Estimates by experts show that at least 200 people die every year in Lagos as a result of collapsed buildings, most of which go unreported.

Amid feasting and dancing at a christening party, July 18, 1985, an uncompleted three-story building on the Lagos Island came tumbling down. Seven children and two women were killed. Three of the dead were kids of the celebrant. As in the Idumota case, the collapsed building was constructed on a small plot of land which hitherto housed a two-room apartment. Similarly, two nearby houses were affected by the falling building. Akeem Mollah, a local contractor, who constructed the sand castle was later charged to court for "criminal negligence and building without regard to public safety."

On May 18, 1985, two months earlier, 13 people were killed when another uncompleted four-story building at Iponri, Lagos, collapsed while casual labourers were putting finishing touches to the decking of the fourth floor at nine o'clock in the night. Neighbours narrated how construction work on the house had progressed at an incredible speed. The foundation was laid just seven weeks before the tragedy and the construction work went on daily, round the clock. Just two days after the Iponri disaster, another house, along Ojuelegba Road, also in Lagos, a walking distance from Iponri, collapsed after a rainstorm.

The public was outraged by these disasters, which happened within 48 hours. The Nigerian Society of Engineers, NSE, quickly set up a panel to investigate them. Newspaper editorials followed. Said *The Nigerian Observer:* "We hope that Lagos disaster will not repeat itself." That was not to be. Three other houses collapsed on Allen Avenue, Bereku Lane and Adeniji Adele, all within the space of a few weeks. On May 9, this year, a two-story building under construction similarly crumbled at Agege, Lagos, trapping and killing the landlord and a woman, said to be his girlfriend. The two had just arrived at the site of the construction in a gleaming new model Mercedes Benz car to inspect the work, when tragedy struck.

Mike Akhigbe, a navy captain and Governor of Lagos State, was livid with anger. He promised to "deal severely with landlords who engage the services of fake builders and draughtsmen who posed as engineers." Akhigbe wished that that was the last of collapsed buildings. But that was not to be. Barely a forthnight later, 20 students of Ipakodo Grammar School, Lagos, sustained multiple injuries when the wall of their school hall collapsed shortly after the closing prayers. It seems secondary school students in Lagos State may have to spend more time praying than studying; if that would save them from rampant collapse of school walls across the State.

A series of collapsing school blocks built during the Second Republic by the Jakande administration has turned some schools into the valley of the shadow of death. Last year, Gbolade Abiodun, a primary three pupil of Jamatal Islamiyya School, Ikoro-du, was crushed to death, when his classroom wall collapsed on him. Only a few months ago on July 15, eight pupils of Bishop Howel Memorial School, Bariga, Lagos, ended up at the National Orthopaedic Hospital, Igbobi, when the wall of their classroom similarly collapsed on them. Christian Mbaeru, one of the seriously injured students, has still not recovered fully, even with the transfusion of four pints of blood.

Outside Lagos, the story is not different. In Enugu, five families residing at a three-storey building along Ona Street, returned from work last year to find in place of their beautiful house, a huge heap of debris. A curious housemaid had averted what could have been a fatal situation. At 8.30 in the morning, Nkechi (the housemaid) was washing nappies at the backyard when she heard some little creaking sound. She turned and noticed yawning gaps tearing right through from the ground floor at several points. Water was splashing out of the wall, plasters and paints were falling off before Nkechi's eyes. Quickly, she drew the attention of another housemaid. All that the two housemaids could take out of the house were little kids, seconds before the whole house buckled and fell apart.

Many people in Ibadan cannot forget October 6, 1971. On that day, 27 people were killed, when a multi-storey building under construction collapsed at Mokola area of the city. Some 48 other labourers sustained serious injuries. In Barnawa Housing Estate, Kaduna, three buildings similarly collapsed in 1981, killing six residents leading to a mass evacuation of the estate. In Benue State, a Briton, Margaret Gusuah, was killed in September 1985, when her family residence in Gboko, collapsed on her shortly after a heavy rainfall.

These days collapsed buildings do not respect mosques or courts of law and their unsmiling presiding judges. In Imo State, Justice J.S. Anyanwu, narrowly escaped death last year, when the whole ceiling of the Isiala Ngwa High Court gave way, a few minutes after the court rose. His Lordship had no choice but to adjourn *sine die*. And in Oshogbo, the seat of Yoruba ancestral arts, two brothers, Sikiru and Ganiyu Nasiru, were killed, May 1986, when the walls of the Oluode mosque caved in, while they were carrying out repairs of God's own house. No prayers could save them. They went straight, obviously, to heaven where there are better mansions that need no repairs.

The question is: What is responsible for this endless calamity? Critics have accused the government; town planning agencies and its corrupt officials. Government has, in turn, accused personnel in the building industry; the architects, building engineers, draughtsmen, etc. Different segments of the building industry have been pointing accusing fingers at one another. Greedy contractors and landlords too, have not been left out of the blame.

Akin Dayo, Lagos-based architect told *Newswatch* that in the past, the Lagos City Council, LCC, was known to be doing a fine job. It made sure that buildings under construction were thoroughly supervised from scratch to finish, using qualified structural engineers to check structural drawings, designs and calculations. The council, he said, was also very strict and uncompromising in its guidelines to contractors, especially in areas of reinforcement and concreting. "Today," Dayo said in despair, "the approving authorities seem to have thrown the good practices to the dogs."

During the Jakande administration in Lagos State, the town planning department, inundated with complains of illegal and sub-standard buildings, appointed 100 uniformed men, called building inspectors. Soon however, another kind of complaint overtook the deparment: allegations of corruption were leveled against the inspectors. It was alleged that they took money to approve even buildings without approved architectural plans. Many developers readily patronized them, brushing aside the town planning department.

At the peak of their lucrative "business," the inspectors allegedly went a step further and set up a fake approval syndicate. Everything went haywire. In 1983, the Nigerian Security Organization, now SSS, was asked to take a look at the town planning department. What they saw was terrible. Three inspectors landed immediately at an Ikeja courtroom on their express way of Kirikiri. When Gbolahan Mudashiru, then a group captain (now air-commodore) became the governor of the state following the overthrow of the civilian government, the air force-man, got angry, and sent the entire inspectors packing.

In their place, Mudashiru appointed 18 young men who hold ordinary diploma in building-related courses. Unlike the Jakande inspectors, the new inspectors had no vehicles to go about their work. In the process, they achieved little or nothing. Said a top town planning official who does not want his name published: "This place is short-staffed and under-equipped. We have made proposals for the government to provide at least motorcycles for the inspectors, but our appeals have not received any attention." He went further to rationalise corruption accusations, constantly leveled against the department. "There is corruption in every big organization in this country, so don't blow our own out of proportion," he said.

But Adekunle Bolarinwa, 32, chairman of Ibadan Metropolitan Planning Authority, IMPA, exposed the ills afflicting two planning departments in Nigeria, with Ibadan as his case study. "A draughtsman can submit a drawing for a three-storey building and get an approval, when, in fact, the law makes it clear that, he cannot handle anything beyond a bungalow," Bolarinwa said. In his one year as the boss of the IMPA, he said, he has seen sufficient irregularity to make him shudder. "One finds that a lot of mishaps have collusion internally," Bolarinwa said.

Town planners alone are not to blame. The dangerous infiltration of all segments of the building industry by non-professionals and fakes is part of the trouble. Said T. Ogu, a building engineer: "The problem is that even the old bricklayer claims to be an engineer, and due to his several years of experience, he quickly dismisses the qualified professional as a newcomer." Femi Majekodunmi of the Nigeria Institute of Architects, NIA, shifts the blame on draughtsmen who by law, are not permitted to design storey buildings. He said evidence of many collapsed buildings, especially in Lagos area, have shown that the drawings of such buildings were prepared by draughtsmen."

Landlords are not helping matters either. In Lagos, it has become a practice for most landlords to complete their buildings before beginning the frantic search for "approved plan." Incredible but true. Besides, they go all out for cheap building materials and labour. Even worse, some obstinate ones among them would not stop building when ordered to do so by town planning inspectors. In the case of the tragedy during a party on the Lagos Island, the town planning department had warned the owner of the house to stop work a month before the incident. He ignored the warning.

Similarly, the report of internal investigations by the LSTPA, now with the police, shows that in the celebrated Iponri disaster, the illegal building was first demolished but the landlord went back immediately to erect another illegal building on the same spot. Said an official of the LSTPA: "Such landlords do not build their illegal structures during working days but at weekends and in the night to evade town planning officers."

Contractors too, have contributed to the incidence of collapsed building. They are known to be hostile to supervision by engineers and architects. They often see professional supervisors as stumbling blocks to their fast bucks. Sometimes, contractors even convince the owner of a building to believe that the supervising professional is out to frustrate his project. There are reported cases of supervising professionals being chased out of sites by clients because the contractor has made him to see the supervising professionals as enemies.

What is to be done then? The NSE, in its investigations following the Iponri disaster, traced the cause of the disaster to inadequate soil investigation on the building site, lack of monitoring of constructions stages and improper mixing of concrete. To avoid further disaster, the engineers want to be allowed to examine buildings plans before they are approved." They also want government to ensure "strenuous certification process" before approving buildings plans.

Following the same Iponri disaster, the NIA also pushed forward a 10-point guideline to the government on how to check future occurrences of collapsed buildings. They recommended among other things that: only registered architects with the Architects Registration Council of Nigeria, ARCON, and registered engineers with the Council of Registered Engineers of Nigeria, COREN, be allowed to present architectural and structural drawings respectively for statutory and planning approvals. They insisted further that the drawings and other such documents for such applications should bear the ARCON and COREN stamps and signatures.

The Nigerian Institute of Town Planners, NITP, has advised government to remove those they called "non-professionals" from the management of planning agencies. It has also called for the involvement of town planning units which approve building designs, as well as structural engineers and architects in the monitoring of construction work at all stages. The professionals in the building industry, themselves have been advised to cut down their exorbitant fees which have served to drive intending developers into the hands of quacks. The public too can help. This, an official of the LSTPA said, can be done by reporting immediately any suspected illegal building or cracks on the walls of any building. "No building collapses without warning. The cracks and crevices we see on houses around us are actually warnings, which must be heeded without much delay," he said. The public, government officials said, must also be less hostile to town planning officials. In 1983, a town planning bulldozer operator was stabbed to death after demolishing an illegal building on the Lagos Island.

The government, said Bassey Inyang, an engineer, has a greater responsibility and must respond adequately to solve the problem. For one, Inyang wants government to mount a campaign on the radio, television and newspapers, to educate and warn the public on the consequences of illegal buildings. He also wants government to impose firm and stiffer penalties on culprits. Government too should recruit professionals to man the LSTPA and provide sufficient equipment and vehicles to town planning departments. *Newswatch* found that the 20 units of the LSTPA have only 10 vehicles, most of them in bad shape.

Bolarinwa, IMPA boss said government can do more. He believes there is "too much bureaucracy" by the supervising ministries, before approvals are given. This he said, tends to force would-be developers into the hands of corrupt and unprofessional officials. "The administrative process must be simplified with a view to discouraging irregularities, which in most cases lead to these disasters."

REIGN OF GEMSTONES BANDITS

For a visitor, Antang is a scruffy, little village of thatched huts, deep in North Central Nigeria. The streets are narrow and dusty. Most natives are shaggy and scraggy. More than one half of them go about without shoes. But Antang, the latest attraction for crooked businessmen, is Nigeria's *El Dorado,* sitting literally on top of huge deposits of precious stones.

Found in confounding quantities in Antang and the neighbouring villages of Nisama, Gidan Waya, Godogodo and Kagoro, all in the Jema Local Government Area of Kaduna State, are precious stones such as diamond, sapphire, quartz, gemstones, ruby, temaline, mica, trona, sicon, topaz and aquamarine. Scratch the soil. A flash. "What you pick," says Sule Ango, a young Senegalese illegal miner, "is a reddish, bluish or transparent piece of stone. That could be diamond."

For years, the villagers had no use at all for these shiny, sparkling stones, which they called "devil stones." The stones, as Aya Musa, an elderly indigene of the area, told *Newswatch*, were considered a nuisance because they posed such a problem in tilling the farm. Soon, foreigners, most of them from Senegal, Cote d'Ivoire, Mali and other African countries descended on the area and picked the stones. They even paid daily "feeding money" to indigenes who gladly helped them get rid of "devil stones."

Suddenly, everything changed. Entire farmlands were ripped off and turned upside down in search of "devil stones." Holes and tunnels were dug everywhere. The population of foreigners in the area soared to unprecedented figures. By December last year, the number of aliens registered by the immigration department in Kafanchan, headquarters of Jema'a local government area, had reached 15,950. Senegalese alone were 3,800. In addition, illegal aliens, according to estimates by immigration officials, were more than half a million. Together, they sacked farmlands and forests, stole and smuggled out of Nigeria millions of naira worth of precious stones.

By October last year, the menace of illegal miners and their barons (who operate in a Mafioso style, like drug barons) had reached crisis proportion. The rank and file of the security agencies in the area, particularly the police, had been deeply penetrated, thoroughly corrupt and weakened. They were clearly incapable of combating the plundering. Accusing fingers were also being pointed at top government officials. They were blamed for "closing their eyes and tacitly encouraging the booming trade" at a time Nigeria's economy needed all the foreign exchange it could muster. Government was sufficiently alarmed. It was time for action.

Late October, Bunu Sheriff Musa, a suave engineer and minister of mines, power and steel, sent a memo to President Ibrahim Babangida. He suggested the establishment of an inter-ministerial committee, comprising the police, customs, immigrations and the mines ministry, to combat the problem. Musa was disturbed by insinuations from registered mineral prospectors that highly placed government officials had a hand in the "plundering of billions of naira worth of precious stones by illegal miners." He said in his memo that the inter-ministerial committee was the best way to stem the tide of illegal mining. The president gave Musa the nod. On November 8, Musa in company of top representatives of the internal affairs ministry met with Mohammadu Gambo, Inspector-General of Police, to explore ways of dealing with the problem. The idea of raid (of illegal miners) was born.

A series of fortnightly meetings by the committee quickly worked out the logistics of the raid. Locations of illegal miners were ascertained. Strategic escape routes were marked down for blockade. The operation was fixed for twelve midnight December 29. At 8.30 pm on the D-day, the crack combined team of police; immigration, customs, security men as well as ministry of mines officials were ready. Fully armed security officials were also drawn from the neighbouring states of Bauchi, Borno, Gongola and Abuja, the federal capital territory. Kept in the dark till the last minute, however, was the Kafanchan police unit. The barons in the business had always boasted that police in Kafanchan "pose no problem" and the committee agreed it could not afford a leak.

By 10.00pm that night, Kafanchan, Kagoro, Gidan Waya, Nisama, Antang (the undisputed headquarters of illegal miners) has been surrounded and sealed up. By 4.00am, the operation was over. Packed in 12 open trailers were about 500 aliens suspected to be illegal miners. The journey to Seme, Nigeria's border town with Benin Republic, for the deportation of the culprits, was about to begin. But one more order was yet to be carried out:

the market-like assembly point of the miners at Antang was to be razed. Shortly after 5.00am, the miners' market was torched. Aided by sweeping harmattan wind, the thatched market, where millions of naira had exchanged hands, quickly went down, burnt to ashes.

After the raid, came the rain of problems. The inter-ministerial committee, it seems, did not quite see beyond the raid. How were the culprits going to be fed? How and where were they going to be kept? How were they going to be treated or sanctioned? In want of what to do, a handful of "overzealous" policemen and immigration officials, who participated in the raid, drove the suspects more than 1,200 kilometres to Seme, in an unbelievably naïve attempt to deport them.

At Seme, Beninois border officials did the right thing. They asked for deportation papers. There was none. Stranded at the border for two days without food were both the culprits and the security officials who arrested them. By next morning, when the BBC and the VOA reported the incident, Nigeria had lost on the diplomatic front. Government was so embarrassed Babangida interrupted a council of ministers' meeting January 5 and dispatched John Shagaya, internal affairs minister, and Bola Ajibola, justice minister, to Seme to order the return of the aliens back to Lagos for proper screening and trial.

"We were all shocked," Musa told *Newswatch* "Something went wrong. There were some problems, problems of decision-making. After the raid, the next step should have been to seek clearance (from the ministry of internal affairs) as to what to do with these people and what sort of procedure should be followed to get them evacuated or repatriated. It was here that the hitch came in.

But Musa said he would not blame the officers who hurriedly escorted the miners to Seme. "They did it in good faith. They may have been hurt by the atrocities those aliens have committed against this country. They must have felt these aliens have no business storming Nigeria's rural areas the way they have done. So, I think they did not want to keep them for an indefinite period and create a problem of accommodating and feeding them," Musa said.

It took the bungled attempt to bundle out the aliens for the attention of the country to be seriously drawn to the blight of illegal mining in Nigeria. A trip to Jema'a local government area shows acute environmental problems of tragic dimensions. Thousands of hectares of farmland have been excavated and transformed into wasteland. Indiscriminate digging of holes and tunnels have also turned farms and grazing lands into death traps for farmers and cattle. Some holes are as deep as 50 feet. At Nisama, *Newswatch* counted more than 100 deep pits on about one acre of land. More than 5,000 diggers, using excavators, shovels and hoes, could be found on the field on a typical mining day.

Last October, the *National Concord* reported that more than 100 paid diggers were trapped and killed in Kafanchan area alone, when the tunnels they were digging in search of precious stones caved in on them. Those trapped are usually abandoned to make the tunnels their graves. "It is a very unfortunate situation to see our farmlands and farmers being destroyed in this way by illegal miners," Ali Madaki, Kaduna State commissioner for commerce and industry. Said in November at a business luncheon organized by the Kaduna chambers of commerce, industry and agriculture. Said P.T.Y. Dalli, another indigene of the State, in a protest letter to the Kaduna-based *Today* newspaper: "My fear is that people in this area (Jema'a LGA) may not go to their farms this year. For God's sake, tell the government to stop these illegal miners.

In Kafanchan, illegal miners live a highflying lifestyle. They own fleets of trendy cars. They hire the best apartments in town and pay rents three or more years in advance. Landlords prefer them to Nigerian tenants because they undertake to renovate the rented houses to their own tastes, at their own expense. Often, they help landlords build the houses they want to rent, right from the scratch. With their affluence, they keep chains of girlfriends, most of whom are still in school, a situation Frank Bala Baba, a councilor in the LGA, told *Newswatch*, is a cause for serious concern for parents. "So many little girls are being put in the family way by alien miners and the boys have abandoned schools in search of precious stones which aliens readily buy off at giveaway prices," Baba said.

Like hard drugs, precious stones fetch big, fast money. Salisu Idris, a young miner, told *Newswatch* he left the Federal Government College, Nassarawa, Plateau State, to join the "gold-rush" in1987. He makes an average of N1,000 a day. "There are days you hit a jackpot and a little piece of beautiful stone fetches up to N4,000," Idris said, smiling. Benson Upah of the *New Nigerian,* who has probably covered the activities of the miners more than any other reporter in Nigeria, reported last October that "some indigenes make as much as N20,0000 in one fell swoop." According to him, "the aliens, who fix prices as well as make the rules, make hundreds of thousands of naira everyday." Said a security sources at Kafanchan: "A fairly big gemstone (the size of a man's fist) goes for about N20,000 here."

The business is also fraught with risks. There are cases of

eliminating by kidnapping, sudden disappearance of dealers and diggers and a whole range of other blood chilling tales. The barons, agents and diggers became fanatically security-conscious, suspicious and fully armed with automatic weapons, soon after government began to post security men to the area. Going to the mining site, for a *Newswatch* reporter, was like "keeping an appointment with death." At Ngawa Malafia, a group of 10 fierce looking miners moved to attack a *Newswatch* reporter.

On October 22, 1988, Sulciman Momoh, a reporter with the *Sunday Champion,* almost lost his life in a similar encounter with illegal miners at Janjala, 40 kilometres from Keffi in Plateau State. "We shall throw you into this abyss below (a 50-feet deep trench) after we find out the bastard who sent you here," a broad-shouldered security guard threatened the reporter. "Drop your camera and bag on the floor and speak up," the guard ordered. It took the intervention and prolonged pleading of a mine supervisor to secure the release of the reporter. "Go away fast," the guard growled, "and don't ever try to sneak into any other mining site or else…"

In Jema'a, the business boomed because the barons made sure they put law enforcement agents, as well as influential indigenes of the area, in their pockets. An immigration officer, who pleaded not to be quoted, said the department has always been frustrated by highly placed officials and indigenes who collude with the barons. "They (barons) have always beaten us to the game. A number of dutiful (immigration) officers are often transferred because they refuse to cooperate with the barons," the officer said.

Isa Muhammadu, the emir of Jema'a, appeared to confirm the allegation made by the immigration officer. Muhammadu told *Newswatch* government was wrong in raiding and arresting the aliens without prior consultation with him. Said the Emir: "The aliens are peaceful and law-abiding people. If they dig the ground, get precious stones, sell and bring prosperity to my people, what is bad about that? You people have driven them away, why do you need my comment now?"

Jema'a Local Government rea is not the only part of Nigeria facing the menace of illegal miners. In Ilesha, Oyo State, the pillaging is on the increase. The metal involved is the king of them all: gold. The main culprits are Nigerians, ably backed by foreigners. In Igun, near Ilesha, where large deposits of gold had been discovered, goldsmiths and dealers are prospecting without licence. An ounce of 18 carat gold (the commonest in Ilesha area) sells for N2,000 at Igun. The same quantity, at the middlemen's centres in Ibadan, attracts as much as N2,400. An investigation by *Insider,* a Lagos confidential magazine, in April last year, showed that the same quantity in Igun and Ibadan exchanged hands for N1,600 and N1,800 respectively.

For the illegal miners and dealers, the market, like in the case of Jema'a's precious tones, is Europe, where one ounce of 18 carat gold sells for more than 500 dollars. To smuggle the gold to Europe, according to *Newswatch* sources, the precious stone, which occurs in dust form, is first taken to conniving goldsmiths at Ibadan. There, the gold dust is melted and beaten into a ring, bracelet or bangle, which the dealer wears or carried as a present on an overseas trip. Abroad, the bangle or bracelet, as the case may be, undergoes a test to confirm its genuineness. Thereafter, the sale is made. *Newswatch* reliably gathered that part of the foreign currency in the black market now comes from this form of illegal gold trading.

The ministry of mines, power and steel says gold was first discovered in Nigeria in 1908. Prospecting by several small companies and licensed individuals quickly yielded encouraging results. By 1940, the annual gold production had risen to an all-time height of 1.36 million grammes. At this time, investigations showed government was not convinced the quantity of gold available in the Ilesha gold mines was worth the investment required. Some Nigerian and Lebanese businessmen, *Newswatch* was told, took advantage of government disinterest and quietly made fortunes out of the mines.

But by early 80s, when the bubble burst in the international oil market and the country desperately searched around for other sources of foreign exchange, government decided to take another look at Ilesha. Now, the verdict is different. Said Musa last week at an interview with *Newswatch*: "In Ilesha area, gold occurs generously in God's given nature. If you scoop the ground, what you get is some yellowish shinning materials. That certainly is gold."

But since 1986 when the Nigerian Mining Corporation moved into Ilesha to begin the mining of gold, not much has been achieved. A small block of offices, called the gold refinery, was built in Osu, a sleepy little village near Ilesha. Constructed with corrugated iron sheets, the "refinery" is surrounded by a thick forest and rusty unserviceable tractors. The miners at Osu, unlike their illegal and affluent counterparts, appear indigent and hard-up. The dreams of the community to have a gold refinery in the area remains what is was in 1908: a dream. The result is the intensification of illegal mining of the Ilesha gold, said by experts to be 99.5 percent pure. Now, virtually everyone who wants to wed in Lagos knows just where to get a gold ring at give-away price: Ilesha.

Musa agreed government was losing "millions in foreign exchange" to illegal miners and smugglers but said it was "very difficult to quantify the loss in terms of Naira and Kobo" because of "lack of statistical information." For now, the atrocities of illegal miners in Ilesha, he said, defy immediate solution because of the wide expanse of land the metal has occurred. For instance, the vast fortune at Ilesha area include the 24-square-kilometre mine at Itagunmodi which is estimated to have about 119,928 ounces of gold. Other unqualified deposits around the area are at Iperindo Iregun, Ibodi, Ijana and Idoka. Said Musa: "This thing is occurring in such a way that you can't fence the place and you can't really say you want to go and harass people until you have an organized mining arrangement."

Illegal miners have probably done worse havoc to tin ore deposits and industry in Nigeria. The London authoritative mining magazine, *Metal Bulletin*, reported in October last year that 50 percent of the tin produced in Nigeria is illegally mined and smuggled out of the country in its raw form to European markets. The magazine puts Nigeria's "correct annual production capacity" at 1,600 tonnes. With the government approved price of N18,000 per tonne, the country losses N172.8 million a year to illegal miners. At the spot market price of N60,000 per tonne, the country's loss a year to illegal miners is put at N676 million.

But Davon Pwajok, General Manager of NMC, says the figures from the London magazine are too low. According to him, the actual quantity of tin ore illegally mined and smuggled abroad is 75 percent of the country's capacity and not 50 percent. The result of this unprecedented boom in illegal transaction is the crippling of official production. It has also led to serious capacity under-utilization of Nigeria's only tin smelting plant, the Makeri

Smelting Company in Jos. The plant, commissioned in 1961, is supposed to process Nigeria's tin ore for export.

Jacob Rwang, Makeri's works director, says that as a result of this problem, the company, with a capacity of 18,000 metric tonnes, was only able to process 100 tonnes in 1986 and 700 tonnes in 1987. The current data from the mines ministry show that in the first half of 1988, the production level further tumbled to a mere 31.99 tonnes. What this means is that Nigeria continues to lose additionally in terms of royalty, customs duty and company tax to smugglers. For the company itself, it means mass retrenchment of workers and inability to pay salaries of a handful of workers left in the company. It also portends that the entire tin industry faces a serious threat of liquidation in the hands of illegal miners.

The bloody clash in 1987 between the police and illegal miners in the tin-rich State, which resulted in the killing of four miners, graphically demonstrated the pervasive tentacles and influence of illegal miners in the region. In a white paper on the report of an administrative panel that probed the clash, the emir of Keffi, Alhaji Mohammadu Yamusa II, was alleged to have "benefited corruptly from the operation of illegal miners" in his emirate.

Although *Newswatch* investigations show that the lucrative business is now on the decline in Keffi, evidence abound that elsewhere in the country, such as Sokoto where gold was recently discovered in Anka LGA, "the business continues as usual." Said Abdullahi Mohammed, chairman of Anka LGA: "So far, not much has been done by security agencies to check illegal mining here."

Lawrence Onoja, a colonel and military governor of Katsina State, has, in the past three years, shouted himself hoarse on what should be done about the criminal assault on Nigeria's mineral wealth. Onoja asked the federal government to treat illegal miners and those found in unlawful possession of precious stones as economic saboteurs. He also said the mines ministry should consider "as a matter of importance," the rapid granting of licences to prospective miners "not only because of the illegality of the act or the loss of foreign exchange, but for security reasons."

Similarly, Nlogha Okeke, president of the national association of chambers of commerce, industry, mines and agriculture, NACCIMA, last month picked holes in the laws governing the mining of minerals. He said they should be reviewed to enable the private sector participate more effectively in the exploitation and development of the minerals. With the present deregulation of the economy, said Okeke, the present mining laws would be a hindrance to private investment in the mining industry if they were not "consolidated and streamlined." According to the NACCIMA boss, the federal government can even take a step further to establish a stock pile of strategic minerals because most of the country's key industries at the moment still depend on foreign imputs and could in emergency would spell doom.

Abdulrahman Ayeni, head of mining engineering and applied geology at the Kaduna Polytechnic, while calling for the overhaul of "obsolete" mining laws, said the Nigerian Mining Corporation Decree No. 39 of 1972 lays emphasis only on distribution and marketing in disregard to exploitation and processing. Said Ayeni: "Necessary and stringent measures should be taken to make the sale of minerals through illegal mining difficult, if not impossible. The illegal but all-pervading ECOWAS market, with the tempting hard currency, should be dismantled immediately to create a healthier atmosphere for the extraction, processing and marketing of solid minerals in Nigeria."

But the mining law, says the government, are not the problem. The problem, the mines minister told *Newswatch*, is perhaps the application of the laws. As the minister put it: "Our laws are quite adequate. If there is anything that can be said to be wrong with the law, it is the application. The police are involved because they are the ones who normally see to the observance of law. The customs are involved in the sense that anything that goes out of Nigeria has to be checked and ascertained that it is the legal thing that should be taken out. Then the immigration people come in because most aliens involved in stealing and smuggling our minerals are not staying under a genuine arrangement."

The penalty for unlawful possession, purchase and smuggling of minerals, Musa says, is life imprisonment under the miscellaneous offences decree. Besides, the requirement for lawful mining, according to the minster, has been made less cumbersome. The mines ministry, in addition, recently published a simplified 18-page "guideline for mining operations in Nigeria" which defines what constitute mining, the laws governing it and how to become a lawful miner. The guidelines, says Musa, sell for a token of 10 naira, to make sure the rules governing the business is accessible to every potential miner. "If you are going to mine something that is worth millions of naira, I don't think N10.00 will pose a problem. And if there is no bottleneck in the issuing of licences, then there should be no reason for anybody to indulge in illegal mining," Musa said.

Though government is currently involved in prospecting and mining some precious stones, the recently approved industrial policy, as well as the privatization and commercialization policies, appear capable of encouraging additional investments in the sector. However, the effort that should go into the exploration of Nigeria's vast mineral endowment appears to be lacking. The entire mining industry seems to be neglected. For instance, in the first half of last year, when Nigeria lifted 48.8 million barrels of crude oil, it exported only 31.99 tonnes of tin. Several other minerals suffer worse neglect and were completely ignored.

After government has spent N25 million in 1987 in futile search for uranium in Bauchi State, it turned around in 1988 to say it was not anxious to exploit vast uranium ore deposits discovered in Kwara State by an independent mining consultancy firm. What is making experts uneasy is the knowledge that while mining holds the key to bailing Nigeria out of the present economic slump, the mistake of the oil boom era, when Nigeria ignored the exploration of other minerals, may repeat itself. As the *Daily Sketch* succinctly said in its editorial: "This great country needs everything it can harness to reshape the battered economy."

THE RAGE OF HEAVENS

As the unusual rainstorm subsided, Usman Aminu, a taxi driver in Kano, drove home. But there was no home. The roof of his house at Sharada, outside the walls of Kano City, had been blown off. The walls also had collapsed, smashing his radio, television and other expensive furniture into pieces. Whatever was left was being swept away rapidly by flood. Luckily for Aminu, his two wives and kids had taken refuge in a nearby mosque together with hundreds of other victims. Wet, drab and shivering, Aminu's family quickly began to cry as the confused man fished them out of the crowd and shoved them into his cab. "Where do we go from here?" One of his wives asked, sobbing.

The two-hour rainstorm, that turned Aminu and hundreds of people in Sharada into refugees, was regarded as a mere drizzle in weeks of torrential rain storm that has taken the State to the edge of a maelstrom. The disaster in Kano State reached its peak August 13, when the multi-million Naira Bagauda dam collapsed under an avalanche of 32 million cubic metres of water. The immediate vicinity of the dam was left in ruins as water stormed its way out of the dam with the force of a volcano. Trees were uprooted. Farmlands were devastated. The Kano-Jos Road at Bagauda and the nearby bridges were ripped off in one fell swoop. Tearing through and excavating the hard arid soil with baffling ease, the gushing water created scenic waterfalls that quickly submerged the Nigerian Mining Corporation's, NMC, brick factory, about half a kilometer away from the dam. Thousands of bricks stacked outside the factory were swept away like a pack of dry leaves. The two kilns in the factory were destroyed along with the factory's wet-pan mills, extruding machines, box feeders, electric motors and two standby generators, crippling operations of the factory.

Office equipment, documents and stationeries joined the high tide that the NMC boss, Godfrey Olayemi, said damaged property of the factory worth more than N13 million. Down the slope, beside the brick factory, hundreds of cattle were washed away as their herdsmen scampered for safety in different directions. Ahmed Suradinki alone said he lost more than 100 cows to the flood.

In just one day of heavenly rage, Bagauda, the holiday resort town of Kano State, popularly known as the "giant in the sun', was ravaged. By late last week, the torrent of water released from the dam had stormed its way through Kano River and several irrigation channels to Gashu, Nguru and Geidam in neighbouring Borno State.

The collapsed dam and the rainstorm, described as the heaviest in 50 years, claimed 49 lives and displaced more than 200,000 people in 3,000 communities. More than 14,000 farmlands were washed away while more than 20,000 houses were destroyed. In Kano township alone, more than 40,000 people were displaced and 6,000 houses were destroyed. In Gaya, north of Kano, Idris

Garba, governor of the State told *Newswatch* more than 43,000 people were rendered homeless, while 5,600 houses were pulled down.

Another seriously affected Local Government Area was Dawakin Kudu, where the governor said about 6,000 houses were destroyed and 49,000 people displaced. Said Garba: "In fact, every local government area in the State has been badly affected by the tragedy in one form or the other. We are looking for something in the region of N100 million to be able to rehabilitate the victims, reconstruct the Bagauda dam and effect repairs on the 21 other dams in the State to avert another disaster'. A breakdown of the estimate shows that the Bagauda dam alone will gulp more than N5 million in repairs, while N50 million will take care of the resettlement of the victims. The balance will go into repairs and maintenance of other dams.

So far, donations and relief materials have been pouring into the State. The federal government was the first to respond to the distress call by Garba. President Ibrahim Babangida immediately authorized the release of N5 million for the purchase of relief materials. On August 24, he flew into Kano and drove straight to the scene of the collapsed dam to have a first-hand knowledge of the situation. Earlier, Babangida had dispatched Gado Nasko, Minister of Agriculture and Water Resources there for an on-the-spot assessment of the damage. Nasko told Garba that the president has, in addition to the N5 million, ordered the release of 10,000 tones of grains for distribution to the flood victims. "This is a very unfortunate destruction of farmlands and irrigational structures," Nasko said. He also announced that the reconstruction of the collapsed dam would be bankrolled by the federal government.

Apart from the assistance rushed in by the federal government, the State's Emergency Relief Fund, ERF, Committee has swung into action. Sahli Ahmed Bichi, the Director-General of the Committee, told *Newswatch* that 26,000 bags of grains have so far been purchased and distributed to the flood victims. A helping hand also came last week from the Niger State government in the form of N250,000. Katsina State donated N20,000; United Bank for Africa, UBA, N250,000; ICON Merchant Bank, N25,000; Continental Merchant Bank, N100,000; MAMSER, N12,000 and the Nigeria Union of Teachers sent in N2,000. Donations also came from Authur Eze, the Onitsha-based businessman, who donated N50,000, while members of the Constituent Assembly sent in N11,360. At the same time, the State also received N10,000 from the Nigerian Air Force Logistics Command; N2,000 from the Directorate of Military Intelligence, as well as 30 bags of assorted grains from the Pan-African Foundation, PAF, a young relief organization established two years ago by Iwok Asuamah, a Nigeria Airways staff.

Shehu Musa, chairman of PAF, who was in Kano, August 19, to make the donation, said it was a "token" effort. Musa, who is also the chairman of the Nigerian Red Cross Society, said the Red Cross was assessing the kind of assistance it would give to the flood victims.

Also in Bagauda to assess the damage, was William Wiklin, Vice-Consul of the United States Consulate in Kaduna. He told *Newswatch* that he was at the scene of the collapsed dam on the instruction of the American ambassador, Princeton Lyman. "The ambassador sent me here on a fact-finding mission in order to assess what we can do to help the flood victims," Wilkin said.

The immediate needs of the victims are food and clothing.

While the relief sub-committees established in all the local government areas of the state were busy last week distributing grains, the ERF headquarters in Kano was combing the market for cheap clothes. "We have just started sending the first batch of clothing materials to victims and most of them in Kano have already been given something to wear. What we are doing now is a short-term measure but a master plan for a long-term solution is being put together by the government," Sahli said.

Part of the short-term measures is the hurried evacuation of villagers from the neighbourhood of dams and river banks. Said the governor: "We are also mounting a vigorous campaign to enlighten our people to settle in areas that are completely outside dams and river banks."

The State government is also considering giving cash assistance to victims who lost their houses in the disaster. "The ideal situation," the governor said, "would have been to provide them with new accommodation but that, you will agree with me, is difficult. The major thing now is to first provide drainages, repair the damaged structures such as roads, bridges, dams and then provide layouts for these people to erect houses of their own choice. But what we are going to do quickly to relieve the accommodation problem is to assist you especially if you have to move out of your original home."

To provide a long-term solution to the problem, government has appointed a powerful technical committee made up of three commissioners and four directors-general, including the director-general of the State Urban Development Board. The committee is to carry out an in-depth study of the disaster and other similar tragedies and advise the government on a "possible permanent solution." The committee will also look into the logistics of resettling victims in safer layout without having to cut them off entirely from their familiar traditional settings and occupation. To back up and implement the recommendations of the technical committee, a fund raising committee headed by Aminu Dantata, one of the state's multi-millionaires, was set up on August 18. The proceeds from the fund raising committee are also expected to help in the reconstruction of the damaged infrastructures. Reconstruction work began last week on the portion of the Kano-Jos road where the damage done to the road had cut off traffic between the two cities.

Barely 48 hours after the Bagauda tragedy, another earth dam in Magago in Gwarzo local government area, about 120 kilometres away from Bagauda, overflowed its banks sending panic-stricken villagers on their heels. The bridge linking the village with Buwawa, a nearby town, was damaged, making it difficult for the fleeing villagers to return home after the flood. *Newswatch* found that the villagers of Magago were to be resettled at a place safely distant from the dam in 1984. Demarcated plots, water and electricity were provided in the new settlement, in addition to payment of compensation to the villagers. But this farming population refused to move, demanding that government build new houses for them before they quit.

Flood disaster in the past few weeks seems not to be just a Kano affair. In Borno State, 26 people were reported killed last week in Fika LGA as a result of torrential rainfall. More than 100 houses were also reported destroyed by rainstorm in Potiskum and Ngadala villages of the State. A total of 50 houses were also washed away in Dekina LGA of the Benue State. In Port Harcourt, capital of Rivers State, hundreds of houses and offices were similarly reported hit by flood last week after 12 hours of continuous rainstorm.

But the most frightening news as at press time still came from Kano State. Tiga Dam, the largest in the state, located a few kilometers southwest of the Bagauda dam, as well as the gigantic Watari dam, west of Kano City, were said to be facing "severe danger" of collapse because of dangerous cracks which had already extended at an alarming proportion in the case of Tiga. Though the cracks in the Watari dam are said to be slightly less, engineers at the site of the dam told a *Triumph* reporter that parts of the spillways of the dam have already given way under the weight of flood. Umaru Kura and Sani Tofa, chairmen of Rano and Dawakin Tofa LGAs respectively, where the dams are located, have sent an SOS to the state and federal governments to hurry and "bring the situation under control." Virtually all major agricultural projects in Kano State and beyond rely on the Tiga, Bagauda and the Watari dams for irrigation. For instance, the Hadejia-Jamare River Basin Development Authority relies entirely on Bagauda and Tiga dams for the irrigation of 60,000 hectares of farmland.

Though most Nigerians remain puzzled at the unusual level of rainfall in a region that normally holds prayers to invoke rain, and some are even tempted to believe a supernatural cause is behind the tragic phenomenon. Experts have, over the years, had shouted themselves hoarse on the lack of adequate maintenance of the dams and the danger that portends for the entire northern states.

Newswatch found in Kano and Kaduna that as far back as 1978, a consultant firm, Haskoning Engineering Limited, had made recommendations on how to preserve the gigantic dams. After a thorough investigation and inspection of the dams, Haskoning engineers observed that the construction of Tiga dam, for instance, was undertaken after poor feasibility studies. As a result, they said, the construction was poor and the dams were already cracking. They noticed poor thickness of the steel lining on the dams; inadequate slope protection, which was done with grass; lack of instrumentation and lack of supervision by local engineers. One other lapse they noted in their report was "failure to write down design and basic technical data decisions, without which tracing of faults and recommendations for remedy became guesswork." Haskoning then recommended that the 50-metre crest of the 5,000-metre long Tiga dam be raised to between 1,740 and 1.943 feet, "to take care of the deficient excess water release system." The state-owned Water Resources Engineering Construction Agency, WRECA, which supervises the dam, was asked to install some vital instruments lacking at the dam. The estimated cost of effecting the recommendation was put at N5.74 million. But little or nothing was done.

In 1986, the six-kilometre Tiga dam showed a longitudinal crack extending one kilometre. The Bagauda dam built in 1968 was also discovered to be cracking. The Nigerian Sub-Committee of Dams, NSCD, was asked to undertake another inspection of both Tiga and Bagauda dams. When the team of NSCD, headed by J. Umolu, submitted its report in November, 1986, they urged the state government to take "urgent remedial actions necessary to properly monitor the developing internal stress and contain the impending hazard." The committee endorsed as "highly sound," the recommendations of Haskoning engineers. It said "the maintenance of the downstream slopes must have been relaxed, hence the neglect of certain areas, which have been deeply incised by erosion gullies."

Short-term measures recommended by the committee, as

shown in the report, included: the installations of piezometers, deformation beacons and seepage measuring weirs at key points of the crack, "in order to gauge the behavior of the dam; the lowering of the reservoir level of the dam for stability and safety, or alternatively the undertaking of underwater investigations to establish the state of the rip-rap and necessary repairs; the carrying out of stability analysis to determine the dams' safety under various water lead conditions: as well as, the exploration of additional outlet capacity by additional land acquisition.

The committee deplored the absence of telephone link within the dams' complex and between the dams and the cities, saying that it was a "serious deficiency which in times of emergency could be the difference between life and death." It further urged the government to act with dispatch as the problems at the dams could degenerate "if appropriate action is not forthcoming."

Again, not much was done to carry out the recommendations of the expert bodies, as government appeared to be discouraged by the cost of repairs and maintenance put at about N27 million. As Adesoye Ettu, a hydro-meteorologist from the federal meteorological department said last week: "Much of this havoc was avoidable had proper maintenance been effected and previous recommendations by experts taken seriously. This negligence, coupled with the disrespect for meteorological forecast and warning were responsible for the collapse of the dam." A few days before Bagauda dam collapsed, Ettu said meteorologists had raised an alarm on the state of the dam during the meeting of the national committee on water resources held at the Bagauda Lake Hotel. But that warning was hardly acted upon and "even the excess water build-up was released too late."

Abdulazeez Umar, engineer and managing director of WRE-

CA, however, attributed the collapse of Bagauda dam to "piping due to activities of millions of termites and ants." He said the dam capacity of 22 million cubic litres of water was exceeded by 10 million cubic litres at the time it collapsed.

He told *Newswatch* that N250,000 had been spent to 'reinforce the dam in July," a month before it collapsed, adding that engineers were at "the very place" the dam collapsed 24 hours before the tragedy. Said he: "It is not fair to say that this particular dam was not properly monitored. In fact, the gauge reading is done at least twice a day and during the rainy season, we read the gauge three to four times a day. What we suspect to be the main cause of this problem is piping due to termite activities."

Whatever the cause of the collapsed dam is, the lesson of the tragedy appears to have been well-taught and rather learnt, the hard way. The choice before the government, said one engineer last week, is "either to repair, maintain and monitor the behaviour of the dams or face the bitter consequences." That is a choice between life and death.

HIS EXCELLENCY THE FARMER

Friday. Another Friday. A convoy of police and military escorts lined the main entrance into the River State Government House ready to speed away with Governor Fidelis Oyakhilome. Half a kilimotre away, at the centre of the Port Harcourt temporary stadium, two Air Force and one Aero Contractors helicopters were standing by. A dozen policemen and half a dozen pilots patrolled the lush lawn patiently.

A governor's aide scampered between the Government House and the stadium and confirmed to the governor that everything was set. The next minute, the governor, accompanied by Agriculture Commissioner, Edward Spiff, emerged from his second floor office, smart in his farming dress, khaki trousers tucked into a knee-high black rain boots. The schedule looked tight. Six farms in seven hours. No ceremonies. No pleasantries. Business.

Same briskness at the temporary stadium. The helicopters whirled into a roaring sound and made a vertical rise into the air as the pilots pulled their airscrew. Off to the farm, with the governor and this *Newswatch* reporter by his side.

Oyakhilome – farmer cum governor of Rivers State - has for the past six months spent every Friday (sometimes going back on Saturday) supervising the 2,600 hectares "School-To-Land" programme, designed to boost food production in the State with the use of jobless secondary school leavers.

Said Boniface Dappa, 52, school headmaster and father of one of the young farmers: "His presence here every weekend is an added motivation, not only to the young farmers but also to us elders. Now everybody wants to own a farm."

Each farm has three palour-size helipads (cemented landing spot for helicopters). At Iriebe farm, where more than 250 hectares have been cultivated and 112 hectares of maize is being harvested, the helicopters circle the farm and perched on the helipads. The governor jumped out, followed by his aides. Some young farmers smiled and waved to the governor from their plots. The farm manager, S.B. Giadom, approached the governor from a small hut. The governor called him by his first name: "How is the harvester doing, Sam? Is it functioning?" Without waiting for a reply he said: "Let's go and see it. Let's see how it works."

Harvesting of maize seems to pose the greatest challenge to the farms at the moment. The land area under maize cultivation at Iriebe is 112 hectares, about 280 standard football field. The 146 farmers working at Iriebe cannot cope with harvesting. Only a few weeks ago, the CFAO donated one single-row harvester to the School-To-Land Authority (STLA), but nobody at the farm seems to know what to do with it.

The general manager of the STLA, Domonyo Douglas, a former lecturer in agriculture at the Port Harcourt University of Science and Technology, told *Newswatch* he had sent for some CFAO technicians to demonstrate how the harvester works. Meanwhile, a young man who tried to operate the harvester ended up spraying the maize into the bush.

"I am not happy. We cannot afford to waste this maize," said the governor. Two decisions were taken on the spot. "Farm manager, get the village women as many as you need. Pay each of them N3.00 a day and make sure all the maize is harvested as soon as possible," the governor instructed. "Don't wait. Start today," he said.

Farm engineer, Rowland Woko, 28, a 1983 graduate of Port Harcourt University of Science and Technology, did not quite seem to be familiar with the harvester. The governor advised him to "try and couple a trailer to the harvester" so that harvested maize did waste anymore.

On the pineapple plot, the man in charge seemed to have made no progress beyond what the governor saw the previous week. "Why. For God's sake, is this man not supervised?" He queried, turning attention to STLA general manager and Iriebe farm manager.

Work on the cultivation of cassava and okro on the farm has progressed rapidly. So far, 40 hectares (100 football fields) of cassava and five hectares (12.5 football fields) of okro have been cultivated. Clearing and tilling of additional area is going on steadily.

At Bunu-Tai farm, where 308 hectares are under cultivation, the problem again is excess maize, begging to be harvested. Though harvesting is progressing at a faster rate, there is the problem of evacuation of the harvested stock. The giant cribs constructed by the farmers were being filled up. "Good job, boys," the governor praised the young farmers. "Welcome sir," they chorused. The governor instructed that a tipper be permanently attached to the farm to ease evacuation of the harvest.

Relationship between the farmers and government officials is very cordial, and, close to being personal. Said an excited farmer: "We don't fear them (the governor and the commissioner), we respect them." Interrupted a female farmer: "We love them, too." The group burst into a loud laughter.

The governor drove round the farm in a Peugeot 504, with the commissioner, accompanied by aides and farm officials. He inspected the newly cultivated yam, cassava and potato plots. On return, he asked for the farm register. Three farmers were absent. "Henceforth, anybody absent for more than three days in a month will be dismissed and replaced immediately," directed the governor.

Replacement is easy. A staggering 22,000 school leavers applied for participation in the programme. A little over a thousand got in and 12,000 are still on the waiting list, eagerly awaiting call-up.

At the Bunu-Tai farm mobile clinic, a young farmer with a black eye was being attended to by nurses. "What happened to your eyes?" the governor asked, with his right hand on the boy's shoulders. As the boy tried to explain, the governor turned to the nurse: "I hope it's not serious?" "No sir," the two nurses replied. "Don't worry, you'll be all right soon," he told the injured farmer, patting him on the back. "Can I get two tablets of Panadol?" he requested. A glass of water accompanied the tablets.

Three newly constructed silos at Kpaa farm are prominent from the air. They have a capacity for 600 tonnes of grains. In anticipation of the bumper harvest, many storage facilities have been contemplated. So far, the total capacity of silos contracted is

2,600 tonnes (one tonne is about the size of a Peugeot 404 pick-up van).

The land area so far cultivated at Kpaa is 187 hectares. Crops planted include maize, cassava and cowpea. Kpaa farm is one of the collection centres where harvest in transit can be dried and stored.

However, young farmers at Kpaa farm, just like in other farms, have a major problem: lack of accommodation. This has dampened their enthusiasm. Said Sampson Loolo, 22, an ex-student of the Birabi Memorial Grammar School, Bori: "If the government can provide accommodation for us, half our problems would be solved."

In an interview with *Newswatch,* the STLA general manager conceded that "our farmers right now are having very hard times, but we try to explain to them that with time, things will be alright." However, Spiff is taking up the problem 'very seriously." He told *Newswatch:* "We are urgently going to provide a dormitory-type accommodation for them." The government opted for the dormitory-type accommodation so that "when the farmers develop and build their houses, we can convert the dormitories into warehouses."

The main reward for the farmers as at now is a monthly stipend of a hundred naira each. But as from next year, each farmer's income will depend on what he produces. Each farmer is allocated a plot of four hectares. It is left for him to produce as much as he can with the help of government input. During harvest, the marketing division of the STLA sells off the produce and pays 85 percent of the money to the farmer's account. Government removes 15 percent – three percent goes to the farm supervisors, while 12 percent is used to defray government expenditure on stipends, training and buying input for the farmers. The commissioner said: "We are not employing them as such, we are creating farmers."

The STLA officials put the harvest per hectare of maize at about three tonnes and estimated that a farmer could make a profit of more than N3,000 in two months. "That is being on the modest side," said an official.

The impact of the STL programme is already being felt in Port Harcourt and Obigbo markets. The STLA maize, which sells at 12 cups a naira, has forced down the price of the commodity in the neighbourhood. In Obigbo market, Madam Amaechi said: "We were selling five-six cups for a naira. We have too much maize in the market now." In Mile 1 Market, Port Harcourt, the story is the same.

The government has moved in to ensure that wastage is minimized. An agricultural commodity committee headed by the commissioner has been set up to buy off excess commodity from local farmers. "If we don't buy off the surplus, they will be discouraged to plant next season," said the commissioner. Government is also planning for food processing factories and the immediate one in mind is gari making factories.

Many people visiting the STL farms for the first time cannot fail to be fascinated by the extent the Rivers State government has gone in tackling the food problem. Said a university professor at Buna-Tai farm: "This is a dream come true."

In an interview with *Newswatch*, after going round the farms, Governor Oyakhilome said: "Our ambition is to supply sufficient food not only to Rivers State, but to other States which for one reason or the other cannot help themselves. If we continue at the rate we are going now, we will achieve our target."

TRAGEDY IN THE CREEK

The riverine people of Nembe, Rivers State, love to begin a journey on Sundays because they hope to have the prayers of the church to preserve all who travel by water. But this fateful Sunday, tragedy came at high tide. Two wooden engine boats: *MV Nembe* and *MV Asfi* collided in broad daylight. *MV Nembe* split into two and sank. Men, women and mostly school children, returning from holidays in Port Harcourt, were thrown into the deep blue sea. Bags of cement, garri, cassava and yams and both pieces of the dilapidated boat, went down to the bottom of the sea. It was a nightmare.

George Fente, a giant of a man, had five children in the boat. Barely three hours before, Fente, oblivious of the looming disaster, had herded his wards into the boat. He wished them farewell. It was the last farewell to two of the kids: Tionpre, 7 and Olali, 5.

Fente's kids were not alone. Ebinyo Amaegbe, 17, also died. So did her sister, Biriyai, 6. They were children of Amaegbe Eremienyo Ogbodo VII, the Amanyanabo of Bessambiri, Nembe.

Ebinyo's story was heart breaking. Peter Brew, a teacher at

Government Girls Secondary School, Nembe said that Ebinyo had first swum to safety. But her younger sister, Biriyai, could not. Weeping profusely and unable to withstand the sight of her drowning sister, she suddenly plunged back into the sea. Together with Biriyai, she was swept away. Fate wrote her a most frightening tragedy and she played it beautifully.

Help was impossible. No communications. No law enforcement agents. The marine police at Degama was too far to hear, not to talk of help.

Seriba, 15, one of Fente's surviving daughters, cried her way back to Port Harcourt to meet her father. Fente grabbed a flying boat, hired two divers and got the assistance of two friends. Off to Sansankiri the zone of death. Diving desperately into the sea, Fente's team picked up the body of Biriyai. The little beauty was trapped between two broken wood.

Night came. Fente returned to Port Harcourt with his team, disconsolate. "There was nothing we could do in the dark, more so, when the current was getting very swift," Fente said. Early morning the next day, the broken-hearted man was back diving deep into the sea. Ebinyo's body was soon to be picked up by Fente. She had no drowning marks to show. She was a picture of a sleeping cherub. Three days after the accident on September 9, Fente found his daughter Tionpre and later, his son Olali. What a pain for one man to endure?

But Fente, the Nembes and their neighbours are trying hard to put behind them the agony of the mid-sea disaster. But what they may not be able to put behind them immediately is their perennial problem of transportation. Said Joseph Dambo, a prominent chief of Nembe: "It is extremely difficult and sometimes very dangerous for us to travel to or from our homes because there are no good boats and we have no road except the sea."

There are no government boats to Nembe. The private transporters are poorly operated and unsupervised. The *MV Nembe*, which sank rapidly after the collision, is said to have carried about 500 bags of cement, several bags of gari, yams and other food items, in addition to an unspecified number of passengers. For a six-year-old wooden boat powered by a 335-horse-power Yamaha engine, the boat carried more load than was safe for it.

Then, there is a great deal of indiscipline among operators. Said Brew, "there is hardly any control in that boat (*MV Asfi).* Passengers have always complained about the reckless attitude of the operators. Though there is a captain, you won't know who is actually in control." Beside, operators have no manifest. In cases of accident just like the one of September 7, it is difficult to say precisely how many people died or survived.

It is the place of the marine police at Degama, say some travellers, to ensure that safety regulations are adhered to. But according to operators, policemen are only interested in taking bribes, "whether we comply with regulations or not." Said Robert Nyalambofa: "we call it toll gate," a euphemism for bribe. "The police just have to get it, and what we do is increase our load so as to cover the "toll gate."

There are other lapses. The *MV Asfi,* for instance, was built for an in-board engine. But it has been operating with an out-board Yamaha engine. That makes it virtually impossible for the operator to have a clear view of his route through the creek. At night when most journeys are undertaken, the boats have no lights except kerosene lanterns, and sometimes small torch lights.

The creek itself is made of numerous narrow and sharp

bends which are veritable death trap for travellers. Dambo, a retired permanent secretary, said the sharp bends have been responsible for previous accidents, one of which occurred in 1984. Nyalambofa accused the State government of paying deaf ears to the entire transportation problem of the riverine areas. "Since ex-governor Diette Spiff left office, other governors and commissioners go to Nembe with helicopters. They don't know and can't understand our problems," Nyalambofa said.

But the new Rivers State Governor Anthony Ukpo said he is quite determined to give the problem a fight. The ministry of works and transport, according to Ukpo, has been instructed to repair all its unserviceable boats for Nembe and other routes. "I am determined that by the time I complete my assignment here, transportation problem for the riverine communities would be sufficiently minimized," he told *Newswatch.*

One way Ukpo may be able to reduce the problem, as Dambo said, is to find out "what went wrong with the Port Harcourt-Yenegua-Koko-Nembe federal road project, for which contract was awarded in the late 70's, at the same time as the Ibadan-Lagos express road." This nightmare just has to stop.

MISSION TO IKO

The Nigeria Airways fight WT 150 did a fast one to Calabar under an hour. In another 90 minutes, the reporter was basking in the warmth of Eket, a little town south east of Calabar, his brand new "adire" jumper, flapping in the soft Eket breeze, whetting his appetite for a calm country life.

"This is where you'll need a cyclist to take you to Iko," the taxi driver announced as he stepped on the brakes of his rickety Peugeot 404 wagon, throwing the passengers off their seats.

Suddenly, a flock of motor cyclists descended on the itinerant journalist, literally pulling him out of the taxi. As he announced his destination, he saw surprise on their faces. One after the other, they sighed and went back atop their cranky motor-bikes, parked some metres away. He told them once again, "I want to charter a motor-bike." Nobody seemed to care. At last someone did, "Ah, you can't get to that place, in this rainy season," said the man sympathetically. Queried another cyclist emerging from a near-by palm wine bar, "Are you from that kind of place?" The journalist was embarrassed but he did not show it. He only smiled, not knowing what to say. The honeymoon is over, he thought. Strange! This is a crude oil-rich hamlet nobody wants to go!

Ten minutes. Twenty minutes, there was no cyclist willing to go his direction. Someone said he might be lucky to find one. So the wait continued. Another 10 minutes, one cyclist arrived and said he would charge N20.00 to a village called Okoroete, less than five kilometres away. From there you can get a canoe to Okoro Mbokho, where somebody can direct you to Iko," he tried to explain reluctantly. Still under-estimating the condition of the road, he agreed to pay the amount the cyclist demanded.

"Remove your shoes, sir. Roll up your trousers," the cyclist said in a commanding tone. "No. never mind" the reporter replied. Perched on the back of the Suzuki 100 clutching a little bag containing a tape recorder and some writing materials, the reporter and the cyclist zoomed off, sprightly acknowledging cheers from a surprised crowd at the road junction.

Behind and in front of them, a thick yawning forest made contact with the winding muddy pathway. Not a human being was found. The thought of cancelling the trip flashed on his mind, again and again. He knew he was embarking on a great risk.

There were many more rivers to cross, he counted twelve in all. But at each point the cyclist now more friendly allowed him to wade through the "rivers" on his feet. When the water was at chest level, he would raise his hands to the high heavens clutching firmly his small baggage of tape recorder, shoes and notebook.

The motor-cycle? Always submerged. But miraculously, a change of plug and a little pushing always did the magic. The reporter wondered why the cyclist ever agreed to make the trip. He thought he should double his fee or rather he should never have tried the trip. Finally, they arrived at Okoroete, the long expected canoe point. There was a small school, a Catholic church, a small market and some mud walled houses around the market place. There were about 23 people in the market at the time.

Just at this time, the reporter remembered the saying of the wise: To travel through the world, it is necessary to have the mouth of a hog, the legs of a stag, the eyes of a falcon, the ears of an ass, the shoulders of a camel, the face of an ape, and a satchel full of money and patience.

A tiny canoe, as deep as a flat plate and paddled by a 10-year-old little girl, ferried him across the river. He was her only passenger. She gave him a small calabash basin. What for? His duty was to fight back and scoop out the water flushing into the canoe violently, as she meandered her way along the creek. Like the cyclist, she was simply ingenious. For this the reporter paid her fifty kobo instead of twenty and she smiled, uttering something in Andoni language, which sounded like "Thank you, sir."

Wet and drab as a sea duck, the reporter, staggered his way up the next village called Okoro Mbokho, asking for the road to Iko. Two boys accompanied him across swamps and swathes, up to a diversion leading to Iko. The swampy pathway was like the dreamland – desolate, dreary and forlorn.

The nightmare came. A heavy rainfall. The flood came surging from left and right. Some plank bridges were washed off. Not a human being nor a shelter. Involuntarily, he broke into a race along the slippery pathway. The sounding cataract haunted him like a devil. The swaying mangrove trees. The deep and gloomy forest. The running flood of lonely dirty water. Their colours and their forms were to him a perfect graveyard of an unbridled adventure.

Running and stumbling, he followed the pathway with fear and dread. He turned around once and twice, and suddenly a flock of sheep passed by rushing one after the other, along the narrow path, then the sound of cockcrow and bees murmuring on top of palm-wine trees. Soon to follow were sheets or rusty and ramshackle roofs. Here is Iko. A church signboard confirmed it.

Like Mungo Park, "I saw with infinite pleasure, the great object of my mission." Some twelve to eighteen oil wells gushing with 9,000 barrels a day. Hundreds of pipelines flushing the oil to Port Harcourt's Shell terminal. But such a wretched village. So poor and full of sick old people. Not a road. Not even a market. The village head, Mbong Ekperikpe, spoke of neglect. He spoke of suffering, diseases and deaths, his house leaking profusely under the rain.

Three hours with Iko village council where the adventurous reporter had some cups of palm-wine to drown his woes. Later he set back along the same route. The joy of being in Iko overwhelmed the dread of a thick swampy forest ahead of him. The true success was the labour. As he lay down in his hotel room in Eket, thoughts of Iko swept his mind. Iko, that wretched oil-rich village. That shady village of crude oil and palm trees. Iko, a reporter's nightmare, the oil man's goldmine.

KILLING THE GOOSE

In the hot afternoon sun of December 5, 1988, five men arrived Iko, a small, oil-rich but poverty-stricken village on the far eastern flanks of Akwa Ibom State. They were drenched in their own sweat and wore the tired looks of people who had been wrestling all day. They had come by sea with a speed boat – the only alternative means of reaching the village from Uyo, the State capital. The only road linking the two places is rough, narrow and impassable all year round. At least there are 12 rivers to cross on that treacherous tract across swamp and swatches. Some rivers are linked to the land only by a wooden plank, just wide enough to accommodate the tyres of one motor-cycle at a time.

But the men with a speed boat are the privileged members of the Akwa Ibom State committee on the use of the state's share of the 1.5 percent federal oil revenue for tackling ecological problems in the neglected oil-producing areas of Nigeria. They met a small and unenthusiastic welcoming crowd of villagers. The villagers, 40 in number, were led by Allison Mbong, a reverend gentleman and supervisory councilor representing Eastern

Obolo (which includes Iko) in Ikot Abasi local government area. Mbong stepped out of the crowd, looked to his left and right, his unsmiling face betraying the subdued anger of Iko people, whose soil has produced at least 9,000 barrels of crude oil per day since 1973 but have benefitted from no basic amenities of any sort.

"We are a greatly distressed people...and we are very angry," he said, clearing his throat to ensure that the visitors heard him properly, as he read through his three-page prepared speech. "The discovery of oil in our village has caused great sorrow and damage to our land and people... our water has been polluted and rendered undrinkable while fishing, our main occupation and sources of income is no more."

The bitter experience of the Iko people is the lot of virtually all oil-producing areas in Nigeria. For the people of these villages, the discovery of oil is a curse. It means for them poverty, hunger and disease inflicted by the immense ecological damage done through many years of oil exploration and scandalous neglect. Although their land had produced this commodity of immense economic value, not much has been done to compensate them for the damage to their environment and the health hazards to which pollution of stream waters – their only source of drinkable water – has permanently exposed them.

In Eruemukohwarien, one of the villages in Bendel State where oil was first discovered, the story is that of untold anguish for the people. They have been dispossessed of their farmlands and little or no compensation paid them. Farmlands, too, have lost their fertility and farming, hitherto a lucrative occupation, has become a fruitless gamble, leaving in its trail hunger and poverty. Eko Idolor, a 55-year-old farmer in the village, who has witnessed all the damage which oil prospecting and exploration has done to the village said the villager's ordeal began many years ago with the arrival of Shell Oil Company in the area. Shell, he said, "took over farmlands and paid compensation only for the crops and not for the land acquired." Idolor said farmers whose farmlands were taken without adequate compensation were persuaded not to take up the matter against the company with the argument that the activities of the company could be of immense benefit to them and their children. That hope, he argued, has also not materialized. "Shell has not done a single thing for this village," he said, the initial smile on his face giving way to the angry countenance of a man in anguish. He had hardly finished making the statement when he remembered one of the efforts of Shell to provide potable water to the community. "I know they dug a borehole," he said, pointing in the direction of what, to date, has been the only attempt by the company to provide water in the area, "but even that borehole has not produced water."

The stalled water project is all the patronage that Eruemukohwarien village has got from Shell. The town now has electric power supply, but Idolor said the facility was provided by the government and not by Shell. He said the hope that Shell would employ indigenes of the village has also been dashed. "They don't give us jobs in the company. As for contracts, they prefer to deal with non-indigenes." There is no hospital in the village and the nearest hospital to the village is in Ughelli – about 15 kilometres away.

Although oil-producing areas of Nigeria have long served faithfully as the sources of Nigeria's wealth, with revenues used in financing the country's numerous social facilities such as airports, expressways, high rise buildings and seaports, these villages have remained the blind spot of Nigeria's socio-economic development lenses. Good roads, pipe-borne water and health facilities remain the lofty but elusive dreams of Nigerians in these villages. Their lot has been unmitigated suffering, bare-faced deprivation and dispossession, in the face of opulence and squandering of the petrodollars from these communities.

In Ekpan, a village on the outskirts of Warri where one of Nigeria's biggest refineries is located, oil has brought a lot of hardship too to the people. Bank Uruejoma, a retired nurse who is now a patent medicine dealer in the village told *Newswatch* that since the establishment of the refinery, life has become extremely difficult for farmers. "We have lost our farmlands to government while what remains under our control now behaves in a way we cannot understand." He explained: "Before our farmlands were polluted, a small plot of cassava farm was enough to feed one family for the whole year. Today, it is no longer so. You need to cultivate several plots to get a little." He said land pollution through oil prospecting, exploration and refining was responsible for this. Uruejoma recalled with a deep feeling of nostalgia, his days as a youth when he accompanied his mother and grandmother to the farm. "Then, even as a seven-year-old boy, I could only carry one tuber of yam home because the yams were always long and fat." But today, he explained, activities of oil companies and the consequent pollution have rendered the land infertile, while waste disposal into the rivers has ruined aquatic lives and turned fishermen into roadside traders and hawkers.

But, unlike Erumukohwarien, the case of Ekpan is not that of total neglect. The village enjoys two main social amenities – electricity and tarred roads, linking it to other parts of the country. The villagers' grudge is against the Nigerian National Petroleum Corporation, NNPC, which acquired their land about 12 years ago for the establishment of the Warri refinery and paid compensation only for the crops and not for the land. Uruejoma, one of those whose land was acquired told *Newswatch* that about N8 million was being claimed for the land by the villagers and that a suit was already in court to compel the refinery to pay. Another complaint of the villagers is the non-employment of qualified indigenes. Uruejoma accused the NNPC's personnel department of "manipulating staff recruitment for the refinery in favour of outsiders."

James Utuedor, a farmer, said the oil companies "have not done enough for the people." Utuedor who is also one of those whose land was taken over for the refinery, said he got no compensation. "I didn't get a kobo for my land and I don't know if they paid anyone else'. Betty Mugidi, his 30-year-old daughter, and housewife is also angry with Shell, NNPC and the Warri Refinery. She argued that facilities being enjoyed by Ekpan villages were provided by government and not NNPC or any other oil company. "What the oil companies should have done for us is to employ our children and that's what they are not doing." Mugidi also spoke of the damage done to the environment: "The cassava we harvest now are unhealthy and are hardly bigger than my fingers." She also said wildlife has been adversely affected. "Noise from the refinery has driven animals which hitherto provided a ready source of protein for the villagers farther into the forest."

Iko in Akwa Ibom State is perhaps, one of the worst cases of neglect. It is bereft of every basic amenity, in spite of 12 oil wells in its backyard. The discovery of oil in the village has not only destroyed its natural source of livelihood, it has ruined whatever gains it had earned from its early contact with missionaries who founded the Qua Iboe Church in Nigeria. In July 1987, a group of

Iko youths, piqued by the silting of fishing creeks by workers of the Shell Oil Company, embarked on a demonstration to protest what Mbong said was "a deprivation of the people's legitimate sources of livelihood." *Newswatch* heard that policemen were quickly dispatched to the village to contain the demonstrations. In the ensuing conflict, 38 houses belonging to the villagers were burnt while properties were looted; women were assaulted and beaten by the police. Many of the villagers whose homes were burnt are still homeless today. The bare sandy banks of the Qua Iboe River on which the village is located was still like a refugee camp in a war-devastated area a few weeks ago when *Newswatch* visited the village. The villagers, unable to build new homes, have turned the river banks into a place of abode.

The Megbede, Ebocha and Omoku communities in Ahoada LGA in Rivers State are not left out in this tale of woes. Their lot has been oil spillages and devastating ecological damages with attendant consequences for agriculture, fishing and the entire economic life of the people. In virtually all the oil-producing areas in Rivers, Bendel and Akwa Ibom States, pollution and physical devastation of the environment by oil spillages are routine. Somewhere in Mgbede, two square kilometres of land has been completely polluted in one of the worst oil spillages in the area.

Gas flaring is another major source of health hazards in oil-producing and refining areas. Apart from physical destruction to plants around the flaring areas, thick soot is deposited on roofs of neighbouring villages. Whenever it rains, the soot is washed off and the black ink-like water running down the roofs is believed to contain chemicals which adversely affect the fertility of the soil. John Ijeh, a roadside trader in Mgbede said the poverty and hunger situation in these villages are attributable to this phenomenon. "Chemicals have ruined our lands and the rivers," he said.

But how guilty are the oil companies? *Newswatch* efforts to talk to some of the companies met a brickwall. In Warri, officials of Shell gave *Newswatch* some brochures which dealt with the company's efforts to reduce pollution and the effects of oil spillages on rural life. Some of the write ups in the brochure contested the villagers' charges of non-payment for land acquisition. "It is an offence under section 98 of the minerals act of 1988," argued one of the Shell's brochures, "for a land owner to refuse the use of his land required for exploration, prospecting or mining purposes," and that "rates of compensation payable for crops and trees damaged or affected by oil are determined after a thorough survey." The company argued that its rates have been "fair and generous and have been defended before law courts, NNPC and state governments." It also said under the land use decree, control of land was vested on the governor of a state and not in any individual, which is to say that no individual has legitimate claim to any land anywhere and can therefore claim compensation for it.

The federal government, on its part, has tried to address the problem of oil-producing areas with the special allocation of 1.5 percent of its revenue to the areas. What remains is for the impact of this allocation to be felt by the people in these areas. In Iko, as in many of the oil-producing areas, the impact of this and other welfare programmes of oil companies are yet to be felt. This is the burden of the federal government and oil companies must shoulder, and fast, before the situation goes out of hand.

IN THE VALLEY OF FEAR

Victor Mugabo, crack reporter of a leading Pan-African magazine was a nervous wreck, as he sat at the departure hall of the Murtala Muhammed Airport, Ikeja, Lagos, waiting for a 45-minute flight to Port Harcourt. His eyes were bloodshot and his voice shook as he tried to pick up discussions with two other reporters. Unable to say much, he recoiled into himself, chain-smoking and gulping some more beer from a tall, white glass by his side. "Please give me another bottle of beer," he said nervously to the waiter, mopping the gathering beads of sweat from his forehead.

Among his peers, Mugabo has a reputation as a tough-minded reporter. But Mugabo is scared stiff of flying. "No I can't stand it. It's hell. I'm better today because I'm travelling at short notice. If my editor had told me I would be travelling in three days' time by air, I would be terribly sick and depressed for the rest of the days leading to the journey," he said, as he lit another stick of cigarette. After his assignment at Port Harcourt, Mugabo did the unbelievable. He opted for the nine-hour journey by road rather than the 45-minute flight to Lagos.

For Joshiah Ellam, a retired army captain who is now a pastor in a Pentecostal church, waiting for a flight to be called is like the last few minutes before firing squad. "To me, the plane is a flying coffin," he said shivering with the mere thought of boarding a flight. On a recent flight from Calabar he sat in the aircraft stiff, his eyes tightly closed as the aircraft gathered speed for take-off. Every time the plane did a variation of route or speed he would hurriedly ask someone what was happening. If an air-hostess went into the cockpit, he was convinced something was wrong. When the plane started to lose height, in preparation for landing, he was 'sure the thing was about to crash." And eventually when the aircraft landed with that horrible noise, "I was cocksure the whole damn thing had finally exploded," he said. During his days in the army, he said, his colleagues never told him he was due to fly until the morning prior to take-off, otherwise, "I would have deserted."

Psychotherapists call this morbid fear of flying aerophobia. Phobia is not restricted to flying alone. One can have a phobia about almost anything from snakes to strings. Among well-known and treated phobias are agoraphobia (fear of open space), aquaphobia (fear of water), claustrophobia (fear of closed or tight places), pyrophobia (fear of fire), ochlophobia (fear of crowd), nyctophobia (fear of darkness) and tocophobia (fear of childbirth). There are even such odd and rare phobias as bibliophobia (fear of books), didaskaleinophobia (fear of school), pogonophobia (fear of shadow), gamophobia (fear of marriage), gynophobia (fear of women), parthenophobia (fear of young girls), genephobia (fear of sex), etc. The sensation experienced in all kinds of phobias, according to psychotherapists, is virtually the same:

pounding of heart, dizziness, palpitation, sweating and a feeling that something terrible is about to happen.

In Britain alone, it is estimated that there are 4.5 million phobics, 300,000 of whom are agoraphobics. Joy Melville has documented the experiences of some phobics in her book *Phobias samplers*: "Seeing a spider (arachnophobia) makes me rigid with fear, hot, trembling and dizzy. My tummy drops, I occasionally pass water, my heartbeat increases tremendously, I sweat, and while the spider keeps still I am unable to move. I just stand there, sobbing and shaking unaware of where I am until I faint." "Mine is churches," said another phobic, "I even have nightmares about them. I feel dizzy just sighting a church and I can faint if I get inside. Nothing will stop me being frightened about them."

A woman who has a phobia about someone touching her neck says she screams in terror "if my husband mistakenly puts his hand on my neck, in fun." Another woman who has a phobia about traffic lights: "I cannot move one foot before the other. I would rather go the longer way around to avoid them." Yet another woman cannot stand a mass of pips. "I can't cut open a melon, tomatoes, pepper or marrows, without my skin crawling with ghost bumps and the knife falling off my hand. I wouldn't go near the kitchen for days." A woman whose seven-years old girl has a horror of buttons decided to take her to the doctor. "We go through tears and recrimination every time she has to wear a buttoned garment."

In Nigeria, phobia is grossly misunderstood and sometimes, misinterpreted. It is often traced to *juju* or charms. A junior staff of Cadbury Nigeria Limited, Ikeja, who usually experiences uncontrolled sweating and palpitation whenever he enters a bus or stays at crowded places once went home to Bendel State to consult an oracle. He was asked to make sacrifices which he did. It did not help him, of course. Eventually, he decided to see a doctor in Lagos who diagnosed his problem as ochlophobia (irrational fear of crowd). He was referred to a psychotherapist at Yaba Psychiatric hospital and before long, he overcame his phobia. Another man who always complains that his office was stuffy even though his air conditioner was functioning well came to the conclusion that he was haunted by witchcraft. He would abandon his cozy office to stay with junior workers in the general office. Eventually, he was persuaded to see a doctor who got his claustrophobia cured.

Phobias are serious illnesses to the extent that they place a burden on sufferers and curtail their activities. Phobias are known to have wrecked careers, marriages and homes, because of the irrational fear of sufferers to do what is perfectly normal. Sonny – Ilechukwu, consultant psychiatrist at the Yaba psychiatric hospital, says the problem is complicated in developing countries like Nigeria because of the stigma the society attaches to seeking psychiatric help. "An American will more freely visit a psychiatrist on any problem that is emotionally stressful than a Nigerian."

The knowledge of how a phobia starts, says Ilechukwu, governs the treatment and explains why there are radically different approaches to treating phobics. However, phobia therapists agree on four main techniques of treatment namely desensitization, implosion, modeling and group therapy. The four revolve around behavioural and analytical instructions on how to control peculiar anxieties and fears. And those who know best how to give such instructions are psychotherapists and hypnotherapists.

WHO OWNS THE LAND?

For some moments, the old man stood, frightened and visibly shaken. Hamza Ibrahim, 65, the district head of Sade, Bauchi State, had sufficient cause to be alarmed. He had just received a disturbing message from Ajiyana Fika, the district head of Fika, Pokistum, Bornu State. "We are going to attack Sade district," the message said, "if we see any Sade farmer on our farmland. The farmland belongs to us. Tell your people to look for another farm."

A timely intervention that morning, March 25, 1985, by the local government headquarters at Darazo averted what could have been the seventh in a series of bloody border clashes between the two communities. "I think we have only agreed to stay in peace together as brothers of the same faith. But the problem has not been settled yet," Ibrahim said.

The problem of inter-state border disputes in Nigeria is not confined to Bauchi and Borno States alone. It is widespread, almost nationwide and by far more serious and intractable in other states than Bauchi and Borno. Clashes break out without a warning and are fought with automatic and sophisticated weapons, in a scenario of full-scale war. At Ikot Umo Essien, one of the border villages between Cross River State and Imo State, villagers were woken up one night, November 1986, to a torrent of machine gun shots. Hundreds of women and children ran into the bush, while their men, armed with charms, poisonous bows and arrows, machetes and all types of small arms, quickly mobilized for a counter-attack against their Onicha-Ngwa neighbours.

The battle lasted for hours. Some 30 people were reported killed and many more injured. The crisis intensified by the third day and transportation between Aba and Ikot Ekpene, the main link road between the two States, was paralyzed. A Mercedes Benz luxurious bus belonging to an Ikot Ekpene-based transporter, Simon Akpan Inyang, which was returning from Lagos, drove into an ambush at Onicha-Ngwa. The bus was burgled and destroyed beyond repairs by Onicha-Ngwa people looking for Ikot Umo Essien people. Rumours immediately spread that all the passengers were killed. But police sources told *Newswatch* that the driver and a conductor were the only persons in the bus. The passengers, who boarded the bus at Lagos were Aba-bound and had disembarked before the incident.

In retaliation, the Ikot Umo Essien side mounted several road blocks along the Ikot Ekpene/Ikot Umo Essien section of the Aba-Ikot Ekpene Road. According to eye witness account, they stopped all vehicles bearing Imo State registration numbers and severely beat up the passengers. Many of them managed to escape into the bush. It took the combined efforts and presence of Ibim Princewill and Amadi Ikwechegh, governors of Cross River and Imo states respectively, to enforce a "temporary ceasefire" so negotiations could begin.

But a few days into the negotiation, another fighting erupted. This time, it spread to other areas along the borders of the two States. It was particularly severe at Arochukwu/Ukwa-Ibom boundary. In two days of fierce fighting, eight persons were officially confirmed dead, while many more were placed on the danger list in various hospitals. At the same time, economic trees, farmlands and other property were damaged.

Reports of border clashes across the country show that the crisis is assuming a very dangerous and widespread dimension. For instance, Benue State has been fighting on five fronts with Plateau, Anambra, Bendel, Cross River and Gongola states. Cross River State fights regularly and fiercely with Benue, Imo and Anambra States. Apart from its clashes with Cross River and Anambra States, Imo State often takes on Rivers State over an oil-rich stretch of land near Ukwa. The clashes, in most cases, do not even respect religious or ethnic affinities. Communities in Oyo and Ondo States have been fighting at the Owena/Igbara-Oke border for several years over the ownership of a little parcel of farmland. Similarly, Imo and Anambra States have been waging a protracted war at Ohaozora/Isielu border; while Kano State takes on Borno and Bauchi States in an unrelenting effort to claim some fertile parcels of land.

In each case, the underlying factor which sparks off the fight has either been political, economic or both. Said Yakubu Hamza, Chairman, Darazo LGA of Bauchi: "Some traditional rulers want to expand their territories so that they can make money from tax collections. Others just fight to control a fertile parcel of land." Ekundayo Opaleye and Tunji Olurin, Military Governors of Ondo and Oyo States respectively, were told recently by community leaders in the border town of Owena that the Obokun LGA of Oyo State has not only been collecting taxes and other levies from their (Owena) villages, but it has been raiding their cocoa farms and seizing the crops.

In some cases, border disputes are struggles to belong or not to belong to a particular community or state. Such is the case of some communities in Abak LGA of Cross River State and Ukwa LGA of Imo State. Last January, parts of the Imo/Cross River States boundary were practically redrawn and three border villages in Ukwa and Arochukwu-Ohafia LGA were handed over to Cross River State in compliance with Decree 23 of 1985. But as soon as the handing-over ceremonies were concluded, the Ukwa people protested against their "forced merger" with Cross River State. They claimed that they had no cultural or linguistic affinity whatsoever with people in their "new" State. Said the chiefs of Ukwa in a protest letter to President Ibrahim Babangida: "The dismemberment of Ukwa community has become unprecedented in the annals of balkanization. This amounts to great injustices and does not augur well for the unity of this country. We humbly appeal to the president to review this truncation of Ukwa territory."

Warring communities never feel satisfied with government solutions to boundary disputes. The case of the dispute between Bendel and Benue States over Ake, a small fishing community, further illustrates this. Just after the Nasir Commission on boundary adjustment submitted its report in 1976, highly-placed government officials of Bendel origin leaked what they claimed was part of the report to Udochi community in Bendel to the effect that the panel had recommended that Ake belongs to Bendel. But when the government white paper on the report was released, Ake was placed in Benue State. Last year, John Inienger, Bendel State Governor, and David Jang, then governor of Benue State, met for three hours after a bloody clash at Ake and decided that the village should continue to be administered by Benue State in line with government decision on it. But the Udochi people alleged in a letter to Babangida last April that "a certain army officer from Idah, who was a member of the then Federal Executive Council, influenced the rejection, in 1976, of the recommendation by the Nasir Commission." Said the Udochi community in their protest letter to the president, after the Inienger-Jang settlement: "The governors claim that the long standing dispute has been resolved. Mr. President, nothing is settled until it is settled aright."

While government finds itself in a dilemma over the problem, tension continues to mount at each of the volatile borders. *Newswatch* learnt that some of the money realized in these areas from so-called community development appeal funds go for the purchase of arms and ammunitions. Cases of kidnapping and mysterious disappearances seem to be on the increase at the border villages fighting over land. Margaret Amoke and Nwoba Aliede were reported recently to have been kidnapped in their farms in the border villages of Ezzeagu and Isu where a dispute between Imo and Anambra States has been going on for years. Sunday Frank, a prominent businessman from Ikot Umo Essien, was also said to have been kidnapped last October and has since not been found. Frank's townsmen told *Newswatch* that their Onicha-Ngwa neighbours are "cannibals" and must have since made "a meat" of their illustrious son. Frank's disappearance led to a recent invasion of Onicha-Ngwa, where the corpse of a chief undergoing some burial rites was hijacked and taken to Ikot Umo Essien.

Police strength in most of the border villages has been beefed up as part of government effort to contain the crisis. In some States, quite some imaginative methods of solving the problem have been devised. Imo and Cross River States government, for instance, decided a few months ago to seize the "zone of death" from the Ikot Umo Essien and Onicha-Ngwa communities. The area, measuring one kilometer (half a kilometer from each side), stretches across the official border line and has been declared a neutral zone for both communities.

Chris Garuba, the governor of Bauchi State, said: "Knowing the causes of boundary disputes and what the natives want, what they are fighting for could help in finding a lasting solution to the problem. "A lasting solution, and a quick one for that matter, has become very pressing, given the cost of the clashes and the resources that are required to keep a temporary peace. Like a senior police officer at Ikot Ekpene said, the problem is becoming "a serious threat to the national security and government must see it that way."

SHOWERS OF SORROWS

It was a New Yam Festival day. The people of Igodor in Ogoja, Cross Rivers State, were in a celebratory mood. Huge balls of hot pounded yam filled mortars, bowls and calabashes, and more was being pounded. Men, women and children dashed about in frenzy, as the pulsating traditional rhythms filled the air, welcoming guests from far and near.

Suddenly, a dark clumsy cloud floated and settled gloomily over the village skies. Before the first traditional rites and sacrifices could be offered to the gods of fertility, the clouds broke and torrential rain descended on the village. Calamity had come knocking. The crowd dashed for shelter. And for good 48 hours, no one dared to set his foot outside, as the heavy and persistent rain led to flood which swept across Igodor and seven other villages in Nkum clan.

Two bridges across Aya River were submerged. Three kids and hundreds of domestic animals were swept off. Hundreds of hectares of rice and yam farmlands were washed away. Houses, schools, churches, clinics, roads and economic trees were destroyed. For another four weeks, the 5,000 inhabitants of the area were cut off from the rest of the world. Igodor, one of the largest producers of yam and rice in Nigeria, stood drenched, virtually immersed and submerged under water. As a result of the flood prices of yam and local rice took a leap. At least, in the last 10 years, this farming village has never seen such rainfall.

Rain, the heavenly showers generally regarded as the harbinger of good, is fast turning an agent of disaster, a paradoxical barrier to the desired self-sufficiency in food production, even in drought-prone Northern Nigerian cities. Across the country, the intensity of rainfall in the past few weeks have left massive destruction to life and property in its wake, aggravating in the process the encroachment rate of gulley, marine and sheet erosion.

Benue, Cross River, Rivers, Niger, Sokoto and Ondo states are some of the worst affected states. Perhaps, unknown to government and many Nigerians, is the severity of the disaster and the fact that many towns and villages in the country, stand a great risk of being completely buried by flood and erosion if a concerted effort is not made to combat the problem.

In Niger State alone, as the steady and heavy rainfalls continue to pound the roofs of villages for days, about 5,953 farmers have been thrown out of their homes and farms. In addition, a total of 65,366 acres of farmland cultivated with maize, guinea corn, yam, potatoes, cassava and vegetables have submerged by the flood. Though only four deaths have been officially acknowledged by government, the death toll is known to have been higher, as about 1,500 families in six local government areas (Luvun, Gbako, Chanchaga, Rafi, Agaie and Lapai) have been marooned by flood since mid-August. It is not possible to get in touch with some of these villages especially in Luvun, except by helicopter, used for dropping relief materials. Susan Suba, the chairman of the Niger State Emergency Relief Fund Committee told *Newswatch*, "the value of property destroyed so far is put conservatively at N20million.

The situation in Niger State which is believed to be aggravated by additional release of excess water from the Shiroro hydro-electric dam, has defied meager relief efforts and resources of Niger State government. As at the time of going to press, the plea for aid sent to the Federal Government about eight weeks ago was yet to receive any response. *Newswatch's* reporters who went round four of the six local government areas by helicopter filed a stunning report of "grave disaster."

Governor David Mark told *Newswatch* that he first dispatched danger signals to Lagos on August 23. The governor followed up with other SOS signals on August 25 and 26 and then a personal visit to Lagos to report the situation. Nothing happened. Said governor Mark in an angry tone: "It is most surprising that it has taken Lagos so much time to react. Honestly, the way Lagos is reacting and the speed with which it is reacting tends to give the impression that this country cannot respond to or withstand any disaster. Imagine, since August 21, we reported the disaster and today, October 8, nothing has been heard from Lagos."

So far the State's Emergency Relief Committee has been able to supply only 1,000 bags of rice, 600 bags of salt and 70 cartons of sugar to victims of flood in the State. Mark said the State needs at least N120 million "fast" to be able to rehabilitate the affected people. "We don't have even one-tenth of the resources required to solve the problem," the governor said.

Analysts say the rehabilitation programme for the flooded villages of Niger and Cross River States may require more than salt and sugar. Government officials agree. Said Michael Ogar, Cross River State Commissioner for Information and Chairman of the disaster relief committee, "the nature of relief needed by the affected farmers is not a token food supply. What is needed is the rehabilitation of their roads and bridges and the supply of farming equipment to help the farmers reactivate their farmlands." Chief Ujoko, the village head of Igodor, supported this view when he said "let them give small and special loan preference to all affected farmers. Something should be done to avoid the repeat occurrence of flood and expansion of gulleys."

The gulleys have been expanding in Ankpa, Benue State. Ankpa town, the headquarters of Ankpa local government area, is facing the danger of being buried by flood and erosion. A heavy rainfall a few weeks ago swept through the town like a hurricane, hauling away and sweeping clean the Ankpa town market. Everything was emptied into the nearby River Umabolo where owners later combed for their wares. A boy of 20, who attempted to rescue his articles, was swept along with the articles. His body was later picked up at the bank of the river. There are five major gulleys in the town named after streets: Idah, Market, Mosque, Zaria and Kano gulleys.

About seven houses have caved into the Idah gulley which has destroyed the whole Idah road. Many more houses are at the verge of collapsing into the gulley. The same gulley is threatening the Ankpa town stadium, standing only 20 meters away from the deep ravine. Contract for the reclamation and control of flood and erosion in Ankpa was awarded early in 1983 to Gyado-Steer Nigeria Limited. The contract was to be completed this year but not much has been done. Many inhabitants of the area believe the contractors are incapable of handling the job. Often, some of the completed portions of the project and heavy concrete slabs belonging to the contractors are swept away into the river. Said the district head, Onu of Ankpa, Halilu Sani: "The control project seems to worsen the situation. I do not understand what they (contractors) are doing. Government should take over the job and award it to a better contractor."

The sole administrator of Ankpa local government area, Daniel Agogo confirmed that "work is not progressing at the rate we like." However, the contractor's spokesman and site engineer, George Okpor blamed the delay on "frequent change of government, delay in payment of contract fees and frequent breakdown of Gboko cement factory," where the bulk of cement for reclamation work is obtained. But the engineer hoped the project will soon be completed.

There is no such hope in Cross River State where nearly all the local government areas are steadily being devastated by menacing marine, gulley and sheet erosion. More than 70 "very serious" erosion sites and a hundred relatively minor but expanding sites have been documented. The worst hit area is Uyo, the second largest town in Cross River State. There is no more trace of the popular Uyo Stadium, as that area of the town is completely buried, leaving behind a gnawing ravine, spanning over two kilometres.

The Uyo gulley is expanding in all directions and is currently at the verge of swallowing the Cross River State University, standing impossibly by the side of the yawning ravine. The Palmwine Club of the University changed its branch name to "Ilya Ravine," meaning Ravine branch of the Palmwine Club. The St.

Luke's Hospital at Uyo, the prisons, barracks and a nearby village, Ita Uruan, are just awaiting imminent collapse into the ravine.

Marine erosion has not spared Calabar, Ibeno, Oron and James Town. In Calabar, the University Teaching Hospital is seriously threatened. The National Museum at Oron is about to collapse. Said Martins Usenekong, the Cross River State deputy chief information officer, "What the marine erosion areas require is not just reclamation from the sea, but the construction of embankment to effectively check further devastation."

But the money to do that is not there. According to Ogar, the State needs about N70 million for erosion control in Calabar town alone and N300 million for the State. "Only the Federal Government can shoulder such responsibilities," the commissioner said.

Eunan Ishabor, a school principal and native of Igodor, wants the Federal Government to take a serious look at these problems especially as some of the most affected areas are the country's bread basket.

Academics and experts in flood and erosion sciences say the ultimate solution to flood and erosion problem lies in the attainment of zero run-off of rain water from each compound and farmland. Un-utilized areas of large compounds should be covered with grass or gardens. Rain water from roofs should be collected and piped into reservoirs for later use or disposed of through deep mud well or pits. According to Sunday Oyegoke, a hydrologist at the University of Lagos, "people should be discouraged, or at least made to realize the risk of setting up settlements within the flood range of a major river.

Governor Dan Archibong of Cross River State, a colonel in the Nigerian Army, has argued that "as a modern society, we have to prepare ourselves for emergencies. We have to guarantee succour to those afflicted and dispossessed through no fault of their own, particularly innocent women and children. We must ensure that in case of any disaster, we as a society will be amply equipped to give immediate relief to victims. This is an invaluable social insurance."

TURNING FARMS TO GOLDMINES

Bankole Oyeniyi, Kunle Olonoh and Ree Adintola returned to Nigeria four years ago after a 10-year sojourn in the United States. The three friends had received degrees in aeronautic engineering, aviation administration and business management respectively. They were gainfully employed in the United States before the urge to return home overwhelmed them.

But the situation they found on their return was frightening. Unemployment was (and is still) rampant, inflation was running wild and basic essential commodities had become a luxury. The situation was enough to send the three of them "checking out." But they did not. At Ibadan, where they lived, the trio took a hard look at the situation and decided to do something for themselves. They set up a farm. Banade Farms Limited at Iseyin, near Oyo, on a piece of land obtained through the Oyo State farm settlement programme. Banade Farms started with the cultivation of 10 hectares of improved yam seedling. But trouble struck in the midst of a bountiful harvest. The yield was more than the young men could cope with. Their efforts yielded more than 300,000 tubers for sale. But buyers were nowhere to be found.

Banade Farms was scared stiff, that it would be stuck with thousands of unsold yam. Advertisements were placed on the radio, television and newspapers, for buyers. Handbills and posters went out. "No order is too small, no order is too big', said one of the posters. When it still appeared there would be no market for the yams in the country, Banade Farms dispatched Oyeniyin to Florida, United States, in February this year, to look for a market.

Oyeniyin's trip was a success. He struck a deal with Florida State Department of Commerce and Agriculture to export the yam immediately. But, by the time Oyeniyin came back to Nigeria with the good news, the adverts had done the magic. Everything had sold out. Some buyers, such as the National Seed Service, NSS, Ibadan, bought as many as 50,000 tubers. The average price of a tuber was about 45 kobo.

Banade Farms' tremendous success was due mainly to the International Institute of Tropical Agriculture, IITA, Ibadan. Said Oyeniyin: "We are lucky to have IITA next door. They made improved seed yam available to us. This is what has made our efforts worthwhile and enjoyable."

Banade Farms is not alone in reaping fortunes from the IITA. The institute has turned farmlands into gold-mines for many others.

Gloria Adebambo, 30, has been nicknamed "wonder woman" or "cassava millionaire." When Adebambo came home from Ghana at the peak of that country's food crisis few years ago, she was virtually a nobody. Soon, she acquired some land in Ojoh village in Akoko-Edo Local Government Area of Bendel State. She quickly developed 300 hectares of cassava.

A year later, the harvest was beyond anything Adebambo ever imagined. Market for cassava in the area was already flooded. For her, there were no advertisements. Her ingenious solution was to establish a cassava factory. Her gari factory now turns out an average of 50,000kg a month and employs a permanent staff of 150. "When I started my cassava farm," Adebambo said, "I went to Ibadan to get good cassava cuttings from IITA. It was very successful and I decided to commercialize it'.

The IITA is one name that may not ring a bell, the way the IMF or OPEC would. But the institute could prove to be as important, if not more important in the economic life of Nigerians. One of 13 international agricultural research and training centres in the world, IITA has, in the past 19 years, directed its efforts towards improving crop yields and food production in the tropics.

In July 1967, when it was established, it became the first international agricultural research centre to be sited in Africa. Nigeria provided a 1,000-hectare piece of land in Ibadan for its headquarters. Principal funding came initially from Ford and Rockerfeller Foundations in the United States. Today, the list of IITA's sponsors has expanded considerably and now includes 24 donor countries, several international organizations such as the United Nations Development Programme, development banks, foundations and several other agencies. The funding is channeled through an international body called the Consultative Group of international Agricultural Research, CGIAR.

The IITA's main research effort or "mandate," as IITA scientists like to put it, is concentrated on the improvement of yield of such tropical crops as yam, cassava, cocoyam, sweet potato, rice, maize, cowpea and soyabean. The institute is also mandated to carry out research into how to improve the framing methods in the sub-saharan zones, so as to ensure efficient land use as well as a sustained production of food.

For experts, government officials and farmers world-wide, who have come in contact with the IITA, the institute has come a long way. The result of its research is set to change the entire picture of tropical agriculture. In Zaire, Tanzania, Malawi, Sierra Leone, Brizil, Columbia Cameroon and several other tropical countries, the IITA's improved seeds are revolutionizing farming. Said Lawrence Stifel, the newly-appointed director-general of the IITA: "We are entrusted with a mission that has profound human consequence. The most direct means of attacking poverty in Africa is to increase food production. The IITA is creating a stream of technologies that (should) give (farmers) the means to start a quiet revolution in the villages of Africa."

Indeed, most of the IITA's research breakthroughs seem quite incredible. The institute has bred several disease-resistant crops. But more remarkable is its development of various methods to boost crop yields about 10 times over. One of such crops is cassava.

Cassava is to Nigeria and other equatorial countries of the world what potato was to Europe in the 19th century. Experts say it is the most important carbohydrate for some 400 million people and accounts for 50 percent of the calories taken in by people living in the coastal zones of Africa. Conscious of this fact, the IITA started working on an improved variety of cassava that would mature faster, yield plenty, and contain none of cassava's dangerous acids such as cyanide, which have sometimes made cassava a "killer menu" for man (and animals alike).

It had been discovered by IITA scientists, way back in the 70's that cassava in the tropics was prone to many diseases such as mosaic disease. They also discovered that the disease was causing yield reduction of up to 60 percent and estimate annual losses of $1.8 billion. Scientists at the IITA led by Sang Ki Hahn, a South Korean, therefore directed their efforts towards developing improved cassava types. Many varieties were developed. Some were even proved to be useful in making bread.

But the most recent and dramatic result is the type called TMS 30555. Tests in Nigeria, Zaire and Malawi have proved that this variety is capable of yielding more than 69 tons per hectare as against four tons per hectare obtained from the traditional varieties. The Ikire community in Oyo State was so impressed by IITA cassava types that they bestowed a chieftancy title on Hahn and nicknamed some of the cassava types *Idileruwa* which means "the load is at the bottom" and *Isunikunkiyan*, which means "not only yam can be used for pounded yam."

One of those who first heard of the IITA's "wonder" cassava was Michael Olawuyi, 54, who hails from Ajibade village, some 10 kilometres from the manicured lawns and tidily cultivated fields of the IITA. A few years ago, he was cultivating less than two acres and barely surviving. But when he began using the IITA varieties, his output increase, and he extended the farm to 200 acres with a permanent staff of 20. He is planning to buy a tractor to boost output.

Olawuyi's townsman, Joseph Adediji, 58, another cassava farmer, earns his living selling the cassava sticks. The IITA cassava sticks are in high demand in Ibadan. Buyers come from as far as Gongola and Benue states with their trucks. Some 100 sticks sell for N50 in Ajibade village. Adediji told *Newswatch* that he makes as much as N16,000 a year from his 30 acres of cassava farm.

Unlike Olawuyi, Adediji doesn't look prosperous. His field clothes seem to be coming part and his black gym shoes do not have laces. But he is a highly prosperous farmer. "The management of the farm is made easy because the foliage of IITA cassava does not permit many weeds in the farm. So the farm virtually does not require any weeding," Adediji said through an interpreter.

Hahn, the man who was behind the development of the IITA cassava, also found the way to increase the yield of yam, which Banade Farms took off with. Traditionally, farmers plant one small piece of yam to get a full-size grown yam. To do that, they set aside about 30 percent of the harvest as seeds for the next planting season. Hahn devised the method of slicing one yam into as many as 20 pieces (about the size of a cube of sugar) each of which could serve as a seed yam. He called the method, minisett technology.

He then pioneered a method of growing the minisetts under plastic sheets (called plastic mulch), whereby the yam does not require tall sticks (stakes) to climb, but grows as a shrub, sometimes just as tall as water leaves on ridges. The plastic mulch makes weeding almost unnecessary, therefore reducing the labour as much as possible. The yield has been stunning. In a short period of five to six months, farmers who have grown the IITA yam, reap as many as 47,000 yams per hectare.

Sometime in 1984, the IITA set aside rules which debar it from dealing directly with farmers, and invited 250-yam farmers in Nigeria to the institute for a field demonstration. At the end of the demonstration, the farmers formed an organization now known as National Seed Yam Growers' association, NSYGA. IITA is helping it to maintain a secretariat and publish a quarterly newsletter. Membership of the association include Banade Farms, Obasanjo Farms and Gloria ("the wonder woman") Adebambo farms. Adebambo is probably one of the biggest growers of the IITA yam in the country. Early in the year, she planted as many as 450,000 seed yam.

The IITA has also made striking progress in the development of a new variety of cowpeas (beans). Normally, traditional beans grow on stakes and take more than three months to mature. But the variety bred by IITA's Indian scientist B.B. Singh, ripens in just 60 days and is called 60-day cowpea. In addition, the 60-day cowpea does not take much labour to plant because it requires no stake. It grows erect, about a foot above the ground, and is resistant to cowpea disease. The yield is as much as 1.2 tons per acre, two times more than the local variety. Moreover, the IITA cowpea thrives even in very dry conditions that would defeat any other crop. It survived Bostwana's drought in 1983, and has become very popular among farmers in Kano, where it is called *Dan Knarda,* after the Kano State Agricultural and Rural Development Authority, which helped in the multiplication and distribution of the cowpeas.

The yield of maize in Nigeria has consistently been about one ton per hectare. The IITA thought the yield was very low and undertook to develop hybrid varieties. B y 1984, scientists at the institute had cross-bred a variety with a record yield of II tons per hectare. Former Rivers State Governor Fidelis Oyakhilome's school-to-land programme was one of the agricultural projects in the country which utilized IITA maize, and the bumper yields earned the programme national recognition last year and led to its adoption by many states this year.

Many farmers think plantain can only grow near the family cooking fire, whose smoke is believed to be beneficial to it. IITA scientists, led by George Wilson, working at the institute's sub-station at Onne, near Port Harcourt, discovered a few years ago that smoke from the home fire has nothing to do with the thriving of plantain. What is responsible is the large quantity of household refuse dump around them which serve as an effective manure.

Wilson, a Jamaican, then came up with the idea of planting the fast-growing, bushy-leaved plant, called Flemengia, between rows of plantain. By pruning, the Flemengia leaves from time to time and spreading them around, a farmer could easily protect the plantain's fragile roots from the sun. Wilson discovered that 2 ½ acres of flemengia could easily support up to 2,500 plantain plants, each capable of producing one bunch a year worth about N10 at current prices.

The news spread fast around Onne, and one of those who heard it was Joe Ebodaghe, a man whose only previous agricultural experience was running a poultry farm. He invested the bulk of his savings in acquiring 100 prime acres of land which he named Ebony farms and hired labourers to plough and plant it with plantain. He felt confident that he could double his investment in the first year. Now, he is thinking of getting into processing where profit would be bigger. Already, plantain chips are being made from Ebony Farms and packaged for sale throughout the country. Ebodaghe said he is looking into the possibility of milling the plantain into flour which could be used for making bread.

The IITA rice, scientists have also developed long grains, early maturing (151 days) and high yielding rice that performs wonderfully both in lowland and upland conditions. The yield for the IITA rice, as shown by tests conducted among local farmer in many part of Africa, is four tons per hectare compared to less than a ton obtained from the local variety.

Although, improving crops is, in some ways, the most dramatic work done by IITA, the institute has taken a close look at the farming systems in the tropics and has come up with good results. A.S.R. Juo, the director of the IITA's farming system programme, sees the key to increased food production in Africa in soil management. Juo, a soil scientist, says African soil, apparently so fertile, is in fact very fragile, once its protective canopy of thick vegetation is removed. Bulldozers, suitable for temperate soil, do a quick job of bringing new tropical land into production, but often do damage that will take more than 50 years for nature to repair. "African soil cannot withstand the impact of heavy equipment and must be disturbed as little as possible," Juo said.

To overcome the problem, IITA, engineers, led by Charles German, developed "appropriate technologies for tropical farmers." They include a system called "no-tillage" agriculture based on the use of light, simple and manually operated equipment for land clearing, preparation, planting and harvesting. Such equipments include the rolling injection planter, farmobile, boom sprayer, cassava lifter and maize shelters.

The rolling injection planter, for example, punches a hole in the ground even through a thick layer of vegetation or debris. Simultaneously, it drops the seeds in the hole. No ploughing or other forms of tillage are required. The tool is now in use in more than 30 tropical countries, and together with other IITA simple tools, are being manufactured by local blacksmiths in Ibadan, Benin and Enugu, some at a price as low as N100.

Despite the proximity of the IITA to Nigerian farmers, investigations revealed that the impact of the institute has not been felt all over the country. Millions of farmers in Nigeria have probably never heard of IITA. But unlike them, those countries like Brazil, Zaire, Cameroon, Tanzania, Sierra Leone and Malawi are believed to have made greater use of the IITA's research findings. Said one scientist at the institute: "Perhaps, only one farmer in a 100 is using IITA" improved varieties and techniques in Nigeria. To that extent, the acreage farmed with new technologies is minuscule."

IITA's public affairs boss, J. O. Oyekan, says the institute is not to blame. "The IITA is not in a seed selling business," he said. As an international organization, the institute is not supposed to deal directly with individual farmers but through government agricultural agencies. In Nigeria, such agricultural agency is the National Seed Services, NSS, Ibadan, to which IITA has constantly donated improved seeds for multiplication and distribution to farmers.

Newswatch was told that the impact of IITA in Cameroon, for instance, owes much to the Cameroonian equivalent of NSS, the Cameroon National Root Crop Improvement Programme, CNRCIP. The CNRCIP has proved to be an indispensable link between the IITA and rural farmers, providing them with the institute's improved seeds. The same, according to farmers in Nigeria, cannot be said of the NSS. Spreading information about these "golden seeds" has been hampered by the country's common malaise-bureaucratic red-tape.

The director-general of the NSS, A. Joshua, has, however, defended the organization's poor records, claiming that "good use has always been made of IITA seeds." According to him the 10 tons of maize and two tons of 60-day cowpeas given to the NSS early this year by the IITA, had already been distributed to state units of NSS for multiplication all over the country. But another senior official of the NSS told *Newswatch* that the NSS extension workers have lost contact with the farmers mostly because some foreign countries that were funding extension services in Nigeria, have withdrawn their support because they think Nigeria is rich. "We have since not done much to beef up the extension services," the official said.

Impatient with the inertia of the NSS, farmers in Nigeria, who are increasingly becoming aware of the IITA, have been trooping to Ibadan to request for improved seeds. One of such farmers is Nigeria's former Head of State, Olusegun Obasanjo. His farm, reputed to be one of the largest privately-owned farms in Africa, is already growing IITA cassava, yam, maize and sweet potato. Said Obasanjo: "I hope there will be more interaction between this great research institute and all levels of practicing commercial farmers in Africa generally, in Nigeria in particular."

SHOWDOWN IN IVORY TOWER

Jibril Aminu, Minister of Education, was visibly angry as he went on network television to make a special broadcast on the strike action embarked upon by university lecturers and the senior staff association. He talked tough and threatened severe reprisals against the aggrieved workers. He said the strike was "ill-considered," "very unreasonable," "wholly unjustified," "seriously reprehensible," "malevolent in conception," "waspish in timing" and above all "not in the spirit of responsible unionism." It was a day, that Aminu did not just flex his muscles as a minister, but proved with his grammar that the minister is a professor.

With angry vocabulary, he ordered the lecturers to go back to their classrooms, and warned that if they failed to do so, they would be "dealt with." Said the minister: "The Academic Staff Union of University, ASUU, and the Senior Staff Association, SSA, are hereby given 48 hours from the time of this broadcast within which to call off their strike action and call on their members to resume normal work in all the campuses. For the avoidance of doubt, if the unions fail to call their members to return to work within the stipulated time, the federal military government will be left with no alternative but to take appropriate measures to deal with the situation."

In ordering the lecturers back to their classrooms, Aminu also instructed university authorities throughout the country to pay "immediately" to the lecturers and other senior staff, the new elongated salary structure. ESS, which was one of the main points of the dispute. He said that other complaints made by the striking workers namely the "gross underfunding of universities, the undermining of university autonomy, and the reopening of shut down universities," were merely used "to becloud" the issue of "padding their pay-packets." Aminu blamed them for ignoring their universities' councils, the National Universities Commission, NUC, and for failing to exhaust all peaceful options before embarking on their protest. He called on the two unions to be "law abiding" and "go back to work immediately," as "this action will no longer be tolerated."

On the campuses, the unions received the message with 'total indignation and outrage." They described the minister's speech variously as "snobbish," "arrogant," insulting" and said the speech could only serve to "inflame" an already volatile situation. "The tone of his speech and his entire attitude go to show the total disregard the ministry of education under Aminu has for the academic communities," Oluwole Ajao, a lecturer in the University of Lagos, said. Desmond Wilson, a lecturer at the University of Cross River State, saw the episode as a "long standing hatred" Aminu has for ASUU. "The man (Aminu) has always persecuted ASUU right from the University of Maiduguri, where he was once the vice-chancellor, what he wants to do now is to further humiliate the union as much as he can," Wilson said. Attahiru Jega, the national president of ASUU in his reaction, vowed that the strike would continue "until the three-point demands are met." Jega described ASUU's demands as legal and legitimate. He said the most important outstanding issues were the 'immediate reopening of the four universities," shut down indefinitely by government and the "restoration of the powers of the senate on matter of closure and reopening of their institutions. All well-meaning Nigerians should prevail on government to listen and heed the legitimate demands of our unions," Jega said. The SSA in a separate statement said it would also continue with the strike, "because of the attitude of government." In other reactions, individual university unions said there was no going back on their protest unit government Maduguri breach of ASUU even turned down an offer by the university authorities to start implementing the ESS ahead of other universities. Saying the measure was 'temporary, inadequate and vague." Students from the University of Lagos and Ibadan, objected to the cold shoulder shown their teachers and threatened to go on sympathy strike said Ekere Emah, a philosophy student of the University of Ibadan: "The demands of the lecturers are very proper and should be handled maturely."

Caught in the battle line are the students themselves. They returned to their campuses only a few weeks ago after a forced six-week holiday imposed by government following their protest against the increase in fuel prices. Four of the 20 closed universities namely, the University of Jos, the University of Calabar, Bayero University, Kano, and Obafemi Awolowo University, Ife, have still not been forgiven for their roles in the April nation-wide students protect, as their students remain locked out for the their month running. The Ahmadu Bello University, Abu, Zaria, has also been closed down following a disputed election result. Some of the universities as the minister noted in his nation-wide broadcast, stand the risk of losing the entire academic session as a result of incessant lock-outs and closure. The current ASUU strike has already disrupted examinations in virtually all the universities.

This issue of incessant closure of universities is at the heat of ASUU and SSA grievances with government. In a press release titled: "Why we are on the strike," the unions had accused government of believing that the best way to resolve crisis in the university is to close them down." They argued that such a method was "not only a waste of resources and inimical to national progress, but does not and cannot offer any solution to the crisis of university education in Nigeria." They said the power to close down universities resides with university senates and the conferment of their powers to anyone else as it is now, is not only "unlawful" but "vindictive and unwarranted. "They are motivated by the 'sordid state of affairs in our universities," arising from "government's general thrust to stifle the university system, frustrate and cow the university to subservience, through chronic underfunding, harassment of retrenchments and dismissals."

This is the first time the SSA is embarking on a strike action. Bola Ajidagba, the chairman of the SSA in the University of Lagos, said the fact that it had taken part in the strike shows that the grievances of the unions are serious enough and demand the urgent attention of the federal government. ASUU, however, has often been at loggerheads with the federal government. About three years ago, the union had to go on strike before the government implemented the university staff salary scale, USS. Last May, the Bayero University branch of the union protested what it described as the "endless harassment, intimidation and deportation of members of ASUU by the federal government."

UNIVERSITY OF CRIMINALS

A burst of gunfire rang through the hall, shattering the midnight tranquility, where scores of students huddled to prepare for their first semester examinations. Commotion and groans of agony seized the air. On the floor, wriggling in pains and bathing in a pool of their own blood, were three students. The gunmen, a gang of fellow students in the University of Nigeria, Nsukka, UNN, dashed across the hall in a guerrilla style, stamped their authority and, in a bizarre act of cruelty, stabbed their already bullet-ridden colleagues with axes and knives.

John Mbaegbu, 30, a disabled second year student studying for a combined honours degree in Biochemistry and Zoology, died on the spot. Emeka Okwum, a student of Philosophy, lay motionless with knife cuts on his head. He was presumed dead until he gave doctors a surprise several hours later. Chika Anyiam of the Department of Religious Studies, received matchet blows on his thigh, bled to unconsciousness and, together with Okwum, were still under intensive care last week at the university medical centre.

Early the next morning, a vicious cult gang which called itself the Ever-Ready-Souls-of-the-Concerned, claimed responsibility for the bloodbath. In a statement issued on pieces of paper smeared with blood, the gang, better identified as the Buccaneers, said its midnight attack was a revenge against "acts of terrorism" by another underground campus cult called the Pyrates. It warned the Pyrates (also known as the National Association of Seadogs) and other members of the university community to be ready to shed more blood and lives "anytime from now." That afternoon, the embattled authorities closed down the university and brought in the police to drive away the students.

The February 22 bloody assault at the UNN was just a mere child's play in the tales of horror, brutality, terror and agony unleashed on the universities and other tertiary institutions in recent times by clandestine students' cults. In April last year, the University of Benin auditorium was jam-packed for a popular campus show called Mr. Kave. Midway into the macho contest, six students, armed to the teeth, stormed the auditorium. 'F-r-e-e-z-e! if you move I shoot you!" the leader of the gang, a half-cast son of a judge, ordered, brandishing an automatic weapon. The auditorium froze. His gang, known as the Black Axe, moved into action. The leader seized the microphone from the MC (master of ceremony) and ordered four students, all boys, to "stand up and move slowly out of the hall." Only one of the boys disobeyed. And in the pandemonium that ensued, two persons, a visitor and students, were shot dead.

On November 15, 1989, a gang warfare broke out between two cults at the Awka campus of the Anambra State University of Science and Technology, ASUTECH. The Buccaneers battled for supremacy with another cult gang called Mgba Mgba Brothers. Gunsmoke choked the campus, driving student and lecturers into hiding. When the smoke cleared, Mba Okorie, a student in the department of applied and natural sciences, was found dead. A statement announcing the death of Okorie, issued by the university authorities, said another student, Philip Ekwempu, a final year law student, was "critically ill (in the hospital) as a result of stab wounds inflicted on him." The statement warned that the activities of campus fraternities were posing a "very grave" problem to the institution and regretted that students sent by their parents to study could turn themselves into monsters, mowing down their fellow students at will.

It sounds stranger than fiction. But the university system in Nigeria is under siege, bombarded, turned upside down and almost ruined by students' fraternities. Majority of students, lecturers and their families now live in perpetual fear. Under the cover of darkness, the gangs torture, rape, kidnap, rob and maim anybody in the campus who crosses their paths. They cheat at examinations openly and threaten lecturers dare open their mouths.

Their names covey awe: The Black Axe, the Black Beret, the Temple of Eden, The Trojan Horse, the Mafioso, the Vikings, the Buccaneers, the Sea Dogs, the Mgba Mgba Brother (meaning brothers in intrigues), just to mention a few. They brook no nonsense from anybody. They carry fire-arms, daggers, axes and knives disguised as walking or swagger stick, and they "baptize' anybody freely with acid. They are the tin gods and sacred cows of campuses. Chiweyite Ejike, 52, Professor of Zoology and Vice-Chancellor of ASUTECH, told *Newswatch* two weeks ago; "Campus cults have assumed the menacing posture of the Frankenstein monster, blood-thirsty and ready to devour our universities."

Early in 1989, two students of the University of Jos arrived in the middle of the night at the Federal College of Education, FCOE, Pankshin, about 150 kilometres south-east of Jos, to initiate some FCOE students into the Buccaneer gang. To mark the occasion and register their presence in the college that night, the fraternity seized a mathematics lecturer and tortured him, allegedly for being 'strict with marks." The man, said one report, "narrowly escaped death'. The next day, the police from Paskshin moved in to rout them. Found on the students were human skulls, buckets stained with blood, matchets and bottles of acid.

A lecturer in the Political Science Department of the Cross River State University, Unicross, Uyo, who thought he was tough, found out too late that he could not withstand the fury of the Buccaneers. After a series of "minor misunderstandings" with the fraternity at the campus, the boys took the battle to his house in the town. They broke into the house and destroyed everything in sight. The man escaped. The lecturer's case, according to *Newswatch* sources, was worsened by the fact that the "gang had identified him as a member of the Sea Dogs, a rival gang. A few months ago, the young man 'disappeared' from campus. Some of his colleagues say he resigned to save his life. Others say he was sacked. The university authorities simply prefer to keep sealed lips.

Another lecturer, terrorized at the Rivers State University of Science and Technology, UST, Port Harcourt, has so far weathered the storm. His office in the two-storey engineering complex was burnt by a clandestine group on a Friday night. The lecturer's trouble is that he is in charge of verification of students' results. When he moved into another office after the first attack, he was assaulted again by a group suspected to be the Vikings.

Although the lecturer and his colleagues would not say why, precisely the gangs are after him for fear of further reprisals, a student of the department of mechanical engineering, who pleaded not to be named, told *Newswatch* how the lecturer's problems began. "After one examination sometimes last year, one of these boys just walked up to him and said: "Look, if I fail this exam, you are finished." They exchanged words and since then, it has been hell for him."

In the last two months, virtually all vice-chancellors have cried out in distress about the atrocities and havoc wrought by the campus gangs. Augustine Ahiazu, Vice-Chancellor of UST, in his matriculation speech January 27, described their activities as "horrifying." ASUTECH's Ejike, also in his matriculation speech February 10, called it a "strange aberration." Gabriel Umezurike, Vice-Chancellor of Imo State University, ISU, last week described the groups as "destructive and murderous." Students are even more distraught. Said Iroegbunam Michael Onuoha, Student Union Leader of ASUTECH: "The whole thing is getting out of hand. They (campus cults) have become so heartless and so callous that students no longer feel safe to pursue learning under an ideal, happy and healthy environment."

Perhaps, in no areas has this callousness been more displayed than in the numerous cases of "acid baptism" and rape in the university. An optometry student at University of Benin woke up early one morning in her hostel last year and decided to go the classroom to read in a quiet atmosphere. On her way, she ran out of luck. The Buccaneers were coming. Her story: "I was a Jambite (first year student) then and didn't know much about them. So, at about 6.00 am, I was trekking alone to the faculty to read and copy some notes before lectures. Suddenly, I saw a convey of cars coming towards me with full headlights on. They were screaming as they came nearer (I was later told they were 'sailing' the previous night). When they got to me, they stopped. I noticed that all of them were dressed in black. As I was about to run, they seized me, threw me into one of the cars, tore my dress. As I screamed, they opened the boot of the car. Inside was the corpse of a boy, with some parts of his body missing? They say I would be thrown into the boot with the corpse if I screamed again. Ten of them raped me, I was so depressed, I went home to Ondo to tell my mother. When my parents came, a lecturer from my area told them my life would be at risk if the boys, who I can still recognize, were reported.

The optometry student was even lucky. Ifeoma of the faculty of science at the UNN has found it difficult to overcome her ordeal. That Saturday evening, she had a visitor, her brother's friend, according to her, who came in from Enugu campus of the same university to visit his friends and dropped in to see her. Minutes later, the boy suggested that they should go have a drink at a bar called Madu, in the Margaret Ekpo refectory, inside the campus. It was about 8.00 pm. As they stepped out towards the bar, a group of boys surfaced from the darkness and formed a ring around the couple. A sharp knife whistled down the boy's left shoulder and he slumped. Ifeoma was seized and dragged into the darkness, raped and abandoned in a state of coma.

Victims of this nature hardly tell anybody their encounters because of the stigma that goes with it. "My friends just knew I was attacked. I couldn't tell them anything in detail, at least up to the point I was still conscious, but it is common knowledge here in Nsukka what girls go through when they fall prey to these vandals," she said. These days, no girl dare step out of her hostel alone after 7.30pm without risking rape. At Nsukka and most other universities, students could only go to classrooms in the night in groups of tens or more. A vigilante group had to be formed by staff and students in Nsukka but that nearly turned the university into a warfront because incidences of gang warfares and clashes escalated. At the peak of these clashes late last year, the Black Axe captured a boy said to be a member of Pyrates, tortured him and almost cut off his genitals. That boy was still at the UNTH last week.

Late last year, the loud cries of a boy forced a University of Calabar, UNICAL, lecturer to stop abruptly at about 11.00pm along one of the campus' major streets. An official of the Academic Staff Union of University, ASUU, and lecturer in the Department of Economics, the man was to get more than he bargained for. The screaming boy, a medical student, running for help, forced his way into his car. But the fraternity gang, hot on his heels, caught up with him just before the lecturer could speed off. They "baptized" the boy with acid and smashed the Peugeot 504 car, property of ASUU. The boy was so badly burnt that UNICAL medical centre had to quickly dispatch him to the university teaching hospital for specialist attention.

Acid attack is the commonest form of punishment meted out by the cults to those who dare to go after their girlfriends. They exercise strict control over their girls and it is dangerous for others to "trespass." Like in the jungle, the fight for females remains at the centre of most blody clashes between the gangs. For fear of reprisals, girls dread turning down their crude overtures. Said a post-graduate student of English at UNN: "Look at my age. Even at my level, if one of the (cult members) stops me now in the campus, no matter how crude he does it, I must stop and pretend to be very nice and ready to go out with him, then allow him to say all the nonsense he has to say, before I venture to move. Otherwise, his gang will blacklist me and make life most miserable for me."

At the height of the havoc wrought by these thugs last year, heads of the seven tertiary institutions in Anambra State met, April 27, to deliberate on how to deal with the situation. In a statement issued at the end of the meeting, the vice-chancellors and rectors said gangs have become the worst enemies of higher education in Nigeria and appealed for a concerted effort and co-operation from government agencies, parents and the public to stamp out what they called 'criminal violence" by the fraternities. As, they put it: "The problem has escalated to warfare and cases abound where clandestine groups from one institution would plan and execute an attack on members of another clandestine group in another institution. They terrorize fellow students, intimidate them in various forms and attempt to bend the general will of the majority to suit their interest. We have such crimes as rape, burglary, thuggery, theft, attacks with daggers, axes and acid. In order to guarantee the proper atmosphere for meaningful learning, it is important to contain the activities of these clandestine groups, immediately.

But there does not appear to be any let up. A gang called the Mafia in the Obafemi Awolowo University, OAU, Ile-lfe, specializes in burglary and robbery. They inform their victims in advance of their intentions and they strike in a way that would make Lawrence Anini, the notorious Benin robbery kingpin, turn in his grave with envy. They go for anything that sells fast and rakes in quick cash. On February 1, 1990, they struck at the ground floor restaurant located at the student's union building, called Forks and Fingers. The Mafia, of course, is not a bunch of hungry students, so they had nothing to do with food. Instead, they carted away several electric and gas cookers as well as nine gas cylinders estimated by Femi Obasa, owner of the restaurant, at more than N50,000.

That was, of course, just one of their minor operations. The previous session, the security department and the office of the vice-chancellor received a note from the Mafia. The gang intimated the OAU authorities of their intention to rob the science faculty of its six computers at a given date and time. Taking the threat seriously, security was beefed up in the campus. But the Mafia knew best just when to strike. Not on the day they promised. Not even that month. Security was relaxed. Then the underground movement went into action. They carted away the six computers in one operation. Said Patrick Obayomi, a retired army captain who heads the security department: "They are tough criminals. The only language they understand is violence."

At the University of Benin, an angry lecturer told *Newswatch* that "there are probably more armed robbers in the campus than outside. He may have painted an exaggerated picture of the situation but the university authorities have had cause to investigate allegations that students were involved in many robberies in the city. During a surprise check recently, security men who searched the boys' hostel at the instruction of Grace Alele-Williams, the vice-chancellor, found seven short guns hidden away in various boxes and wardrobes. One of the young men found with a gun, *Newswatch* gathered, "had an unexplained and serious wound on his leg."

What had actually led to the surprise check was the arrest in the government reservation area, GRA, of a group of boys said to be members of the Black Axe, in a case of attempted burglary. The student who led the thieves to his father's house was said to be unhappy with the father for withdrawing a car from him. He connived with his fraternity friends to steal the car but ran out of luck when the night guard fired at them. In panic, they scaled the walls into the next premises, the home of a top police officer, and found themselves in police hands. At Nsukka, laboratory equipment, video recorders, lecturers' and visitors' cars are constant targets of gangsters. Said a Zoology lecturer: "You hear these boys talk about 'deal'. Deal is outright stealing and robbery."

No doubt, universities' authorities have punished some members of evil gangs caught in the act. Three institutions (Unical, Calabar Polytechnic and Imo State University) have, in the last three weeks or so, dismissed 50 members of the underground gangs. But the way members of these societies get away with their act and continue to thrive without much hindrance raises the question of just who they are, what they look like and what makes them so pervasive.

Chineye Mba Uzoukwu, an alumnus of UNN and son of a professor at UNN, has spent almost his lifetime at the campus and has a low down on the fraternities. "A Buccaneer or a Pyrate does not look like a hideous, grim-faced caricature, as their name suggest. They are children from what you may call rich homes. You may ask me why it is that they are so few and yet have so much clout on the system. The answer is that they feel protected. They see themselves as 'the untouchables' and nobody is going to tell them anything or do anything to them," Uzoukwu said.

Casmir Chuks Ani, a doctorate student of philosophy of law, agrees. "They are fraternities of affluent families that have gone astray." According to Ani, the fraternities were meant initially to serve as a link between children of elites in high institutions but like any other mafia group, Ani said, they started defining their territories and, from that point, violence and gang warfares began. "Rarely can you find a poor man's son in these secret fraternities, and that is a scientific statement," he said.

Uzoukwu, who now works with an advertising firm in Enugu, put the problem in a sharper perspective: "It is a kind of identity crisis, an ego problem. First, they are over-pampered at home and they come to school hardly prepared for the task and challenges of academic endeavours. They gain admission, in most cases, through the back door. They wear designer clothes and are more interested in impressing on other students that they are special. They want to be seen in the best parties in town. In an academic community, where the majority is too busy to notice them or pander to their wishes, they tend to react adversely."

Ahiazu, the vice-chancellor of UST, Port Harcourt, worried about the adverse effect of these vicious gangs, undertook a thorough study and investigation of the fraternities in his university. His aim was to get to the roots and source of the dare-devil mystique surrounding the fraternities. He successfully penetrated the groups and through agents, witnessed their dreaded meetings and initiations. Here are his findings: "They meet only at midnights at very odd places (valleys, hill tops, cemeteries, forests) dressed in dreadful apparels. They drink some sort of diabolical concoction which contain human blood and the blood of other animals and eat certain dirty, smelling substance. They engage in strange body movements which are generally similar to that which the fairies of Queen Titania of Shakespeare's *Midsummer Nights Dream* do, while sending their fairy queen to sleep."

In addition, said the vice-chancellor, "during these meetings, they don't talk normally but use certain sounds and symbols which are only intelligible to their members. They behave in a manner, as if possessed or as if they had become transformed into extraterrestrial beings." While initiating members, the vice-chancellor found, to his horror, "they subject them to gruesome bodily torture, to the extent that the weak ones, who cannot withstand the excruciating pains, may die in the process." The university itself, Ahiazu confirmed, has "recorded such incidents of death in the past, as in other universities."

The explanation for this bizarre ritual by students may be found in drugs. Ejike is seriously worried about this possibility. This ought to be thoroughly investigated and if drugs are part of the problem, then we have got a real monster in our midst," Ejike said. A staff of UNN in the students' affairs department, who requested not to be named, is certain that drugs are in use by the fraternity members. "Drugs are very much in use. It is not just grass or indian hemp. That is something that has been there for as long as I can remember. But the boys have now gone into heroin and something they call 'Chinese capsule." One student described to *Newswatch* the effect of "Chinese capsule" on users: "You swallow it with water or alcohol and in a few minutes, you will be on top of the world. Nobody can mess around with you."

But the cover and protection given these fraternities by some university authorities border on scandal. *Newswatch* found that the majority of students publicly expelled or rusticated find their ways back to school. The son of a former adviser to President Shagari was expelled last year from the UNN. The young Buccaneer returned to school in a matter of weeks. There is another case of a police officer's son in the Department of Mass Communication at Oko Polytechnic. Popularly call A. B. Nigeria by his friends, the boy, a Buccaneer, was expelled for organizing the raid and robbery of the off-campus hostel. Some stolen properties were recovered from the boy. The school said he was expelled but the young man never missed lectures for more than a week.

There is also the son of a professor in the agriculture department at OAU, nicknamed "Don." "Don," ironically, spells terror. He has been identified as leader of the Mafia in the university. Together with another son of a former vice-chancellor called "Kete," they rule OAU. But they are untouchable. In UNN, for instance, the numerous cases of cult members charged to court for various crisis are "settled" out of court because, as one mass communication lecturer puts it: "One person's father knows that person's father who is a judge, a magistrate, a dean of faculty or a vice-chancellor."

Onuoha, students' leader at ASUTECH, put the problem at the door of university authorities. "Take, for instance, the kind of case we had at the Awka campus (of ASUTECH). The university senate took a decision to suspend some students and the deputy vice-chancellor in charge of the campus somehow went back on that decision and the boys were recalled before their term of punishment expired."

Law enforcement and security agencies, accused often of high-handedness, appear to be fed up and tend to look the other way while the universities stew in their own juice. Early in the year, for instance, fraternity bandits went beserk at ASUTECH, Enugu and ransacked a nearby hotel. The owner of the hotel rushed to a nearby police station to call for help. The police refused to help. Said the owner of the hotel: "They told me the boys are big men's children. "If you shoot them, their parent will make sure you (the policeman) face the music. If you go there with a baton, the boys will shoot you down, and you will die and nothing will happen."

Concerned university administrators, sociologists, psychologist, criminologists, jurists, parents and students alike are caught in the vortex of this calamity. Many tend to say "violence begets violence; let us give them a dose of their own medicine." For now, that is the situation in some campuses such as the ISU, Okigwe, where culprits are paraded naked in female hostels, beaten and bruised before being handed over to the police. As Ani put it, "it is a way of saying: to hell; enough is enough.

But asked Nnamdi Onugha, Attorney General and Commissioner for Justice, Anambra State: "Can we do something sane now to avert this calamity?" In his speech January 22, while opening the 1990 legal year in the state, Onugha had dedicated a major part of his address to the issue and warned: "If nothing is done and pretty soon, the situation will get worse and become dangerous to the extent that no rational parent will feel safe enough to permit his child or ward to continue his studies in any of the affected institutions.

The Attorney-General, to be sure, is a victim. His second son, a 22 year-old final year law student at ASUTECH, was shot four times in the leg May 22, 1989, during a gang warfare. The National Orthopaedic Hospital, Enugu, performed what Onugha described as a "marvelous job" to restore the boys leg. But the boy is still limping, nearly a year later and maybe forever. "Take the case of my son," Onugha said, "If he had lost his leg completely, he would have wrecked his life, all for nothing." He pleaded: "If you people (in the press) can arouse the conscience of the nation to this tragic affair in our higher institutions, you would have saved many lives and the future of our country." He called for a "national round table, comprising relevant sectors of the society, to tackle the subject and recommend solutions to government.

Ejike, one of the very few university administrators prepared to speak out on the subject, said a careful study and analysis was required since the problem touches on the very fiber of Nigeria's youths and leaders of tomorrow. "That is why I am pleading that the society must look at the problem with sympathy, so that we, the elders, don't end up handing over the future of the nation to a new generation that we will be scared of." Parents, he said, hold the ace in any successful attempt to solve the problem. "If we do not have a big anchor on parental care, we cannot even start making some headway."

Onuoha believes the academic programme in tertiary institutions is not tasking enough to occupy students, leaving room for ugly situations like campus cults, to rear their heads. He said the fraternity problem would become more complicated if the cults succeed in their current attempt to win and hold students' union offices. To overcome, he said, academic programmes should be more rigorous, examinations should be based on a high percentage of roll call and expelled members of cult gangs should not be re-admitted in any other university or be allowed to pursue their education abroad. "The situation now is that if it gets worse, their parents fly them abroad to complete their studies. That should be made impossible," Onuoha said.

The security system in the campuses came under security of Udobi Ikeje, president of IMECS Nigeria Limited, Lagos. He said security is very loose in campuses, with security men virtually powerless. He suggested a campus police force, because "university communities cannot pretend to be islands, separate from the larger society, nor can they be allowed to remain lawless."

Ani wants Wole Soyinka, Nobel laureate, held responsible for the entire problem. "He started it all. He founded the Sea Dogs and all these other groups are factions of his creation. He must have an idea on how to chain these mad dogs."

The activities of campus cults, Uzoukwu said, is a symptom of a sick society and cannot be treated in isolation. There are hardly any role models for the youths to emulate. "These gangs we are berating and trying to stamp out are the typical offsprings of our type of society. These young men have seen outright rouges and embezzlers of government funds, who are supposed to be in jail, being hailed as pillars of our churches and communities. A chap in the university has an idea of the father's salary and knows that the fleet of cars, buildings and summer holidays abroad are made possible by dishonest means. He absorbs that value, that wealth is might and might is right. He knows the father is a Buccaneer in his own way. So, what he talks about is money. If you do not have money, you are nothing to him, degrees or no degrees."

BAD DAY FOR BAD BOYS

Tension mounted as the suspects jumped down from a police van and marched, head bowed, into the stuffy, little court-room. Anxious parents, students and friends of the suspects, looking gloomy, crowded into the room and spilled onto the courtyard. In the dock, facing a stern-faced chief magistrate at Uyo, capital of Akwa Ibom State, were seven students of the Cross River State University, Unicross. They were the third batch of 16 suspected members of the National Association of Adventurers, otherwise known as Vikings, a vicious campus cult that has, for months, unleashed a reign of terror on the university community and its environs. But this morning, they looked like bullies with clay feet: the intimidators are today the intimidated, visibly scared stiff and shaken by the prospects of being jailed. It was such an unfamiliar scenario for them, their eyes glancing over the Spartan courtroom pitiably as if begging everyone to have mercy and beg the judge for them.

A short legal battle ensued. Ansalem Eyo, the prosecuting state counsel, read the charges of assault, willful damage and other atrocities against the hungry-looking and emaciating suspects. He argued that the suspects be returned to police custody in view of the seriousness of the case. Dominic Okon, one of the defending attorneys, objected and pleaded that the court should grant bail to the bad boys "because the offence is a bailable offence." Chief Magistrate Orok took a calm look at the scruffy young men crammed into the dock in front of his table and mercifully granted them bail in the sum of N2,000.00 each and surety in the same amount. He adjourned the case till April 3, 1991.

Outside the courtroom, the suspects, some of whom had spent five weeks in detention, hugged their friends and managed to smile, having seen hell face-to-face in police detention. But most of them were visibly sick – coughing constantly and wiping their running noses. "Cell is hell-fire. That is a satanic kingdom. My back, waist and ribs are hurting badly. We slept half-naked on the bare floor, with hardened criminals. I don't want to go back there," Dan Akpovwa, a final year communication arts student, said.

For months, secret confraternities in the university had waged a running battle with students, lecturers and the neighbouring Afaha Oku and Ikot Akpan Oku villages where the university is located. There were cases of rape, axe and acid attacks with the campus. But the climax began a few months ago when two separate "hit" operations by the Vikings shook the university community to its foundation and sent the authorities scurrying for the police. The first incident was November 29, 1990. Aniefiok Akpan, a law student, and Iwat Umoren, another student, were attacked in the middle of the night and almost killed by members of the Vikings. In that bloody brawl, the two students received multiple matchet cuts and almost one half of Akpan's buttock was chopped off. The following night November 30, the Vikings continued the rampage. They visited the shop of Akpan's mother across the campus and destroyed everything at sight.

Information pieced together by *Newswatch* indicates that the clash between the Akpans, Umorens and the Vikings actually began in a forest in Afaha Oku. Akpan and Umoren, said to be members of the rival gang, called the Klansman Kon- franternity, KK, were believed to be attending the KK nocturnal meeting near the same "island" where the Vikings were meeting. Vikings sources said the morning after Akpan and Umoren were attacked, the KK carried out an indiscriminate reprisal attack on suspected Vikings boys. "And this was why we had to mount a counter-attack at the shop of Barry's (Akpan) mumsy where the crazy KK boys were using as their den," one suspected Viking said.

As the inter-gang clashes escalated, it became nearly impossible for even the neighbouring villagers of Ikot Akpan Oku and Afaha Oku to go out of their homes once it was night. Said Enefiok Okpon, village head of Ikot Akpan Oku: "The normal lives of the villagers were completely disrupted. Once it was 8.00 pm, nobody could move because these boys had carved out territories for themselves in our village. I receive reports of axe attacks almost on a weekly basis. Those residing directly behind the school could not even get motor-cyclists to take them home in the evening. So the village council met and set up a task force that mounted security checkpoints on our roads."

That task force succeeded, to some extent, in containing what Okpon called 'this stupid game." But gansters did not take kindly to the audacity of the native task force. They marked out some "stubborn members" of the task force for attack.

The attack came on February 1, 1991. A noted member of the

task force was to bury his father, who was a respected community leader. At 12 midnight, February 1, amidst the vigil night festivities, the gang of Vikings arrived the premises in a Mercedes Benz car. In what Vikings sources tagged "Operation thunder Storm" the gang opened fire at the crowd of dancing villagers. Three people were gunned down with serious injuries. The panicky crowd ran for safety and never returned. "That was the turning point," said Okpon. "This incident was a complete humiliation and violation of our people and rites. And we vowed we could not tolerate it any longer."

The villagers were said to have mounted a counter-attack in which one student was killed. It was in the midst of this tension that the police moved in, in full force. The local task force was expanded to include police anti-crime squad, still stationed in the village primary school.

A police raid a few days later, at the homes of suspected Vikings chief, was to pay off. At the off-campus residence of Udeme Obot, a final year Fine Arts student, police carted away the entire secretariat of the gang, with membership forms and photographs. Known as the executioner (official title of the head of the Vikings), Obot was among the first to be arrested. Among the 16 students later arrested was Sanja Bhatia, an Indian who is a final year marketing student; Emmanuel Okpokam, Etop Ikpe, Aniefiok Newton and Robert Ulaeto (department of fine arts); Okechukwu Ike and Ofem Owai (department of accounting); Ndueso Akpawa, Nse Ibok, Emmanuel Ebe and Samuel Ebe (department of business administration). But one man the police could not arrest was the founding executioner of Vikings in Unicross, Charles Ndanyongmong, a third year chemistry student. One of the bailed suspects told *Newswatch* last week that their tough mate was "simple AWOL (absent without leave)." Said one investigating police officer: "That (arrest of Ndanyongmong) will be a big catch."

Savouring the success of their operation, the police, March 6, decided to carry out an identification parade of suspects, in an effort to track down those who took part in the attack on Akpan and his mother's shop. The victims were taken to the police station to face the suspects. Only one suspect was picked out: Obot, the incumbent executioner. Armed with all the "incontrovertible evidence," as one State Security Service, SSS, official put it, the university authorities rustication notice, signed by M.O. Dickson, Registrar of the University, said the suspects could reapply for admission after "you clear your case with the police and bring a written clearance for the attention of the vice-chancellor."

But getting the police clearance is "next to impossibility" and suspects, including Akpovwa, who have protested their innocence, have already missed their first semester examinations. Godfrey Essien, the university spokesman, explained the university's position in the case: "It is more or less an external problem that happens to involve our students. And the policy of the university is that any student that is involved in a police case stands suspended until he sorts himself out with the law enforcement agency."

With the escalation of atrocities by campus cults in the last few months, the federal government recently issued an order to university authorities to bring their students to order or get shut down.

THE ARTS OF EXAMS MALPRACTICE

Undergrads in many Nigerian universities have elevated the 'business' to a new art form. Diverse and ingenious strategies have been invented, finetuned and deployed by students, to outsmart lecturers and score underserved marks in examinations.

But the wheel of Justice appears to be grinding faster than expected. The chickens are home to roost across campuses nationwide. The University of Calabar struck first with a bang, big enough to scare even the brave. In one fell swoop, 24 Malabites, as Unical students are fondly called, were expelled. University of Jos, Unijos, was to follow suit. It announced the expulsion and suspension of 32 students. The University of Lagos, Unilag, took the cue from both Unical and Unijos, as it announced the rustication and dismissal of 54 students. The previous week in Katsina, a "lover boy" lecturer in the Federal College of Education was sent home on indefinite suspension. His crime: assisting his "sweetheart" in examination fraud. Earlier in the year, the wife of a commissioner in Ogun State cabinet, who is a student at the

Federal college of Education, Abeokuta, returned from the Christmas break to receive the bad news of her indefinite suspension from the teachers' college. Her crime: examination fraud.

This week, as the second semester examinations begin in nearly all the universities and 84 other tertiary institutions in Nigeria, campuses are tense and school authorities alarmed more than ever before by the prospects of massive and systematic examination fraud, perpetrated and perfected by students, lecturers and non-academic staffers. Said Para Mallum, Professor and worried Vice-Chancellor of Unijos, in an interview with *Newswatch* last week: "Examination malpractice is breaking new grounds and fast becoming a culture in Nigerian institutions. Regardless of what the school authorities are doing, students are becoming more sophisticated in perfecting the (art) of cheating."

Inside the engineering school examination hall of the Calabar Polytechnic last October, a drama was acted out before an audience of more than 200 students. Few minutes after the examination started, Bassey Utin, a Mechanical Engineering lecturer, spotted a student copying copiously from a fullscap sheet he had smuggled into the examination hall. The lecturer walked quietly up to the student, stood by his side and demanded for the sheet of paper that students here nickname as "bullet." In a flash, the boy folded the paper and threw it into his mouth. In an attempt to swallow the "bullet' he choked as the bulge of paper struck in his throat. "Get him a glass of water, hurry please, get him a glass of water," the frightened lecturer called out. There was pandemonium. Minutes later, the water arrived. As soon as the culprit washed the "bullet" down his throat, he took to his heels to the amazement of the lecturer and other students. Security men gave chase. He was caught.

In the University of Cross River State, Unicross, Uyo, where another student swallowed "bullet," the lecturer was not so kind. Ukana Ikpe, a young political science lecturer, went straight for the student's neck. He grabbed it with all his might. "Bring it out, now, now." He succeeded and dangled the damp piece of paper openly for other students to see. But at the Federal polytechnic, Ilaro, the lecturer was not so lucky. The student almost bit off his finger in the struggle to extract the paper from the culprit's mouth. Students who prefer this method of cheating have found out that a white tissue paper is easier to swallow than rough fullscap sheets.

When the Unijos Senate Committee on Examination malpractice sat last month to consider a similar case against J.Y. Salihu, a student of Management Studies, and D.C. Atori, a Zoology student, it had no alternative than to punish the two students. Said the senate committee's report: "Salihu (like Atori) went to the examination hall with tissue paper which contained information relevant to the examination and when invigilators tried to examine them, Salihu (like Atori) snatched, chewed and swallowed them. The committee considers the destruction of evidence a serious matter and in line with earlier decisions on such cases, expulsion is recommended."

In most universities, rich students simply hire their brilliant counterparts with mouth-watering fees to write the examinations for them. In the University of Benin, Uniben, last semester, a third year sociology student dressed in a colourful native caftan took permission mid-way into the examination to visit the toilet. Two minutes later, a different boy dressed in the same caftan emerged from the toilet. The examination attendant who accompanied the boy to the toilet did not notice that it was a different person that emerged from the toilet. So he escorted him back to his seat. But the invigilator could not be fooled. He approached the new boy and requested for his identity card. The game was up. Said Patrick Igbinovia, Associate Professor of Criminology, and chairman of the University Examination Malpractice Committee: "The two students had to be dismissed from the university.

In the University of Lagos, six of the 54 students sent home last April were found guilty of impersonation. Ola Showunmi, a third year Actuarial Science student, was found guilty of impersonating Adekunle Adelabu, a third year business administration student. O. Aderinwale, a fourth year computer science student, was caught impersonating Oniwinde Adeniran, a first year business administration student, A. A. ogunjobi, a third year student of the same department, was caught impersonating B. D. Edward, a second year student of the same department. In all cases, the punishment was dismissal.

In the Obafemi Awolowo University, OAU, Ife, five of 14 students punished, three months ago, were on grounds of impersonation. Joseph Adewunmi was dismissed for impersonating Okechukwu Owelle. Owelle was suspended for two sessions. Jika Adudu was suspended for one session for "procuring one Adebayo Sanniowo to impersonate him" in a first year mathematics course called MTH 101. Makinde Abiola was suspended for two sessions for "procuring Adebayo Patrick Ajayi to write a physics examination for him." Ajayi, who took to his heels when apprehended during the examination, also earned a two-session suspension for the crime.

Unlike the University of Lagos, where such crimes earn outright dismissal, OAU culprits earn just a two-session suspension.

Owelle, who was an exception and was dismissed, earned a heavier punishment because the Disciplinary Board for Examination found that "he had been involved in examination malpractice for three consecutive sessions. In Unijos, the penalty, like in Unilag, is stiff: expulsion. Last month, a third year Political Science student, A. Owobu, was expelled but his co-conspirator left no traces and went scot-free. Owobu, in two separate examinations, had "smuggled the question papers minutes after the examinations began to another colleague outside the examination hall. The unknown student sat back and wrote excellent answers to the questions, then sneaked into the hall during the usual melee that follows the end of examinations and submitted the well-written scripts while Owobu submitted nothing. Said the report of the Senate Committee on Examination Malpractice: "When Owobu's handwriting was compared with (his previous scripts), incredibly there was dissimilarity in POL. 315 and 318. He is found guilty and expulsion recommended."

More bizarre episodes abound in many other higher institutions. There is a case in the University of Lagos, where an associate professor in the biochemistry department of the medical school was alledged to have answered, in his handwriting, "part of some questions for a female student." A senate committee which was set up to investigate the matter unanimously concluded that "the allegation made against the lecturer is proven." Similarly, there is the case of Sunday Isah, a student of the College of Education, Kafanchan, who was caught writing examination for his wife, Attracta, during a Grade II Teachers' Certificate Examination. And early in the year, security agents in Benin quizzed a final year female student of the Bendel State University, Ekpoma, for writing examination for her mother, a school mistress and final year National Certificate of Education student of the University of Benin. The dutiful daughter had successfully sat for a paper the previous day, before she was arrested the next day as she was writing another course on education curriculum.

For more than one year now, the institute of Physical Education of the OAU has been rocked and virtually brought to a standstill by examination fraud. Seven lecturers, apparently led by Samuel Salokun are pitched in a battle of wits against Joseph Fawole, the acting director of the institute. Both factions are pointing accusing fingers at each other in the celebrated case of examination fraud allegedly committed by Jane Williams, a star handballer and final year student of the university. During the 1989/90 rain semester examination in the university, Williams was said to have answered a particular question in the *psychology of coaching* examination, which was not in the final question paper, but was in the original draft questions submitted to Fawole for vetting. The course, PED 468, was taught by two lecturers, Salokun and J.T. Ogundari, who jointly set the examination.

But the big question of who leaked the draft question to Williams or whether it was leaked at all became a puzzle. Salokun fired the first salvo. In a protest letter to Fawole, September 14, 1990, he said he discovered while marking the answer scripts that the answer booklets of Williams bore some "irregular features" that suggested that 'the candidate had a foreknowledge of the questions before the actual examination took place." An internal three-man committee within the institute was set up to investigate the matter. The committee was bedeviled from start to finish. First S. Adeniran, a lecturer appointed as chairman of the committee, turned down the offer. All other committee members threw back the job at Fawole, saying almost in every case, that the case was too complicated and "requires the care and thoroughness which may be beyond the capacity of the panel." No one in the institute wanted to touch the case, even with a 10 feet along pole.

By October, the case had gone to a powerful probe panel of seven headed by T. O. Fasokun, deputy dean of the faculty of education. The case against Williams was that the offending question she answered was not related to or among the questions asked. The colour of a blue pen used in answering that particular question was also alleged to be different, meaning she brought prepared scripts into the examination hall. Williams mounted a spirited defence that left the probe panel confused and still puzzled. She said nobody apprehended or caught her in the examination hall cheating. On the controversial No. 3 question, she said she answered the question the best way she understood and it was the duty of the examiner to judge whether she was wrong or right. On the different colour of blue pen used on her script, she said that was a non-issue, as students go to examination halls with more than one pen in case of problems with the pen of first choice. On the inconclusive word on one of her scripts and the changing positions of pin on her script, she said time was against her and such inconclusive words are common under examination conditions. The committee got stuck. Said one of William's friends: "It will be interesting to see how the Gordian knot of this celebrated case will be untied in the coming months."

Last February, as the probe panel's work ground to a standstill, a group of students, who called themselves "Concern Students," sent a petition to Adeniyi Osuntogun, the vice-chancellor. They said the William's case was the handiwork of Fawole, the acting director of the institute. Said the protest letter: "We have seen this head of department (Fawole) running for shelter under your (VC) canopy; but we know you will give a good account of yourself and that of your stewardship to the Almighty God. Justice must prevail. You have to tell the committee set up on this matter to let you know who, out of the lecturers, leaked the question papers to this student." The petitioners said it was "not the first time (similar) things have happened in the institute."

Two months after the students' petition, academic staff in the department wrote also to the vice-chancellor. "We are no longer ready to perform any functions in the Institute of Physical Education under the leadership of Fawole," the petition dated April 18, said. Last week, *Newswatch* could not reach Fawole but the man defended himself enough in the probe panel set up by the vice-chancellor.

Probe Panel: Do you keep photocopies of lecturers' question papers?
Fawole: I have not done that once.
Probe Panel: We want to know your opinion, whether or not a leakage had occurred?
Fawole: I want to strongly believe that the exam was not leaked.
Probe Panel: Do you think the candidate answer the question that was asked?
Fawole: Mr. Chairman, sir, I have not got the marking guide. You did not give me time to read it.

Newswatch investigations showed that Fawole and Salokun, the man who blew the first whistle on the alleged malpractice, have a long history of bitter relationship. In a 1988 internal memorandum to Fawole, Salokun had accused his boss of falsification of 1986/87 rain semester result in his course and putting pressure on him to alter grades. "Remember also that during the 1987/88 harmattan semester examination, you again pressed me to change the grades of two female students," the memorandum said.

Female students appear to be at the centre of the storm in many cases of examination fraud. Most care-free female students, from *Newswatch* investigations, spend more time scheming, planning and perfecting how to entice examiners and literally sweep them off their feet. And they appear to be always one step ahead of the authorities. From a method called 'super-print," whereby girls copy expected examination answers on immaculate white underskirts, they have graduated into a method called "tattoo," whereby they copy the expected answers, deep on their smooth, delicate thighs. Said Felix Ajoku, head of department of mass communication, Calabar Polytechnic. "They put (or write) these things in the innermost places on their bodies, where you cannot reach in examination halls. So, you often see a girl sitting in a very unbecoming position in the examination hall (her loose skirts all pulled up nearly to her waist, her things bare) and she is not alone."

One lecturer at the University of Nigeria, Enugu campus, told *Newswatch* his encounter with the "tattoo' method of cheating: "I had stood in for a colleague as invigilator. As the examination got underway, I spotted a girl looking down and twitching on her seat constantly. I walked up to her and noticed her thighs were uncovered and a wide apart. I said to her in a stern voice: 'Sit as a woman', she just took another look at her near nudity and looked straight back into my eyes, smiling. I was embarrassed. When I looked away, I noticed nearly half a dozen girls round that part of the hall were sitting in that curious position. I simply walked away. I didn't want to be dragged into any unnecessary controversy by a probe panel."

That apart, "unholy examination alliances" between brilliant male students and their freaky, bubbling and gum chewing female mates are common place. At the University of Port Harcourt, brilliant boys are the toast of their female "subscribers" who pay with food, money and of course sex. Most lecturers interviewed told *Newswatch* they have been enticed by girls, "though unsuccessfully" to quote them, for sex, usually a few weeks before or after examinations. Here is one incredible story told by Ajoku. "Sometimes, a female student goes to a guest house, hires a room, comes back and tells the lecturer: "Here's the key, take me out," Aba Onukaogu, English lecturer in Calabar Polytechnic, said lecturers are actually the ones being sexually harassed by female students. "The student comes to you and say, sir; I must pass this your course by all means." Of course, that is a clear enough for you to know what 'all means' mean.

For the boys, they pay cash, most times; to get question papers in advance or substitute their poor answer scripts later with another written in the comfort of their rooms. Last month, when examination fraud scandal rocked the Ahmadu Bello University, ABU, Zaria, a committee set up to investigate the scandal found out that more than 40 students had prior knowledge of the examination questions on political science and international relations. The committee also discovered that the students paid between N200 and N500 to obtain the examination questions. One lecturer told *Newswatch* that "some shameless lecturers" even go to the extent of demanding for fixed sums of money. Most lecturers, *Newswatch* investigations show, are on the payroll of some rich and influential parents. Richard Ekanem, rector of Calabar Poly-technic, told *Newswatch* his lecturers are being "induced with cash" and it is not impossible a few bad eggs among them are falling for it.

Even the prestigious and only Nigerian Law School in Lagos has not gone unsmeared by examination fraud. The myth of the purity built around the legal institution was dented when two law school students were caught last year making frantic efforts to substitute some bar examination answer scripts with fresh one in the director's office. "The problem is endemic in all school campuses in the country. Those who are caught and punished are just a tiny fraction of the culprits. They are regarded by students as the unfortunate ones," said one student of agric economics in OAU.

Some few years ago, examination malpractices were rare and isolated occurrences in Nigerian universities. Now it is, from ev-ery indication, the new normal. The statistics in Unijos, for in-stance, tells a story. In the 1988/89 session, only three students were suspended and a student warned. The following session, the number rose from four the previous year to 52. Among them, four were expelled, 47 suspended and three warned. In the cur-rent session, 36 students have already been punished, while more than double that number of cases are pending in disci-plinary committees. Among the 36 so far punished this year, 23 were expelled, nine times more than the number expelled in the last three years.

At the secondary school level, the situation appears to be worse. Three years ago, Nigeria ranked No. 1 in examination mal-practices in the General Certificate of Education, GCE, conducted by the West African Examinations Council, WAEC. Concerned educationists, university administrators, lecturers and government officials are asking themselves the question; why is the problem getting out of hand?

At the tertiary level, shortage of facilities such as classrooms, hostels, recreation facilities, as well as lack of books, adequate manpower and poor feeding have been identified as part of the root cause of the problem. Said Robert Itam, deputy rector of Calabar Polytechnic. "The condition under which students study and write examinations is conductive for malpractices. Proper examination must be conducted under specified conditions and when that is not done, you create the room even for a saint to cheat." In the Calabar Polytechnic, for instance, no new classroom block has been built since the institution started in 1973 with 250 students. Now the polytechnic crams up more than 5,000 students under the same facility.

Mbuk Mboho, lecturer in the communication arts department, unicross, talked about books and library. "Most universities in Nigeria today are making do with substandard and overcrowded libraries. Books are scarce and where found, are very expensive. It is common to find a student using one or two notebooks for all his courses because he cannot afford more. This is certainly not a conducive atmosphere for serious study." Mike Ibezugbe, sociology lecturer at the University of Benin, blames the problem on shortage of manpower. "There is little or no invigilator in the true sense of the word because the size of students easily outnumbers the lecturer or examiner. One lecturer may be supervising more than 300 students, who may not even find a desk to write with," Ibezugbe said.

Then there is the problem of low morale and morals of lecturers. "Lecturers have suffered status degradation and their commitments have plummeted. The close monitoring of students is not even there, partly because it is very difficult to even recognize and monitor students closely when you have more than 500 faces in a crowded hall," Etannibi Alemika, a senior lecturer in Unijos said. But the words of lecturers, too, are a write-off. The University of Ilorin, in 1988 punished three lecturers for "serious malpractices with regard to the assessment of examination scripts of female students, the falsification of examination results and improper intimacy with the same female students."

The same year, the Federal Polytechnic, Idah, Benue State, suspended a head of department and six other lecturers for examination malpractices bordering on intimacy with female students and aiding them during examination. Similarly, two lecturers of the Federal College of Education, Gombe, Bauchi State, were sacked in April 1988 for "submitting inflated course work marks for the female students." A third lecturer was warned and demoted. And in 1989, the appointments of three senior lecturers of Kaduna Polytechnic were terminated, while two other lecturers were retired, "on compassionate grounds," after a probe panel found them guilty of various degrees of examination fraud. But as one student in the University of Port Harcourt said: "More than half the number of guilty lecturers goes unpunished.

Most academic staff of universities blame the problem too on dubious admission processes. Said Sam Alamika: "There is so much corruption now in the admission processes. The Joint Admission and Matriculation Board Examination, JAMBE, question papers are leaking and being paid for by influential parents. Some parents get their wards admitted by all means, even when they had failed the entrance examination. So the universities are saddled with materials of low quality who know they cheated their ways into the university and are poised to cheat their way all through to the end." Sam Egwu, Political Science Lecturer in Unijos, agrees. "The autonomy of the departments over admission matters has been eroded by too much concentration of powers in the hands of the vice-chancellor. In the process, the vice-chancellor, in league with corrupt JAMB officials, actually overburden the universities with academic invalids, "Egwu said. In addition, Igbinovia of Uniben traces part of the problem to frequent and indiscriminate closure of universities. "Each time the university is forcible closed down, semesters and course works are condensed and students become panicky and start to explore the best means to pass their examination," Igbinovia said.

Perhaps the best explanation of widespread examination fraud in Nigeria is that it is clearly a reflection of the larger society. Muzali Jibril, Professor and Dean of Postgraduate Studies, Bayero University, Kano, BUK, articulated the problem succinctly. "Examination malpractice is the product of a society that nurtures cheats and mediocres and turns them into celebrities. It is a reflection of the moral decadence of our country. In this country, we have pen robbers, armed robbers, smugglers and drug barons who are glorified by the grace of their ill-gotten wealth," Jibril said. Modegths Uwalaka of Unilag, in a *National Concord* story, says Nigeria is a "haven of cheats." As he puts it: "The society has (turned the blind eye) to the accumulation of these cheats in our polity. Okechukwu Onuoha, a student of the UNN, throws a challenge: "Let that vice-chancellor, let that commissioner or minister of education, let that politician, governor, top military or police officer, or even journalist who has not cheated his way through in various ways cast the first stone."

Last week, as some concerned citizens talked about the problem, many more were worried about the solution. Mallum, the vice-chancellor of Unijos, advocates a "de-emphasis of paper qualification." Gabriel Umezurike, vice-chancellor of Imo State University, in a recent matriculation speech, recommended that the problem should be handled with a 'firm hand and ruthless approach," which includes severe punitive measures. The Sogbetun tribunal set up in 1977, following the first major mass leakage of WAEC examination, made three major recommendations, namely: "Tightening loopholes in the present system of examination; abandoning examination completely and replacing it entirely with a continuous assessment method: and reducing the 100 percent weight placed on final examinations; and conducting examination based only upon the objective types test."

The Decree No. 2 of 1984 stipulates a 21-year jail term for culprits as a deterrent. But university authorities look at the decree with scorn. Eno Usoro, Professor and Dean of the social science faculty at Unicross, compare the punishment in decree 20 to "killing a fly with a sledge hammer." While other institutions and persons are worrying about the solution, the Sokoto State Polytechnic, Birnin Kebbi, has found a solution, albeit comic already. Mohammed Gulma, rector of the polytechnic, decided last year to paint black all desks and tables in the school to prevent examination crooks from writing answers on them ahead of time.

But this problem goes far beyond comic and cosmetic solutions. Said the *National Concord* editorial: "Examination leakages make nonsense of educational qualification and discredit the institutions and the nation as a whole."

TOP COPS AT WAR

It is a battle royale. Three top cops in Nigeria are at each other's jugular. It looks like a fight to finish. Who will finish who, is not clear at the moment. What is clear is that money is at the centre of hostilities.

The bitter duel of who controls the millions of Naira accumulated by Umanah Umanah, the Port Harcourt moneyman, has saddled the police command not only with an internecine war but with a considerable burden. One major burden is credibility. This problem appeared last week to have sown some wild seeds of distrust and bitterness within the rank and file of the police in Rivers State, with ripple effects fast spreading across the entire police sixth zone, comprising Rivers, Cross River, Akwa Ibom and Imo State.

For a while, the police force appeared to look like an atomistic formation, in constant bombardment with itself. Top officers are pointing accusing fingers at one another. Missiles in the form of petitions and queries, *Newswatch* found out, are flying left, right and centre, as top officers battled to stay afloat the murky water of scandal surrounding their roles in the lucrative venture of keeping stockpiles of money that is not theirs.

Last week, two camps were discernible in the internal wrangling. On the surface, it appears the face-off is between officers who wanted the court order to release Umanah on bail obeyed and officers who opposed the court order and wanted it disregarded. Deep down, however, money appears to be the crux, and some officers may have already gotten their fingers soiled and burnt.

A few weeks ago, Bello Ahmed, the Assistant Inspector-General of Police, AIG, in charge of Zone Six Command, was suddenly transferred to the training department in Lagos, far away from the Port Harcourt money. *Newswatch* was reliably told in Port Harcourt that Ahmed, whose operational base was in Calabar, consistently opposed the detention of Umanah against court orders. However, Owens Onoge, the Rivers State police commissioner, did not see with Ahmed and refused to comply with the wishes of Ahmed, his immediate boss. Onoge hinted to some of close aides that he can only take instructions solely from Godwin Abbe, a colonel and governor of the State.

Ahmed, according to police sources, took the case to Aliu Atta, the Inspector-General of Police, IG, and No.1 policeman in Nigeria. Atta authorized compliance with the court order and the release of Umanah, whose magic bank had left all commercial banks in Port Harcourt cash-strapped and reeling in shock. The next day, Ahmed summoned Onoge, in company of the accused persons (Umanah and five of his staffers), to his base in Calabar. Though he did not go ahead to effect the immediate release of Umanah, he issued fresh instructions to Onoge and tried to take over control of the matter, on the ground that the case extends far beyond Rivers State to other states in the zone.

Back in Port Harcourt, Onoge fought back and apparently got the IG on his side. A counter order from the IG was issued late in the night the next day, cancelling his previous orders to the AIG to release Umanah. The counter order, *Newswatch* was told, put the AIG on a tight spot. It said the IG was "not properly briefed" on the matter and queried whether it is true that the police has been "sold for the sum of two million."

"We were very angry," one police officer told *Newswatch* in Calabar. "We knew someone had blackmailed us, possibly from Port Harcourt. What the signal said indirectly was that we in Calabar had collected a bribe of N2 million from Umanah," the officer said. To worsen the situation, *Newswatch* was told, a query for misconduct signed by Potter Dabup, a deputy inspector-general of police, DIG, for IG, was sent to the AIG on June 24. The query did not, however, mention the N2 million, but alleged that Ahmed, the AIG, on June 13, 1991, attempted to release Umanah from detention, using the court order as a "springboard and smokescreen," a move, the query said, would have aided Umanah to "escape to Cameroon." Furthermore, the query said the alleged action amounted to insensitivity, fanning social insecurity and encouraging the breakdown of law and order. However, police authorities in Lagos last week denied any query was ever given to Ahmed. Said Frank Odita, police commissioner and force public relations officer, in an interview with *Newswatch:* "Ahmed Bello was never queried. Neither is his transfer connected with the case of Umanah."

Nonetheless, investigations by *Newswatch* show that a query was, in fact, issued to Ahmed. Impeccable sources in Port Harcourt and Calabar last week said Ahmed's reply to the query was to open a can of worms. The AIG, *Newswatch* was told, informed the IG that Onoge, the Rivers State commissioner of police, was hand-in-gloves with Umanah. The AIG is believed to have documented the extensive relationship between Onoge and Umanah and parceled it to the IG. For one, the AIG is said to have disclosed that Onoge was receiving a monthly "protection fee" of N50,000 (fifty thousand naira) from Umanah.

The reply of the query, dated July 8, also alledged that Onoge was a customer with Umanah's company and as at May 20, had a deposit of N500,000 (five hundred thousand naira) with Resources Managers. The deposits, a different source said, was usually sent through a staff of Radio Rivers who is a close friend of Onoge. Then, the AIG is said to have also thrown a bombshell. He revealed to the IG that while Umanah was in detention, Onge allowed Umanah to sleep at the Presidential Hotel, Port Harcourt, from where Umanah travelled at about 11.00 pm in the night of May 20, to Calabar in his BMW car and returned in the early hours of May 21, to the police station where he was supposed to be detained. Umanah, it is believed, was secretly permitted to go to Calabar by Onoge to instruct his staff on what to do and "tidy up certain things."

Investigations at the Presidential Hotel, Port Harcourt, show that Umanah actually checked out from his Room 128 on May 22, two days after he was officially detained. Besides, the AIG, in his reply to the IG's query, is said to have made references to police regulations and the IG circular which forbid state police commands from investigating cases above N100,000. He is also said to have argued that he stepped into the matter to quell the rising tension and determine the extent of the Rivers State command investigations, moreso, when the zonal command found out that even the officer in charge of the Special Investigations and Intelligence Bureau, SIIB, in the State had not been brought into the picture of the case.

Some police officers in Port Harcourt and Calabar argued that the secret permission given Umanah to move about alone in the night, as far as to Calabar, could have created a chance for the moneyman to escape to Cameroon if he had wanted to. Top police officers in Port Harcourt believed a thorough and independent investigation of the police role in the matter would expose the real culprits in the scandal.

For instance, there are allegations that procedures were not followed during the police take-over of the offices of the Resources Managers, as they (police) did so without search warrants. Some officers also alleged that the police command in Port Harcourt is covering up the case of a sergeant who was arrested with a Resources Managers' bag containing N600,000 (six hundred thousand naira). Though the sergeant is in detention, the police command was, at press time, yet to acknowledge the case.

When *Newswatch* met with Onoge, the police chief in Port Harcourt, last week for an interview, he refused to discuss any of the issues. Said Onoge: "I won't say anything. The Umanah matter has been exhausted by the press."

DAY OF THE LONG KNIVES

This afternoon, May 20, 1991, Port Harcourt, the proverbial Garden City of Nigeria, was soaked in tention. For weeks, speculations were rife that government may decend on Umanah Umanah, a popular businessman, whose finance company was paying a whopping 720 percent interest rate per annum to customers. The gold rush, as it were, had left virtually all commercial banks in Port Harcourt and beyond, empty as customers withdrew their monies embloc in preference for Umanah's Resources Managers Nigeria Limited, RMNL.

Umanah, the magic banker and Managing Director of RMNL, had become something of a folk hero in town, courted by monarchs and tycoons and showered with praises by traders and students everywhere he went. Top government officials were among his premium customers. Left to hold the short end of the stick, commercial banks were crying out for more than a year and now it seems their tears had reached powerful quarters in government. Something must be done about this magic bank. To be or not to be!

Today is the day of reckoning. Inside the EXCO chambers of the Rivers State Government House, at about 1.15pm, 15 top government officials sat pensive, to begin the extraordinary Security Council meeting summoned that afternoon by the governor. Godwin Abbe, Colonel, Governor and Chairman of the meeting, sat at the head of the table.

Flanking Abbe were S.K. Dagogo-Jack, Deputy Governor; A. T. Badey, Secretary to Government; Sam Oniyide, Colonel and Brigade Commander of the 2 Amphibious Brigade, Port Harcourt; Owens Onoge, Commissioner of Police; J.A Agbebi, Navy Commander of *NNS Okemini*; E.B. Sule, a squadron leader and commander of the airbase; O.C.J. Okocha, the Attorney-General; and A. Dosumu of the State Security Services, SSS. Impeccable sources told *Newswatch*, there were also some six unusual faces specially invited for the extraordinary security council meeting: O.C. Isiakpona, Manager, Port Harcourt Savannah Bank; D.P Iyabi, Manager, Pan African Bank; J.S. Imhoede, Controller, Central Bank of Nigeria, Rivers State Branch; Andrew Egbelu, Commerce Commissioner; E.O. Denenu, the finance commissioner; and S.M. Oruseibio, a director-general in the governor's office.

It became clear immediately to the select audience that the matter at stake was monetary matters. Abbe, looking severe and stoic, confirmed this when he told the council the sole agenda was the legality of the financial operations of RMNL, which has been giving the state financial institutions a run for their money. According to inside sources, the governor wanted the meeting to determine (i) whether RMNL was operating legally or not; (ii) if they had contravened any banking laws, even though their operation was legal; and (iii) if their operation had directly or indirectly affected adversely the economy of River State.

The questions were first directed at the bank managers. Iyabi, the Pan African Bank man, said the company was operating legally but stated that its interest rate of 60 percent amounted to 720 percent per year. As a result of the high interest rate, Yabi, according to *Newswatch* sources, also said deposit that commonly should have gone to the banks went to RMNL and the bank vaults stood empty without deposits. Furthermore, he said RMNL was not supposed to receive deposits, since it was not a licenced bank. In his final submission, the banker said it was not mathematically possible for any financial institution in the country to trade on 60 interest payments to customers and make a return on its investment.

Isiakpona, of Savannah Bank, reportedly said he disagreed slightly with Iyabi but concluded that RMNL was "not doing anything illegal." He expressed concern however, about the high interest rate of RMNL and marveled about its sources of money supply and the use to which the money collected from customers was put, so as to yield so much profit. Imhoede of Central Bank, was emphatic in his contribution that RMNL had violated banking laws. Okacha, the Attorney-General, gave his legal opinion and stressed that RMNL had violated banking laws by receiving deposits and paying interests on them.

Besides, the Attorney-General was quoted by inside sources as saying that the very high interest rate paid by RMNL was "out of tune" with Central Bank guidelines. For Denenu, the finance commissioner, his major concern was "how to collect legitimate tax money on the profits of RMNL, if it turned out to be a legitimate business." Dagogo-Jack, at a point, reminded the bankers of RMNL's new method whereby customers paid deposits through the banks and also received their certificate from the bank. The bankers reportedly replied that the deposits were supposed to be kept in the bank for a minimum of five days, with no charges for the services.

At that point, *Newswatch* was told, the governor thanked the non-members of the Security Council for their expert opinion and requested them to take their leave. Then, Abbe sought the opinion of each of the Security Council members. Onoge, the police commissioner, first narrated his efforts in "quiet investigations" of the activities of RMNL, with regards to its legality, source of money supply and the end use of the money collected from customers, "with no good results." Oniyide, the brigade commander, expressed concern about the fate of customers and argued that RMNL had been operating for more than one year without complaints from customers.

According to *Newswatch* sources, the brigade commander said he was worried about how the huge amount deposited would be recovered should RMNL be closed down. He stressed the security implications of closing down the company in view of the fact that "almost everybody in Port Harcourt city has deposits with RMNL." He wondered also if the right of the company would not be violated if it is stopped from further operation and emphasized the "dilemma of recovering deposits" from the company. Badey, the secretary to government, referred to the letter from the Central Bank which said RMNL had faulted provisions of the decree, "although it did not spell these out to make investigations fast."

Having reviewed the situation exhaustively, Abbe wanted members to suggest what line of action government should take. Dosumu of the SSS advised that immediate action be taken by arresting Umanah. Badey supported the idea and said the operations of RMNL should be suspended while police investigations continue. Agbebi, the navy commander, spoke in the same vein. However, Onoge, the police chief, advised against arresting Umanah. According to inside sources, he "felt that RMNL was a legal limited liability company (registered) to do business in financial investments and thus had not broken the law so far."

Continuing his submission, Onoge said "nobody had so far complained of being cheated." He, according to impeccable sources, "elaborated on his concerns about the security of the state and feared that, because of the millions of naira invested by the public in RMNL, chaos might ensue, resulting in a breakdown of law and order should the arrest be made." Rounding up his submission, he advised for "more time to carry out thorough investigations before effecting arrest." The governor was not impressed by Onoge's argument which, apart from anything else, was a minority opinion.

The governor directed Onoge to arrest and detain the Director-General of RMNL and his lieutenants before 4.00pm that day (May 20, 1991) and asked Badey to write a formal letter requesting the commissioner of police to arrest and detain the Director-General of RMNL and his lieutenants in police custody before 4.00 pm of the same day. He also asked his deputy to write letters to all bank managers in Port Harcourt to freeze accounts of RMNL and copy the commissioner of police and the governors of Cross River and Akwa Ibom States.

The extraordinary security meeting took a recess shortly after 3 o'clock "to effect the arrest of the Director-General of RMNL and his lieutenants." The meeting reconvened at about 6.00pm, said *Newswatch* sources, "to deliberate further and take directives from the governor" and finally wound up at 7.30pm.

THE REAL McCOY IN THE SADDLE

In most parts of Nigeria, he is fondly called "the workshop man." His reputation goes far beyond the shores of Nigeria. Late last December, the appointment of the "workshop man," at the age of 60, as minister for science and technology, took a rather unprepared nation by surprise and sent several of his admirers jubilating. Academics and scientists around the country proclaimed he was just the perfect choice. Newspaper editorials and commentators dubbed him a genius and praised President Ibrahim Babangida for choosing Gordian Ezekwe, scientist and foremost Nigeria inventor, for the science and technology portfolio.

Ezekwe is a Nigerian Mechanical Engineering professor with a difference. He strikes everyone who meets him for the first time as a rugged roadside motor mechanic: rough and charred hands, greasy and worn-out overall, Spartan and virtually uninterested in and bereft of the basic comfort of life. In Enugu, his permanent base, he converted his official residence into a workshop and lived in the boys' quarters with his family. His antecedents marked him out as the man who could be relied upon to usher Nigeria into the much desired technological age.

He was a top notcher at the renowned Biafran Research and Production RAP, outfit, which, in a mere 15 months, fabricated and manufactured a wide range of weapons, ranging from armoured personnel carriers and tanks to rocket launchers and remote-controlled missiles. In the past 15 years, Ezekwe has, as the boss of the Project Development Agency, PRODA, a copy-technology outfit at Enugu, presided over the invention and development of more than 100 products, including the first made-in-Nigeria car exhibited late last year. He has personally made two inventions: a mechanical cassava-peeling machine and an egg-turner for small incubators. Not surprisingly, Ezekwe's appointment has suddenly shifted the issue of Nigerian technology into the front burner of national debate.

Last week, looking a bit uneasy behind a large oak desk in his palatial Victoria Island office, Ezekwe told *Newswatch* he would require more than his inventive ingenuity to pull Nigeria out of the morass of technological backwardness. "No one man does it. It is going to be a combine thrust of the best hands and brains, in all the sectors of the society and of all and sundry in this country, including the clerks," Ezekwe said. Appointed on the eve of the 21st century, Ezekwe appreciates the task placed before him. In Ezekwe's hands, many believe, has been placed what is indisputably the most relevant and significant portfolio in the land today.

This week, barely a month after officially assuming office, Ezekwe will lock himself and 24 directors of the country's research institutes into a room somewhere in Lagos in a bid to "map out strategies' for Nigeria's "fast attainment of technological capability." The top level meeting is expected to produce a detailed 'document on what technological goals Nigeria wish to attain at a given time." Naturally, the nation anxiously awaits the outcome of that meeting. The country also anxiously awaits every single step Ezekwe and his colleagues scattered all over the university, polytechnics, colleges of technologies, industries and the armed forces will take to extricate Nigeria from the jaws of total and deadly dependence on foreign technology. The cause for anxiety is obvious. Nigeria is in danger and no matter the price and barrels of oil it sells daily, faces a grave future if it cannot put itself on the road now for rapid technological development and self-reliance.

Caleb Olaniyan, Professor and President of the Nigerian Science Academy, NSA, among others last week, in an interview with *Newswatch*, took a dispassionate look at the state of the Nigerian technology and concluded it leaves no room for cheers. Edmund Kaine, copy-technologist and successor of Ezekwe at PRODA, agreed with him. "I can say we have not even started', Kaine said in his Enugu office. In September 1988, Ezekwe and his friend, Saka Nuru, Professor and Director of the National Animal Production Research Institute, NAPRI, Zaria, sent a memorandum to the Constituent Assembly at Abuja demanding for a constitutional provision for technology acquisition in the constitution. In the memorandum, they placed before the law-makers a thorough assessment of the state of Nigeria's technology. "When we think that there are no industries in Nigeria today that mass-produce ordinary hammers and chisels, not to talk of common machine tools, then we realize what our true size is in this technological age," the two professors said. The two friends told the law-makers that a country that cannot mass-produce basic production tools, talk less of mechanizing their work processes, cannot produce surplus food, cannot have functional transportation and information transmission, cannot provide social services, cannot even guarantee its national security nor master and exploit the land it calls its own for the betterment of its people. Said the memorandum: "Simply put, social and economic development on a national scale is next to impossible outside the context of use of machines in massive number."

Unfortunately, such national problems in Nigeria as food and debt crises are discussed in high-sounding fiscal terms. But even laymen in Nigeria are fast coming to grips with the fact that most of the economic problems besetting the country today stem, in the main, from crass technological illiteracy. Even then, very few Nigerian top functionaries appear to discover this crucial link, let alone show any serious commitment to issues of indigenous technology.

Nigeria's quest for technology is a pathetic story of fumbling in the dark. Available records show that since independence in 1960, Nigeria has spent a staggering N23 billion in try to "transfer technology" from industrialized countries, but with nothing to show. Not a surprise. There is actually no such thing as transfer of technology. The country allowed itself to be fooled. As Oliver Mobission, one of the best Nigerian computer scientists and head of computer development programme at the Anambra State University of Technology, ASUTECH, put it: "what Nigerian (decision-makers) call transfer of technology is at best equipment transfer, which we have no feel for how it is made or how to modify it to suit our environment. Technology can only be acquired and this can be done in many ways: you can develop on your own, you can copy, adapt or modify and you can steal. You cannot buy it."

In the frenzy to "transfer" foreign technology, Nigeria actually stopped at nothing, simple or sophisticated. Even contraptions that had not functioned anywhere in the world were "transferred" to Nigeria. One was called aerostat balloon. It was supposed to "revolutionize" tele-communications in the country. Nigeria spent more than N200 million for that junk. It never functioned for one day. The length and breadth of the country is littered with such white elephants.

While the "transfer" boomed, thanks to oil boom, research breakthroughs and prototypes of inventions within the country remained abandoned in the cooler and were completely ignored. The neglect continues. Research institutes remain embarrassingly starved of funds. Right now, virtually all the research institutes are in the red. Said Olaniyan: "The money the research institutes have is just enough to pay salaries. They do not have funds for proper projects. The scientific staff draw up very attractive programmes but that is where it ends. I am a member of the board of the National Fisheries Research Institutes, so I know what I am talking about."

A glance at the science and technology budget in the last five years tells the story better. In 1986, the science and technology ministry got N7 million out of the country's capital expenditure of N5.9 billion, representing 0.1 percent of the capital expenditure. The ministry's allocation dropped the following year to a mere N6.9 million (0.3 percent), in spite of the increase in capital expenditure to N6.7 billion. Though there has been a steady improvement from 0.3 percent in 1988 to 0.6 percent in the current budget, the science and technology vote remains dismal compared to other developing counties and the United Nations, UN's recommendation that at least five percent of national budgets of developing countries be set aside for science and technology.

Newswatch gathered, for instance, that until last year, the National Science Academy, NAS, was receiving an appallingly low N25,000 as its annual subvention from the government. They got N50,000 last year, thanks to Emmanuel Emovon, Professor and Ezekwe's predecessor. With that paltry grant, NAS is expected to pay staff, publish research findings, monitor research institutes and cross-check claims of inventions.

About a year ago, an international seminar on the implementation of the science and technology policy was held in Ibadan. The seminar, co-sponsored by the International Research Development Centre, IRDC, Canasa, and the Nigeria Institute for social and Economic Research, NISER, among others, took a look at the funding of research and development, R&D, in Nigeria and dismissed it as "cosmetic." The seminar noted that Nigeria was yet to comply with either the UN recommendations that developing countries allocate at least two percent of their Gross Domestic Product, GDP on R&D, or the Organization of African Unity, OAU's, Lagos Plan of Action recommendations that member-states should commit at least one percent of their GDP to science and technology.

The paradox of it all is that most scientists and African countries still pin their hope in Nigeria. Said Anya Anya, Professor of Zoology at the University of Nigeria, Nsukka: "Given the sheer size, population and resources (oil money), any relevant and successful redirection of Nigeria's technological development will catalyze African development in appropriate manner." But the sleeping giant, it appears, is reluctant to wake up from its slumber. Its oil money is pumped into extravagant and damnable lifestyle of a few government and ex-government officials. Oil money is channeled into the hands of contractors for the construction of fly-overs, Shakespearean theatres and multiple Olympic stadia sometimes in the same city. Oil money erects traffic lights in Nigerian towns where hardly a hundred cars are found. Oil money is building multimillion-dollar mosques and cathedrals. It cannot fund research.

Between 1985 and now, Nigeria's percentage of GDP committed to R&S hovers between 0.1 and 0.6. Industrialized countries such as Britain, Japan, West Germany and USA, that can be said to have already attained development, devote not less than 2.5 percent of their GDP to R&D. The expenditure of South Korea and Taiwan for the same purpose, at a point, was said to be as high as 15 percent. Said the Ibadan seminar on the Nigerian situation: "it is difficult to comprehend Nigeria's lukewarm attitude toward implementing the (well-intentioned) recommendations initiated and signed by our governments years ago."

The attitude of the government towards funding R&D has, of course, been emulated by the private sector, largely made of multinational companies. Records show that less than 20 percent of companies in Nigeria have budget allocations for R&D or do even care to set up research departments at all. Some multinational companies would rather sponsor sports competitions than set up research departments or contribute to science and technology fund. Emovon told *Newswatch* summit last year that out of the N13.6 million donated at that time for the science and technology fund, the private sector had only contributed N3.6 million. It is a pointer to the things the industries hold dear.

There are other serious handicaps. Bureaucracy is not the least. Olaniyan told *Newswatch* that the science and technology policy which, thanks to Emovon, became a reality in 1987, was in the bureaucratic mills for 23 years. Said Olaniyan: "An attempt to develop a science and technology policy dates back to 1964. The government would set up a body and, after a few years, it would give it another name. First, we had the council for science research, then it kept changing without really achieving its goals. Is that the best way to tackle a serious problem?"

In December 1988, Babangida turned the sod of the National Science and Technology Village in Sheda, Abuja (a place where scientists and technologists were to hibernate and carry out their research free from distraction) and was praised for 'taking a significant step forward for the advancement of science and technology." There was a great deal of fanfare about the place. Shortly before Babangida's visit to Britain last year, a British film crew arrived Nigeria to produce a documentary on Nigeria. At Abuja, the film crew were attracted by a huge signboard advertising the national science village. The visitors changed their route and headed for the village. At the end of the long trip, a wide expanse of grassland was all they saw.

The problems dogging the steps of serious technological endeavor in Nigeria are volumes. They range from scarcity of basic textbooks to complete absence of laboratory equipment for science students. But, perhaps, the most telling handicap is the problem of commercialization or mass production of useful research results. In the last 10 years or so, Nigerian researchers have individually and collectively made breakthroughs in the invention and development of various products. They range from computers (by ASUTECH) to fake drug detectors (by Oleka Udeala). Udeala's effort has received recommendations from the World Health Organization, WHO, but remains disused and unpatented in Nigeria. Researchers, obviously, have no capital to commercialize prototypes and are not known to be the best of businessmen. But the private sector that is best suited to commercialize prototypes are not short of excuses.

Olusoji Awodapo, assistant director of the Nigerian Chambers of Commerce, Industry, Mines and Agriculture, NACCIMA, told *Newswatch* that adequate information on prototypes are hardly brought to the attention of industries. Besides, he complained about indiscriminate research, and said industrialists and potential users are not involved in the development of prototypes from the initial stages "so that we can make inputs relevant to our specific needs." Still, some prototypes are simply dismissed as *juju* inventions and their developers said to lack necessary educational qualifications to make sense. Damian Anyanwu, who uses herbs to invent radio shortwave transmitters and body-contact microphone, said to be the first of its kind, falls under this category.

Nigeria's first-ever science week, held in October 1988, featured with fanfare seven kids from Government Secondary School, Eket, Akwa Ibom State. They made headlines by using 100 percent local herbs to prudce a tooth-past. They named the tooth-paste Abbe, after Governor Godwin Abbe of their State. The herbs, excited government officials confirmed, grow in abundance in the State. But the Abbe tooth-paste is nowhere in the market. Many are weighing the impact of such a neglect on the Abbe and other Nigeria kid-inventors.

The American Newsweek magazine of September 30, 1985, ran a cover story on a young man called Steven Jobs. It detailed how Jobs and his friend, called Wozniak, started the now famous Apple computer in the garage of Wozniak's house. Jobs was just 20 years when he began toying around with the idea in 1975 and by 1977, he was selling the first generation of his computers. In 1980, Apple went on the stock exchange, with each share selling at $22. Jobs' shareholding alone was worth $432 million. Jobs was now 25 years old. There are many Steven Jobs in Nigeria stifled and frustrated by an insensitive environment.

A prototype of a yam pounder invented in Ibadan and rusting on the shelf for years was taken up by a Japanese company some years ago. Nigeria is now spending huge foreign exchange importing the same product from Japan. The Federal Institute of Industrial Research, Oshodi, FIIRO, a few years ago, invented and patented the use of sorghum for beer brewing. Nigerian brewers refused to touch it, even with a 10-foot-long pole, relishing instead in the use of imported barley. German brewers at Hamburg bought the sorghum beer idea and perfected the technology. In 1985 alone, the Germans received order worth N100 million from Nigeria breweries.

Virtually all breweries in Nigeria, thanks to the structural adjustment programme, SAP, rely now on local sorghum for their products. But the lesson appears hardly learnt. Said Ukandi Damachi, Professor and industrial relations consultant: "this situation is very unfortunate. It is sad for Nigerians to ignore what they originated only to turn around and import same from abroad." But even in Damachi's home state of Cross River, the government, in these days of SAP, has turned its back on the efficient and manually operated water pumps manufactured by the Calabar Polytechnic in favour of similar water pumps imported from India, at about thrice the price of the locally-made pumps. Said a lecturer of the Polytechnic on the government's repeated calls for technological take-off: "It is all noise and politics. They are not serious."

How to move forward on the path of technological growth and what direction to go has engaged the minds of scientists and laymen alike in the past few weeks. The basic, though sometimes misleading, question is: how did other developing countries do it or how was Biafra able to make its modest technological achievements in such a short period?

Kaine, a leading player in the Biafran effort, explained: "Biafra knew it had no alternative. It knew it could not rely on importation for long. The body of scientists and engineers (RAP) were given necessary support and funding. It followed that almost every problem was referred to RAP and would be solved, though often in a crude way. Some of the equipment and weapons were not even properly tested before they were deployed. Often, they worked to our disadvantage, exploding in all directions, killing and wounding us but they were improved with time. We should be able to start something close to that now."

Ifedayo Oladepo, university administrator and former president of NAS, said countries such as Japan, South Korea and India were not forced by circumstance of war to develop their technology. "All they did was make their market inaccessible to the outside world, importing only what was needed to teach them to master a particular art." Their success, he said, rested on determined and co-ordinated national effort, rigid self-discipline, dedication, self-denial, huge financial investment in R&D and the adoption of science and technology as the centre-piece of national planning. As the professor put it: "While SAP has made the country look inward, it has liberalized trade. We must shut our doors for sometimes to the outside world if we are to be an industrialized giant'.

Success, it seems, is all tied up to money. "Ezekwe would have to be as aggressive and forceful as possible to be able to secure sufficient money for Nigeria's technological take-off. Without money, he will just be warming his seat," Olaniyan said. Worried about money, Roland Osagie Ainabe, a commentator, suggested in the Daily Champion two weeks ago that Ezekwe should set up "a powerful lobby group" to run after top decision-makers for increased allocation to science and technology. Left on their own, Aniabe is sure; the country's decision-makers would pay nothing more than lip service to the problem. The lobby group, he also said should also ensure industries pay their mandatory contribution to the science and technology fund.

PRODA has shown some capabilities in the area of military technology and there has emerged suggestions that the research institute and other relevant research projects could be bankrolled by military budget. Though the Defence Industry Corporation, DIC, in Kaduna has failed to meet up with its Brazilian counterpart established about the same time, the might of the military budget of R&D was demonstrated last year when the Nigerian Air Force successfully developed a training aircraft called Air Beetle. What is needed now, said a contributor at a recent army engineer seminar in Jos, is the "fostering of military-academic link." To make any headway, Kaine said, there is need for what he called executive authority to back all science and technology programmes in the country. "An authority must be clearly charged and empowered to work. The president should be the mover, and the chief executor should report directly to him. There should be a clear mandate and authority and total commitment at all levels. There should be set target and strict surveillance."

One other way, says Charles Ndiomu, retired major-general

and former Director General of the Nigerian Institute for Policy and Strategic Studies, NIPSS, Kuru, is to improve the patenting system in Nigeria, which is bogged down by red tape. Said Ndiomu: "In a situation where inventors fear that their intellectual properties cannot be protected, they will be wary of disseminating their secrets (which can lead to) improvements and commercialization." The liberal patenting system in America is said to be one of the major sources of inspiration for technological breakthroughs in that country. By 1987, the US patent and trade office was issuing more than 75,000 patents a year and will soon issue its five millionths. As Thomas Jefferson, inventor and third American president put it: "The issue of patents for new discoveries has given a spring to invention beyond my conception."

The best way out of Nigeria's technological backwardness, many have suggested, it to steal and copy, at all cost. Technologists call it adaptive research, defined as "genuine imitation, exploiting every loophole in other people's industrial fortress – by means which are lawful, overt or covert – for expanding the frontiers of one's technology or furthering a business enterprise." Those who belong to this school of thought include Onwuka Kalu, multi-millionaire industrialist (who practices what he calls "copy engineering" at his Nails and General Steel Manufacturing Industry, NAGSMI). Ezekwe himself and a host of technology starved Nigerians agree. "That is how Japan did it: copy, improve and mass-produce. Why can't we do it?" That is what everybody seems to say.

But most advocates of copy technology do not often realize that the country even lacks the infrastructure which is required for the copying to be done. In their memorandum to the Constituent Assembly, Ezekwe and Nuru underscored that problem. For Nigeria to copy and mass-produce a common machine such as car, they said, the local market must first sell cast iron billets, used in building vehicle engines. That is absent. The market also must supply adequate alloy steel billets required for the making of crank-shaft, connecting rods, steering links, bolts etc. That, too, is absent. The market must provide, in abundance, so many other relevant materials and semi-finished components and accessories used in making cylinder, gaskets, spark plugs, fuses, cables, lamps, seats, etc. They are not just there.

This crucial area of provision of basic engineering raw materials and infrastructure for copy technology, it appears, will occupy the immediate priority of Ezekwe if his colleagues give him the go-ahead later this week and if government allocates sufficient funds for science and technology development. According to the OAU committee of technology ministers, 'experience indicates that no country has attained any breakthrough in its economic development without the development of (this) science and technology base." Here lies the success or failure of the workshop man.

RETURN OF THE STORMY PETREL

For more than eight hours, the surging crowd laid siege on the Aminu Kano International Airport. They drummed and danced and shared kolanuts among themselves. And when the Kabo Tours aircraft that brought their famous son from Lagos touched down at exactly 3.21 pm, the people of the ancient city of Kano went wild with jubilation as they literaly rolled out the red carpet to give Abubakar Rimi, former governor of Kano State, jailed by President Babangida, a triumphant re-entry into the State he governed for four years before he was sent to jail.

The detachment of police posted to the airport and other strategic points in the city had a tough time taking charge. A police bomb disposal van conspicuously parked at the tarmac to scare away the surging crowd was of little or no help. As the light skinned handsome ex-governor stepped out of the aircraft to the loud ovation from the crowd, he smiled and waved; evidently satisfied that he still lived in the hearts of his people. By the side of Rimi was his wife, Sadatu, and close friend and political associate, Paul Unongo, whom Rimi had referred to jokingly in the aircraft as "the governor of Benue State who never was."

The journey to Rimi's house at Durnin-Hadejia Road was even more colourful. Kano people, old and young, lined all major streets to cheer and welcome their charismatic son. Thousands of those who couldn't catch a glimpse of him and those who did immediately descended on Rimi's residence – it was jam-packed by singing and dancing crowd. In the struggle to get into the living-room, where Rimi sat with his close friends, the main door was pulled down, forcing Rimi to come out and talk to the crowd.

Looking trimmer and boyish in his flowing *babanriga* and grinning broadly most of the time, Rimi tried to speak atop the bonnet of a car, but got drowned by the shouts of his admirers who merely wanted to see him. Pestered by reporters, who kept a vigil in his house for interviews, Rimi addressed a press conference the next day, November 3, in his house. Rimi spoke on various national issues, including the leadership and the conditions of Nigerian prisons.

"If I have my way, I will send every potential Nigerian leader to prison – every judge, every police officer, every soldier, every traditional ruler etc. They need to be there to learn at least for a month, Rimi said. This, according to him, is necessary because most of the elite do no appreciate the plight of the common man, and one month incarceration would drive home the need for prison reforms. Rimi, who had spent three years in six prisons in Nigeria – Ikoyi, Kirikiri, Benin, Kaduna, Kano and Yola – said, he left many people in prison, who had been there for 10 years without trial, either because officials say their flies are missing or there is no vehicle to take them to court or, still, policemen are not available to take them there or the judge is too busy to try the case.

Turning attention to leadership and the political situation in the country, he said Nigeria, since independence, has been ruled by groups of reactionary elements and those who attempted to change the *status quo* suffered persecution and all forms of tribulations. In his own case, he said, he was sent to prison because of his political belief and conviction. "The idea was to make me conform and thereby mellow down my views. But they have failed. I have become more hardened in those views. I have no intention of foregoing my political beliefs to serve the interest of the ruling class. If I were to become the governor of Kano State again, I will do what I did, all over again."

Rimi, unrepentant and irrepressible, insisted that he was not corrupt as the tribunal that sentenced him suggested. "If I was corrupt, I would not be in jail at all. Those who stole money either showed up briefly in jail or were not in jail at all. I have never believed I was in custody. I never lamented my fate. I am ready more than at anytime to serve the Nigerian people. I will not be deterred in the pursuance of this goal. If necessary, I am ready to go back to jail for my beliefs." Rimi also predicted victory for the "progressives" in the coming local government elections. "I know and believe and by the grace of God, the government of Nigeria from this local government elections to 1992 and forever will be in the hands of the progressives."

Rimi was sentenced to 44 years in jail, September 15, 1984, for allegedly receiving the sum of ₦593,000 as "kick-backs" from Dantata Sawoe Construction Company. The sentence was to run concurrently for a total of 21 years. Rimi's lawyer. Afolabi Lardner, was so outraged by the judgment that he told the Special

Military Tribunal point blank that its judgment was based on "hearsay." Later, the government decided to reduce the jail term to five years based on the recommendations of the Bello Review Committee, which looked into the cases of jailed politicians.

In September last year, a group which called itself "The Free Rimi Committee" emerged. They argued against the "injustice" meted to Rimi and prayed the government to release him. Bashir Ibrahim, the secretary of the committee, said the imprisonment of Rimi was the "most mysterious" of all those tried by the tribunal. They were rounded up and brought to Lagos where they had a brief chat with security men.

The campaign must have helped Rimi's case. A few months later, the government said it was granting a release to Rimi, after the repayment of the alleged "kick-back." Rimi said he was not paying any kobo because that would mean he was guilty of the offence. Suddenly, government decided November 1, to throw the gates of the Ikoyi prison open and set him free. Said the jubilant ex-governor: "Now I am out. This is the judgment of posterity."

A GOVERNOR'S NIGHTMARE

The office is small; smaller than most governors' offices in Nigeria. The walls are not visible, until the door is pushed open and a light wind elbows the curtains to float gently against each other. Just like the curtains, the carpet is wine colour. There is enough space to take in more furniture but it seems the occupant care less. A small flower pot sitting on the floor to the left and a little green-white-green flag standing to the right, combine to create a sense of reluctant grandeur. This is the office of Colonel Dan P. Archibong, 38, military governor of Cross River State.

On New Year eve, he had, as he does every working day, walked briskly into this office, acknowledging compliments from his aides. Right from the entrance, he was greeted warmly by staffers, some of whom were his former school mates at St. Patrick College, Ikot Ansa, Calabar. He enjoys the rare advantage of being the least controversial and one of the most likeable governors to govern his home State.

However, despite Archibong's seemingly comfortable position and disposition, he has plenty of headaches: the many problems of Cross River State. Talking with his hand constantly cutting a quick stroke of the air, Archibong said the business of government in Cross River State is marred by privation. "The biggest business here is the civil service. Everybody depends on government. It is either government gives or nobody takes," said the governor.

His government must come out with about N10 million monthly for salary, yet what it can generate from internal sources is less than half of what is pays out. The industrial base of the State is weak and this is, in spite of its great potentials as a source of raw materials. Industries operating in the state are down and almost out. The Calabar Cement Company, Calcemco, for instance, which is one of the most modern cement factories in the country, is virtually closed down because of spare parts and import license problem.

Archibong said he is trying to get some repairs done at the factory so that it can re-open its production lines. The stumbling block, however, is finance. According to the governor, the Federal Government had approved a five million naira grant to the company when former head of state, Muhammadu Buhari, visited the state last year. That was easier said than done. Federal officials have made it difficult for the money to be released to the company, even as a loan. "Now we are saying, please give us the money as a loan, but they are dragging their feet," the governor said, his voice suffused with anger.

Archibong's anger is further heightened by the problems of the Asbestos factory at Oron, which is now fully on its knees. The company produces pipes for water project. Somehow, sufficient market survey for the product was not done. Soon after the company started production, it became clear that only Cross River

State may have need for the water pipes. But the State had no money to embark on any water scheme, and nobody else needed the pipes. According to the governor, apart from the management problem, "the conception of the industry was misguided."

But government, he said, is not going to give up. A diversification programme is now being put together at the factory to enable it produce some marketable products. The problem again, the governor said, is money.

If money is the problem for the asbestos and cement factories, it ought not to be for the State plywood company, Seromwood Limited, because N3.5 million was provided for its operation in 1983. But the money simply vanished into thin air. Now the plywood company, the governor said, does not even have a saw to cut down the abundant trees in the State's forests. Not surprising, production has fallen to less than 30 percent of installed capacity.

Similarly, the Sunshine Batteries Limited at Ikot Ekpene, which Archibong commissioned November 1984, is now operating with a skeletal staff, while the general manager has been asked to stay home until investigations into financial mishandling in the company are completed.

As if the problems of dead industries were not enough, erosion menace has assumed such a magnitude that Archibong called it "a major catastrophe." While he was taking a walk with his poppy down the Calabar beach just behind his house last December 26, Archibong had discovered to his dismay, that the former House of Assembly complex, a stone throw from his house, may soon be claimed by a yawning gulley. He went back feeling helpless.

There is virtually no part of the State that erosion has spared.

The Cross River State University at Uyo is seriously threatened. At Oron, it is the national museum, while in many other parts of Itu and Abak, many villagers have vacated their homes for fear of being buried alive by gulleys. Said Archibong: "I have said this many times but it appears nobody is listening. Let me repeat that this erosion menace is beyond the capacity of any State to handle."

One percent of the federation account is allocated for solving ecological problems including erosion. In the 1985 State budget, N0.5 million was put aside for erosion. That money, Archibong said, was not even enough for the study of erosion problem, talk less of controlling it. For the federation account allocation, *Newswatch* learnt, the modalities for sharing the fund have not even been worked out by Lagos. Archibong hopes those responsible for disbursing the money will act before it is too late.

Yet, what makes the governor more worried is that telecommunication and information facilities in the State are far below tolerable standard. The equipment at NTA Channel 9, Calabar are obsolete and the station hardly monitors network programmes without tears. The radio station in Calabar cannot cover more than 30 kilometers radius outside the State capital. The telephone system is even worse. It is so difficult to make a call within the State that callers hardly attempt other places outside the State.

Archibong is not taking things lying low. He said "Cross River State is too strategic for the country for one to start playing around with telecommunication system."

With such a catalogue of problems, Archibong refused to count his blessings. But he may eventually do so when many of the problems affecting the State are solved once and for all times.

A SPLIT DOWN THE SEAM

The jubilation came to a halt abruptly. A stoutly-built middle-aged man, sweating profusely under the scorching afternoon sun, in his three-piece suit, walked up to the cultural group at the edge of the field and instructed them to immediately stop their acrobatic display. Another cultural group standing by to entertain the audience received similar instructions to return to their dressing room. Placard-carrying women in Nigerian Labour Congress, NLC, T-shirts who had sung and danced round the field for hours, returned to their seats under the 12 canopies erected in the main bowl of the Ogbe Stadium, Benin. Gloom was on every face. Most NLC officials stood in small groups, heads bowed, chatting in whispers and looking constantly at their wrist watches.

"It's 11.30 already. Something must be wrong. This conference is not going according to plan," one impatient invitee in the state box said loudly. For more than two hours, NLC officials, delegates and invitees to the third quadrennial conference of the NLC had waited for the official opening of the conference, to no avail. Ali Chiroma, the incumbent president seeking re-election, who was scheduled to arrive at 9.00am, was nowhere to be found. Takai Shamang, his opponent, had not shown up either. Abubakar Umar, minister of labour, employment and productivity, who was scheduled to arrive at 9.25am, was yet to do so. There were no signs or sirens heralding the arrival of John Mark Inienger, the host governor (of Bendel State) who was scheduled to arrive at 9.40 am to give a welcome speech.

At 11.45am, Yahaya Hashim, NLC's assistant general secretary in charge of industrial relations, reached for the microphone. He said the conference can go on "with or without" the absent officials. He called on Lawrence Peterside, Chiroma's deputy, to read the prepared "presidential address." About 20 minutes into the speech, Chiroma surfaced. A loud ovation welcomed him. Before he could alight from his car, he was on the shoulders of his jubilant supporters. But the man himself was not excited. He looked withdrawn, angry and could barely wave back at his numerous supporters. Peterside stopped half way into the address. He looked even more confused over what to do.

"Go on. Go on. Read the speech," a section of the crowd shouted from the canopies. "No. No. The president must speak. Up presido! Up Chiroma! Up Presido!," another section of the crowd shouted. The hefty men carrying Chiroma took him straight to the wooden rostrum placed at the edge of the field. An argument ensured for a while among the executives over who should read the speech. All the while, Chiroma waited for his aides to make the decision. The decision went in favour of Chiroma. But the man seemed to have lost interest in the presidential address. He abandoned the speech and went straight to tell a strange story of his encounter with the authorities that morning, which kept him away from the conference.

By about 9.00 that morning, when he was about to leave for the venue of the conference, Chiroma said, he got "a message" that Inienger, the governor of Bendel State, wanted to see him before the conference. Quickly, Chiroma proceeded to Government House. According to him, he was "put in a room," to wait for the governor. Thirty minutes later, a protocol officer ushered him into the governor's inner office. Together with the governor already were a cross-section of his cabinet, Umar, the labour minister, David Isang, the commissioner of police, Sam Elaiho, Attorney-General of the State, "some top military people" and "surprisingly," Shamang, Chiroma's opponent, accused by Chiroma's camp of working with the government to destabilize the NLC."

The governor, according the Chiroma, brought out a court order and "without reading it, started interpreting that the court order is stopping me or restraining me from holding the conference." Chiroma said he stoutly told the governor and those present that they were misinterpreting the court order. The court order to Chiroma was at the instance of David Emovon, the chairman of the Bendle State council of the NLC. It said Chiroma and his Bendel caretaker committee, which had removed Emovon from office weeks before the conference, should stop conducting themselves as the state council officials. The court also required Chiroma to stop dealing with the committee. In addition, the court said Chiroma could go on with the conference but should not stop Emovon from participating in it as chairman of the state council.

Chiroma said when the governor and his team could not bend him on the court issue, "the governor and the minister insisted we should keep the court order aside and look at the NLC constitution on the issue of who should organize the conference. The NLC constitution empowers only the state council, as host, to arrange for and organize the conference. But in the weeks leading to the campaign and the emergence of ideological camps, Chiroma and some members of the Bendel council loyal to him had allegedly forced the state executive council out of office in "unusual circumstances." Chiroma and his supporters had, therefore, taken over the responsibility of hosting the conference. The governor, according to Chiroma, felt he (Chiroma) cannot host himself.

Chiroma remained adamant. He said he told the governor that the matter was already in court and "whether I had put aside the state council or used them, is for the court to decide and the court wants us to come on April 6, 1988." (Meanwhile the governor, according to a source in Government House, "may have wanted to settle the matter" out of court since the two camps had "made direct contacts" with government. So they attempted to persuade Chiroma. He became more militant and "challenged the governor"). According to Chiroma: "What I told the governor was "since you are now an expert in NLC constitution, why didn't you stop a meeting by the purported faction (Shamang's group) of the NLC? It is only my own you want to stop."

Angry at this point, the governor sent out Chiroma and Shamang to wait in a separate room, while he tried to reach a decision with other top government officials present. "After about 40 minutes," said Chiroma, "the chief protocol officer came and told us the governor said 'you people should go away'.

At the end of Chiroma's story, his supporters shouted, "S-H-A-M-E TO THEM." Particularly enraged was Hassan Sunmonu, the fire-spitting secretary-general of the Organisation of African Trade Union unity, OATUU. He stepped forward and seized the microphone in a combatant stlyle and, in ten minutes of explosive verbal warfare that was cheered from beginning to end, Sunmonu tongue-lashed both the Shamang faction of the NLC, called "Social Democrats," as well as the military government of Inienger. He said the "Social Democrats" are nothing but demonic rats, "anti-labour, anti-democrat, anti-Nigeria, anti-Africa masquerades and mercenaries'. He urged workers, therefore, to support Chiroma. "Comrades," he called twice in loud angry tone, "if you are patriotic Nigerians, if you support economic independence and liberation of Africa, if you support the destruction of apartheid in South Africa, suppot Ali Chiroma and his people."

He said he was "disappointed" by the "attitude of the Nigerian government." He said the major international labour organizations, including the International Labour Organisation, ILO, the Organisation of Trade Union of West African States, OTUWA, and the Commonwealth Trade Union Council were represented in the Chiroma camp. "Who has gone to them (Democrats)? It is regrettable that the Nigerian government is not represented here." The crowd roared again

"S-H-A-M-E TO THEM."

The OATUU secretary-general said government will fail if it attempts to destabilize the NLC. "They (government) can destabilize students' union, they can destabilize any other group; but the day anybody, and I repeat, anybody, any government, attempts to destabilize the Nigerian Labour Congress, they will set this country on fire," Sunmonu said.

Steve Faulkner of the Commonwealth Trade Union Congress, spoke next. He said he viewed "with great concern the increasing tendency of African governments to restrict the legitimate role of trade union movements." All the while, Michael Imoudu, the

87-year-old labour veteran who came all the way from Lagos, sat speechless, watching the NLC at war with itself.

Some five kilometres away, the Shamang-led faction of the NLC squeezed themselves into the small conference hall of the Metro Holiday Inn, along Agbor Road, Benin City. The hall could hardly contain one-tenth of the "Democrats." Unable to contain the heat in the hall, a decision was taken to hold the conference outside the hotel premises. Chairs were hardly enough. But the 20 unions represented appeared determined to carry its "cause" to a logical conclusion. Canopies and chairs were immediately sent for and hired. Hundreds of delegates packed quickly under three canopies, while the rest scattered everywhere on the premises, waiting for the next canopy that would be erected. The members of their new National Executive Council, NEC, constituted the previous day, sat under the shed of a large almond tree.

A motion was tabled for all the unions present to identify themselves. Abubakar Seidi, the acting general-secretary, said only unions with both their presidents and general-secretaries would be recognized as fully belonging to the group. Twenty unions met the requirement. They were splinter groups who belong to both factions. Each of their presidents was given a chance to speak. Newton Eruobodo, the president of the National Union of Automobile, Boatyard Transport and Equipment Allied Workers, said: "We have been called neutralists by the press. But this afternoon, we are here as Democrats." The crowd stood up and clapped. Kabir Yar'Adua, the national president of Radio, Television and Theatre Workers Union of Nigeria, RATAWU, said: "There is no going back on our grouses against the so-called Marxists. We believe in the cause of the Democrats, and we are Democrats, come rain, come shine."

Some unions went a step further. They issued press releases attacking the Chiroma-led Marxists, while declaring their support for the Democrats. R. O. Iduwmajogwu, J.A Ladeji, D. O. Onodjecha, president, national treasurer and deputy secretary-general, respectively, of the Agricultural and Allied Workers Union of Nigeria, AAWUN, said in their release, dated April 24, that "we belong to Social Democrats. Our union supports social democratic principles and are part and parcel of the struggle to purge the Ali Chiroma-led NLC of their high-handedness in suppressing other unions." C. K. Odikpo, the president of the Non-Academic Staff Union of Educational and Associated Institutions, NASU, said the stand of his union is that "it is either democrats or there will be no NLC."

Shamang, 42, in his speech, said he saluted the courage, dedication and determination of the Democrats. "Even in the face of great difficulties, under the sun and without water or soft drinks, I am proud, brothers and sisters, for find that we remain solidly together and very adamant." He said the Democrats should ignore the name-calling and "false accusation" made against them, as it is meant to destabilize them. "They have called us names. They have said we have taken money from government, from America, Britain and, of late, Israel. I urge you to ignore them. They are the culprits. Chiroma should first explain why he went behind the door to demand for N250, 000 from the governor of Bendel State. It is no more a secret."

Shamang, in his "victory speech," called on both factions to close ranks. "There comes a time in the history of a movement," he said, "when old hatchets have to be buried, entrenched prejudices forgotten and past mistakes brushed aside. That moment is now." But no hatchtes were being buried as political greed, intrigues and undue flirtation with government successfully tore the NLC down the line. Shamang said his group, which he said is the legitimate NLC, is finished with Chiroma because they are "too corrupt and too rich to understand the problems of Nigerian workers and cater for them."

The case of the alleged demand of N250,000 by Chiroma from Inienger was given prominence by the Democrats camp "to show how corrupt they are and how they flirt with the government." Emovon, the Bendel State chairman who is the new national deputy treasurer of the Shamang-led NLC, told *Newswatch* the circumstances surrounding the N250, 000 scandal.

According to Emovon, at a stage during the preparation for the conference, his council wrote to the government requesting for accommodation, vehicles, security and cocktail party by the governor for the expected NLC delegates. Government replied that they are short of vehicles and accommodation and, instead, would give the council N50,000 to assist them in arranging for the conference. On January29, Emovon said he received a phone call from the governor's office. He thought the cheque was ready. But the caller, instead, said he wanted to know where Chiroma was lodging. "We were surprised and we said he was not in town because we would have known. The caller asked if it was possible for the man to come here without our knowledge." Until Chiroma left, he did not see Emovon.

Later Emovon was told by another person close to Government House that a cheque of N250,000 was being prepared "for you people." Emovon told the person it was only N50,000 and not N250,000. The person insisted it was N250,000. Emovon then smelt a rat. On February 5, he and his secretary went directly to the governor "to find things out." "He (the governor) told us he was expecting Chiroma to come and collect a cheque of N250,000. He (the governor) also asked us whether we were not aware of it and we said we were not. He (the governor) was surprised and asked us if we were opposed to it. We made it clear to him that it was not proper for Chiroma to come behind the scene and collect the money."

The governor did not appear to be convinced. But Emovon said he told the governor what obtained in the previous congresses. In 1981, at Kano, it was at the conference that Abubakar Rimi, then the Kano State governor, announced that he was writing off the expenses incurred by the state NLC in hosting the conference. In 1984, at Enugu, when Allison Madueke was the governor, it was also at the conference that he announced the donation to NLC. "I said how can it be that in Bendel State, this man (Chiroma) is coming behind the scene without even informing us," Emovon said. There and then, Inienger promised Emovon he would not release the cheque when Chiroma shows up if the state council officials, led by Emovon, were not present because it would amount to betraying the Bendel State workers.

That same afternoon, Chiroma arrived Benin and approached the governor. No dice. At about 8.30 pm, Emovon said, he was watching television when the telephone rang. The caller said Chiroma wanted to see him urgently. "I told them I'm not coming because I usually don't go out of the house after 7.00pm. Besides, I said, how can the president come to this town since morning and did not ask for me up till this time. I refused to go." Emovon believes that was the reason "the Marxists led by Chiroma engineered my purported removal from office when we had already gone far with the arrangements." Shamang corroborated the story and said the issue was raised by the governor and the minister that morning. "Chiroma did not deny it," Shamang said.

In an interview with *Newswatch* February 23, Chiroma was evasive for most of the period the interview lasted. He simply said: "I approached the governor for assistance. That's all I can say about that." One of Chiroma's assistant general-secretaries told *Newswatch* that Chiroma did approach the governor "not on his personal capacity, but on behalf of the NLC." Throughout the Benin congress, the issue jolted the Marxist camp seriously and tended to spoil the more popular positions and cause of the Marxists. Said a member of the Nigerian Union of journalists, NUJ, a strong member in the Marxist camp: "This case of N250,000 is a spoiler. This is Chiroma's albatross."

But the Democrats, too, had a fair share of scandals in their camp. Most unions in its ideological camp, according to Chiroma, are dues defaulters. This was destined to affect their electoral chances come the Benin conference, since the number of delegates to the conference would be based on the level of remittance of dues. A day to the deadline, all hopes were lost, at least by the NLC secretariat officials, that the heavily indebted unions can do anything about their financial situation. Naturally, the Chiroma camp were happy because their victory in Benin was certain, since the "Marxist" unions owed little or nothing.

Just three hours to the end of deadline on January 31, the "Democrat" officials arrived at the Surulere branch of African Continental Bank, ACB, with their car boots loaded with money. Before the close of business, they quietly paid into the NLC account "N221,280" cash. Off, they went, celebrating. Minutes later, when Chiroma's aides arrived to finally scrutinize its accounts for purposes of accreditation, it was dazed by its sudden affluence. Said Lasisi Osunde, then the *bonafide* NLC secretary-general: "We could not believe that some unions that had not paid their secretariat staff for five months could come up with such a backlog of dues."

The NLC's fears were confirmed when Mustapha Zakari, national president of the Nigerian Coal Miners' Union, NCMU, whose union's backlog of dues had been paid up by the Democrats, wrote February 8, to complain that he was not aware of the N12,480 paid for his union. Said Zakari in the letter: "It has come to our knowledge that the sum of N12,480 was paid by some unknown persons, purportedly acting on our behalf, as our outstanding affiliation dues, we wish to state that the N12,480 does not represent 10 percent of our monthly dues nor is it from the union's account." However, Zakari said "the said amount should be regarded as a donation to the NLC by this unknown group, on behalf of the Nigerian Coal Miners Union."

Deeply perturbed by the incident, Chiroma, in a letter dated February 12, wrote to Ismaila Gwarzo, the director of State security Service, SSS. He complained bitterly about the huge payments. He listed the names of the unions involved and the amount in each case. He attached photocopies of the bank teller and the letter written by Zakari to deny knowledge of the money. Said Chiroma in the letter: "The money came from the same source, was paid on the same day, at the same bank and from the same teller by the same person. The money was also in the same denomination. This has never happened in the history of trade union movement before." Chiroma called on the SSS to investigate the matter. "Our appeal to you, dear sir, is to look at these development from the perspective of the long-term interest of the country," Chiroma said.

Though some labour officials and watchers believed Chiroma went too far to involve the government in the matter, the big question still remained: where did the Democrats get such a huge sum of money from? Was it from America, Britain or Israel, as some Marxist sympathizers said, or was the money from the security vote of the Nigerian government as has also been alleged? Sunmonu suggested the Democrats got the money from Israel when he said at the Chiroma-NLC conference: "Anybody who is supporting the agents of imperialist countries who are supplying arms to South Africa is not a friend of the NLC and is not a friend of Nigeria."

Newswatch asked Shamang, in Benin, where he got the money from. Shamang began his answer in parables: "Here you have debtor and the creditor. The creditor has been using this debt to kill all the debtor's children for over 10 years. One day, it got to a stage you, the creditor, are looking for the head of this debtor. This man rushed, by all means, and got money to pay you. Have you, for God's sake, any moral justification asking to know from where he got his money?" Shamang asked.

Now, talking in plain terms, Shamang said the Social Democrats became "tired with this group (Marxists), and we said we are going to take the bull by the horn." He said the delayed payment of dues was a grand strategy which his camp deviced after series of meetings on how to wrest power from the Marxists. "I can now tell the world what happened and I want myself quoted. These people (Marxists) became too fraudulent. We put our heads together and we said if you pay this money too early, they will withdraw it and spend all. If you take a cheque to them, they will delay it and play a game by saying the cheque bounced. If you take cash to them, they will spend it and if you take the cash to the bank earlier, they will use the record just as they have done now to manipulate the figures. We were hiding these strategies because we were preparing for conference. Now that the conference is over, the public should know what happened."

He continued: "These unions that were suffering (Democrats) took the decision that we should watch these idiots till the last minute. So we moved to the bank about three hours to the closing of the cut-off time for payment. During the process, some mistakes were made. Somebody, instead of paying for the tin miners, paid for coal miners. This was how it happened." Shamang said it was "stupid" of the Marxist camp to "invite the government security to come and probe us." He said the actual amount involved was N235,000 and not N221,280 as published by the Chiroma NLC.

Outside the campaign of slander and foul tactics adopted by both camps, the two camps have traditionally found it convenient to breathe down each others neck, instead of working as a team. The only thing they ever agreed to do was to disagree. The Marxists, for instance, have always accused the Democrats of being too pro-establishment and, therefore, incapable of protecting the interest of workers. The Democrats, on the other hand, always accused the Marxists of being too "dictatorial," "oppressive" and "confrontational" in their approach to issues and problems. They alleged that the NLC, under the Marxists, knows next to nothing except strikes whenever a problem arises. This approach, the Democrats argue, does neither the worker nor the government nor society any good because it constitutes impediments to progress.

In the separate resolutions adopted by the two camps last week, each side tried to win the sympathy of the workers. Both sides called on the government not to remove oil subsidy. In addition, the Democrats appealed to government to overlook the anomalies arising from recent payment of revised fringe benefits. They asked the government to regard overpayments already made to workers as "made in good faith" and refrain from making deductions. The Democrats also called for a high-powered probe into the finances of the NLC "in view of several discrepancies detected" by the Registrar of Trade Unions. Both sides said they will resist any attempt to split the NLC. The Democrats, at the end of their conference on February 24, had 20 unions on their camp out of the 42 industrial unions in the NLC. The Marxists had 22. They said they had 18 of the former 19 state councils in their camp and they constitute 67 percent of the NLC.

As the warring camps left Benin last week with two different National Executive Councils, NEC, the gulf between them remain as wide as ever. Eskor Toyo, Professor of Economics and renowed Marxist, told *Newswatch* the crisis is normal. But some other experts say the furture is fraught with signs of danger.

The loser, at the end of the day, they all agreed, is the Nigerian worker. Said Moris Adeyemi, a labour analyst: "As it is now, all of them are ready to sacrifice the workers for their selfish interests. So there are no options as of now for the workers. It is either they lose or they lose."

RAY EKPU IN THE DOCK

As early as 8.30am February 4, 1986, the old National Assembly's Committee Room B5 was bursting at the seams. About 200 journalists, lawyers, businessmen, trade unionists, ex-politicians, students, law enforcement agents and friends of *Newswatch* crammed themselves into the small first floor conference room that normally would not take more than 50 people. And up till 1.39 pm, when the court rose, the crowd kept swelling. It was an unprecedented scenario. *Newswatch,* the authoritative and respected news magazine, was on trial before the military government tribunal headed by Justice Samson Uwaifo.

Only the previous day, some fierce-looking mobile policemen and plain clothes officers had called at *Newswatch,* premises to drop six summons from the Uwaifo tribunal. Ray Ekpu, Deputy Editor-in-Chief; Nosa Igiebor, Associate Editor; Dele Olojede, Assistant Editor; Dare Babarinsa, Senior Staff Writer; Soji Omotunde, Staff Writer and Joyce Osakwe, Reporter/Researcher, were summoned to appear before the tribunal at 9am the next day, to show cause why they should not be charged for contempt of the tribunal for their stories in the February 3 edition of the magazine concerning the panel's verdict on former president Shehu Shagari and his deputy, Alex Ekwueme.

D-Day. lmeh Umanah, chairman of the board of *Newswatch* Communications Ltd, clad in white trouser and a windcheater, with white shoes to match, sat quietly at one corner of the room. Tony Momoh, Journalist and Lawyer, General Manager (publications) *DailyTimes* was also there and a crack team of 12 lawyers from Gani Fawehinmi Chambers, backing *Newswatch* was in place. Segun Osoba, *DailyTimes* managing director, was among top journalists present.

Fawehinmi walked briskly into the Committee Room followed by a young man who carried a large trunk box containing voluminous law books. *Newswatch*and other top journalist left their seats to welcome the "people's" lawyer. On his return, Ekpu had lost his seat to Yakubu Mohammed, *Newswatch's* executive editor. "Let him be on his feet, he is the accused," Giwa joked - "Please, move over to the dock there, it's kept for you" Agbese jibed. There was a prolonged laughter. Soon, Ekpu was not only to lose his seat, but his freedom too. He was to stand for 2 hours and 29 minutes as the legal battle raged on.

Uwaifo and members of the tribunal entered at 9.35 am, about 35 minutes behind schedule. The judge proceeded immediately to produce a copy of the February 3 edition of *Newswatch* from a large brown envelope.

Judge: "Mr. Ray Ekpu, come forward,"

Ekpu: "Yes sir."

Judge: "You are the publisher of this magazine?"

Ekpu: "The magazine is published by *Newswatch* Communication Ltd."

Judge: "This is the article you wrote (opening to page four article titled) *A Hollow Ritual*
Ekpu: "Yes"

Standing about three feet away in front of the judge, Ekpu and the judge engaged in an eye-ball to ball exchange for about 90 seconds. The judge blinked, Ekpu won. That was the last battle Ekpu won in Uwaifo's tribunal. Uwaifo, his voice shaking constantly, read out some portions of Ekpu's article and said almost every part of the article was "damnable." Uwaifo followed up by giving Ekpu a thorough dressing down.

Whenever he cited his favourite legal authorities like Lord Mansfield and Lord Denning, he would say in a ridiculing tone, "I doubt whether that would make any sense to Mr. Ray Ekpu." There was graveyard silence in the room except for the non-stop chorus of the clicking cameras.

Uwaifo said he would have overlooked Ekpu's article as an "idea of a foolish man," but "you are a journalist of high regard so I would not," adding "you must be held responsible for what you have done."

He asked Ekpu whose interest he was "serving' – your own, your magazine's or the nation's." Citing a 1770 quotation from Lord Mansfield, published in Lord Denning's book *Laudujarks in the Law,* Uwaifo re-echoed. "Let justice be done, though heavens may fall."

Cold sweat began to trickle down Ekpu's forehead. His white handkerchief kept running from his forehead to his neck and face. Soon, the collar of his sky-blue suit was soaked with cold sweat. But like Paul of Tarsus, he stood firm, taking every bombardment with philosophical calmness. Uwaifo told Ekpu: "If you want to destroy your enemies, you pray for rain, you pray for rainstorm or probably you pray for thunder. And that will help you to strike them down." Uwaifo was poised to punish Ekpu. Giwa, Agbese, Mohammed, Osoba and others wore worried looks.

Police Commissioner Emmanuel Ugowe, a member of the tribunal, took his turn wondering why Ekpu should dabble into areas he does not have training. He said Ekpu had demonstrated his "incompetence." Ugowe said he did a research and discovered that Ekpu was good in writing about "marriage affairs, coffee shops and sports." There was a prolonged laugher. He said Ekpu did not have the "monopoly of foul language."

Earlier, Fawehinmi had announced himself and 11 other lawyers defending Ekpu and Newswatch. They were Tony Momoh, Dele Awokoya, Christine Umole, H. A. Odetoyinbo, Tessy Akpeki, Iyabo Fawhinmi, Chima Ibe, O.A.R. Ogunde, Tayo Oyetibo, Simon Nweke, Dr, Tunji Abayomi and Rolly Dairo. Fawehinmi had also said he represented the Newspapers Proprietors Association of Nigeria, NPAN, and the Nigerian Union of Journalists, NUJ, which he said were "constitutionally and psychologically present here."

Suddenly, Uwaifo stunned the hall when he announced that Ekpu would be sent to prison custody "until the tribunal had time to try his case."

Fawehinmi was on his feet immediately. A heated argument ensued between him and Uwaifo "My Lord," shouted Fawehinmi impatiently and stridently, at the top of his voice "I am amazed, I am amazed My Lord." Citing several portions of the constitution rapidly, Fewehinmi argued that "it is constitutionally wrong to send the accused persons to prison custody when no charge had been preferred against them." Uwaifo replied quickly and surprisingly that "I am not following any constitution." Looking astounded, Fawehinmi warned that if it was the judge's desire to punish the accused outside the law of Nigeria and in a minor offence that could only attract a maximum of N20 fine then, "I hand over the accused to you to do whatever lawless deed you like with him."

Yet, Fawehinmi pressed on. He said if there were any persons to be punished, they were Shehu Shagari and Alex Ekwueme, arguing that in some countries, they would have been shot. "Where would they be shot, in communist countries?" Uwaifo asked. "In Ghana," replied Fawehinmi sharply.

When the judge insisted on his decision to detain the journalists, Fewehinmi packed his law books and was about to leave when the judge said the case would be dealt with at 12 noon. Simultaneously, the defence lawyers and the scores of journalists present staged a walk out on the judge, in protest against the detention of Ekpu and others. There was a mild drama and confusion as mobile policemen scampered up and down looking for Soji Omotunde, one of the accused, who had joined his colleagues to walk-out on the tribunal.

12 noon. The afternoon session began in a more than tense atmosphere. Apart from NUJ president George Izobo, more media executives had arrived from neighbouring States. *Tribune's* editor-in-chief, Felix Adenaike and *Sketch's* Managing Director, Peter Ajayi had come. While the crowd was waiting for the tribunal members, journalists continued to make lighter matter of the trial. "Ray, the jail bird," Giwa called from one end of the room. And there was a guffaw. Said another media executive to Ekpu's wife, "Uyai, touch your husband for the last time."

The heat in the room became unbearable. The air-conditioners had all packed up. There was only one standing fan behind the tribunal members. Ekpu's wife kept wiping the husband's face, as the man would not stop sweating. Then Uwaifo and his men came in. Same court room ritual. Pulling the *Newswatch* copy again from his brown envelope, Uwaifo called on Fawehinmi to make his submission. He ordered that the defence counsel should restrict himself to defending Ekpu's reference to the tribunal as a "kangaroo court." Ekpu, in his articles had said the trial of Shagari and Ekwueme was "contrived in the manner of a kangaroo court."

Fawehinmi argued that the reference to the tribunal as a "kangaroo court' should be looked at in the "totality of the article." Fawehinmi went on to cite several sections of the constitution to defend the accused but Uwaifo cut in to repeat that "the constitution does not apply to this tribunal." Fawehinmi insisted the tribunal "must find its tap root in the constitution."

After a heated argument, Fawehinmi proceeded to submit that the accused were "not guilty of any contempt." He read portions of section 12 of the Tribunal of Inquiry Act to support his argument and cited several legal cases where "high pitched criticism, permissible under the law" had been used to disagree with public officials. For anybody to be found guilty of contempt, the counsel said, there must have been a publication; the publication must relate to an inquiry of any proceedings therein; such inquiry must be in existence or pending at the time of the publication and the publication must be calculated to prejudice an inquiry that was in existence during the time of publication. The defence argued therefrom that, in the case of the accused, Uwaifo had completed the trial of Shagari and Ekwueme and the article published by the accused cannot be said to prejudice his judgment and therefore, not contemptuous.

Arguing further, Fawehinmi said, the tribunal cannot deal with the matter "in isolation of the past" and wanted the tribunal to say whether it did not complete the trial of Shagari and Ekwueme before the said article. "If so you can go on trying the accused" the lawyer submitted. Fawehinmi said even if the tribunal was still sitting on Shehu Shagari, the tribunal should take note that the matter was of "serious national importance and of serious political magnitude that there is noting a member of the press, in effectuation of his constitutional rights and duties can say that can be casually regarded as contemptuous.

Fawehinmi further argued that any issue affecting Shagari is a public matter since his government had affected the lives of every Nigerian. Uwaifo, however, cut in to say "we were not asked to inquire into how he ran his government." Fawehinmi replied, "my Lord, you cannot run away from that at all because you had already inquired into some aspect of Shagari's government."

In support of his submission of "no contempt at all," Fawehinmi said Nigerians have made a more serious, more vitriolic and more damaging attacks on public officers and the court of appeal had held that when those attacks go into the realm of public matter, the court must be very wary in treating such criticisms as contempt. He cited several similar cases including that of Nwankwo Vs the State; Onagoruwa Vs Araka; Ishola Vs Azikiwe (Ishola was accused of trying to debase a legend in his article); National Assembly Vs Tony Momoh, etc, all of which were decided in favour of the accused persons.

Uwaifo asked "what has that got to do with this panel?" Replied Fawehinmi, "The panel must accept criticism, that is what I am saying. You are public officers, sir, paid from public funds, with deductions from their salary." The crowd was again tickled into a long fit of laughter. The judge warned Fawehinmi to watch his words: "Mind what you say: don't use this as a forum to attack other people." Fawehinmi countered, "My Lord, if I have to attack other people within the laws of this country, pardon me, Sir."

Defence counsel changed tactics. Quoting Lord Denning, whom he said is "my lord's favourite," Fawehinmi referred to a stinging criticism against a court by *The Punch,* a British publication of February 14, 1968, where the magazine said: "The recent judgment in the federal court is a strong example of the blindness which now descends on some of our judges. The legislation has been rendered virtually unworkable by the unrealistic, contradictory and erroneous decisions of the court. So, what do they do? Apologise for the trouble judges have put us to. Not a bit everyone seems out of step in that court.

Lord Denning in his judgment in that case said: "That article is certainly critical of this court, very critical. It is admittedly erroneous. This court did not give any decision which was overruled as the article said. But judges cannot continue to consider allegations against themselves. It is a jurisdiction which undoubtedly belongs to us, but which we will most sparingly excuse, more particularly, as we ourselves have an interest in the matter. We should never use this jurisdiction to uphold our dignity or suppress those who speak against us. There is something far more important at stake. It is no less than the freedom of speech itself. It is the right of every man in parliament, out in the press or over the broadcast to make fair comment even outspoken comment, on matters of public interest. We cannot enter into matters of public controversy, still less into political controversy."

Lord Denning's injunction made little impression on Uwaifo.

Finally, Fawehinmi pleaded with and urged Uwaifo to take

cognizance of the views of the federal government on the Shagari controversy and freedom of press, and abstain from meting out punishment on the accused persons in order not to embarrass the federal government. To punish the defendant for contempt, Fawehinmi said "would further bring the tribunal into public ridicule." He urged the tribunal to take judicial notice of how the federal government has reacted to the feelings of the public by listening to the complaints of the public, including the defendants.

Said Fawehinmi, "I submit, therefore, sir, bearing this in mind, that you must take judicial notice that the federal military government acted on the comments of the Nigerian people, through the press and the accused must not be seen to be guilty of contempt. If you punish them, it will not only be an embarrassment to government policy, but a total dislocation of the government stand on this matter."

Uwaifo cut in: "Chief Fawehinmi, note that, that does not concern us at all." Fawehinmi went on to refer Uwaifo to the Digest of the Supreme Court Cases 1956-1958, volume 2, page 365, which says that "the court must take judicial notice of the declared policy of the federal military government of Nigeria."

Forty minutes of legal fireworks later, Fawehinmi ended his submission with a plea: "please, my lord, spare us the embarrassment of punishing the accused, whom I know are very patriotic and well-meaning Nigerians."

Hush fell on the room. Uwaifo began consultation with members of his tribunal. Whispered Dapo Aderinola, chairman of Lagos State NUJ, "what emerges from that consultation now will make or mar this tribunal."

Uwaifo wrote his judgment. Members of tribunal read and

signed it. The hall waited in silence. Then, Uwaifo cleared his throat. The moment everyone dreaded had arrived. He discharged the five *Newswatch* reporters in only three sentences. Then, he settled on Ekpu. He found him guilty and fined him N20.

Outside the Committee Room, George Izobo, NUJ president, instantly called journalists off their beats from all tribunal throughout the country, for one week beginning same day, saying "judges must stop taking journalist for a ride."

Of course, Ekpu backed by Fawehenmi vowed that afternoon that Uwaifo would not take him for a ride. Within 24 hours, Ekpu struck back with an eight-point appeal against the decision. Fawehinmi, who filed the appeal on his behalf, submitted that Uwaifo's tribunal erred in law in convicting the appellant of contempt when he was merely exercising his fundamental right of freedom of expression on a matter of extreme public importance and interest.

Furthermore, Fawehinmi argued that the tribunal misdirected itself in law when it held that the article, written by Ekpu, was calculated to prejudice the inquiry or proceedings before it.

The battle continues.

KILLED BUT ALIVE

With pop tunes and poems; in paintings and sculpture; Nigerians mourned the murder of Dele Giwa last year and sought in every possible way to immortalize his name. His death has touched off such a tidal wave of mementoes: T-shirts, bumper stickers, umbrellas, calendars, notebooks, jotters, caps, nylon bags, photographs, badges and posters. Painters went to work, reproducing Giwa in colour. Sculptors came in handy with statues and busts.

In Lagos, the Nigerian Union of Journalists, NUJ, changed the name of its conference centre to Dele Giwa Hall. The union also instituted a roll of honour and gave Giwa a post-humous award, the first journalist to be so honoured. In addition, the union immediately lifted the ban on the *Concord* newspaper's chapel, an amnesty "in honour of Giwa's memory as a man of peace." Similarly, the suspension of Bola Adedoja, a former president of the union and now commissioner for information in Oyo State, was revoked, all in honour of the slain editor.

In Abeokuta, the Ogun State council of the NUJ renamed its press centre, Dele Giwa Memoral Press Centre, 'for his immense contribution to the development of journalism." In Jos, Alex Fom, a well-known medical practitioner also renamed his hospital blocks after the slain journalist. He said he was making the gesture "as a practical demonstration of the need to immortalize the name of a prolific writer." In Shendam, Plateau State, the Youth Agrarian Enterprises, similarly renamed its 1,000 hectare model farm after Giwa "to ensure that his ideals as a model journalist and tireless advocate of social justice, as crystalized in *Newswatch,* survives." The department of mass communications of Calabar Polytechnic on its part instituted the "Dele Giwa Memorial Award," for the best student reporter.

Samuel Oyebanji, an Ilorin-based artist painted a life-size portrait of the fallen hero. He took it all the way from his workshop to the Kwara State Council of the NUJ, where he presented it to Bayo Osagbemi, chairman of the council. "This man was a superstar," Oyebanji said, and left in tears. Similarly, Bamiji Lawal of Lap Artistic Products, Ibadan, painted a beautiful portrait of Giwa and presented it to Ray Ekpu, *Newswatch's* editor-in-chief. So also did Kunle Arts, a Lagos-based art studio. At the National Museum, Onikan, Lagos, Giwa was mourned on stage in a drama titled *Yelling for Dele,* which ended with the artists breaking down on stage. And in Benin, Bendel State, David Omonhimin, a sculptor, made a full-size bronze statue of the assassinated editor. Henry Onwufuju, a Lagos-based businessman paid N30,000 for the statue.

The teeming population of school children and youths, who saw Giwa as their model and folk hero, were not left out of it. They littered kiddies pages of newspapers with rhymes and drawings captioned "Dear Dele Giwa." At the government school, Akamkpa, Cross River State, the Press Club changed its name to 'Giwa Club" and members are now fondly called "Giwarite." At nursery and primary schools in Eket, Akwa Ibom State, little tenderfoot children replaced the wordings of their favourite songs with Giwa's name and made it a point of duty to sing the song every morning before marching into the assembly hall for prayers. Teachers loved it and sang along with them.

Talk about songs! Professional musicians cashed in on it too. Orlando Owoh, was the first to come out with a long playing (LP) album on Giwa. The record was a runaway sell-out. The Mandators, in their chart-bursting reggae LP, *Crisis,* sang to protest "letter bomb in Nigeria." And only last week, just as preparations for the anniversary of Giwa's death were in top gear, a talented young musician, Ottong Peterside, released a six-track LP, *Senseless Killing.* In two tracks, "Senseless Killing," and "Last Laugh," the reggae artist sings emotionally about the death of Giwa and the inability of the police to track down the culprits. The album is rated by critics as "one of the best reggae albums to be made in Nigeria." As Peterside sings in his album: "Jah, let not the wicked laugh the last."

A TALE OF TWO EDITORS

On a busy Wednesday afternoon, February 3, 1986, George Okoro, 46, had just breezed into his office at the Imo State Newspapers Limited, INL, along Egbu Road, Owerri. As the editor of the *Nigerian Statesman,* a government-owned tabloid, his mind was fixed mainly on the packaging of the next day's paper. He had barely taken his seat behind his desk when his secretary came into his office to deliver him a letter. The envelope showed the letter originated within the INL. He tore it open immediately. The message was baffling. Proceed immediately on your annual leave.

The letter was signed by Eyioma lgbokwe, the managing director of the newspaper house. Okoro was not amused. The official roster had scheduled the editor to take his annual leave in September. Besides, the sudden annual leave letter did not state when the editor would resume duties. Something must be wrong. Yes, it was the editorial just published that Wednesday morning, titled *The Question of Spartans Deal (1).* The editorial had criticised government decision to hand over the ownership of the

Spartans Football Club of Owerri to a private businessman, Emmanuel lwuanyanwu.

As Okoro cleared his desk, downcast and ready to go home, the editor-in-chief of the newspaper, Nduka Onum, was directed to act as the editor till further notice. Onum agreed but defied instructions to discontinue publication of part two of the same editorial. The next day (February 13) he published it. And before he arrived his office that morning, his annual leave letter was also waiting. Onum was furious. He tendered his resignation letter on the spot. Again, another acting editor was appointed and that added up to three editors in about three days. In the dramatic twist ofevents that ensued, Okoro lost his job. He says he was fired, but government officials at Owerri claimed Okoro, like Onum, "panickly resigned."

'The saga of Okoro's exit from the *Nigerian Statesman* began only a few months after he left his prestigious job as the production editor of the *Daily Times*in Lagosto become the editor of the Owerri tabloid. One Friday morning, Okoro recalled, he had just entered his office when his phone rang dissonantly. He reached for the receiver and the voice on the other side said he was the commissioner of industries, and he wanted to find out why his picture was used for a news story published that day on abandoned projects.

Okoro explained that it had to do with the fact that the matter fell under his ministry and that the commissioner need not worry since most of the abandoned projects reported were there ever before the commissioner was appointed. The commissioner quickly diverted the course of discussion and queried the veracity of the story. He was obviously not happy with the report, at least, from the tone of his voice. But matters became worse when the editor advised the commissioner to "simply write a rejoinder" if he disagreed with the facts of the story. Okoro said the man slammed the phone on him. The next thing Okoro knew was that the matter went to the commissioner of information. "Then the governor came in too, and they decided to do something about me," Okoro told *Newswatch*.

But Okoro was not afraid either to step harder on government's sour toes provided he had sufficient reasons to do so in line with acceptable practice. The opportunity came during the IMF debate. Okoro was on a short holiday when his paper wrote an editorial title, *Let Kalu be*. That editorial was a reaction to 'The Punch's editorial which had asked for the deployment of the then minister of finance, Kalu Idika Kalu, over his stance on the IMF debate. Okoro told *Newswatch*, the *Let Kalu be* editorial was in bad taste and was inspired by Kalu himself who hails from Imo State and influenced the employment of some senior staff in the editorial department. "They would have found it difficult to get that editorial into the paper if I were around," Okoro fumed. So when he (Okoro) returned from his holiday, he decided "with the editorial board" to publish what he called "a definitive statement on the IMF debate which clearly kicked against the previous editorial in support of Kalu." Said Okoro, "We knew we were playing into the hands of some powerful officials, but we thought it was an act of patriotism to cry against the acceptance of the IMF loan."

Okoro said those he called the "Lagos group" comprising some very top federal government officials from Imo State, became hostile towards him since their attempt to put the *Nigerian Statesman* in their breast pockets had been rebuffed. "Sometimes, they summoned us (Okoro and Onum) to their offices in Lagos or to their hometowns whenever they came to the state.

They complained we were not giving them the necessary home support and publicity. At a point, in January 1986, they gave us two weeks ultimatum to change or be fired. But I personal said, I am not going to be anybody public relations officer," Okoro declared.

But government officials at Owerri told *Newswatch* Okoro was someone else public relations officer, and that always brought him in confrontation with government. Temple Benson, the state commissioner of information himself a veteran journalist, said Okoro allowed himself to be used by some influential businessmen and politicians outside the state. For instance, Okoro collaborated with a newspaper baron (name withheld) in promoting a weekly paper at the expense of the *Nigerian Statesman.*

So, government developed cold feet and feared that the editors can portray them a very bad light, given the chance. The February 12 and 13 editorials on Spartan FC had obviously confirmed government fears and thrown its officials off gear. Only on December 9, 1985, the *Nigerian Statesman* with Okoro's imprint had written an editorial praising Emmanuel Iwunyanwu for taking over the Spartans FC in the face of dwindling government finances. Just three months later, another editorial on the same issue completely reversed its earlier stance. "What suddenly happened?" Benson queried.

Okoro was still on his "annual leave" when on February 22, the board of directors of INL, headed by Ralph Opara, a veteran journalist, sent for him. The "holidaying" editor told the board bluntly that government was interfering too much in the running of the paper. Opara said "nonsense had been made of the editorship of the *Nigerian Statesman* and the whole business of news gathering and dissemination in the newspaper house."

Apart from the OIC issue, the state government, Okoro said, had ordered censorship on stories concerning the controversial Imo State airport project, the new campus of the University of Imo State and a common matter like the UPE. "I told them at the rate we were going, the paper might have nothing to publish in future. I told them I was quite fed up and if things did not improve, I would quit." That was Saturday, February 22. On Monday, February 24, two days after appearing before the board, the clash between the editor and the state government reached a theatrical crescendo. Okoro got a letter from the management which said the board had accepted his resignation. The man was flabbergasted. He told *Newswatch* "I never resigned."

In Owerri, Igbokwe had no written proof of Okoro's resignation in his office. Said a senior newsroom staff at INL: "Okoro had his say, but government had its way."

THE PEN AGAINST THE GUN

Onome Osifo-Whiskey, managing editor of *Tell* magazine was on his way to the church two Sundays ago, in the company of his children, when trouble struck. Three cars forced his car off the Ajanaku-Opebi Road junction, Ikeja, Lagos. It turned out to be government security operatives. He was arrested.

Two weeks earlier, Soji Omotunde, Editor of *African Concord,* was arrested in a similar Gestapo style along Adeniyi Jones Avenue, Ikeja. Lewis Obi, Editor-in-Chief of *African Concord* and immediate boss of Omotunde said "Omotunde tried to find out why he was being arrested, but the agents would not oblige him. He requested to drive his car to wherever they were taking him, apparently for fear of losing both his car and freedom. That too was turned down. Then his abductors turned violent. They shoved and dragged him. He fell down right at the middle of the road. They bundled him into their car and gagged his mouth as he was shouting to attract public attention."

Like Osifo-Whiskey's arrest, no official explanation has been given so far for Omotunde's arrest and incarceration. Last March,

Ladi Olorunyomi, wife of Dapo, editor of *The News* magazine was picked up at her home and detained for months in the hope that her husband would resurface from his hide out. But the frightened editor has sneaked out to far away United States. Some days ago, on November 3, security agents returned to the Olorunyomi's home and arrested her again, this time in place of Bayo Onanuga, the magazine's editor-in-chief, who had become adept at beating security dragnets.

Similarly Arit, wife of Nosa Igiebor, *Tell Magazine*'s editor-in-Chief, was reportedly arrested when security operatives went for the husband recently. Igiebor scaled a high fence on sensing the arrival of his "customers" and has since resurfaced in London.

With security operatives hot on the heels of many journalists, some publishers literally publish on the run, moving from one hide-out to another, in a new regime of underground journalism.

But has the media really been under siege during the Abacha four-year strangle-hold on power? The answer is yes and no. Yes, because as the fierce-looking general clocks four years in power this week, there are more journalists in detention than at any other time in the history of Nigeria. Some, who are not in detention are underground and those who are not underground are not sure when they will take their turn in detention or underground. And those who don't want anything to do with detention and underground are trooping out of the profession in search of greener and less turbulent pastures.

Chris Anyanwu, Editor-in-Chief of *The Sunday* magazine, *TSM*, Kunle Ajibade of *The News magazine*, Charles Obi of Classique magazine and George Mba of Tell magazine are serving 15 years jail term each for being "accessories" in an alleged coup plot against the administration of Abacha. Anthony Uranta of the defunct *Abuja Newsday* is serving 12 months imprisonment at the Kirikiri medium security prison, in Lagos. He was jailed by the Lagos State Task Force on environmental sanitation for an undisclosed offence. Jenkin Alumona, editor of *The News* was picked up in the premises of the Nigerian Television Authority NTA, Lagos barely a week ago, shortly after he stepped out of the NTA studio where he also anchors a sports programme.

A good number of other journalists have been briefly detained, suspended, assaulted and even whipped in the last few weeks. Those detained included Akpandem James, and Chris Ikwunze, *The Punch and Vanguard* correspondents respectively in Port Harcourt, Babatunji Wuse, of *The News,*Reth Ateloye of *Fame,* Segun Olatunji of the *DailySketch*, Demola Abimbola of *The News* and Gbenga Alaketu of *Tempo.*

In Imo State, Oby Agbai the chairman of the state council of the Nigerian Union of Journalist, NUJ, was on September 3, thoroughly flogged by security men in Government House, Owerri and later hospitalized for multiple injuries. Agbai who works for the state-owned tabloid *The Statesman* had a few days earlier criticized the state government for poor funding of *The Statesman* at a luncheon organized by government for media executives. That seems to be her offence.

In Yobe State, John Ben Kalio, military administrator of the State last month ordered the Yobe State Television, YTV, station shut down and the staff on duty flogged mercilessly by his aides. Eight members of staff of YTV were arrested and taken to Government House where Ben-Kalio, a wing commander, allegedly supervised their canning. Their crime? They had aired a documentary on the tenure of Dabo Aliyu, former governor of the State.

Media watchers predict tougher days ahead as government tries to steer the political transition train out of misty clouds. Sensing danger, wives of journalists are dragging their husbands ears every morning about what they write. Said one reporter: "My wife is now my editor. If she says strike out that sentence, I do not hesitate because I understand that to mean I will not follow you to Kirikiri o!"

But if the four years of Abacha administration have been a tale of woes for the press, pressmen cannot escape blame. The state of the media and the practice of the profession has left most professionals gasping for breath.

Lai Oso, head of mass communication department in Ogun State Polytechnic believes that the ethical conduct of the press in the last four years has become a matter of concern not just for public officials and the general public but even for practitioners of the profession. "Ethical codes which are expected to guide journalism is anything but respected by a cross section of practitioners" he said. Ikechi Nwosu, a Nigerian scholar, says that adherence to code of journalistic conduct by Nigeria journalists is in reality very minimal. "Political partisanship, outright bias, wolf crying and distortions are not uncommon," he said.

At the biennial convention of the Nigerian Guild of Editors in 1996, Abacha summed up his impression of the press in a speech many regarded as "acerbic." Said Abacha: "the rational dimension of the practice was jettisoned for the more salacious variety that came dripping with the sectional and putrid tinge of unprofessional and gutter practice." He said journalists have forgotten the underlying demands of objectivity, respect for facts and existence of different view points. His complaint, it was clear to editors, was not directed against the entire Nigerian press but a section that Oso said, "has decided to see the Nigerian social reality from the different perspective opposed to the officially approved one."

But Abacha's observations, it must be admitted, were not too far from the truth. Objectivity, fairness, truth, balance, and neutrality, which are the cardinal creed of journalism have in the last four years of Nigerian political crisis been almost completely sacrificed by a large section of the Nigerian press, in favour of subjectivity, bias, lies, outright insult and resentment of key players of the Nigerian political saga. Perhaps, worse than any other time in Nigerian history, most of the Nigerian press in the last four years has displayed a hitherto unknown capacity for manipulation and distortion of news for political and personal ends. This has in most cases won the press disrespect even from casual readers, who are becoming increasingly wary and fed up with bombshell headlines that is anything but true. For some media watchers, the issue is not just a matter of junk journalism, it is guerrilla journalism, a moral equivalence of war. This is perhaps understandable, given the painful injustice that attended the annulment of the June 12, presidential election, which MKO Abiola clearly won in every geopolitical zone of Nigeria.

Relations between Abacha and the media have not always been cat and mouse. When Abacha came to power four years ago, he waved an olive branch at the press. He deproscribed the *Punch, Concord, and Abuja Newsday* proscribed by Ibrahim Babangida, the former president. Said Abacha in his maiden broadcast: "On the closed media houses, government is hereby lifting the order of proscription with immediate effect. We however appeal to the media houses that in the spirit of national reconciliation we should show more restraint and build a united and peaceful Nigeria."

Many thought the prospects and foundation of a good government-press relations had been laid. It was not to be. The honeymoon was over in a mere 10 months.In September 1994, Abacha wielded the big stick. He banned *the Punch, National Concord and The Guardian* for six months. Alex Ibru, publisher of *The Guardian* was then Abacha's minister of internal affairs but that was immaterial. For 18 months, the three media houses and all the titles in their stable were forced out of the news-stands. The collision course charted by both the administration and the press became difficult to reverse. In 1994, alone, the Nigerian Union of Journalists reported 110 cases of press freedom violations. These included the arrest and detention of leading Nigerian journalist such as Ray Ekpu, Dan Agbese and Yakubu Mohammed all of *Newswatch* for publishing an interview with David Mark, a retired brigadier-general.

In 1995, the Paris based *Reporters Sans Frontiers, RSF,* in its report of the world press situation said Nigeria was"one of the countries with the worst press freedom violations in recent times." It was in that year that government also revived the newspaper registration board set up by the Babangida regime. Each publication was expected to pay an annual subscription fee of N250,000 and a non-refundable deposit of N100,000 before making the newsstands. But the press has fought that plan to a standstill, at least for now.

To the credit of both the government and the press, Nigerian journalism remains in the words of *London Times"* surprisingly ebullient." Under the Abacha administration several new titles such as *Thisday, Post Express, The Diet, The source and National Post* have joined the newsstands. It is also under Abacha that Nigeria has seen the emergence of private radio and television stations, which now include African Independent Television, AIT, Ray Power Radio, DBN Television, Channels Television, Minaj Television, Murhi International Television, MIT, among others.

Inspite of recent spate of arrests and detention of journalists, none of the media houses has been shut down in recent times. Even his worst critics would give him credit for his tolerance of many adversarial publications against his person and government. *Newswatch* was told last week that left for some of his officials in the ministry of information, nearly half a dozen titles would have been proscribed by now.

But to date, Abacha remains the most distant and remote of the Nigerian leaders to the press. In four years as head of state, he has not granted a single interview to any Nigerian newspaper or magazine. That, in itself, speaks volumes.

OFFICER AND A RADICAL

Alozie Ogugbuaja jumped from his seat and punched the air fiercely, as he dropped the black receiver of his telephone set. His lanky frame stiffened a bit and his eyes shone with happiness at the news that he had won the first round of a legal tussle against his dismissal from the police force. As his friends began to troop into his bungalow at the Housing Estate, Calabar, Ogugbuaja dashed into his disheveled study and updated his diary with a typewriter: "Wednesday, November 2, 1988 – A Lagos high court presided over by Justice Olushola Thomas rules that Alozie is still a policeman until..."

What the Lagos high court offered Ogugbuaja was a chance to defend himself against the serious charges of sedition, incitement and treason leveled against him by his bosses, a chance his lawyer, Gani Fawehinmi argued, he was not given by the police authorities, before he was hurriedly dismissed. His dismissal, Fawehinmi told the court was a violation of section 33 of the 1979 constitution, which has not been suspended, modified or defaced by any decree. Said Fawehinmi: "If a Nigerian citizen, either in public service or not, is accused of any criminal offence, his service in any employment cannot be terminated on grounds of being accused of a criminal offence, until he has been formally charged, tried and convicted in a court or tribunal established for that purpose under the constitution."

Ogugbuaja's latest trouble began September 27, 1988, in a rather innocuous setting of the Calabar police officers' mess. The police community relations committee, Calabar, was billed to make a donation of N10,000 to the Cross River State Police Command. Ogugbuaja, in his capacity as the divisional police officer, DPO, Atakpa District, in Calabar metropolis, was invited to the ceremony which was to be presided over by Parry Osayande, the state commissioner of police. After the ceremony, a young man walked up to the DPO, introduced himself as Armstrong Abangson, a student of mass communication at the Calabar Polytechnic, undergoing his internship at the *Nigerian Chronicle,* a government-owned newspaper at Calabar.

He said he wanted to write a profile and requested Ogugbuaja for an interview. Ogugbuaja, reportedly turned down the request and refered Abangson, instead, to the *Chronicle* "backfiles" for all he needed to write a profile. Ogugbuaja drove off, thinking that was the "end of the matter." It was not.

On October 8, eleven days after the Abangson-Ogugbuaja encounter and barely three weeks after Abangson began his internship, the *Chronicle* went to town with a half-page "profile" on the police officer, it was Abangson's very first story for a newspaper and it landed with a bang. In the story, Ogugbuaja was credited with the statement to the effect that the military has failed the country as an agent of revolution but has "only succeded in entrenching themselves as members of the ruling class."

Ogugbuaja according to the story, also declared that "we have to look elsewhere for an alternative source of revolution." That alternative source, he suggested, could be found in the workers, market women, students, journalists, the unemployed, the underemployed and the police force. Said Ogugbuaja in the story: "I am talking about the people's police force and not the Dodan Barracks or government police force, which is what we have now." Finally, Ogugbuaja asserted in the story that "the people's policeman should turn his gun on the government rather than on the people," if the inspector-general of police or the president contradicts the will and aspirations of the people.

The story was so explosive, *Newswatch* was told, the governor of Cross River State, Ibim Princewill quickly telephoned Osayande to "complain." But Osayande had to wait till October 10, to commence action against the officer because October 9, was a Sunday. By 10.00am, October 10, a police signal was dispatched to Ogugbuaja, posting him "with immediate effect" to the state police headquarters at Diamond Hill. Sam Onuko, another superintendent of police, was posted to replace Ogugbuaja as the new Atakpa DPO. Ogugbuaja heard the news first from Onuko, who arrived early enough to take over his job. A mild drama was to ensue as Ogugbuaja refused to vacate his seat for the new DPO. His argument, according to reliable sources was that "the procedure was irregular." The drama dragged on till 2.00pm, when a wireless message finally got to Ogugbuaja, ordering him to hand over "within 24 hours."

The next day (October 11) as Ogugbuaja was busy writing his handover notes, the telephone rang. He was immediately summoned to Diamond Hill. For about three hours, Ogugbuaja waited in Osayande's secretary's office, a rare situation, since the young officer was close to the commissioner and usually saw him "at very short notice." At about 1.30pm, he was finally ushered into the commissioner's office and without any delay, Osayande handed Ogugbuaja a two-page query personally signed by him, in the presence of Ezenwa Ifejika, the state deputy commissioner of police.

Osayande, in the query, said the publication was "undesirable," "seditious," and had the intension of "bringing into hatred or contempt or inciting disaffection against the federal government of Nigeria and exciting the citizens of Nigeria to attempt to procure the alteration or overthrow of the federal military government."

Osayande, according to *Newswatch* sources, also blamed the young officer for not seeking or obtaining permission before granting the interview as stipulated by civil service rules. Angry, the usually friendly police boss, gave Ogugbuaja two hours "to show cause why your conduct should not be reported to the inspector-general of police for severe disciplinary action."

Newswatch sources at Diamond Hill said the tone of the query for once threw Ogugbuaja "off balance." The source said when Osayande arrived in the Cross River State command in 1987 from Benin where he presided over the end of the Anini saga, he sent for Ogugbuaja, "who was in a kind of exile at Oron" (now Akwa Ibom State), after his "pepper soup" doctrine. "Such a brilliant officer should not be allowed to waste away," Osayande was quoted as saying before transferring Ogugbuaja to Calabar. He created a 45-man special duty strike squad called research unit and put Ogugbuaja in charge. After the special squad completed its task of lowering the rate of armed robbery in the State, the commissioner dismantled it and named Ogugbuaja a DPO. Now, the tone of his query as "shocking" even to some senior officers who thought the commissioner would eventually pardon "his boy."

But if Osayande had had any intensions of pardoning the superintendent, the reply the young officer sent back "made things very difficult," a *Newswatch* source said. Ogugbuaja in his four-page reply denied granting Abangson an interview. He said all the materials used for the "profile" was what he had said before both at the Justice Akanbi tribunal and in his "several memos" to police authorities. "In some," he said, "I confirm that I had propounded the doctrine of people's police force variously but not at any formal interview. If implemented, it would build a more efficient and effective police force. It would evolve a society that treats the causes rather than the symptoms of crime. I should be commended not condemned."

But what irked police authorities in Calabar most, according to *Newswatch* sources, was the digression in Ogugbuaja's reply, which took a better half of his four-page letter. In the "offending digression," Ogugbuaja accused not only the police authorities but the government, of double standard. He said the government has found it easy to "harass" him all the time because he is not from a privileged family. "I wonder if my father had been the Ooni of Ife, the Alafin of Oyo, the Oba of Benin, the Obi of Onitsha, the Emir of Kano, the Emir of Gwandu or if I had been the son of one of the bourgeois families or a well-connected military officer, (whether) I would have gone through what I am going through now." He gave his boss the example of Abubakar Umar, a former governor and lieutenant-colonel in the army.

He said Umar, as a major and sole administrator of the Federal Housing Authority, FHA, used the *National Concord* forum to "viciously attack and discredit" a military government. "Yet," he said, "He has nothing more to offer this country than Alozie Ogugbuaja does. This country belongs to all of us. I shall question any overt or covert action that suggests, implies, denote, or connotes that some Nigerians are second or third-class citizens in their own country."

When the letter got to Osayande, shortly before the two-hour deadline, *Newswatch* was told, "the man couldn't hide his anger and disappointment." On October 12, he forwarded his recommendation to Lagos. A copy was sent to Porter Dabup, the Rivers State commissioner of police, who is doubling as the boss of Zone 6, since assistant Inspector-General Usman Adeyemi retired about five months ago.

While Ogugbuaja spent about a week idling away at Diamond Hill without any specific job, except to await the decision of the IGP, the Cross River State government turned its eye on the *Nigerian Chronicle* that published the controversial profile. Okon Eyo, secretary to the Cross River State government, dispatched a protest letter to Patrick Okon, acting General Manager of the newspaper corporation. Okon, in turn summoned Joshua Okpo, the features editor and Abangson, the author of the profile. Okpo told Okon he instructed Dennis Utang, the entertainment page editor to help edit the story because he was busy performing other important editorial functions, since the paper has been operating in the last four months without an editor or deputy. On October 17, Okon wrote to suspend Okpo and Utang while Abangson's internship was terminated.

As the unfolding crisis began to snowball, Abangson quickly sent a letter to Princewill, Gambo, Osayande and E.D. Akpan-Iquot, his head of department at Calabar Polytechnic. According to Abangson, in a letter written on the same day he was sent packing at the *Nigerian Chronicle*, the profile was not based on any exclusive or press interview. Said he: "In order to put the record straight, I want to state categorically that the publication was not based on any exclusive or press interview rather it was a flashback on things he said predominantly at the Justice Akanbi panel two years ago. I, therefore, regret any embarrassment caused partly due to the misinterpretation and misconception of the write-up."

On October 21, as Ogugbuaja reported at Diamond Hill to await posting, he got something else in turn: a signal saying he was suspended with effect from October 8, the date the profile appeared in the newspaper. Part of the letter said he was placed on half pay. It was another October blues for the radical officer, as he had suffered his first suspension on October 6, 1986. He did not stay long enough to collect the "half pay" as his dismissal letter was to follow quickly. Signed by Musa Yahaya, deputy force secretary (II) for the IGP, the letter said the officer was dismissed for making "incitive, seditious and treasonous statements against the federal military government of Nigeria." Curiously, the dismissal letter was dated October 20, a day before the suspension, suggesting as one of Ogugbuaja's brothers said that "Alozie had been dismissed even before he was interdicted."

Ogugbuaja's friends and relations say his latest trouble is a carry-over of the 1986 "pepper soup" palaver. As the spokesman of the Lagos State police command at that time, Ogugbuaja had told the Akanbi tribunal probing the 1986 students' crisis that the Nigerian armed forces "are the unregistered party of Nigeria," whose members are overpaid, drink beer and pepper soup quite early in the day and do nothing else but plan coup." Police authorities had denied then that his suspension was connected with the testimony before the tribunal, but rather to an illicit affair with a female member of the National Youth Service Corps. On November 19, when Ogugbuaja was serving his suspension, he said some unknown men tossed a grenade under his car, as he drove home from a social visit. The grenade failed to explode and was later detonated by bomb experts. The police said it was a smoke bomb.

Ogugbuaja signed and collected his dismissal letter October 21 and turned up later to surrender his police warrant card, firearms and other police property in his custody. Late in the night of October 30, he sneaked into Lagos, (avoiding the airport) behind the wheels of his jeep and told Fawehinmi, to challenge his dismissal in the law court because he was wrongly dismissed without proper investigations. The legal action paid off, at least in the first round. Ogugbuaja returns to the court for the substantive suit November 11. One of his numerous friends who refused to be named called it "a moment of respite." For now, the fearless policeman lives to fight another day.

THE COMING REVOLUTION

"My name is Golden Sekibo. I am a Niger-Deltan. I hold a Bachelors Degree in Political Science and a Masters degree in International Relations. Right now, I am an Okada rider (commercial motorcyclist) in Port Harcourt." The audience froze to a pin-drop silence, as the young man paused to fish out a piece of paper from his breast pocket.

"When I heard about this conference through one of my passengers, I promised myself that I would make it to Uyo, even if it meant riding down here on a motorcycle and that is what I have done. I am glad that this conference is a reality. We, in Niger Delta, are a people conquered. We are a people robbed and spoiled. We are enslaved, snared in holes and fair game for all. And there is none to say 'enough-is-enough.'" A loud applause seized the hall, as he waited almost calmly for the uproar to subside. "Let those who have ears listen to me: Revolution is not made, it comes. It is coming soon in Niger-Delta. Those who make peaceful change impossible make violent change inevitable." Anger was palpable in his tone and the same feeling permeated the entire hall.

Nothing in Sekibo's carriage or comportment had suggested he was educated and nothing about him prepared the packed hall of academia, politicians, diplomats, businessmen and journalists for the dynamite the young man would unleash. He looked haggard like a typical motorcycle-taxi driver. His trousers were faded and his shirt thread-bare. He had only managed to get the microphone when a chance was given to the audience to ask questions at the end of a paper by one of the key speakers. In only three minutes, he x-rayed the despoiled condition of the Niger-Delta, blasted the leadership of the region for the historic betrayal of a people in exchange for personal crumbs and provoked the consciences of not a few. He was not alone.

Thrice, when George-Hill Anthony, President, Commonwealth of Niger-Delta youths for peace spoke and when James Essien, a lawyer and Mrs. Victoria Udoh, an American-based educationist spoke, I saw men fighting back tears with little or no success. Anthony told a story of a Niger-Delta village, where local folks sneak early enough in the morning to scavenge garbage heaps of oil company workers and are depending solely on these left-overs to feed their children. He narrated a sordid story of blood and death in the hands of cruel security agents posted to ensure free and uninterrupted flow of crude oil in Bayelsa villages. Ben Chuke, the Minister of Special Projects in the Presidency could not help but acknowledge " the reality of this suffering" of the Niger-Delta people. Though not a Niger-Deltan, he himself told a story of how he visited the home town of Bayelsa State governor, Alamasiagha from Yenogoa, the capital city and how what could have been a one-hour return trip became seven-hour ordeal on impossible road. Yet, I can say, these were just the appetizers.

The stage was the first international conference on Niger-Delta held last week in Uyo, the serene capital city of Akwa Ibom State. I would not have forgiven myself if I did not find time to be at that conference. It was for many the singular most important event in the Niger Delta region in recent years. For three straight days, breaking of oil pipelines, uprooting of drilling installations and kidnapping of oil company workers gave way to breath-taking intellectual interpretation and repositioning of the oil-rich but poverty stricken region.

Not that thousands of Niger-Deltans that thronged the venue of the conference thought little of the courageous role of militant youths but that they needed to back their struggle with a sound and well-articulated blue print for integration, development, co-operation and sustainable peace in the region. Sponsored by the governments of Akwa Ibom, Bayelsa, Delta, Rivers and Cross River states under the auspices of Integrated Development Initiative, a non- governmental organisation, it drew the best of minds in various development issues from as far as United States and attracted the officials and interests of UNDP, UNESCO and Ford Foundation.

The first day was akin to walking the political minefield. Senate President Pius Anyim and Speaker of the House Representatives, Ghali Na'Abba, who sent strong delegations led by Senate Deputy Whip, Ibok Essien and south-south caucus leader in the House Ndueso Essien; washed their hands off the problem of the region and pointed accusing fingers instead on the Presidency. Anyim said, the National Assembly had made every attempt through the NDDC Act as well as in past and present Appropriation Acts to ensure that the region receives its legitimate entitlement but for the Presidency which claims to be wiser than all the membership of the National Assembly put together.

Governor Victor Attah of Akwa Ibom State, the chief host, in a keynote address, warned against the danger of divide and rule. Waxing metaphorical, he said: "The broom is a fitting lesson in the concept of unity and strength. A broom stick is easy to break, But any energy (directed) at breaking a bundle of broom is dissipated, We must remain bound in this struggle, no matter the odds."

Yet nearly half of the governors in the core Niger Delta were neither present at the conference nor represented. Speaker after speaker blasted the absentee governors for either lack of seriousness and loyalty to the cause of the region or being lackeys of some vested interest. Apart from the Bayelsa State governor who had representatives throughout the conference, Delta State made strong representation with a delegation of House of Assembly members. But Rivers State, one the closest neigbours of Akwa Ibom was visibly absent at governmental level. Angry delegates and participants from the state could not resist the temptation to speak about their government with unkind words. After Senator David Dafinone, a prominent son of the region delivered his paper on "Niger-Delta: Yesterday, Today and Tomorrow," someone queried him on the leadership problem" in the region. His answer was sharp and terse. "All I can say is that Jesus came to serve and Judas came to steal and betray." Chief Harold Dappa-Biriye, Chairman of that session agreed with him and said some governors of the region were gambling with the destiny of the region, a not too disguised reference to governor Peter Odili of Rivers State, who many said preferred his closeness to President Obasanjo over and above the Niger Delta cause.

The conference went ahead to deliberate on oil companies and the regions environment; human right violation; options for prospective investors. In a session chaired by General Edet Akpan (rtd), former NYSC Director General, Dr. Esohe V. Molokwu, the Regional Coordinator of UNESCO in Nigeria, said all the four ecological zones of Niger-Delta "have been systematically degraded and in some cases destroyed." Molukwu, like all other key speakers, out-lined detailed options and solutions available to the region in the short and long term.

Mike Ozekhome's paper on legislating for integration, development and growth, was one of the star papers. But beyond that, it almost caused an instant uprising as delegates especially those from youth organisations rose up and loudly demanded for an end to injustice in the region. Said one angry contributor from the audience: "If the oil wealth of Nigeria was in Sokoto, Ogun or Zamfara, how many people in Niger Delta would be allowed to get to the top."

It was the same session that Professor Akpan Ekpo, Vice Chancellor of the University of Uyo, presented another star paper on Investment Opportunities: Options for Perspective Investors, while Professor Calestine Bassey of the University of Calabar presented a paper on Imperatives of Federalism, Resources Control and Grassroot Economic Empowerment. The subject of resource control became explosive. Professor Bassey said resource control was at the root of war in Katanga and Columbia. He reduced the constant political battle in Nigeria between the three majority tribes to a fight for the control of oil wealth. "If there is anything that the three major Nigerian tribes have agree, it is the federal control of crude oil money."

Other issues such as capacity building and skill acquisition as well as education for survival in Niger Delta were tabled and discussed by such international speakers as Dr. Uduak Udofia, Dr. Amaechi Nzekwe, Dr. A. A. Ikoiwak and Dr. Ekeng Anam-ndu.

At the end, virtually all the multifaceted problems of the region were examined, documented and solution proffered.

At least 10 consultation committees were set up to fine-tune the blue prints and draw up the work plan on specific development issue. This should be a treasure to the region as it struggles to free itself from the stranglehold of indigenous colonialism.

EZE GOES TO VILLA

He walks fast, talks fast and acts fast. To keep pace with this nimble 49 year old tycoon, his consorts and aides are literally on their toes round the clock.

But nestled in his ninth floor presidential suite at Nicon Noga Hilton Hotel, Abuja, this Wednesday afternoon Arthur Eze, prince of Ukpo and millionaire-businessman, appeared shut off from the dust raised by his all-out campaign to persuade head of state, General Sani Abacha, to run for the 1998 presidential election.

In the company of half-a-dozen personal staff, he looked so disarmingly simple, you wouldn't know who is the boss here. But in this disguised atmosphere of leisure, the big boss was doing what he likes to do best: staying one step ahead of others.

Hitherto thought to be apolitical and hardly known for anything else except philanthropy, Eze, an American-trained engineer, sprang a surprise three weeks ago, when he arrived Aso Rock Villa, Nigeria's seat of power, with a retinue of 150 paramount rulers, from the nine eastern States of Nigeria, with a mission that astounded political observers. Be our next president please, they pleaded with the taciturn general.

This came at the time politicians and, indeed, the nation were trying hard to read the lips of Abacha just after the independence anniversary speech. A better part of the political class was livid. Others gasped helplessly in resignation. For many, one thing was certain: Eze's move, backed up by the entire traditional institution of eastern Nigeria was yet the most serious and spirited attempt to draft the Head of State into a race that has been remarkable for lack of racers.

At an exclusive interview with *Newswatch* last week, Eze, a wrestling enthusiast, challenged politicians to come into the ring with Abacha if they are macho enough. "I have looked around, I have not seen any challenger. Have you seen any? Where are the presidential candidates? The fact is, we have no alternative to Abacha, we have to draft him. Other presidential candidates have abandoned us. He (Abacha) cannot abandon us now," he said with mischievous determination in his tone.

For a man who hardly speaks to the press and holds no known view on any national issue, his emergence and the opinion he expressed in his interview with *Newswatch* last week might engage the political class and analysts for some months to come. "I don't want another civil war. Any mistake now can lead to an unpalatable scenario like in Congo Brazzaville. So we must support Abacha. General Abacha has direction. He has (already) won peace for Nigeria. Without peace and security, I cannot be here and you cannot be here. Everything will crash," he said.

According to Eze, all those talking about the presidency in southern Nigeria are confusionists. "Those talking about a president from the south are spoilers. They are faceless people. They don't want to be president, they want to cause confusion. They will not succeed," he added.

In addition, Eze pointed at Abacha's achievements on the economic front and said Abacha must be given a chance to consolidate on them. "Even his enemies will agree with me that Abacha has succeeded in achieving stability in exchange rate and a restoration of sanity to the banking sector through the failed banks tribunals. We have witnessed reduction in the incidence of 419 and money laundering, elimination of fiscal indiscipline and enforcement of accountability in the management of public funds. These are gains we cannot allow some faceless politicians to come and squander," he told *Newswatch*.

Only the previous day, Tuesday October 28, a youth organization known as National Association of Igbo Youths, NAIY, had appeared on network television at prime time to back Eze and Abacha. Said Chidi Okolo, national coordinator of NAIY: "We condemn in totality the clandestine activities of some faceless and self-acclaimed Igbo leaders called *Ohaneze,* who (are trying to) malign Prince Arthur Eze. We declare our support for Prince Arthur Eze and endorse the candidature of General Sani Abacha in next year's presidential election."

Another organization, known as Youth Earnestly Asked for Abacha, YEAA, headed by Daniel Kanu, son of the proprietor of Agura Hotel, Abuja, also took turn the same night on network news to re-echo and intensify the pro-Abacha campaign. Preceding YEAA and NAIY declarations, tension had descended on the nine eastern states particularly the core east. In Enugu, capital of Enugu State, various socio-political organizations staged mass rallies in support of Eze and Abacha. One group known as "Concerned Igbos, CI, led by Alex Ezike, stormed the Enugu press centre, carrying placards which praised Eze and castigated *Ohaneze,* the pan-Igbo group led by egg heads of the core east.

The CI, which had representatives from Anambra, Imo, Enugu, Abia and Ebonyi States later drove in a convoy to the Government House in Enugu, where Sule Ahman, a colonel and military administrator of Enugu State, promised to look into their complaint and advised them to avoid confrontation with opposing groups. "If democracy is to thrive in the country, nobody should persecute another because he holds a contrary opinion," Ahman said. It was in the same vein Alozie Dike, an academic spoke: "He (Eze) has the right of choice and the right of association. Why should those who have exercised their right to oppose Abacha think Prince Eze has no right to support Abacha."

All arrows seemed pointed at *Ohaneze* and possibly Igboezue Cultural Association, ICA, said to be controlled by Emeka Ojukwu, who is speculated to be quietly longing for Aso Rock. But neither the *Ohaneze* nor ICA, responded as a body last week. Lnstead, *Ohaneze* met behind closed doors in their Enugu GRA office and expressed shock over the activities of Eze, who they berated for using Igbo people to feather his business nest.

Pini Jason, newspaper columnist and vocal Igboman condemned Eze and his mission with Eastern traditional rulers as foolhardy, disgraceful and ridiculous. Said Jason: "Between Prince Arthur Eze and the garishly plumed traditional rulers, I can see a common ground. They are all traders. For Arthur Eze, this project is another contract." Jason argued that Easterners need no traditional rulers to make a choice between the boat and the shark. "Those who purport to speak for the Igbo, when they know they don't, must stop sending the wrong signals to other Nigerians," he said.

The signal sent by the visit of Eastern traditional rulers was received with anger elsewhere. Felix Oboagwina, a public affairs commentator described the traditional rulers as spineless fellows. "What is incomprehensible is the unwholesome posturing to stampede General Abacha into believing that Nigerians earnestly wanted him, when it is obvious that the odds of sustainable democracy are against him," Oboagwina said.

Sanya Anayoade, a political analyst raised questions about the credibility and acceptability of the traditional rulers in their domains. "It may be necessary to find out in this calculus who the traditional rulers who made the trip to Abuja were representing. Who did they consult? Who were they speaking for? It is pretty certain that they were speaking for traditional rulers, not the overwhelming majority of the eastern people," Anayoade said. He said he was convinced that northern traditional rulers and their western counterpart could not be drafted to join what he called "the dirty campaign."

Prominent Igbo leaders *Newswatch* spoke to, refused to speak on record for fear of being seen to be opposing the Head of State. Said one Igbo leader in Lagos last week: "This is a matter of great embarrassment to us. *Ohaneze* has to do something fast about it and publicly."

Coincidentally, documents on Eze's contracts with Enugu State government began to make the rounds last week in Enugu after *Ohaneze* meeting. Believed to be circulated by *Ohaneze,* the documents centred around alleged $796,774.95 paid to Triax Group in 1991, for the supply and installation of Harry transmitters for which, Eze's opponent allege, the contract was not performed. They insisted that what Eze's company did was to supply Enugu State Broadcasting Service, ESBS, with part of the items contracted for by old Anambra Broadcasting Service, ABS. They also allege shaddy deals in the multi-million dollar African Development Bank, ADB – assisted project.

But Eze dismissed the allegations last week as "lies by faceless politicians." Said Eze to *Newswatch*: "Go and find out from Enugu State government. They are still owing me $1.3 million dollars on the ESBS job. And on the ADB project, government is owing me $17 million. But those faceless politicians will never tell you the truth."

Indeed some politicians, in the east are clearly agitated about Eze's adventure into politics. If not anything else, the way he has deployed money to ensure victory of his candidates has left his opponents flat on their backs. They spoke about what they call "massive corruption and blatant trade of votes sponsored by this money man." This, according to his opponents, has led to "unpopular and dubious characters stealing their way to office." It has also notched the political temperature several degrees near boiling point.

But Eze told *Newswatch* he is surprised about such accusations because he is not a politician, neither does he habour sympathy for any political party. He, however, said young people who approach him for assistance whether in politics or business often smile back home, because he is on the side of the younger generation. "Some old politicians wanted to keep themselves permanently in office. I said no, you must allow young people to survive" he said.

According to Eze it is against the same backdrop that he patronizes the Ndigbo Progressive Forum, NPF, seen as the archrival of *Ohaneze*. "*Ohaneze* is made up of old people, we told them please hand over the baton to us, so that we can supplement what you are doing. But they want to take oxygen from us."

Similarly, the Eastern Business Forum, EBF, funded by Eze visa-vis the Enugu Chambers of Commerce, Industry, Mines and Agriculture, ECCIMA, is said to have the same undertone. What has become a visible trait in all organizations sponsored by Eze is the zeal with which these organizations are pursuing the pro-Abacha campaign.

Last week some political observers began to sketch a meeting-point between Arthur Nzeribe's campaign to transform former President Ibrahim Babangida to a civilian president and (Arthur) Eze's replay of his kinsman's script. "From Arthur to Arthur, what a curious coincidence," one editor said in a discussion with his colleagues.

Highly endowed with money both Arthurs are engineers, hail from the same ethnic group and are in their own rights gems in political cybernetics, controversy and generosity. Worth millions in pounds sterling, with investments across the world, Nzeribe, literally held Nigerians hostage after the June 12 elections with his Association for Better Nigeria, ABN, which dominated Nigeria's political theatre in the last days of Babangida regime. Said Nzeribe then: "The Third Republic would witness gross instability if IBB is not returned as civilian leader."

If Nzeribe is a chief, Eze is a prince. His late father was one of the longest serving paramount rulers in Igboland, having become the royal father of Ukpo, Dunukofia LGA, Anambra State, at the age of 20. At his death, Eze's elder brother Robert, a German-trained doctor succeeded him. Eze himself studied mechanical engineering in California US. On his return from US in 1979, he set up the Triax Group of Companies which has now become a business empire comprising Triax Airlines, Orient Bank, Telecommunication and Broadcasting Company, construction and engineering concerns. He also has substantial investments in breweries. He owns more than 90 percent share in Premier Breweries, Onitsha.

Though the rich prince is publicly staking his enormous wealth for the first time in politics, he has been a pal of virtually all Nigerian government in nearly two decades. He told *Newswatch* he hit his first jumbo contract during the Shagari administration when three governors, Sam Mbakwe of Imo state, Solomon Lar of Plateau State and Abubakar Rimi of Kano State, awarded him contracts to build their radio and television stations.

During the Babangida regime, he was very prominent in military cricles and was believed to have made a lot of money in the process. In one of his numerous philanthropic acts, he built and equipped a hospital at Wushishi, Niger State and named it Iyani-wura Hospital, in memory of Babangida's mother. Similarly he attended and donated generously at all Better Life Programmes, the pet programme of Babangida's wife, Maryam, that invitation were sent to him. He has extended a similar gesture to Family Support Programme, championed by incumbent first lady, Mariam Abacha.

With an accountant wife, Victoria and five children, Eze has managed for years to steer clear of public glare. Now in the affray, there seems to be many questions on the lips of his friends and foes alike. Can Eze weather the storm and walk the slippery terrain of Nigerian politics? Will this Arthur succeed where another Arthur failed? Asked last week by *Newswatch* what he would do if Abacha declined today to contest for the presidency. "If he says today that he is not contesting I will leave Nigeria tomorrow" he said.

A DESPOT AND THE POPE

The Pope never bargained for such. It was purely a pastoral visit to Catholic Church in Nigeria. But the old man was to discover, to his chagrin, that Nigerians from all faiths and denominations, choking under the draconian rule of General Sani Abacha, were pinning their hopes on him to persuade the iron fisted ruler, to let go the jugular of the nation.

As Pope John Paul II drove through the streets of Abuja, Nigeria's new, shining capital city, enthusiastic spectators held up copies of the newspapers for him to see. POPE OUR LAST HOPE was the screaming banner headline of *The Vanguard*. Virtually all the newspapers cast SOS headlines and wrote passionate editorials and features appealing to the Pontiff to persuade the head of state, General Sani Abacha to do the right thing: hand over power, not to himself, but to a democratically elected government; to release all politicians and journalists and respect human rights and human lives.

"Bail us out, Holy Father! Bail us out!" a group of youths cried out as the "Pope Mobile," his transparent, custom made SUV approached the city centre. Simultaneously, welcome billboards, banners and posters placed by government along the expected routes of the Pope gave a different impression of a country practically under siege. Both the government and its critics were eager to gain the Pope's ear and plead the merits of their case.

The first group was the association of Roman Catholic bishops and archbishops called the Catholics Bishops Conference of Nigeria who had already, on the eve of the pontiff's visit, urged Gen. Abacha to free political prisoners and make amends with opposition groups. They told the Pope that they were not comfortable with the situation on the ground as the "Nigerian nation is critically ill" and suggested that in his meeting with Abacha he should stress the importance of dialogue and reconciliation. They also requested him to entreat the government to "release all political detainees and prisoners and allow them to participate fully in the transition process." The Conference submitted to the Pope a list of 150 detained and imprisoned politicians, unionists, activists and journalists for onward delivery to Abacha, with a request for him to release them.

The Pope also received a long memo from a group in the US known as the Nigerian Pro-Democracy Network, NPN, a coalition of pro-democracy organizations in various parts of the US. It told the Pope that, since Abacha came to power in November 1993, the entire country has been held hostage by a "systematic silencing of every dissenting voice," including that of MKO Abiola, the winner of the 1993 Presidential elections. "Beginning with the political class, the regime has targeted labour leaders, intellectuals, journalists, students, human rights activists and environmentalists," the memo said. It cast doubts on the genuineness of

Abacha transition to civil rule programme. The Pope would be doing the will of God to intervene, the NPN said.

An international group of journalists, *Reporters Sans Frontiers* told the Pope Nigeria was "one of the most repressive African countries with regard to freedom of the press"; that more than 90 journalists had suffered repression last year and "at present, six additional journalists are being detained without official reason. Some of them are waiting to be tried and their health is said to be poor." The group asked the Pope to intercede on the journalists' behalf.

The Nigeria Civil Liberty Organization, leaders of Protestant churches and families of detained activists, also placed their hopes in the Pope for a solution of Nigeria's problems. And a group of women pleaded in their letter: "The rest of the world seems to have abandoned us in the hands of merciless soldiers. We have exhausted every means of securing the freedom of our husbands. Don't go home, please, Your Holiness, without securing the release of our husbands."

The government, however, also had every intention of taking the utmost propaganda advantage of the Pontiff's visit even naming two streets as Pope John Paul II Street andPope John Paul II Crescent. Loquacious Foreign Affairs Minister Tom Ikimi ensured that the Vatican envoy in Nigeria gave the Pope its side of the story. He was told of the "peace and stability" which the Abacha administration has secured for Nigeria since taking power.

Pope Pius II lived up to expectations. With no direct reference to the regime, the implications of his homilies were transparent. He repeated the same message publicly on two separate occasions, in Onitsha and Abuja, before a combined audience of more than five million.

At his reception ceremony and at the two outdoor Masses he spoke against injustice, dictatorship, military rule and abuse of human rights. With reference to the official motives of the visit, the beatification of Father Cyprian Michael Tansi, the Pope declared: "The testimony borne by Father Tansi is important at this moment in Nigeria's history, a moment that requires concerted and honest effort to foster harmony and national unity, to guarantee respect for human life and human rights."

He recommended an "attitude of reconciliation" on the part of the government and the people as well as a "return to constitutional order and democratic freedom."And in what was perhaps his closest sailing to the wind, he declared there could be no place "for intimidation and domination of the poor and the weak, arbitrary exclusion of individuals and groups from political life, misuse of authority or the abuse of power. Justice is not complete without an attitude of humble, generous service."

In anticipation, the answers had no doubt been well rehearsed. To the Pope's call for "honest efforts to foster harmony, national unity and guarantee respect for human life and human rights,"General Abacha said his government needed "prayers to persevere in our task without discouragement." To the call by the Pope for an "attitude of reconciliation" and "restoration of constitutional order and democratic freedom," the dreaded General said his administration abhorred dictatorship; and the transition programme which was being midwifedby him would give birth to "a new era of stability."

Behind closed doors at Aso Rock, the head of state's official residence in Abuja, the Pope followed up with a list of 60 names of people who should be given freedom, perhaps the same names that had been given him by the archbishops and bishops. The list includes Chief Abiola; General Olusegun Obasanjo, former head of state; Frank Kokori, president of the oil workers' union; Olu Fa-lae, former Secretary to the Federal Government, and dozens of other politicians and journalists. Joachin Nevalro-Vaal, the Vatican spokesman, said the 60 names were "compiled by the Holy See" based on information from international organizations, detainees' families, journalists and the government. In Pope John Paul's 82 missionary journeys outside Italy, this was only the second occasion on which he had presented such a list. The first time was to President Fidel Castro of Cuba who had acted upon it immediately.

That the Pope would succeed in Nigeria where other world leaders had failed remained no more than a hope. Pleas in the past for the release of political prisoners by Commonwealth Heads of State and others have been received with indifference. Abacha's announcement last October during Nigeria's Independence Anniversary that he was releasing political prisoners turned out to be a non-starter; not one political prisoner was released except General Shehu Yar'Adua, former deputy head of state, whose body was "released" for burial after he died in prison in suspicious circumstances last November.

Abacha-watchers and political observers believe the General may not listen to the papal supplications, except possibly on the issue of self-succession. But Catholic leaders in Nigeria were optimistic that the Papal pleas would not go unheeded. "His requests have never been rejected by any world leader nor by any faction or rebel leader. Nobody is known to have turned down the Pope," is the sanguine reminder of Father Matthew Kukah, Secretary-General of the Catholic Secretariat in Nigeria.

But there was no immediate flinging open of the prison gates either during or in the immediate wake of the Pope's departure.

THE MAKING OF A SAINT

On a misty morning, one week before Pope John Paul II touched down in Onitsha on the banks of River Niger, for a historic mission to Nigeria, a group of 12 men, made up of two Nigerian priests, three Vatican clergy, five gravediggers, a cameraman and *Africa Today's* Regional editor for West Africa, Anietie Usen, filed into a tranquil cemetery, where 37 catholic priests are buried inside the sprawling premises of the Holy Trinity Cathedral.

The newest grave was barely 24 hours old. It belonged to the Rev. Fr. Vincent Nwosu, a parish priest and member of the Protocol Committee for the Papal visit. He died suddenly after serving Mass the previous Sunday. But his grave was not the destination of the 12 men. Instead, they made for that of Fr. Cyprian Michael Iwene Tansi, the Nigerian monk who died in Leicester, England, in 1964.

The gravediggers went to work immediately to exhume Tansi's remains. The soil was hard and unyielding. "The remains are needed for the beatification Mass by the Pope next week," explained Monsignor Hypolite Adigwe, Director of Catechetics,

Onitsha Diocese Pontifical Mission Society. It took four-and-a-half hours to crack through six feet of soil, concrete slabs and red bricks to reach Father Tansi's grey, iron coffin. As it was lifted, the crowd of devotees outside the fence jumped for joy, rapidly chanting prayers, some in Latin.

From the cemetery, the unusual coffin was carried into the residence of Archbishop Albert Obiefuna of Onitsha, trailed by a curious crowd of church members. The Vatican priest, led by Father Paulino Quattrochi, the Postulator General for the Causes of Saints, took over. Assisted by two other Vatican specialist doctors, the iron coffin was slowly and carefully opened. Inside, there was another brown wooden coffin held together by four giant screw nails and red ribbon tapes. On top of it was a metal plate bearing Tansi's name. The archbishop cut the tapes. The Vatican clerics opened the inner coffin.

Lo and behold, inside a glass case, Father Tansi's skull and the major bones were intact. There were also a silver crucifix, missal and rosary with which he had been buried. More prayers were chanted as the selected audience of clerics crowded around to touch the coffin.

With Father Tansi literarily back from the grave, the tempo of activities to welcome the Pope increased. Even non-Catholics and non-Christians as well as top government officials were to some degree affected by the awe and mystique surrounding an otherwise obscure man whose life the Pope was coming to celebrate and proclaim as saintly.

In life, Tansi had stood resolutely for righteousness, sincerity and the relief of the oppressed. Thirty-four years after his death, the Pope would deliberately emphasize those qualities because of their particular relevance to contemporary Nigeria.

Tansi, as the Pope would announce, is the first Nigerian in the Catholic Church's history to be officially proclaimed "blessed"; the first African in modern times to be beatified. Saint Augustine of Hippo (present day Algeria) was elevated to sainthood in about 354 AD for his philosophical treatise. Saint Monica, mother of Saint Augustine, was proclaimed a saint for her prayer life and role as a model Christian mother, also in 354.

Between 1885 and 1887, Charles Lwanga, a Ugandan catechist and 15 other Ugandans such as David Mulumba were either beheaded or burned at the stake because of their faith and sermons against the corrupt and perverse rule of King Mwanga of the Kabaka dynasty. These men were later proclaimed saints by the Vatican.

As Father Michael Golden, an Irish priest and Church historian, explained, Tansi was "the first in Africa to be raised to the rank of the blessed, not because he was martyred, but because he lived a life of unique holiness."

Ironically, Tansi was born a pagan, in 1903 at Aguleri, and Igbo community on the banks of the Anambra River just a few kilometres from the River Niger. He rebelled against paganism yet became a hero for pagans and non-pagans alike. In life, he was hardly known beyond the rural confines of his community. In death, he is an acclaimed model of holiness. Throughout the catholic world, prayers can now be made in his name. On March 22, 1998, the day he was formally proclaimed "blessed" by the Pope, the Pontiff also decreed that January 20, Tansi's birthday, be marked henceforth as Father Tansi's Day in the Catholic church worldwide. This is part of what could be called the Father Tansi paradox.

I spent one week in Aguleri, Tansi's village and diocese just before the Pope arrived Nigeria and pieced together the life and times of this self-effacing man, directly from men and women who knew and interacted with him at close quarters. "He was remarkably short and some people used to call him Father Little," said Chief Gabriel Chiatula, the 70-year-old Onolueze, (deputy king) of Aguleri. "Now, he is standing so tall you could call him "Father Large."

Paul Manafa, a retired civil servant recalled how Tansi had a stammer and how, in 1937 – 38, he taught him the Catechism. "He also taught me, when he was the headmaster of this school. He hated laziness and lateness in arriving at school or Mass. He would hide behind one of the mango trees to catch latecomers. Some people thought then that he was too rigid, too uncompromising, with his church and Bible doctrines."

Patrick Chinwuboba, a retired agronomist, remembered Tansi for his life of fasting and prayer. "He was always starving and praying. One day some church women cooked him a very delicious chicken meal. He just looked at it, then addressing himself, said: 'This flesh can cry till tomorrow, I am not giving you any food for one week' and he gave the food away to others."

Chinwuboba remembers that even then, in the '30s and '40s, villagers had nicknamed him "the holy man" and "if a young man behaved very well we would nickname him 'Holy Tansi.'"

Hillary Anisiobi, now a 60-year-old Catholic priest, was 12 when he met Father Tansi who baptized him in 1940. It was from his baptism certificate signed by Tansi that he got to know his age. It was also his admiration for Tansi's "pious and simple lifestyle" that later inspired him to join the priesthood. Today, by virtue of his posting to St. Joseph parish in Aguleri, Father Anisio-bi sleeps in the same bedroom where Father Tansi used to sleep. "I want to be holy like Father Tansi and I want to do much for this community like he did," he said.

Cardinal Francis Arinze, head of the Vatican's inter-religious department was among hundreds of young men inspired to join the priesthood by Father Tansi. He explained: "He was near God, not just a priest. After I saw him, I said 'I want to be like this man'. Nobody preached to us that we should become priests. Just seeing him was enough."

These days Aguleri and the Catholic world in Nigeria seem to think and talk about nothing else except Father Tansi. Some remember him for the schools he built and his zeal to ensure that more children received Western education. Yet he himself was not a particularly bright student at the schools and seminaries he attended. When he was in his late forties in Nigeria, his bishop wrote of his "mediocre intelligence." Later, at the monastery in England, St. Bernard Mount Abbey, his theology was so bad that a fellow monk compared it to that of a "poor catechist."

Yet, Father Tansi has become a subject of more than a dozen books published in many European languages by eminent scholars. Said Elizabeth Isichei, professor of history and author of *Entirely for God. The life of Michael Tansi.* "What made him remarkable was the iron strength and tenacity of his will which was from boyhood directed entirely towards God. He never compromised with things which paralyzed most men's potential for holiness."

Father Tansi at his ordination took a vow of poverty and self-denial. In his life, both in Onitsha diocese and at the monastery in England, nothing would distract him from what he considered the path of holiness, neither food nor tradition nor earthly belongings. This was when Catholic priests, at least in Nigeria, were the No. 1 citizens in rural communities, riding in cars, living in the best houses, eating roasted chicken, drinking beer and whisky and observing celibacy only in the breach. Gregory Wareing, monk and colleague of Tansi at Leicester, wrote in his biography of him that he "nearly died of fasting." His only surviving brother, Pa Nneke Tansi remembers how "somehow he found joy and strength in a lifestyle that appeared like punishment to us. Everything that appealed to every other young man did not attract or appeal to him."

While a priest in Nigeria, instead of the Ford van provided by one of his parishes, Tansi preferred to trek through swamps and bushes to the 50 out-stations assigned him. I was told a story of how a new priest was sent to replace Tansi at Dunukofia, near Onitsha. On his first Sunday at the parish, the new priest mounted the pulpit, spread his hands wide and said to his congregation: "I am not Father Tansi I must have a cook." It was "Father Tansi's mortification and self-denial" that was "beyond the normal," according to Aloysius Adimonye.

He had only one good soutane (cassock); the other three were a network of self-sewn patches. He slept on a plank with just a mat over it. During Lent, he slept on the bare floor and walked on bare feet.

He had already worked in three parishes when in 1949 he was posted to his home parish of Aguleri. Every priest, especially the Europeans, dreaded Aguleri which was "paganism in all its ugliness and horror." Bishop Joseph Shanahan, one of the best known Catholic priests in Eastern Nigeria, once said: "It would take six generations to form a genuine Igbo Christian." New-born twins were instantly thrown into "evil forests" as food for soldier ants and wild animals. Frail old women were regarded as witches and killed if a younger person in their family died, no matter what the cause of death. Father Tansi's mother was killed for just such a reason while he was away at school in Onitsha.

He was so uncompromising and hostile to traditional animist religion that the community petitioned for his transfer. Masquerades he regarded as symbols of Satan; he told women that they (masquerades) were not spirits but their husbands, sons and brothers in disguise and even announced the names of men in the village who were mask carriers. One day one of his women leaders seized a masquerader by the mask, an offence punishable by death but Father Tansi ensured nothing happened to her. Instead, the case went to the White man's court where the four men behind the masks were forced to pay the woman four pounds each.

In addition, Tansi stood up against the practice of consulting diviners and made his friends swear never to take traditional titles because he considered them to be an initiation into satanic priesthood. But now, said one Aguleri Catholic, "masqueraders roam about freely and all the men of means in our churches have taken traditional titles."

Phisically, the Aguleri of Father Tansi's days does not appear to have changed much. It is a beautiful village amid red earth, sparkling clean brooks, valleys and hills. But it is very much the home of paganism: groves, shrines and idol worshippers. Most families own their own personal gods, personal shrines and personal diviners. Outside Father Tansi's family house, which his only surviving brother and nephews now occupy, there were no fewer than five shrines including one filled with the heads of various animals recently sacrificed. Another shrine was built over an ant hill.

A book called *Christ, the Ideal of the Monks* lent to him by a missionary kindled Tansi's strong desire and prayers for monastic life. He came to the conclusion that "the steady services of prayer and self-denial will contribute much more to the increase of the church and to the salvation of human race than those who work in the external direct services of the Lord's Vineyard."

Father Tansi entered the monastery at Mount St. Bernard Abbey, Leicester, in July 1950 and for the next 13 years he was an enclosed, contemplative monk, living, as he put it "entirely for God."

One month after the Silver Jubilee of his ordination in December 19, 1963 (actually on January 20, 1964) Tansi died of an ulcer related illness.

As Father Emmanuel Nwosu, the Postulator for the Cause of St. Tansi, put it: "The fame of his sanctity among the priests, the religious and the laity led to the application to the Vatican in 1979 by Cardinal Arinze, who was Archbishop of Onitsha, for his beatification. Cardinal Arinze's application was supported by the Bishop of Nottingham, where Father Tansi spent his last years, and by all the Catholic Bishops of Nigeria."

The investigation of the life of Tansi by the Vatican and the process of canonization began in earnest in 1986. A tribunal of inquiry called the Diocesan Information Process was set up, at the end of which the Vatican set up another tribunal known as the Vatican Sacred Congregation for the Cause of Saints Tribunal, to examine the documents on the proposed saint and vote for or against his beatification. The vote of the Vatican Tribunal was positive and the Pope was advised to beatify Tansi.

But before this, a miracle credited to the candidate for canonization was required. In the case of Father Tansi, an apparently incurable fibroid patient, Philomena Emeka, claimed she was miraculously healed after she touched Father Tansi's coffin in 1986. No less than 15 other phenomena credited as miracles have been reported since, including two that took place during the Papal visit.

THE ABIOLA TRAGEDY IN CONTEXT

Not since the eve of the release of Nelson Mandela on February 11, 1990 had the world been so happy in anticipation of the imminent freeing of an African political prisoner. No less a person than the Secretary-General of the United Nations had altered his schedule to hold interviews with MKO Abiola, the world-famous Nigerian political prisoner. So had the Commonwealth secretary-general, who later posed for pictures with the prisoner himself and the Nigerian Military Government's number two man, Admiral Mike Akhigbe, in a meeting, transmitted worldwide by the CNN and BBC. He was moved from his solitary confinement to a "respectable" villa so that foreign delegations from the US and British governments, as well as top officials of the Nigerian government and members of his family could meet him.

Finishing touches were being put in place for the triumphant homecoming of the winner of Nigeria's freest and fairest presidential elections in 1993, who had been deprived of the throne and thrown instead into jail by the military junta led by Sani Abacha. In Lagos, his huge mansion had been refurbished. Journalists were sleeping in Lagos Airport in anticipation of his arrival from Abuja, a free man at last. The nation was in a festive mood. The one person whose electoral victory defied all traditional, regional, religious and tribal calculations was worthy of a hero's welcome.

Then a shocker! The unthinkable and completely unbelievable happened. In the very presence of the US government delegation, headed by the under-secretary for foreign affairs, Thomas Pickering, MKO Abiola collapsed, rushed to the hospital and incredibly died. He died. The man died.

The shock waves reverberated around the world. Within Nigeria, the grief exploded into a gale of violent protests that swept through most parts of The South-West, with death toll in tow. At least two palaces of Yoruba paramount rulers, known for their support for Abacha, the military dictator, were set ablaze. Several houses and vehicles of suspected military apologists were reduced to ashes. The anger spread beyond the five predominantly Yoruba States to the southern minority but oil-rich States of Edo, Rivers, Akwa Ibom and Delta. Throughout the country, ethnic tension approached dangerous dimensions. There was even an open talk of disintegration. In The South-West, protesters carried large banners and posters declaring an "Oduduwa Republic" and chanting "We want freedom ... We want Independence."

Stephen Wole Oke, secretary-general of NADECO (the opposition National Democratic Coalition) in Kwara State announced to the press that secession is on the table. "Since the death of Abiola, there has been a clamour from our people that, if there is no possibility of living together harmoniously, everybody should find their own way. Those in authority, especially the northern cabal, should recognize that nothing can stop Nigeria from going back to its pre-1914 status." It was a tragic irony that the sudden death of a man who had used his legendary wealth to weld ethnic and geopolitical cracks of his country was now the reason for splitting up the country.

Highly embarrassed, Nigeria's new military leader, General Abdulsalam Abubakar, quickly went on air, hours after Abiola's death, to share the "understandable grief" of Nigerians. He pleaded for calm as he promised to give Abiola a dignified burial. He lamented that MKO died on the brink of his freedom, following a series of consultations between his government and the representatives of the international community and his family. He disclosed that the meeting of the Provisional Ruling Council, the country's ruling body, had actually been scheduled to convene on July 9 (the day after Abiola died) to formally approve his release. "For me personally and for the nation at large, this must be one of the saddest moments of our lives. I never envisaged that I would be faced with such a momentous tragedy within the space of one month (in office)," the general declared.

The Abiola family and close associates could not accept the initial statement by the government that Abiola had died "apparently of cardiac arrest." They angrily voiced suspicion that he could have been poisoned by agents of the military. NADECO deputy leader, Senator Abraham Adesanya said: "I haven't any doubt in my mind that the military cannot absolve itself from blame for the death of Chief Abiola. Who prepared the tea he was drinking when he had this cardiac arrest? Are the dregs in the cup still available?"

Wuraola, one of Abiola's daughters, told CNN: "The military had my father incarcerated and he died in their care. Regardless of the technicalities of his death, they are responsible." Emmanuel Inwuanyanwu, multi-millionaire publisher and politician from eastern Nigeria, told the *Punch* newspaper. "Any sign of foul play in the sudden death of Chief Abiola would have devastating consequences on Nigeria's future. That would be a big problem for all of us."

Because of these widespread misgivings and demands by the Abiola family and pro-democracy groups, The Head of State agreed to fly in expert pathologists from the US, Britain and Canada to perform an independent autopsy. Sources close to Aso Rock, Nigeria's seat of power, told *Africa Today* that General Abubakar had actually reckoned on Abiola's release being the crowing point of his fledgling administration and was as keen as anybody to know the result of the autopsy. He could not be certain that Abiola's death had not been the work of supporters of the late General Abacha within the security services, intent on embarrassing him.

The preliminary result of the autopsy announced by Dr. James Young, Chief Coroner for Ontario, Canada, the leader of the international team of pathologists, showed that Chief Abiola had "a long-standing history of heart disease" and evidence of hypertension. Toxicology tests were also to be carried out in Ontario to find out whether there was any possibility of poisoning. The preliminary autopsy report, while not having the desired effect of calming reactions to Abiola's death, did increase public confidence democracy.

While Abiola was being buried in front of more than 20,000 mournful supporters, the government itself knew that the June 12 issue, the very cause Abiola fought and died for, was very much alive and would be decisive in determining the future of

Nigeria. As Dr. Peter Obans, a university lecturer in Lagos, put it. "Some people made the mistake of thinking that if Abiola was out of the way, the June 12 crisis would go away. But those people need to be educated: the issue of June 12 is beyond individuals. It is a people's cause, a liberation struggle to free out people from years of domination by a cabal in northern Nigeria."

Obans' view was echoed by various groups and leaders throughout the country. To Taribo Davies of the Democratic Alternative (DA): "The June 12, 1993 election, in which Abiola won a landslide victory in every state of this country but was denied power by some Northern Nigerian soldiers and their mentors, was an expression of the fundamental principles of justice, equality and fair play. It was not about Abiola per se; it was a moment when Nigerians of all ethnic origins with one voice voted for their freedom and a change of destiny. Such a principle does not and cannot die. Not a thousand battalions of soldiers can kill it." For Solomon Lar, former governor of Plateau State, "because June 12 is a struggle for equity, justice, fair play and democracy, this is the time for everybody to embrace it."

There is a feeling of "collective victimization" in some of the comments in the wake of Abiola's death. Said Olusegun Obasanjo, Nigeria's former head of State, who himself had just been freed from the trauma of two-and-half years in prison: "Abiola's tragedy is our tragedy, the tragedy of Nigeria. We must accomplish what he died for."

Most Nigerians realize that his death is bound to push Nigeria to a new reckoning and change perceptions of the way the country should be governed. According to Reuben Abati, a political commentator with *Guardian* newspapers in Lagos, the principles Abiola championed and for which he had to pay the ultimate sacrifice, such as "the inviolability of equity, justice, openness and fairness as the hallmark of a good society and as the barest minimum of peaceful co-existence," are bound to endure. Abati said June 12 is about the emancipation of Nigerians from internal colonialism, emancipation from continuous misrule and from the dictatorship of the military and a privileged minority.

Northerners have governed the country for 34 of the 38 years of Nigeria's existence as a sovereign nation. Except for two brief periods of democratic governance lasting 10 years, the remaining 28 years witnessed a military dictatorship that acquired its most baleful image under the despotism of General Abacha. This has left the vast majority of the people in The South and scores of minority ethnic groups in The North with a deep sense of marginalization. Under Abacha, virtually all the key and sensitive political, military and diplomatic postings were given to his kinsmen, who also headed 34 of the 36 major government parastatals in the oil, gas, banking and maritime sectors. This shameless nepotism and the sheer cruelty that was the hallmark of Abacha's five-year tenure were major contributory factors in the reversal of what happened on June 12, 1993 becoming almost a crusade, with Abiola its captive champion.

Some analysts are now conceding that the ethnic imbalance in the political equation was overlooked by UN Secretary-General Kofi Annan and by British envoy Tony Lloyd, when they interceded last month between the Nigerian government and Abiola, as they reduced what was in fact a crisis of nationhood to a matter of just holding another election. As Suliman Dauda, a political analyst, put it *to Africa Today* in Abuja: "A country of 250 ethnic nationalities and more than 120 million people cannot surrender its fate and accept the dominance of political power by just one ethnic group. That is a recipe for disintegration."

After Abiola's death, Colonel Abubamkar Umar, former military governor of Kaduna State and a prince of Sokoto Caliphate (northern Nigeria), warned of dire consequences if northerners insisted on ruling Nigeria alone, even when defeated in elections. Said Umar, who resigned his commission because of the nullification of the June 12 election: "Whatever are the feelings of some people in the north, it is crystal clear that, unless the presidency is conceded to The South as a panacea to heal wounds, I do not foresee peace in Nigeria."

As tension mounted, Dr. Sunday Mbang, a luminary of the Methodist Church of Nigeria, told northern leaders at a press conference: "I make bold to say that the people of the northern part of the country must forget about ruling Nigeria for now so as to enable others to think they can belong and feel together. There must be a spirit of give and take. If there isn't, then the reconciliation we are looking for will elude us and this will never be the kind of country we want."

Analysts project various reasons for the pathological fear of some northern elders of having a southerner as President. According to one observer, they have made governing an industry. A Jos-based magazine, *North*, in an article entitled: "The crux of national reconciliation," maintained that every developmental index had revealed that The North is decaying and slipping into irrelevance, in spite of the fact that it has ruled Nigeria for 34 of its 38 years of independence. The magazine queried: "With the 34 years of northern domination, infrastructural development (in the north) is stunted and the literacy rate is collapsing. If mechanics from southern Nigeria were to stop work and depart to their States of origin, most vehicles in The North would be off the road. Whenever the Igbos (of The East) close their shops in most northern cities, common Maggie cubes (spice) become a scarce commodity. Where then does the benefit of political domination lie?"

The magazine also pointed out that The North fared better economically and politically during the regime of General Obasanjo, a southerner, than under the northerners, Generals Babangida and Abacha. Its editorial also asked whether The North really had the right to benefit from the oil in The South if it continued to condemn southerners to second-class status. "It has become very obvious that the continuous rule of The North over Nigeria is not just being resented but has become the most destabilizing agent in our country," it said. The magazine called on General Abubakar to ignore "the chauvinists, whose insistence on political supremacy has brought the country to the brink of disintegration." It concluded its editorial by noting that "the world no longer opposes secession."

Widespread and deep-seated resentment against the monopoly of power is part of the reason Abiola won an unprecedented victory, which broke down every known tribal, religious and sectional tendency in Nigeria, signaling an end to tribal politics. It could have afforded the country the opportunity to build a modern society on a new foundation. For some political observers, both within and outside Nigeria, the June 12 election was probably the most significant political event since independence. The shocking annulment of that election actually confirmed southerners' long-held fears that the Hausa/Fulani ruling class was bent on holding on to power in perpetuity.

Said Dr. Tobi Lawson of the University of Port Harcourt: "It became clear to all of us in The South and to other smaller ethnic groups in The North that, if the northern ruling class would not concede power to Abiola, who was their friend, who has spent his fortune sponsoring their political and religious causes for years and who, as a leading Muslim, contested the elections with another Muslim and northerner as vice-president, then they would not concede power to anyone else, no matter how much they smiled at you and sermonized about national unity." At that point, Lawson said: "Some of us came to the conclusion that we will either take power on the streets, as in Indonesia and the Philippines, or sit down together at a sovereign national conference to renegotiate the terms of our co-existence as distinct ethnic nationalities.

The Abacha administration made sure a sovereign national conference was impossible. Instead, it opted for a National Constitutional Conference (NCC) which, as it turned out, Abacha had merely designed to buy him time to consolidate his hold on power. He pretended he would allow power to rotate around six major constituents of the country, beginning from The South. On the strength of that posture, his five political parties (later dubbed the "five fingers of a leprous hand") went ahead to elect chairmen who were all northerners, a clear signal that the president, as agreed in the NCC, would emerge from the south. But, when it was time to talk about the presidency, Abacha scared away all the southerners and forced all the five parties, headed by northerners, to adopt him as the sole presidential candidate.

Such blatant arrogance and insensitivity to the feelings of southerners had provoked drumbeats of secession even during the NCC in October 1994, as delegates from the southern minority states of Delta, Akwa Ibom, Rivers, Cross River and Edo, home of Nigeria's oil wealth, threatened to pull their people out of Nigeria. They demanded that genuine conditions of federalism be enshrined in the constitution. They named these as equitable sharing of power, a better revenue-sharing formula, a rotating presidency and federal adherence to principles.

Even before Abacha's game plan was clear, these oil-rich southern minority states accused certain "hidden forces" in The North of manipulating delegates and the draft constitution to ensure the continued marginalization of their wealthy region. The region, which voted heavily for Abiola, remained restive for most of last month and its leaders have continued to say that, in spite of the arrests and execution of some of their leaders, including Ken Saro-Wiwa, they would not be intimidated any longer.

The oil-rich "south-south," as the region is now known, was a major battleground during Nigeria's three-year civil war with Biafran Igbos in The South-East, in which more than one million people were killed. The Igbos have not stopped complaining of marginalization by the government. Most of their top leaders, including Emeka Ojukwu, the ex-Biafran leader, and Alex Ekwueme, former vice-president of Nigeria, were at the NCC and insisted that zoning and rotating the power base was the only way to keep a multi-ethnic society like Nigeria together.

Ekwueme, who has consistently been in the vanguard of democracy and in the campaign for freeing Abiola, warned again at the burial ceremony: "Nigeria cannot be a nation unless and until every part of the country has a sense of belonging. In spite of the vicissitudes and setbacks we have experienced, we should not relent in our efforts to build a nation where all Nigerians will have a sense of belonging. We have a sacred duty to do this, not only to ourselves but to the entire Black race in Africa, America and the Caribbean."

He was speaking as a statesman. But his younger generation kinsmen in the Eastern Mandate Union put it in the following way (rather as Dr. Nnamdi Azikiwe, Nigeria's first president, might have done to White colonialists in the 1940s or 1950s): "We refuse to be slaves or second-class citizens in our country. We have been colonized for three decades now by a feudal clique in The North. It is time to draw the line so that our children will have a country where the principles of justice, equity and fair play will not be a luxury."

However grave the political implosion is considered to be, the more human face presented by General Abubakar's administration so far has been a source of hope that there will be a peaceful and just outcome of the present impasse.

Political analysts are in agreement that, if the general moves fast along the route to genuine democracy, he might resurrect the soul of Nigeria from the ashes of political injustice and victimisation. If he fails, some are predicting an already charged situation may become even more inflammable. They recall chief Abiola's homily a few days before his arrest and incarceration: "The day a people are told that they are destined to be perpetual drawers of water and hewers of wood, good only for permanent enslavement and domination, that is the day the journey to their freedom begins. The road might be long, rough and tough. But freedom, justice and equality are too precious to surrender. This is the meaning of June 12. This is why June 12 will remain significant for now and for tomorrow."

BACK FROM THE BRINK

The maiden speech by the new Nigeria head of state General Abdulsalam Abubakar was short: only five minutes. Abubakar paid tribute to his predecessor, General Sani Abacha: "We salute his honesty, resoluteness, fearlessness and total commitment to the preservation of Nigeria as a united, stable and prosperous entity." He said his administration would stick to Abacha's programme for a transition to civilian rule: "we remain fully committed to the socio-political transition programme of General Abacha's administration and we will do everything to ensure its full and successful implementation."

But he did not say what Nigerians wanted to hear.

They wanted to hear that Moshood Abiola, detained winner of the 12 June 1993 presidential elections, and scores of other political prisoners, were to be released. They wanted to hear about the demolition of the political structure Abacha had created to ensure his election as a civilian president on August 1, this year. They wanted to hear that the 1993 election, whose annulment began Nigeria's continuing political crisis, had been revalidated and a national government of reconciliation formed. They wanted to hear that the 1995 constitution has been approved and promulgated into law. They expected a change of direction.

The military top brass who form the Provisional Ruling Council (PRC) had laboured long and hard over the speech, in the hope of carrying the country and international opinion with them. The text was changed three times. But what they came up with was widely criticized as merely new wine in an old bottle.

The word "we" appeared nine times, indicating a move towards collective leadership. It was clear that Abubakar had chosen discretion as a better part of valour, and opted for wider consultations before embarking on any changes. The PRC, like the rest of the Nigerian people, was believed to be divided on most of the thorny issues. But virtually all ethnic, religious and human rights organizations gave the new government the thumbs down.

"This speech by the new Head of State shows clearly that the people around Abacha and Abuja have lost touch with the reality of our situation," the National Association of Nigeria Students (NANS) said in a statement. "How can anyone say that he wants to continue with Abacha's policy, when the rest of the country and the world are against it and when those policies are the same line of action that has brought Nigeria to its knees?"

The Supreme Council of Islamic Affairs said that, instead of continuing with Abacha's policies, Abubakar should release Abiola and other political prisoners. The Christian Association of Nigeria (CAN), the National Democratic Coalition (NADECO) and the Congress of Northern Youths for Democracy (CNYD), among other groups, urged Abubakar to set the tone for reconciliation by first freeing Abacha's captives.

On Abubakar's fourth day in power, police arrested scores

of prodemocracy protesters marking the fifth anniversary of the June 12 elections. Most of them, including Gani Fawehinmi, a leading Lagos lawyer and government critic, were quickly released. A leading northern figure close to some of the military chiefs told *Africa Today* that it was unlikely Abiola would be released soon, although other political prisoners might be: "I guess what they would do is release those that pose little or no security risk, and see how it goes."

After just one week in office, Abubakar showed that, although he might be a man who acted cautiously, he was prepared to act, ordering the release of nine political prisoners and detainees. They include former head of state Olusegun Obasanjo, journalist Chris Anyanwu and human rights activist Beko Ransome-Kuti, all jailed three years ago on controversial charges connected with an alleged plot to overthrow Abacha.

Also let off the hook were Ibrahim Dasuki, revered former Sultan of Sokoto, who was deposed, detained and banished by Abacha; Bola Ige, former Governor of Oyo State, detained for participating in a May Day rally; Frank Kokori, general secretary of the oil workers' union, detained since 1994, as well as pro-democracy activists Chief Olabiyi Durojaiye, Uwem Udoh and Milton Dabibi.

The chief press secretary to the head of state David Attah said the action was taken on compassionate grounds. Although Abiola was not included, the gesture signaled what political observers described as a genuine move towards reconciliation. It also suggested that Abacha had personally been the main obstacle to reconciliation and the only man on the PRC lacking in compassion.

On the same day, the popular military governor of Lagos state, Colonel Muhammed Marwa ordered the unconditional release of 20 pro-democracy activists arrested during the demonstrations marking the anniversary of the June 12 elections. "In the spirit of reconciliation as enunciated in the maiden broadcast of His Excellency, the head of state, I have directed that the State attorney-general should drop charges and allow those arrested in connection with the rally to go free," Marwa announced in a state-wide radio and television broadcast.

The two events sent positive signals across the country and won some support or respect for the new administration. Said Fewehinmi: "I am extremely happy and delighted. Freedom is the greatest spice of life. Now tension will begin to reduce, chaos will begin to evaporate and we want to see the other political prisoners released. The president-elect, MKO Abiola, must be released for the joy to be final and total." Adamu Ciroma, a prominent political figure in The North said: "We are very happy. We want to see more. We (referring to the group of 34 leading Nigerians who recently wrote to Abacha to advise him against self-succession) are still expecting Abiola. It is one of the most important ingredients for reconciliation. We are happy government is moving in the right direction."

Most watchers of the Nigeria political crisis agreed that the move by the new administration was a good omen. "It is a major step to pull Nigeria back from the brink of disintegration. Clearly, this has shown that government intends to usher in a new era," said businessman and senator-elect Dr. Ime Umana. There were strong indications as *Africa Today* went to press that the government had made contacts with Abiola.

However, Isa Mohammed, the chairman of the United Nigeria Congress Party (UNCP), the leading party that master-minded Abacha's self-succession, told voice of America that Abiola should not be released to head the interim government because Abacha had almost concluded the formation of a democratic government.

His was very much a minority voice. Worried about the consequences of further political stalemate, the former military governor of Kaduna state and popular northern opinion former Colonel Abubakar Umar wrote to the new leader. He advised him to dismantle Abacha's transition programme, even at the cost of extending his tenure by one year, and to bring Abiola into a new future for Nigeria.

Ohaneze, the socio-political organization that speaks for the Igbos of eastern Nigeria, held a press conference on the same issues. Its leaders, Chief Chukwuemeka Ojukwu, the former Biafran leader, and Professor Ben Nwabueze, advised the government to dissolve the Abacha transition agencies and constitute new ones that would command the confidence of Nigerians. It rejected, however, the idea of a government of national unity and any postponement of the military's exit date.

Clearly, there is a groundswell of opinion in favour of discontinuing the discredited political programme of the Abacha administration. As the Committee for the Advancement of Human Rights and Law (CARL) put it: "There is nothing in the transition programme of the former head of state to be followed (because) that programme was dead even before the death of General Abacha."

The reason is clear. The five political parties under Abacha's regime were for all practical purpose, "five fingers of a leprous hand," officially sanctioned by the government and set up to do Abacha's bidding. His supporters teleguided every move made by the parties, ensuring his emergence as the only presidential candidate in an election that had been scheduled for August 1.

Even Ebenezer Babatope, former minister of transport and aviation and an Abacha loyalist, has added his voice to calls for Abubakar to initiate a new short political programme. Babatope, a member of UNCP, and an elected senator, said in a statement announcing his withdrawal from Abacha's transition programme: "Our decision of April 1998 (the adoption of Abacha) has rubbished any argument that the existing political parties will undoubtedly be acceptable to a substantial section of the Nigerian people. The socio-political problems of Nigeria will be deepened rather than lessened or healed."

This line of thinking suits most military officers, who are now frank enough to admit that the Abacha transition programme was built on a foundation of fraud and dishonesty. But most of the army officers in government who favour abandoning Abacha's political structures are believed to be using this as a bargaining chip for prolonging military rule by an extra year. "The military cannot go on October 1, as scheduled, if new parties have to be formed and proper elections conducted at all levels. To be able to do a good job, an extension of the transition schedule by at least one year should be expected," one officer told *Africa Today*. According to another source close to government: "It is almost certain that the political programme of the Abacha era will be jettisoned because it has been widely rejected and shunned by well-meaning Nigerian leaders across the length and breath of the country and by our traditional friends overseas. But what is not certain for now is whether government will buy the idea of a government of national unity that would supervise a genuine transition or go it alone."

No one is quite sure what Abubakar will do. He is still keeping everything close to his chest. The political parties, whose leaders met the new leader on June 14, to ask him to continue the discredited transition programme, found him inscrutable, a good listener, but a man who betrayed no emotion on which way he might swing.

The political parties' argument was that a break with the transition programme would mean jettisoning everything that the late head of state had done. Four of the parties advised the dissolution of the existing political and electoral agencies as part of urgent action needed to sanitize and restore confidence in the transition programme. They also suggested the replacement of most ministers and military governors who openly identified with the favoured party.

How these developments are impacting on the military, especially the core officer ranks, is difficult to say. Close watchers of the military have expressed fears about the future. "I don't think that they will be supportive of each others," said Ghana's President Jerry Rawlings. Rawlings believes there may be cracks in the army at a time like this. "Let's pray for the commanders to realize that they shouldn't do anything that would lead to the disintegration of that nation." Alhaji Abdulkarim Daiyabu, a political analyst, says the military could be further factionalized, at Nigerians' peril. "Go and count how many officers have been changed, retired prematurely, dismissed or killed since Babangida and Abacha came to power. The number will outnumber those serving. Others are being suspended and monitored. And for every military officer retired, dismissed or killed, there are die-hard loyalists in the military behind him. You cannot read it in their faces. All these are pointers that all is not well."

It is indeed true that all is not well with the military. It is discredited and polarized, with officers not trusting one another. In fact, since Abubakar was appointed head of state by the PRC, there have been speculations about dissention within their ranks and the possibility of an attempt to oust the new ruler. The ministry of defence dismissed the speculations as the work of "a few disgruntled elements," but according to observers the mere fact of denial was in itself an admission that something is wrong.

However, increasing concern about Nigeria's political crisis has led western nations and even key opposition figures in Nigeria to adopt a conciliatory approach towards the new government, in the hope that a solution can at least be found. US State Department spokesman James Rubin said the Clinton administration considered Abubakar as better placed than Abacha to conduct a true democratic transition. "We generally regard him as someone who is capable of taking this historic decision and we very much want him to do so," Rubin said. US president Clinton telephoned Abubakar to ask him to move quickly towards civilian rule. The White House said Clinton had "underscored our desire for improved bilateral relations in the context of Nigeria taking swift and significant steps toward a successful transition to a democratically elected civilian government."

Political leaders who have been on the offensive over the years have cautioned pro-democratic groups to exercise some restraint and give the new leader the benefit of the doubt. "I think we have choices in Nigeria, but we should take the most reasonable one, and that is to give the new leader room to make the right decisions," say Abiola's daughter Dr. Wuraola Abiola.

Some opposition figures seemed prepared to give Abubakar time to establish himself, in the hope that the military elite will move in a more democratic direction. Others were less forgiving:

"These things are cosmetic," said Fawehinmi. "Abubakar has not made any fundamental statements, has not made any fundamental changes. He hasn't taken a step to convince anybody he wants a new Nigeria." The coming hours will determine whether the new administration will use the window of opportunity opened by the death of Abacha to engineer a true political and economic reconciliation in Nigeria.

COLUMNS

MIRROR ON THE COAST

My wife has not found it funny having me stagger into the house at 2.00 am every day, at least for the past two weeks. She has not said so. But the blank expression on her face is a study in silent protest.

I guess she's certain that I am back to my crazy *old* days at *Newswatch*. Those were days of no nights; and nights of life at the edge. Those were days and nights of raw zeal and sheer bravado.

But I have grown by far more grey hairs in *The Pioneer* than *Newswatch*. In *Newswatch*, grey hairs ran in the newsroom but here, it is something close to epidemic. With about 150 staff cocking their guns at me, there is no place to hide from grey hairs. You need to see my head.

And the last two weeks has been quite testy for everyone in *The Pioneer* as we were confronted with the task of designing, packaging and publishing a weekend edition literary with bare knuckles.

Media and publishing consultants who do such jobs speak a lot of big grammar and go away with bags of money. But a handful of 12 staff just sat there at our board room, sweating and gazing at the ceiling as I breathed down their necks. The result is the newspaper you are reading now.

I flew the kite September 5, 1996. It was the first official briefing the Ministry of Information and its parastatals had with the new military governor, Navy Captain Joseph Adeusi. Sunday Ekpo, the Commissioner of Information led the team comprising Mr. Monday Idiong, then information director general, Dr. Mbuk Mboho, general manager, Akwa Ibom Broadcasting Corporation, Mira Idem, director of the Centre for Arts and Culture and myself, general manager/CEO of Akwa Ibom newspaper Corporation. We sat in a cream leather settee inside the palatial office, partially encircling the governor.

After about 30 minutes, my chance to speak came. My Commissioner had already articulated the problems of *The Pioneer* and I needed to sell just an idea which I had canvassed in the past in vain. "Your Excellency, we can publish a *Weekend Pioneer* within your 100 days in office, provided...." I got a quick attention. A proposal with provisos followed days later. The nod was given. And today, Adeusi, a man whose home in Lagos used to be a beehive of journalists, is the midwife of journalism newest baby in Nigeria – the *Weekend Pioneer.*

As the maiden edition of this newspaper shall be officially presented today, Adeusi shall also be commissioning for *The Pioneer* four units of Desktop publishing computer, fitted with scanners and LaserJet printers, possibly, the most sophisticated computer system in the State today. This was one of the provisos.

In design, concept, outlook, and style, *Weekend Pioneer* as you can see is refreshingly different, not just from *The Pioneer* but from other newspapers east of the Niger. *Weekend Pioneer* shall go from coast to coast strictly for news behind the news, particularly in The Eastcoastal states of Akwa Ibom, Cross River, Rivers and Bayelsa, which is why we are called "Mirror on the Coast."

The Eastcoastal states of Nigeria are not only rich in crude oil and fish, but in people, events, culture, arts, entertainment, sports, business and of course, churches. With churches sprouting like mushrooms, it does appear the eastern shores of Nigeria is at the threshold of a spiritual revival, just as the prophets (excluding Peterside Ottong) said it would be. And so we have assigned ourselves the task of mirroring the boom and bumps, the cheers and jeers as well as the cries and laughter of this strategic economic nerve centre of Nigeria.

We aim to strike a professional balance between the seriousness of unserious issues and the unseriousness of serious issues.

Government, I insist, has a right to be heard. I don't know what my *Newswatch* and *Tell* friends would make out of that but *Weekend Pioneer* shall at least, hear out our governments especially those of our target audience.

These, you may agree with me, are no mean tasks; which is why we cannot do without your backing. It is not on the day or month or year a baby is born that the helpless little one is abandoned to cater for himself. That would be a case of abandoned baby, which is not a joke. A baby would need to be helped until he can sit, crawl, walk and find his footing before he is allowed to fend for himself. This we expect from our readers, advertisers, and governments.

Last Sunday, I almost jumped out of my skin when the governor told me in company of Obiota Ekanem, acting editor, *The Pioneer* and Ekaette Ekpo, acting editor, *Weekend Pioneer* that he was planning to cut subvention to our company. For a while I lost my composure and when he noticed the horror on my face, he came to my rescue. "Don't give yourself unnecessary high blood pressure. Before I cut the subvention, there are some measures we are going to take to make sure you stand firmly on your feet."

Stand by us too. *Weekend Pioneer* shall not let you down. And that's not a political promise.

POISONOUS PEN

This is the season of brickbats. Our sharp shooting ground troops must be having a field day launching their legendary missiles with spiteful ease and skill.

If you think I am speaking Greek, you must be new in town and may not have known that the art of petition writing, this part of the Niger has gone nuclear. It is not just a thing done by an aggrieved lazy man, who has squandered his legitimate entitlement and opportunity. It is not just a sporadic foray of a man with halting English. It is a crusade, an industry, a well-organized project, by means of cheap sleaze and verbal banditry.

Which is why I don't envy public servants: and in this very season, members of the just dissolved Akwa Ibom Executive Council. That they have survived for three months despite the sheer tons of missiles unloaded on them at the arrival of the new governor, Navy Captain Adeusi, is proof both of their thick skin and Adeusi' knowledge of our ground troops.

Now that the men we sought favours from and sometimes got it, appear to be slightly outside the corridors of power, some of the ground troops who were camouflaging as good friends and loyal staff, will emerge from their ambush. I can see laser guided Tomahawk missiles with fixed names and addresses.

How do I know? I have understanding of times and seasons. This is the season of brickbats. Here in the land of promise, it comes on the wings of new administrations. It comes when opportunists want to smear and write-off the out-going administration they had just served and praised. It comes when job seekers are jockeying for plum positions. This is the season of brickbats, missiles and projectiles. Beware!

Thank God, Adeusi has scaled a hurdle or two. He has shuffled his directors-general just as he appointed four new ones. Plum ministries have been won and lost at least for now. So contenders for DG's job and their army have beaten a tactical withdrawal by now. But with the cabinet and board seats still up for grabs, and with "inspired" staff praying for disaster against their terrible bosses, this is the season to undo men; o yes, by all means.

If you ever thought petition writers are mere nattering nabobs of negativism, you must be joking. Their strategy is charming. If you want to petition my staff who misquoted you in spite of brown envelope, here is how: first, get a beautiful writer with flowing prose an generous adjectives.

Second, start the letter by congratulating me for being a genius, the people's general manager, the best manager of the year, a God-fearing officer; a rare gem of inestimable value to the state and the nation.

Third and this is critical; unleash a chilling half-truths and falsehood on the brutality, barbarism and roguery perpetuated by my brown envelope reporter, which if not checked will blow up the newspaper house. Forth, suggest your brother as a better reporter who cannot touch a brown envelope even with a 10-feet long pole. Then conclude by whishing me everlasting tenure in office. The objective is simple: even if the truth is found out later, the allegation is enough to paint my staff black, knock out my confidence in him, put question mark on his integrity and throw him into public odium for a while.

Did you hear or read the story of the N300 million dash to Akwa Ibom government by an oil company which could not be accounted for? Did you hear the story of a commissioner who sold three government cars to himself? What about the commissioner who back-dated cheques worth millions of naira to cover large-scale fraud? They were inspired by by nothing else but overnight palmwine and pepper soup. Simple.

But careers have been cut down mid-stream. Reputations have been ruined. Families have been saddled with stigma and stains. Take a look at the federal bureaucracy and count how many names are Akwa Ibom. Most of those that would have made it were shot and pulled down by sharp shooters for no offense or minor offenses that are corrective rather than punitive.

Make no mistake. Petition writers, have their place in the system. They have come to stay and since they are thriving they must be made to take some responsibilities.

I advocate stiff sanctions where allegations are proven to be untrue or half-truth. A friend of mind says that's unnecessary because the menace of petition writers should be regarded as a hazard of public office. What a hazard! My puzzle is that people are still lining up to face such poisonous hazards. There must be a better hazard than being turned into a dart board.

THE MAGIC ECONOMY

Did you notice that last Christmas was the first Christmas in many years that Nigerians didn't have to cope with fuel scarcity? It was truly merry Christmas for all of us but miserable Christmas for profiteering petroleum dealers. They may never forgive government for pulling the rug from under their feet and pulling out all the stops to give Nigerians a crisis-free Christmas. It was a victory of many helpless Nigerians over their few greedy countrymen.

Did you also notice that quite unlike what obtained in the past, where price hikes usually accompany the fanfare of Christmas, prices of consumable items, this time around, remained low and in most cases actually plummeted, down the mountainside to the ground below. Despite the usual frenzy of sales and purchases of this period, such surge in market activities, did not translate into commensurate skyrocketing of prices.

Rice, that non-negotiable Christmas dish, witnessed a price crash. I confess my wife bought a 50 kilo bag at Aba for N3,100 way back in November in lieu of the usual price hikes in December, but to our surprise the same rice was sold at N2, 500 on Christmas Day. Less competitive varieties all over the country went for cheaper prices. Some Nigerians who thought rice would only be available for all in the year 2010 were forced to change their minds.

The prices of other food items such as beans and groundnut oil also behaved themselves properly, keeping a rather low profile. So were prices of electronics. Although prices of some products have continued to decline since the new imports guidelines packaged by finance minister, Tony Ani, were published, dramatic falls surely were not expected this season.

You may think my fascination is unusual but what seems unusual to me is the light glimmering in the distance. It looks faint and unsteady, but it sure thrills me. Only three days ago, Ani announced a new tariff structure, lowering at the same time prices of locally produced brands of cement. Ani said the decision to cut cement prices were actually reached voluntarily by the manufacturers, confirming reports last September that the Cement Manufacturers Association of Nigeria, CMAN had actually tabled such a proposal before government.

The good news is that all brands of cement are now to sell between N285 to N327. As I was writing this column just before press time, I dispatched two of our staff separately to look up cement prices at Ewet market. From N460 early in the week, the product price has taken a dive to N430. Fillip to the building industry.

Don't rush for conclusions, you may say. But you see, I don't think all that government deserves at every point in time is a cane at the back. Those of us who have the calling and courage to berate government when it goes wrong as it is wont, must also be sufficiently large-hearted to commend and encourage government, when it does well.

When last November, I read in *The Economist* of London, a rare positive commentary on the Abacha Administration and the Nigerian economy, I reckoned things could be getting better. But I have had real trouble with a colleague here in *The Pioneer*, who is not happy the value of the Naira has appreciated against world's major currencies. The value of the Naira which stood over time at about N80 per dollar went up by Christmas to N67 per dollar, and for my colleague this is bad news because a few dollars she receives regularly from her sister in US will no more fetch a house full of Naira. Selfish interest!

The value of the Naira vis-à-vis selfish interest of a few Nigerians is the real issue of the 1997 Budget being awaited by Nigerians. This is one issue that can make or mar the gains so far made.

Naira is still regarded by economic analysts and market operators as grossly undervalued and lacking in militancy to effectively reflate the economy. That is big grammar. For laymen like us, the present exchange rate of the Naira only favours very rich Nigerians with a lot of foreign money outside Nigeria.

To that extent, only this tiny percentage of privileged Nigerians may have an axe to grind with an enhanced Naira value, mainly because an enhance Naira will slash their profit from currency trade. Naturally, this group has been very vociferous in their demand and insistence on the exchange rate status quo. This group, made up of top government officials and their collaborators, are also direct beneficiaries and sponsors of the present dual exchange rate, whereby one dollar exchange for N22 for a selected few, while the rest of us including the productive sector are made to struggle for a dollar at the rate of N75 at the autonomous market. Nothing could be more unfair.

Predictably, this has damaged the productive capability of average businesses, made nonsense of the purchasing power of many Nigerians, increased unemployment and possibly the social temperature of the country.

With his trade mark iron hand, General Abacha should take the bull by the horn and called off this expensive bonanza, by abolishing the current dual exchange rate. He should not allow a small percentage of Nigerians to frustrate the significant and near magical turn around he has ushered into our once reprehensible economic landscape. Certainly, somebody's ox will somehow be gored. But how to sustain the momentum and trajectory of his economic recovery programmes should be the preoccupation of his 1997 economic goals. Nothing more, nothing less.

GATES OF HELL

Eschatology, if I must tell you, is the teaching on how the world will come to an end. I know you don't like good things to come to an end, which means I must be careful not to spoil your appetite this weekend.

But there is this man called Finis Jennings Dake. Dake, one of the world's most famous authorities on Biblical dilemma, has put in an amazing 100,000 hours in 43 years researching and searching for keys to unravel tons of prophecies, parables, fables, allegories, visions and alleged contradictions on such mind-bending topics as Armageddon, hell-fire, raptures, tribulations, the millennium and antichrist.

There is another man called Auka Obi. Obi is a Nigerian lawyer, based in Enugu, but very frequent in Europe and American bound aircrafts. He shares something in common with Dake, namely, a passion for eschatology. I know Obi only by reputation. My hope of listening to him last year crashed. A group of Christian businessmen who promised to bring Obi to Uyo last year lost him to others in America. I only managed last October to speak with Obi's wife and daughter on telephone, at the request of my businessmen friends. It didn't quite help matters.

Majority of Christians, maybe ninety-something percent, do not hide their perplexity, when it comes to these mystifying issues replete in the Book of Revelations. As a matter of fact, most preachermen, even in the celebrated Pentecostal hierarchy, admit little knowledge and prefer the bread and butter issues to such posers as antichrist, etc. I have bought volumes of Dake's books but have been largely unsuccessful in cracking through them.

Somehow, I had a chance encounter last year, with Ynot Rednas. Rednas is a preacherman and top computer operator with an American oil company. He scared me stiff with his analysis on antichrist. He said the antichrist, an opponent of Christ, the great opposer of Christianity, who is expected to topple the world and make life a hell for all those not raptured, is here with us already. He fingered the Pope and William (Bill) Gates Jr. 40, the richest man in the world, as possible candidates. He painted a mysterious picture of Gates, a man without known parents, a recluse and working hard quietly underground to put the world in his pocket. I became curious since that day about Gates and made an ambush for every possible information on Gates with scanty result.

Early this week, the lead came off Gates. *TIME,* the iconic American weekly news magazine, perhaps the best known magazine in the world, went in search of the real Bill Gates and published an outstanding cover story on the man it says is "shaping our future," obviously as "one of the most important minds and personalities of our era."

Gates has parents, afterall. *TIME* showed pictures of Mary, Gates' mother with Gates himself at age three as well as those of

Bill Gates Snr, and Bill Clinton, American president, golfing with Gates. Gates even owns a wife Melinda and a daughter, Jennifer. But *TIME* barely stop short of saying Gates owns the world, which should be frightening.

Of course Gates has the world literally in his breast pocket. As at last Friday, Gates had amassed a fortune of $23.9 billion (don't bother about the naira equivalence, which should be in zillions). Last year, he made $30 million a day. "That makes him the world's richest person, by far" *TIME* says.

His computer company, Microsoft, is standing like a colossus ready to swallow the world. It keeps $8 billion in cash. According to *TIME;* "Gates' success stems from his personality, an awesome and at times frightening blend of brilliance, drive, competitiveness and personal intensity." That is not quite comforting either.

Besides, we are told "Gates remains personally elusive to all but a close circuit of friends. Part of what makes him so enigmatic is his nature of intellect. He has incredible processing power. He can be so rigorous as he processes data that one can imagine his mind may indeed be digital. He shows little curiosity about other people even President Clinton, whom he played golf with recently. He is analytically rigorous and emotionally reserved. He rarely looks straight at you. He can lack human empathy."

Well, that's what *TIME* says about Gates. But what does Gates himself say about himself, humanity and perhaps God? "It's possible, you can never know, that the universe exists only for me. It will be hard to deal with me from now on unless I am incharge," he said.

You can fathom whatever you like out of that, but listen; Gates does not have much regards for human intelligence. "I don't think there is anything unique about human intelligence," he says. "All the neurons in the brain that make up perceptions and emotions operate in a binary fashion. We (Microsoft) can someday replicate that on a machine. Eventually, Microsoft will be able to sequence the human genome and replicate how nature constructed intelligence in a carbon-based computer system. It is like reverse-engineering natures product in order to solve a challenge," he told *TIME*.

But isn't there something "special or divine" about human soul *TIME* asked Gates. "I don't have any evidence on that. We (Microsoft) will understand the human mind someday and ex-plain it in soft-ware terms" Gate promised. That's not a mere threat by Gates. After all, the prophecy of end times in the book of Daniel (12:4) clearly stated that, come end times, "knowledge shall increase." So God is not surprised, you may say.

Which reminds me of church! What does Bill Gates say about Church? "There is a lot more I could be doing on a Sunday morn-ing," he says. Gates obviously worships technology. Wait a min-ute; is this truly the end of the world as eschatologist says? Could this be the Biblical Gates of hell? Shall it prevail? I hope your weekend is still intact!

THE FEAR OF BOMB

In 1988, I was among scores of international journalists drafted to cover the withdrawal of Soviet troops from Afghanistan. That assignment was a nightmare.

From the comfort of Geneva and serenity of Zurich both in Switzerland, where I jetted out, I spent my first two days in Asia imprisoned in quarantine arising from frivolous queries on my international vaccination certificate. That was in Karachi, the permanently furious and highly temperamental city of Pakistan. The day my ordeal ended, a military truck rammed into the sleek Ford Mustang of the American diplomat who secured my freedom, and turned it into a wreck but we escaped unhurt. The rest of the week was like walking a mine-field as news and scenes of bomb blasts and explosions kept everybody in what a Canadian journalist called bombdage.

You had to take inventory and position of things in your hotel room and crosscheck them when you are back to ensure that your mattress and pillows are still same in size and that nobody

THE FEAR OF BOMB

left behind a strange parcel in your absence. Ditto for the buses and cars assigned for your movement.

At Peshawar, the border town between Afghanistan and Pakistan, we returned home one evening to discover to our shock that part of our hotel complex had been ripped off and brought down by a bomb. The bomb did not come from the sky. It came from a hair salon on the ground floor of the rebels infested hotel.

Away from the highly inflammable border region and now in Karachi, the commercial capital of Pakistan, you would have thought things would relax a bit. No. At the airport, security personnel are near mechanical in their relationship with passengers. After our luggage had been x-rayed and checked-in and we walked into the departure hall, a colleague from Kenya left his hand bag on his seat and walked towards a duty-free shop. He was quickly apprehended and returned to pick his bag. Why? You just don't leave your bags behind because the security people suspect it could be a bag of time bomb.

Nigeria has not gone anywhere near such a scary scenario yet but security consciousness may have to occupy the minds of Nigerians a bit more this year than ever before. And that's not without reason. The frequency of bomb blasts and explosions of late, at the airport, fly-over bridges and even in the heavily guarded convoy of the affable military governor of Lagos State, Colonel Mohammed Marwa, seems to send a strong signal to Nigerians, that the issue of security will have to move up our front burners and grab the attention of not just security agencies but average Nigerians.

I have noticed at our airports that security checks have doubled, maybe tripled, especially since the mysterious crash of the

ADC airline and the bomb at the Lagos international airport that claimed the life of its chief security officer. And since the Marwa convoy and Army bus bomb blasts, I have also noticed a pall of fear descending on Nigerians as even the most innocuous parcel is looked upon with suspicious. My secretary Elizabeth Daniel has suddenly developed cold feet opening even some of those juicy and well known PR parcels from multi-national firms.

I returned from a three-day trip to Lagos last weekend to find a parcel of fruit wine from a friendly company, curiously and unusually unopened and isolated on top of my file cabinet. And then, as I was writing the column, Alice Udoma, our dutiful administration staff had to bring, rather unusually, an official DHL parcel for me to open. Of course, I refused. I couldn't belief my ears when I heard her say "I open you in the name of J-e-e-s-s-u-s-s." A similar scare first gribbed Nigerians, at least temporarily, in late 1987 when Dele Giwa, my boss at *Newswatch,* was murdered with a letter bomb.

But the actual security we must begin to think about may have to go beyond the confines of airports and the temporary scare arising from specific or sporadic incidents. This critical issue will have to be taught, drummed and inculcated into the sub-consciousness of not just uniformed and security operatives but the ordinary Nigerian. And this may begin with real and deliberate creation of security awareness.

Security awareness or consciousness is the totality of a persons' knowledge and understanding of the great need to protect himself at every point in time against possible danger to his life and property. This leads to a spontaneous prevention, avoidance and or elimination of perceived sources of danger and risk to himself, his family, community and by extension country.

While such a life-and-death matter should not be taught to uniformed and security operatives alone, the uniformed and security operatives will have to show and lead the way. Security is compromised when a uniformed operative manning a check point at the airport, see port, expressway or government and company premises, forgoes his critical duties in exchange for a dirty N10.

A uniformed friend of mind says the difference between journalists, judges, bankers, civil servants and his organization is that his colleagues collect their *"egunje"* openly and without scruples at roadside check points whereas the rest of us do it in our offices.

But the difference is beyond that. The difference is life and death. A uniformed man at check point who ignores a truck-load of unverified consignment for a ready tip may have exchange the lives of many Nigerians with peanuts.

If tecent bomb blasts have political connotations as it is widely believed, it also explodes with economic miscalculations. The security man who calculates what goes into his pocket at the expense of what goes out to the unfriendly world as widows, orphans, handicapped, is a security risk.

In order not to have security risks dress up in uniforms, the economy of the uniform men must receive serious consideration as part of our security fortification. But beyond that, education holds the key to our collective security. That might sound simple but it's certainly not a day's job.

The people who send bombs to kill just anybody, man or woman, adults or children, guilty or guiltless, may actually be Oxford-trained professors and prosperous but not educated. Good education, anywhere, takes time, patience and money. We had better start now than later.

WAR FRONT BY ANOTHER NAME

Unlike other inventions, the original idea of a motor vehicle cannot be attributed to an individual. Custodians of car history however agree that Nicolas-Joseph Cugnot of Lorraine, France, was the constructor of the first true, self-propelled motor car. That was in 1769.

I have seen the pictures of Cugnot's steamer in books. It is a huge, steam-powered, three-wheeled artillery tractor. It was said to have run 20 minutes only at the speed of about three kilometres per hour. These early vehicles were so much a thrill that early writers such as Alexander Pope described them as possessing wondrous to tell instincts with spirits, rolling from place to place, self-moved (and) obedient to the beck of gods."

Men like Carl Benz of Germany were of course not impressed by these violent steamers but persisted in an all-out effort to build a petrol-fueled vehicle in the face of many obstacles such as poverty and bitter objections by his associates who considered him "unbalanced." Benz day of triumph came on July 3, 1886, when his first car was driven in public. The three-wheeled vehicle with a steel frame was built in the shape of a horse shoe and a speed of 15 Kmph was reached in its first outing in Mannheim, Germany.

As the story goes, Benz himself drove the car beside his small factory, his wife running, clapping her hands, as the little machine rolled, before a broken chain stopped it. Fifteen years later, on March 31, 1901, Benz launched what was then regarded as a "revolutionary high performance car named Mercedes after his daughter. The new remarkable Mercedes Benz with a maximum speed of 53 mph was sold to a diplomat in Nice. But the first best known commercially successful car was the American Oldsmobile, made by Ransom Olds, who sold 425 cars in 1901.

Through commerce, motor vehicles made its way to Nigeria in the 20's. I cannot really recollect the first car I ever set my eyes on. It must have been the car of a European doctor who worked at Qua Iboe Mission Hospital, Etinan, in the mid 60's. Whenever the car approaches, children of my age, and adults too, would run and take vintage positions to see the beautiful object roll pass. Immediately the car passes, we would run to the sandy road and walk or lie down on the tyre marks. It was great fun. Then my grand-mother and other women would collect the sand around the tyre-marks and sprinkle it on crops with the hope of bountiful harvest.

Later three men from my village, who were working in, I think, Port Harcourt or so, came home with *Morris Minor, Vauxhall and Peugeot 403.* It was a major spectacle.I and many children could not sit in the church that Christmas day. We stood outside staring at those cars, longing to touch them and praying for the moment church would be over so that the owners would drive the cars and send us running after them.

Before that Christmas was over, I got a chance of riding in

the *Vauxhall.* I couldn't belief my eyes. The trees were running backwards; the skies; everything was on the move. I just perched there on the back seat grinning from ear to ear; wishing everybody in the world was seeing me inside a car. I wondered whether the car was forking right when the steering turned left or vice versa. When the man blew the horn, I wished I knew the particular button he pressed. I thought the speedometer was the car clock and I was sure the gear lever was the brakes. When the short, five minutes journey ended, I almost exploded in ecstasy. It was a thriller.

But vehicles on Nigerian roads these days don't thrill. They kill. Last week, the short distance of about 30 kilometres between Uyo and Ikot Ekpene recorded seven motor accidents in one single day. Worse hit was the Peugeot J5 bus, which crashed into a Mercedes bus at Utu Ikpe, exploding in fire and killing 21 persons.

A few days before that day, I was at the University of Calabar Teaching Hospital to see my pastor. I met him with a POP on his right leg. Again, it was a J5 bus which crashed into an army truck killing 10 passengers. In a similar incident two weeks ago, 25 persons were also killed in Owerri in an accident involving a J5.

I have heard those who know complain about the general shape of J5. Mechanics say the idea of positioning the engine and electrical components in the bonnet of the bus causes congestion and create constant contact and friction between batteries, kick-starter and fuel tubes, resulting in rampant fire whenever J5 is involved in a collision.

Another defect of J5 has been identified as its wheel hub, bolts and nuts. They are said to wear out easily leaving the tyres to do a solo race. J5 is said also to be a front-wheel drive, without a back axle and therefore not suited for the pressure of mass transportation.

If this is true, J5 should be withdrawn from public transportation for checks and necessary re-engineering. There are countries that their transport unions and traffic agencies would since have ensured that is done. The priorities of our transport unions and traffic agencies are however obtuse, making road transportation and driving in Nigeria a nightmare. And this is beyond J5.

Where are the road safety men? What are they doing about the new fad by truck drivers of mounting powerful hunter's light on their bonnets, which render other road users totally blind in the night? What are they doing about the booming sales of alcoholic concoctions in our motor parks? What are they doing about the steady disappearance of road signs on our roads? Beyond this, what is government doing about the influx of fake motor spare parts and lubricant into our market?

Nigeria records 27 times more accidents than the US which has the largest number of vehicles in the world. Nigeria tops the chart of road accidents in the world by 1993 figures recording a staggering 293,000 deaths in 2.2 million accidents within three years. Nigeria loses an average of N1 billion yearly on road accidents. This looks like casualty figures straight from the war front. Is Nigeria a war front?

THE GRANDEUR OF POLITICS

This is the week of Harold Laswell. If that sounds Greek in your ears, I am here to give you a helping hand. For your information, we all owe Harold Laswell a glass of red wine, this weekend. You want to ask why. Well, this is the austere man, who in just six simple, graphic words gave politics its truest meaning; namely that politics is "who gets what, when and how."

Better belief it, this is the most popular and widely accepted definition of politics by eggheads, even in the moon, where Americans have conducted elections via satellite.

You see, politicians must thank their stars. And Dwight Eisenhower too. Eisenhower, 34th American president, thought so highly of politicians, he nearly forced the world of Thomases to believe that politics is a serious, noble profession. I know, some of you don't think so highly of politics and politicians. Not a problem, you have a good company.

Do you know a man called Charles De Gaulle? You would have head also of Ambrose Bierce and Nikita Krushchev. These were men who had very low opinion of politicians. De Gaulle, French general and statesman thought "politics is too serious a matter to be left to the politicians." I hope you can read between the lines. Ambrose Bierce, American journalist and author of sardonic stories said "politicians are people who conduct public affairs for private advantage." And Khrushchev, that celebrated Russian statesman, said "politicians are the same all over. They promise to build a bridge even where there is no river."

Our five great political parties DPN, UNCP, NCPN, CNC and GDM have done a dazzling job of their short campaign. Politicians, you know, are eternal optimists. And all five have promised with equal zeal to win landslide victory. Which is why I got an axe dangling over the heads of two of my editors during the week for daring to suggest that NECON would whack out one of our great parties. NECON did not. All the parties are battling inch-for-inch for control of the State.

What must however be worrisome a bit is the spate of litigation, in-fighting and cross-carpeting in virtually all the parties. One critic says this is a sign of political immaturity. But I think someone must tell Nigerian politicians that winning is not the only word in the dictionary of politics. May be politicians have forgotten already that this spirit of nothing-but-victory has been our undoing even in recent past.

In all political contests, someone must be defeated. What is defeat? "Nothing" says Wendel Phillips, renowned American reformer, "but education, and the first step to something better." Defeat is not the worst of failures, so goes the saying by sages, but not to have tried is the true failure. Indeed, politics has become so expensive and grueling that the defeated is equally an import man as the elected. French moralist Michael De Montaingne

wrote many years ago that there are some defeats more triumphant than victories.

I was watching the American presidential elections live on
CNN with my wife Stella in November, 1992. With substantial
percentage of result undeclared, George Herbert Walker Bush,
the incumbent president and the man who had just made American proud in the Gulf War, suddenly accepted defeat, telephoned
Bill Clinton, congratulated him and a party ensued at both men's
headquarters till day break. I was so touched I just found tears
rolling down my check and my wife couldn't understand why. It
was the majesty of democracy.

Mature politics and politicians admit one fact the good victory is one-handed but peace after elections give victory to both
winners and losers. Sometimes, we discover to our chagrin that
the quality of the man elected is by far inferior to the man defeated. Well, that is the fun or folly of democracy. It is the right to
make even the wrong choice.

At the end, every freely elected government, as 20th American President James Garfield said, is managed by the combined
wisdom and folly of the people.

This is my way of wishing politicians a good outing this weekend.

THE SCHOOL OF NOTHING

My college days were fantastic. Make no mistakes, mine was not the best secondary school in this wide world. Not Kings College; not Hope Waddel; not Etinan Institute nor HOTRICO or HOFACO. Just a backyard school somewhere in the palm tree belt of Akwa Ibom called Apostolic Secondary School, APOSCO.

But what made a world of fantasy for me was going to school at all. I was not expected to. I came from one of the most impoverished backgrounds imaginable. At two, I was already an orphan. At eight I was adept in the farm. And before I could make my primary six exam fees of about N2.50, I had to weed expanse of cassava farms and construct a native fence for a palm produce trader in my village. So finding myself in college via a scholarship was magic.

Oh! I can't forget the first day I arrived the boarding house, sitting astride on the back of a bicycle, strapped between my locker, six-spring bed, grass mattress and the cyclist. I thought the world was in my pocket.

The school was young, barely five years old, when I enrolled.

Student's population was probably below a thousand. Teachers were mostly school leavers. The principal, Mrs. Ayo Udo, a strict Yoruba woman and the vice principal, Mr. E. O. O. Akpabio were the only university graduates. WASC results were usually poor. Until my set, no student had passed in Division Two.

But we made waves in football, music, cultural dance and drama. I was the college prefect and goalkeeper for two years. Some of APOSCO's footballers like James Etokebe and Ini Udoi-dung wound up in Nigeria's national team, the Green Eagles. I and a dozen other represented the Cross River State in several national cultural festivals, winning medals and trophies, not just for our school but for our State.

Some of our girls even toured America to dance (forgive us) bare-breasted. Thereafter a lot of them wound up at FESTAC '77, to dance (again forgive us) half-nude. My class mate Oku Ikang Ita, is still a member of Nigeria's national troupe, dancing around the world. So what we lost by flunking exams badly, we made up by entertaining the world.

But last weekend, I came face-to-face with a pathetic school and school children that seem to have lost the best of both worlds; flunking exams habitually and without the minimum comfort of a playground to compensate for school blues. I am talking about the Christian Secondary Commercial School, CSCS, right here in the heart of the capital city of Uyo.

For three weeks or so, this school had put pressure on me to preside over their inter-house sports competition. So last Saturday, I headed to the school to sit back and enjoy what I thought would be a keen sports competition. But my first shock came just before I drove into the school compound. I was diverted midway to another school in town. Why? We have no football field or playground of any type. A 27-year old government college in Nigeria without a football field? You must be joking! I am not, sir. Please don't let Captain Adeusi, the governor or Moses Essien, the commissioner of education, hear this story, I warned my guide.

Shock Number Two. This is the first inter-house sports competition in this school in six years, I was told. Adorned in green, yellow, blue and white colours outside a borrowed football field, hundreds of excited students began the day with a march past, just as I was called to take the salute. But the crowd of parents, friends and guests almost laughed their heads off as this array of confused legs scattered all over the field kicking everywhere, hobbling, dancing, and limping, right, left, right, left all in the name of marching.

The parade was executed with a flare of unintended comic and I would have loved to laugh, if it were not such an unlaughable matter. They couldn't just march better than that. They have no field of their own to do rehearsal. For me it was one emotional moment that depicted in a rather poignant manner the festering sore of our public schools. It was one scene that truly underlined the absentmindedness of our educational system. Here, I have borrowed some phrases from Ray Ekpu to me announcing one of my many awards,

CSCS has a population of more than 2,000 young Nigerians. It is one of the four schools in Akwa Ibom, I am told, that operate morning and afternoon shifts, with two different principals. The morning school alone has 1,011 students in 25 classes of 470 boys and 541 girls. They have never played football at school; never played basketball, volleyball or any ball for that matter. They are cut-off entirely from sporting life and recreation even, as we are busy seeing visions of the 21st century.

If the condition of these young Nigerians is not finding expression already in various forms of deviant behavior, then educational psychologists should dump their theories in the Mississippi.

Can you imagine a school without a playground of any sort, without a football team and without heroes of track and field events. Is that a school? Well, one of the principals in his speech tried to console the students by saying the school has in stock some footballs, jerseys, javelins, shot-put, discus, etc. But I am sure I wasn't the only guest who wondered whether these games are played on notice boards.

One of the primary reasons education changes people is that students admire colleagues who tower over them in prowess, charisma, talent, experience and intelligence. Often the single greatest influence during college years does not come from the classroom but from the playground. These opportunities, the students of CSCS are denied and I hope that's fair enough.

Where you choose your children to attend college is a decision that will affect you and your children for a life time. If you agree with me, let me go a step further to say that where a community or a country chooses to train their children is a decision that will affect the community or country for a life time. This is my country and this is my worry.

When I was confronted with this sad picture last Saturday, my immediate instinct was that the school is short of space and should be relocated. But the PTA chairman Prince Joseph Okpon was quick to correct me. This school that has no playing ground of any sort actually has a government approved land mass of 4.420 hectares, enough for four football fields. But "powerful individuals" have encroached and snatched the land for their own houses.

I confess, this matter touches my heart. And this column is an SOS not just to relevant government departments in charge of these serious issues, but to voluntary organizations, corporate citizens and individuals with hearts for children and education. Send your love to those confused and tensed up children. Let's rescue this school. It is possible.

THE SILVER LINING

Here's a story that amazes me. Edgar was fired from job after job: cowboy, policeman, law clerk and stenographer. Then he failed when he tried to make a living selling door to door. Not to be denied, Edgar started his own business, an advertising agency – and went bankrupt. An eternal optimist, he decided to start a correspondent school to teach people how to succeed in business. That failed too.

He was thirty-seven years old, nothing but failure, a flop. Perhaps out of desperation, perhaps because fantasizing was the only thing he felt he could do well, he wrote a story about a man in the jungle of Africa. Two years later that story became a book, *Tarzan of the Apes.*

I don't know why Edgar Burroughs had to fail so much before he found success, but I do know that his failures were necessary to keep him from settling down before he found the career that has produced more than 36 million books in thirty languages.

Have you failed once? May be twice? That's Ok. Make another run at success. It's the only way you'll get beyond failing.

Abraham Lincoln, one of the best known and heroic American presidents started life as a bundle of failure. He failed in business (1831); defeated for legislature (1832); again failed in business (1834); lost his sweetheart (1835); had a nervous breakdown (1836); defeated for Congress (1845); again defeated for Congress (1848); defeated for senate (1855); defeated for vice presidency (1956); defeated for senate (1858) and ELECTED PRESIDENT OF USA (1860). How would you describe Lincoln's feat? One writer has compiled Lincoln's feat under a tittle "Salute To Courage."

There is an Old Norwegian story about a fisherman and his two sons. One day they went out to sea to fish. As they headed home with a big catch, the sky blackened and a severe storm caught them. And they were lost and faced with death in the middle of the sea. They had no idea how to find their way back home.

Suddenly a dim yellow glow appeared on the horizon. As they headed toward the light, it grew brighter. They thought someone was burning a fire signal, a beacon for them. When they came in closer, they rejoiced to see their hometown and their friends yelling to them from the dock.

As they pulled in, the fisherman's wife cried out in tears, "Darling, the most terrible things has happened. I'm so glad you are home. We have lost everything; fire has wiped out our house." The fisherman replied "what happened? "I was cooking in the kitchen and the fry-pan caught fire and I dropped it and our whole house caught fire and burned down."

The fisherman climbed out of the boat and didn't say a word. His wife asked "Darling, didn't you hear me? We've lost everything." The fisherman put his arms around her. Let me tell you the other side of the story. The same fire that burned down our house saved our lives.

All failure is relative: relative to the perspective of side and of time. From the shore, the fire seemed a tragedy. From the sea, the fire was salvation, hope and life.

Willie Stargell was for years one of best American baseball players. He played in seven all-star games, won the National League's Most Valuable Player Award, and played in the World Series twice. In the surface, it all seemed like success. However Willie also has the unenviable record of committing the worst foul shots (1,936 times) in baseball history.

But given the perspectives of time, Willie has written: "I feel that to succeed one must fail and the more you fail, the more you learn about succeeding.

To be obsessed with failure or disappointment is crime. If you learned something, if you were moral, if you kept perspective, no event is a failure. See what you can learn and discover about yourself through failure. Then it will be a success.

Don't quote me. Quote Rodney Laughlin. Happy weekend.

THE COST OF DYING

The most Rev Dr. Brian Usanga caused a celebration in The South eastern coast of Nigeria last week. By the powers conferred on him as the Archbishop of Calabar Ecclesiastical Province, comprising Akwa Ibom, Cross River and Rivers States, the revered Catholic priest decreed an end to extravagant funeral.

In the new burial regulation known as Calabar Ecclesiastical Province Special Burial Regulation, the archbishop abrogated various forms of burial jamboree including serving of alcoholic drinks during funeral rites. The new canonical proclamation, tinted with a tone of papal infallibility, described expensive burials as a "shameless parade of sins."

Accordingly, the regulation prescribed that (i) burial must take place within 14 days of death (ii) coffin and grave must be simple (iii) vigil consisting of prayers must end before midnight, without drinks and entertainment.

On the burial day the regulation stipulates that (i) only snacks may be served (ii) provision of soft drinks is optional and (iii) on no account should alcohol be served. Stiff penalties await violators of any aspect of the regulation and Catholics are expected to comply, of course, religiously.

Did I hear somebody say hallelujah? Give His Eminence a hand *s-a-m-b-a-d-y.* I can bet, even the protesting protestants are applauding the archbishop, even if *Nicodemus-ly.* Not because we are broke (I rebuke) but because all of us badly needed someone to bail us out of a pre-historic fad that now threatens to push bereaved families into the abyss of bankruptcy and starvation.

Writings of pre-historians like J. Maringer and E, Bendam shows that ancient people buried their dead with food, furniture, ornaments and tools which they dumped in the grave in the belief that the dead still needed those items in the world beyond.

In some societies, the burial of the dead was even accompanied by human sacrifices with the intention to provide the dead with companions or servants in the next world. Maringer tells one story in which twelve young Trojans were slaughtered and burnt on the funeral pyre of the Greek hero Patroclus. Similarly royal graves excavated at the Sumerian city of Ur, dating 2700 BC revealed retinues of servants burial with their royal masters.

The Zoroastrian custom is however simpler but scary. Their dead is exposed on a raise platform to be devoured by birds of prey, in a bid to expedite their transition to heaven above. In India, the corpse is burnt in fire. As the smoke goes up, the soul is believed to be released to ascend the sky. Moslems world-wide dispose their dead within 24 hours of death.

Some other customs dismember the dead before burial. The Egyptians and Romans at various stages in the past removed the head, the viscera and fingers before burial. In medieval Europe, the heart and entrails of important people were buried in separate places. William the conqueror, for example, was buried in St.

Ettiene, but his heart was left to Rover Cathedral and his entrails interred in the church in Chalus.

Similar practice exists in Nigeria. Five Obas of Ijebu land, Ogun State, three weeks ago met on Easter Monday at the palace of the amiable Awujale of Ijebuland, Oba Sikiru Adetona. The singular agenda was review of burial rites of Obas. At the end they decided they don't want to be buried the traditional way past Obas are buried. In the traditional way, Oba Adetona disclosed, the corpse of an Oba is cut into pieces, the heart is specially prepared and eaten by other Obas. Other pieces of the body are buried at various locations within the town but the head is reserved and given to the Oba's family for veneration. Said Adetona to the press at the end of the meeting. "We want waivers, we want decent burial according to our religious beliefs. This is better than the older primitive cutting of the body and mutilation of the organ. Please bear with use," the Oba pleaded.

A few weeks ago, I listened to a man in Calabar lament how he sunked in millions of naira for the burial of his mother. He sold his house, sold one of his two cars, sold a plot of land and still had to take a loan. Why? He had to build a house in his village, buy a designer casket, fly-in musicians from Lagos, buy cows, publish obituaries in newspapers, TV and radio, print posters, invitation cards, programmes, assorted souvenirs not to mention choice food like salad, coconut rice, fried rice and co.

For eight months, the body of the mother roasted in the mortuary with mortuary fees put at more than N100,000. On burial day, as legion of friends descended on his village, half the villagers and relations stayed away in protest. The few available ones vented their anger openly and police had to be invited.

What a price to pay! Enough to jar the nerves of bishops. Enough to rattle royal fathers. And the message must be drummed home: **give your ageing parents a more befitting welfare than a befitting farewell. Dead men don't eat salad nor drink big stout. It should not cost more to die than to live**.

THE 21ST CENTURY COUP

Britain has a way of cloning America or vice versa. Take a look at the recent past: Jimmy Carter and James Callaghan; Ronald Reagan and Margaret Thatcher; George Bush and John Major and now Bill Clinton and Tony Blair. Like America, Britain is not just phasing out old computers, they are equally flushing out old, weather-beaten politicians.

Americans were the first to flash a red card to pre-World war men in politics when they elected a 44 –year-old strikingly handsome yuppie as President in 1992. Then, as if they were thumping their nose at Britain, they re-elected the charming Democrat for a historic second term late last year.

Britain became jealous. They could hardly wait for the May 1 elections. Now, they have not only given the world Bill Clinton's alter ego, they have given Clinton his high school junior, who can speak in the lingo of the new generation. So you see, fashion is not just about jeans shirt and trendy sneakers, but also about yuppie presidents and trendy governors.

Perish the thought? Well, at your own risk. Make no mistakes about it, this issue is not a matter of jeans and sneakers, it is all about the 21st century, which, by the way, is around the corner. No country, it seems, wants to begin the next millennium with waist pains, walking sticks and snuff boxes, much less with a jolly good uncle who does not understand the difference between cobwebs and websites.

Blair, the Oxford educated lawyer and the youngest British Prime minister since Lord Liverpool in 1812, arrived Downing Street a week ago at the age of 43. Attractive and accompanied by his cute, cheerful wife, Cherie, and three kids Eaun, 13; Nicholas, 11; and Kathrynne, 9; you could pass him for any middle-class worker in Britain.

Last Sunday, the new Prime Minister showed how modern and how really a man of the people he is when he ditched his official Daimler limousine and opted for a 7-seater Ford Galaxy, for his drive to the morning mass with wife and children. And the country, may be the world, was tickled.

Casually dressed in khaki-like trousers and tie-less, (open-neck) light blue shirt, he waved aside a sixty-seven thousand pounds worth official car in favour of a Twenty-seven thousand pound Ford, commonly used by average urban families in Europe. Jubilant Galaxy dealers reckoned Blair has sent Galaxy sales into multiple digits.

The *Independent* newspaper, caught up in the excitement, announced "Everything has changed." Each word was painted in different colours, in case less literate readers fail to gather the thrilling significance of the words. Dreams are to be fulfilled. A new face for the new millennium, hopes are high.

Wonderful! Wonderful! Wonderful! Blair's cabinet is positively bristling with talent and youthfulness. The average age is forty-some-thing. His closest ally, Peter Mandelson, 43, the architect of the election triumph, has been rewarded with the job of minister without portfolio, believed to be a very powerful position that make him Blair's ear in every cabinet committee. He would not only assist in the strategic implementation of government policies and their effective presentation to the public, but will have a powerful role in keeping Blair's modernizing crusade on track.

Modernity is the word. One thing that struck all those who watched the British elections on TV was how many of the rejected tory candidates were old and past it. In contrast, the labour candidates were youthful, enthusiastic and full of promise. They are new faces in politics and they include an incredible 120 women, the highest number of women parliamentarians in British history. Some 101 of them are new and members of the Labour Party.

While Blair is the youngest prime minister in 185 years, Clair Ward, 24, Labour parliamentarian for Watford, is the youngest of all the law makers. "The reason I was elected is not because I have long hairs and whatever it takes to be a babe. I want to be seen as a serious politician who has something to offer," she said in an interview with the *Mirror*. In the last 100 years of British politics, there have been 4,500 male parliamentarians and only 169 women.

Women were not eligible to sit in the English Parliament until 1918. The first was Nancy Aster, a Tory. One of the reasons behind the influx of young women parliamentarians, according to reports, is the positive discrimination by the Labour Party. Lorna Fitzsimmon, 29, one of the "Blair Babes" as they are called, put the incursion of young people into politics in perspective: "The reality is that we have achieved a lot for our age and broken through the glass ceiling of politics, which has been an older man's preserve for a long time."

Yet another striking feature of the Labour victory is the mother and son who won in different constituencies and have written a new chapter in the history of British politics. Ann Cryer, 56 widow of radical politician, Bob Cryer and her son, John, 33, a journalist, are symbols of the historic landslide won by the Labour Party.

The ousted Conservative Party certainly did not just pay the price of fielding ageing candidates. They paid the price of over-staying in power. For 18 years, they ran Britain almost like a one-party State. Clair Ward, 24, the youngest parliamentarian was just six years old, when Thatcher defeated Callaghan after the "Winter of Discontent" in 1979.

For over-staying and for misreading the political temperature of the world at the turn of the century, the Tories won a paltry 135 votes, the lowest since 1832, while Labour, fortified with new age candidates, won 419 of the 659 seats, the party's most impressive victory in history.

A sign post to 21st century politics? I don't know. What I reckon is that Blair's resounding victory, coming on the heels of America's Clinton, signified a great demand for change from the old, worn-out generation to the new, vibrant era.

I hope when the euphoria in Britain is over, Blair will be brave enough to champion his 21st century agenda.

NOSTALGIA FOR SIERRE LEONE

I was speaking with President Joseph Momoh of Sierra Leone in Freetown in April, 27, 1991, when he told me: "Nigeria can't sit by and see things go wrong in Sierra Leone and not show concern." (Newswatch May 13, 1991).

Six years later, Momoh's prophecy came to pass when Nigeria along with other brother-West African nations refused to sit by, as happy-go-lucky corporals took their bazookas to the State House last week, and drove away the man properly and popularly chosen by the people to govern Sierra Leone. As the bloody saga in Freetown plays out on TV screens round the world all week, I found myself overwhelmed by rhapsodies of Sierra Leone.

For the better part of 1990 and 1991, I covered and reported (to quote Dan Agbese, editor-in-chief of *Newswatch*) "bloody wars and political crisis in Africa more than any other Nigerian journalist." I was in Benin Republic when democratic movements rose up and sacked Mathieu Kerokou. I was back in Contonou to watch the Presidential elections and went on record as the first Nigerian journalist to interview Nicefore Soglo, who won the election shortly after Kerekou was forced to step down.

I was in Liberia, the day troops of Charles Taylor set their feet on Monrovia, interviewed a lonely President Samuel Doe and filed the story on the *Last Days of Samuel Doe* that won the Nigerian Union of Journalists Award of Excellence in features writing in 1991.

It was actually my adventure in Liberia that introduced me to Sierra Leone. That weekend I was on my way to Lome, Togo, when my bosses recalled me to head instead for Monrovia. I left Lagos for Conakry, Guinea with Nigeria airways in the hope of flying *Air Guinea* to James Spriggs Airfield in the heart of Monrovia. Robertfield Airport on the outskirts of Monrovia had already been shut because of bombardments by invading rebel forces.

At Conakry, I found that Air Guinea had just suspended flights to Monrovia. The only option open to anybody crazy enough to go Monrovia was to go to Freetown by road, find his way via Bo to Kenema, the border town between Sierra Leone and Liberia and then head to Monrovia across the Mano River Bridge.

Which is what I did. The rest of the story was bloody. Two of my colleagues Kris Imodibe of the *Guardian* and Tayo Awotusin of the *Champion* were killed. Frank Iwuebueze, still in the *National Concord* was rescued by Burkinabe troops and later flown into an American ship and ferried to Freetown.

The Sunday morning I escaped, Kris and Frank were with me up to a point where Kris gave me a letter to his boss Lade Bonuala still the MD of the *Guardian* promising me he would join me later.

Now back in Freetown along with hundreds of refugees, on a Monday, I discovered the only flight to Nigeria was Wednesday. Unlike the refugees, I checked into the Paramount Hotel, probably one of the best in Freetown, poised to savior my narrow escape.

I was at the Reception Desk of the hotel that night when I saw a long convoy, obviously, of a very important person drove out of the adjacent white storey building. As I stepped out of the hotel the next morning, that simple white storey building, to my surprise turned out to be the "Office of the President of Sierra Leone", according to a signpost in front of the building. Why can't I go and talk to the president, I said to myself. I walked across the road, made my way for the huge gate and in 10 minutes I was already seated before the Press secretary. He promised to get back to me. It wasn't a political promise.

The next morning, at about 11.00am he drove me up a hill to the president's residence where I met a relaxed, bulky man in light blue French suit. For one and a half hours, I was the only guest of the president. When his kids kept running past the palour, interrupting our pre-interview chat, he took me upstairs to his private study, besides his bedroom which was littered with souvenirs, gifts and books. Life-size and other portraits of then Nigerian President Ibrahim Babangida was all over the place. "We have known each other for 29 years" he told me when he noticed my curiosity about IBB pictures.

Afterwards, Freetown became second home. Not just because I had become guest of the President but because Freetown in the early 90s was so much like Calabar in the 70s, where I grew up. Narrow roads, rusty roofs, wooden houses, hospitable visitors hugging people, familiar names, and familiar manners.

If you have seen Hope Waddel Institute, Calabar, you have seen Fourah Bay College, Freetown. I couldn't believe there could be such identical people and cities, yet so far apart. And so every time I arrive Lungi airport and drove a few kilometers to take a ferry to Freetown, it was like crossing from Oron by ferry to Calabar. Then you enter the shops or visit the market: fish, coconut, Bournvita, Lipton tea, Omo, Key soap, plastic plates most of them brought in from Lagos.

Some "proud" Nigerians are often tempted to think Sierra Leone is simply another Nigerian State unseparated even by distance. Even President Momoh told me that much. "Quite honestly, I am happy because it is a good thing to have a big brother, so that when it gets to a point where things get tough, you can go to your big brother, "he said.

This is the point Western critics of Nigeria's action in Sierra Leone are missing. Nigeria is Sierra Leone's big and blood brother. America is not, Britain is not. A big brother runs to the rescue of his sibling in distress. A big croaker runs away in time of need and watches from safe distance just like The Western nations have done in Sierra Leone. That is the difference.

We Nigerians must begin to thump our chests, not our noses, whenever we do the right thing, the outcome and the rest of the world notwithstanding. As at press time *CNN* and *BBC* were trumpeting "Nigeria's humiliation" in the hands of coupists in Freetown. But I'm so proud we put our right leg forward. Not going to Sierra Leone would be risking Liberia. That will be too much of a risk. I am so proud Africa is speaking with one voice. The coupists have found no friends outside. They have found no friends inside either. I bet Sierra Leone is not Nigeria's Vietnam. This is not Pierre Bouyoya's Burundi. This is not even Tejan Kabbah's last days. This could possibly be the last days of coups in Africa.

Well if you miss this column next week, I could as well be heading for Freetown. At last, my cumulative leave is taking off Monday. Do send me some *Leones* if you can. Don't forget there is no free lunch even in Freetown.

GOODBYE TO LIBATION

A quiet combustion is consuming the fabrics of our tradition and nothing may ever be the same again. Can you believe it: that libation, the fetish arts of dining and wining with the dead is fast being consigned to the cemetery?

You dare not try it here in the can-do city of Uyo or risk the wrath of irate new generation, who think nothing could be more barbaric in these last days of the 20th century.

Now, to make things worse for those cranky old wizards who think they can manipulate us with their deadly rituals, quite a number of local government areas are putting official seal to the anti-libation crusade.

Stella Effiom, the iron lady who runs the municipal government in Uyo, says she will not brook any libation during her tenure. And that's official. Instead of spending hard-earned government money to lavish some totemic ancestors with cows and gins, she will seek to feed the living, some of whom have not received legitimate entitlements such as pensions for years. And she said this in a rather Thatcherite fashion to the discomfiture of those traditional priests who were dressed up, towels and all, for a feast with the dead.

A week earlier, at neighbouring Etinan, Ime Inyang, the popular youth leader, who won elections to govern the Oxford of Akwa Ibom State, had openly given a thumps down to connoisseurs of libation, during the swearing in of his councilors, his first official duty on the job. Apparently, the manifesto of the United Nigeria Congress Party, UNCP, on which platform Efiom and Inyang ascended to power, did not include buying cows and gins for evil spirits.

But the angst against this fetish practice has not just begun: the wind of change is merely sweeping deeper into the crevices of a State, where, since its creation nearly 10 years, ago, hundreds, maybe thousands of cows, along with drums of gin have been sacrificed, with official nod, to evil spirits and deities, to the utter detriment of the spiritual and material wellbeing of the people.

In the newly created Ibesikpo-Asutan council, libation has never and may never be poured, the way things are going. Right from the very first meeting of the traditional rulers' council, the crusade against libation erupted from the most unlikely trajectory. Chief Ita Etuk, lawyer, village head and perhaps, the best known atheist in Akwa Ibom State stood up, just as libation was about to be poured and moved a motion that libation should not be poured in the new local government area for seven years, in order to test the power of the Christian God vis-à-vis ancestral gods. The motion was unanimously adopted. To quote Ita Etuk: "I stopped that libation and everybody was happy."

So what's the big deal about libation that's generating so

much fuss among the younger general? Or what has made libation so leprous that nobody wants to touch it even with a long pole?

I have watched libations being poured at many levels, including the ridiculous level of enacting such brazen wizardry at public functions. From my observation, I can define libation with some authority, primarily as an act of communication and communion with the spirits of the dead for the purpose of invoking and deploying them to supervise, manipulate and control the living. You will not find that in any book.

To be sure, and just to satisfy my curiosity, I went for the dictionary meaning of libation and it said it all: viz: "the pouring forth of wine in honour of a god." Note the small "gee." I decided to check up the meaning of "god" and found out it means "idol," and I decided to find out the meaning of idol. Here is it: "a figure, an image, a semblance, a phantom; a counterfeit (of God), a false motion or erroneous way of looking at things to which the mind is prone." That is Chambers English Dictionary.

Those who understand libation will readily agree that it is a practice of dealing with evil spirit. Jenning Dake, the American scholar who spent 100,000 hours in 43 years to write one of the best known study bibles, define witchcraft precisely in the same words as the practice of dealing with evil spirit.

Again, those who are familiar with libation will not hesitate to agree that libation is a means of communication with the dead. Dake also explains that communication with the dead is a kind of divination known as necromancy. You may reach any conclusion at your disposal but you won't be too far from the truth if you say that libation is a level of witchcraft and necromancy.

Libation cannot be poured just by any face in the crowd. If you dare it, you can as well sing your *Nunc Dimittis* and suddenly join your ancestors to become an ancestor yourself. To be sure, libation can only be poured by ordained traditional priests of good standing. Those highly anointed traditional priests can hold an entire stadium spell bound once they step onto their invisible pulpits.

Be it in marriage ceremonies, dedication of new-born babies or commissioning of factories, etc.; this practice is performed in the belief that we mortals cannot supervise, control and guide our paths and affairs properly, but must submit to the supervision and guidance of the spirit of dead men. It is not on the same premise that believers in Almighty God predicate their prayers?

Often at public function, both the priest of the Almighty god and the priest of the devilish god are invited to pray, one after the other. Usually, the priest of the Almighty would casually go to microphone to read mere sanctimonious platitudes written on a piece of paper, without any thought to it or impact.

But the anointed ancestral priest would step out with enchanters, drink offering and kola-nut. With studied artistry and display of oratorical prowess, he would invoke all known deities of the land, casting a spell on his audience, who soon respond with deafening applause. With vernacular, native wisdom and deeper insight into spiritual realms, this fetish priest easily outwits and overwhelms our American phonetic preacher. Not a surprise that so many factories, electricity and water projects commissioned under the spell of fetish unction have quickly become a ghost of themselves, ready to join some destructive ancestors.

My surprise however is that many of us still drink with relish the left-over drinks served to the dead, unconscious of the fact that we are boozing with the dead in the same cup.

Scales are just beginning to fall from the eyes of the younger generation and it is becoming clear that drunken ancestors have caused more harm than good to our well-being and it is high time we starve them.

SIREN OF GOOD TIDINGS

It was a little after eight o'clock Thursday morning last week. I was already on the third page of my write-up and racing. I had arrived the office quite earlier than usual, unnoticed even by some security staff. As the early morning harmattan haze faded reluctantly to make way for a distant, obscure sun emerging seemingly from Ikot Akpan Abia, I burrowed my head into heaps of files stacked by the left side of my metal desk.

My mission this morning was to complete, before my routine duties, a self-imposed task of writing an annual report for the company. Spread across the rest of the table were additional files, figures, graphs, tabulations and reports submitted by various head of departments. As I took a quick look at the bottom line (summary) of every report, I beamed occasionally with smiles, very much thankful to God for the modest achievement recorded by the company in the last six months.

Suddenly, the wailing of a powerful siren seized the air. Elizabeth Daniel, my secretary, who was helping with the files dashed to the window, to take a look. Then without warning,the siren tapered and terminated as if someone had strangled its jugular.

"It's the governor, it's the governor," she screamed almost uncontrollably referring to Lt-Col. Yakubu Bako, the state military governor or administrator as they are now called. I flew off my seat and raced down the staircase like Ben Johnson, the fastest man on earth. His Excellency was already at the foot of the staircase leading up to my office, sandwiched by a retinue of security guards. "Good morning Your Excellency. Pleased to welcome you, Sir," I greeted him several stairs away from the stern-looking soldier. "Yes, Yes, good morning," he replied as I led the way straight into my office. "Seat for you, Sir," I said, "No, No," let's see your facilities. Show me this place first," he said.

Nothing much to show or see. Two-storey residential building rented six years ago; a newsroom with three typewriters; a photographic unit inside a kitchen, bereft of the simplest photographic equipment; a stationery store that goes by the name of a library; unserviceable distribution vans. No printing press, no lithographic equipment, no page or plate maker. Nothing, "So how are you producing the newspaper? He queried, looking quite surprised. "Literally with bare hands, bare knuckles, Sir," I said grateful for the question. "Well done," he said. Then the siren came back to life and the convoy zoomed off with the tall, soft-spoken and respectable officer.

For about half-an hour after his departure, I and my colleagues stood there almost transfixed and breathless. It was a classical surprise visit. Not even his personal staff including the press corps and protocol had a clue. He took off straight from his residence and drove straight to *The Pioneer.*I wondered what could have been, I was not at work. How proud I was all my key staff and heads of departments were on seat. But some of our departments were caught pants down. Worse hit was the photo unit. There was not a single photographer to record the visit. Trust Obiota Ekanem, the acting editor, queries have been flying like scud missiles since the early morning visitor left.

The distinguished visitor, I dare say, was a harbinger of good tidings. Don't ask me what tidings he brought because, wait a minute, I don't speak to the press. But for a State governor to drive privately to see the uncompleted Pioneer House, then pay an official visit to its temporary base and entertain series of briefings on the newspaper project, all within two weeks of his appointment, speaks volumes about his interest in the project. I salute His Excellency.

Just six months or so ago, *The Pioneer* suddenly took a new shape, completely redesigned and repackaged to meet standards of modern newspapers and whet the appetite of increasingly well-informed and thirsty readers. We introduced extras such as cartoons, juicy columns, soft-sale pages, serious analytical features, etc. Our readers liked it and showered us with encomium. Our people felt proud, to have one of the best newspapers east of the Niger. First, sales figures went up, advert support multiplied and our revenue (hope the tax men are not reading this) showed modest improvement. For this I want, on behalf of *The Pioneer* clan, to say a big thank you to our readers, advertisers and critics. Criticisms have helped us a lot in our attempt to give our audience a respected and fast selling newspaper. And let me say this (but don't quote me) one of our valuable critics is Lt.-Col. Bako, who has already sold us very useful and unbelievable ideas that will begin to manifest soon and will surely add to our credibility and sales figure.

I know that the one big question in the minds of our readers is: when are you going daily? I am dreaming of three to six months. In reality, I can assure you that Bako will surely make a difference. Not just in breaking the jinx of publishing a Daily *Pioneer* but in the quality and spread of the newspaper. Quote me.

We, on our part are very much on our toes criticizing ourselves, reassessing our focus and thrust and aiming to be the best. Yes, you don't believe government newspaper can be the best? But let me repeat what I said in the maiden edition of this column six months ago which I believed is still relevant today: "A jaundiced government newspaper that does not win the confidence and respect of its readers, no matter how beautiful, cannot serve the purpose of packaging its government and people no matter how good the government and people are. For this reason, *The Pioneer* shall be balanced, critical, analytical, fair, firm and at all times shall try to reflect the views of the broad spectrum and cross-section of the government and people that own it." Stay with us.

IN LOVE WITH FISH AND OIL

For whatever reason, France has never hidden its aversion and phobia for Nigeria. As a student of international relations a few years ago, I was on the receiving end of various theories on why France prefers, at the slightest or no provocation, to bare its fangs at Nigeria.

In 1967, France was the chief sponsor of Biafra, fuelling for three years the bloody civil war that killed approximately three million Nigerians; maimed and orphaned several thousand others. In 1973, when Nigeria successfully spearheaded the formation of ECOWAS, France became a stumbling block, and master-minded the establishment of the CEAO for Francophone West Africa, in a bid to checkmate and frustrate perceived Nigeria influence in the region. Back in 1961, France's insistence on testing its new atomic bomb in the Sahara, right in Nigeria's backyard, resulted in a diplomatic row that almost saw the closure of French embassy in Lagos.

And now, for the "love of Cameroun and it impoverished black people," France is back at Nigeria's jugular. In an otherwise minor and natural squabble between two neighbouring brothers, France has marshaled its arsenal, complete with frigates, fighter helicopters and paratroopers into the Limbo region of Cameroun ready, for a showdown that is not only totally unwarranted but completely uncalled for.

As a prelude, France, has launched a full-scale diplomatic war against Nigeria, and while masquerading as Cameroun, has dragged Nigeriato the World Court, the UN Security Council and the European Union, all for a peace of African soil. What a great protector and friend Cameroun has found in France!

Make no mistakes, France has no such love for Cameroun or any black nation for that matter. It had only a few weeks ago ensured the devaluation of the CFA in Francophone West Africa, making life unbearable even for Cameroun. The truth is that France is going into this war simply for the love of oil and fish. The oil and fish of the Bakassi Peninsula are the mouthwatering dish that lured the "Frogs" into this veritable trap. Nigeria therefore must be prepared to make France pay dearly for this irresistible delicacy. In the oil-and-fish-rich waters of Bakassi must lay in wait a waterloo for France.

The latest news coming in from Cameroun is that Yaounde, urged by France, ordered last week the stock-taking of assets and bank accounts of Nigerian business in the country. If these reports are anything to go by, Nigeria cannot turn the other cheek. A census of French (not Cameroun) businesses in Nigeria must commence as a tit-for-tat.

French businesses and investments in Nigeria range from oil exploration and marketing to banking, construction, automobile and distribution companies. The last count by experts in 1992 showed that there are more than 180 French companies operating in Nigeria. This makes France the second largest foreign investor in Nigeria.

In the area of oil exploration and marketing, Elf and TOTAL are the two leading French companies. Elf which came to Nigeria in 1962 as Safrap (Nig) Ltd, had by 1984 increased its oil production level to 38.8 million barrels per year. Elf marketing as at 1989 had about 103 petrol stations nationwide and has since veered into marketing of kerosene, diesel and industrial lubricants. TOTAL with more than 300 petrol stations nation-wide is clearly the leader in oil marketing business in Nigeria.

France also has a strong foothold in the banking sector. These banks include UBA, AFRIBANK, Societe Generable Bank, Universal Trust Bank, UTB, Merchant Banking Corporation, MBC, etc. UBA alone has more than 100 branches in Nigeria. The combine assets of French banks in Nigeria as at 1985 stood at N8.5 billion. Yet another area which France has milked Nigeria is in the automobile sector, through the making of Peugeot cars, regarded more or less as the official national car of Nigeria. In 1981 alone, Peugeot Automobile of Nigeria, PAN, produced nearly 60,000 Vehicles for the Nigerian market alone.

France is not left behind in the construction business in Nigeria. French construction companies that have become household names because of multi-billion naira contracts include Fougerolle, Bouygues, Dumez and Spibat. Figures made available by NIIA researchers show that in 1981 alone, French construction companies won 65 contracts with 10.4 billion French Franc. Other notable French companies in Nigeria include the CFAO and the SCOA, which are giants in the distributive trade.

Maybe for obvious reasons, France now appears to be thumping its long nose at Nigeria. France it seems is quite aware of the economic crisis which may have weakened Nigeria. France is also aware that the political class has rubbished Nigeria, virtually turning it into a banana republic, with little or no respect in the committee of nations. And so this is time to deliver the knock-out punch.

Well, France is making a big mistake. Nigerians must prove France wrong. If for the love of Bakassi oil and fish, France is prepared to forgo its investments in Nigeria, then Nigerians must be prepared to make France forgo both.

IN SEARCH OF A MANDELA FOR NIGERIA

The last few weeks have been very agonizing for Nigerians. The resounding success of The South Africa polls, which sent the whole world into wild jubilation, turned out to inflict on the Nigerian psyche a moral admonition, bordering on international ostracism.

Suddenly, the full impact of The South African breakthrough, their maturity, their honesty and sincerity of purpose, their determination to enthrone justice and the world-wide acclamation that followed, became a Nemesis of sort for Nigeria, haunting our collective conscience, cutting us down to Lilliputs, taking the shine off our political pranks and making us look more and more like a banana republic.

Suddenly, it dawned on us Nigerians that South Africa has done what "Napoleon" could not do. It became clear to us that what South Africa has done has catapulted the hitherto notorious country head and shoulder above the self-styled giant of Africa. It became so crystal clear that democracy, justice and fair-play, could and will make a world of difference between the fortunes of the two countries. The scales fell off our eyes and we began to appreciate that South Africa would reap bountifully the goodwill of countries who hold democratic values dear to their hearts, namely: US, UK, Japan, France, Germany, India, Pakistan, South Korea, Brazil, name them.

A friend of mine, Udo Okon, broke down and wept when the news came that F. W. De Klerk had conceded defeat and congratulated Nelson Mandela even before vote counting was over. It was a somewhat unseemly sight for a senior government official like Okon. But the man was not weeping for De Klerk. He was crying for his beloved country, Nigeria. Nigeria, it must be admitted, is a political nightmare. It is in short supply or put it bluntly, bereft of men like De Klerk: men with large heart, men of virtue and sincerity of purpose and men who are truly men.

If De Klerk were Nigeria; he would have sat tight at the State House, contrived and frame mischief, spun out decrees like cobwebs, to entangle, ensnare and incapacitate every serious presidential contender. He would have singlehandedly disqualified and banned Mandela from contesting the election, maybe for the sin of growing grey hairs or spending too long a time in jail or divorcing Winnie or for speaking haughty English that most Nigerians do not comprehend.

If however, Mandela managed to beat the trap and contest the election, the result would be forfeited with impunity, either because of the colour of Mandela's necktie on Election Day or for having as friends such bearded men like Fidel Castro and Sam Nujoma. De Klerk's propaganda man would tell the whole world that the colour of Mandela's necktie is not in the national interest and could set fire on Niger Bridge. Ridiculous country!

Certainly, Nigeria is short of men. Men like Mandela: men of principles, valour and guts; men of their words; men of honour, upright men; selfless men; reliable men; men who can pledge their lives for a just cause and stand by it. This country has leaders who are nicknamed Maradona (Trickster, Dribbler, Cheat) and they are proud to answer the name. We have men who are elected governors but gang up to reject another man elected president in preference for a military despot.

This country can boast of men, "big men" (emirs, obas, obis, obongs, senators, judges, lawyers, journalists) who would readily look the other way and sell their birth rights for a mess of porridge. This country can boast of fickle-minded men, the-neither-here-nor-there men; the-more-you-look-the less-you-see men, the-i-have-a-family to-feed-men.

Yes, we have men, who do not stand for anything except their bellies, indeed men, whose stomach is the centre-piece of their domestic and foreign policies. So we are saddled in Nigeria with men, who are committed "stomachcrats" and advocates of "stomachcracy": the government of the stomach, by the stomach and for the stomach. And as long as their stomach is filled, others can jolly-well burn to ashes.

This point must be made. We Nigerian men have failed this country and shamed our people. We must admit responsibility for the insipid woes of our fatherland. We must admit that for a mess of porridge, we have turned our backs on the suffering and anguish of our people. Very important, we must admit that if elections could not be conducted in Nigeria successfully but could be smoothly conducted in what was regarded as an apartheid enclave, a pariah State, then what is going on in Nigeria is possibly worse than apartheid. Which is why we need Nigerian Mandelas and De Klerks to bring sunshine to our faces and return us to the path of sanity.

PILGRIMAGE NOT PICNIC

The dark cloud was in the morning. And that was a bad omen. One of the ramshackled buses, conveying Akwa Ibom pilgrims broke down right here in Uyo, just along Ikot Ekpene Road. That was five minutes into the two-hour journey to Port Harcourt Airport, where an aircraft was waiting to complete the journey. Not quite a surprise. Pilgrims who saw the smoking vehicle crawl in to convey them had no difficulty writing off the contraption. Somehow they had no choice, but to file into the wobbling wagon.

After a few minutes of fiddling under its belly, the mechanic came out with a partial bill of health. Well, you can proceed to Port Harcourt, he said. But that was not to be. The bus, property of Uyo Capital City Transport Services, UCCTS, finally ran out of oxygen and dropped dead. Time was 11.am. That was at Ikot Ekpene. And that was that.

Stranded pilgrims, who had bade farewell to their loves ones as early as six in the morning, littered the road, fumming and uncertain whether they could still make the flight, rumoured (yes rumoured) to take off at 12 noon. You could see frustration in capital letters written boldly on faces of pilgrims. Some were simply beside themselves with rage.

As livid pilgrims carpeted officials responsible for the poor arrangement, Pastor Ubong Udoh, a member of the pilgrim's board travelling in the Ill-fated bus rallied round to raise funds for another bus. Then Rev. Idara Ideh, secretary of the Pilgrims Board, arrived to the rescue. Squeezed inside small Toyota buses, picked from a roadside motor park, the stranded pilgrims finally made it to Port Harcourt Airport at 3.25pm. A journey of two hours had tuned into a nightmare of five hours.

Exhausted and visibly upset, the unsmiling pilgrims trudged into a Hajj Camp (yes Hajj Camp) at the extreme right flank of the Port Harcourt Airport. But the Hajj Camp offered no comfort either. It was like jumping from frying pan into fire. The camp is more or less a warehouse; just the roof, four walls and bare floor. No chairs, no fan, no railings, no water, no restaurant. Nothing, except hunger and anger.

The check-in formality was slow and chaotic, worse than the Nigerian Post Office . And that's being polite. Then someone tossed a couple of mats on the floor. Pilgrims (some of them high society persons) in their Sunday best, at first snubbed and ignored the mats. That was a big mistake as they later found out. As minutes turned into hours and the sun slowly withdrew itself to usher in the night, those mats became hot cakes. The high and the low hustled for mats and those who weren't lucky enough had to hit the bare floor, waiting for OKADA AIR, the official airline contracted for the journey.

By about 10.00 pm, OKADA AIR, finally flew into Port Harcourt. At about 12 midnight, the aircraft choked with 295 pilgrims, shot into the dark, humid sky as if it was heading for the golden ball of moon hovering in the horizon.

Thirty-minutes in the air, the Fasten-Your-Seat-Belt light went off just as the dong of an electronic bell sounded. We relaxed and floated our seats into a more comfortable position. The air hostesses, almost a dozen of them, sprang to their feet. Some passengers, who were used to the luxury of international flights, began to expect some pampering and feasting. But the unsmiling girls in blue skirts and white blouses gave them thumbs down. They simply went about throwing, rather furiously, trays of rice, bread and cakes in front of pilgrims.

To accompany the meal was pineapple juice in small waterproof sachets. As I took a look at my wrist watch, it was 12.35am. For many pilgrims, who had left home before 6.00am the previous day, it was their first meal in almost 24 hours. They simply attacked the meal with speed in spite of the unappetizing and unattractive content of their plates.

For pilgrims, who had travelled Swiss Air, KLM, Ethiopian Airlines or any other airline on international routes, the in-flight service was a far cry, an embarrassment: bread without butter or jam; dry and barely cooked jollof rice with a piece of saltless dry meat (the type shared to the general public at funeral ceremonies); fruit juice without a straw, and a polite request for water was like asking for a mighty favour. Request for tooth picks were completely ignored.

Apparently, Okada hostesses had long concluded that pilgrims were inconsequential people whose airfares were after all paid for by government, and who may never have boarded an aircraft before. And they went about their jobs without the slightest courtesy. No "drinks for you, please"! No pampering. No gesture of courtesy whatsoever. Were they recruited from Outer Mongolia or the jungle of Malaysia, I asked myself constantly. The three-course meal I was expecting faded into a mirage. No ear-phone for stereo channels. No movie to entertain passengers. No blankets to warm your feet a bit, just there like a frozen fish. I ventured to ask one hostess for the in-flight shop. The overworked young woman simply snubbed me and hobbled down the aisle. Who knows, she may have been conscripted in the last minute to do the journey. Who knows, may be the airline had not paid her salaries for the third consecutive month. This is Nigeria, you know!

Of course, the fight went on. All in the dark. Total darkness. Literally and metaphorically we were in the dark. There was a complete lack of information on our movement. Where the hell on the planet could this aircraft be flying now? I kept asking myself. Boeing 747s have facilities that show passengers on a screen, a map of their flight path, speed, altitude, mileage and every major city, country, river or mountain the aircraft is flying across.

This facility usually make international flights very captivating for passengers, who get glued to the screen enjoying at the same time intermittent commentaries and jocular remarks by pilots. In this case, it was like flying in the Ozone layer: blank and lost.

Seven hours later, we discovered ourselves at Ben Gurion Airport. Hallelujah, it's Israel. We sang and clapped and danced and rejoiced. The agony of the last 26 hours faded into insignificance as we were simply overwhelmed by the hospitality of the Israelis. Right from the tarmac, where a fleet of luxurious airport shuttles drove us to the arrival hall, it was SHALOM (PEACE BE TO YOU). Customs and immigration officials were so polite and kind even in their effectiveness, thoroughness and efficiency.

As we left the airport for our first stop at Bat Yam, a suburb in Tel Aviv, we were wondering, whether we had actually been checked or some unseen electronic gadgets did the magic. "Unbelievable" Sir Valantine Ndah said to Sir Maurice Ebe, trying to compare the situation back home.

At Bat Yam, we ran into the warm embrace of Sun Hotel staff, who ushered us into the hotel lobby with a smile and chilled orange juice. We betted it was going to be a picnic. Soon we cruised in an air-conditioned bus, fitted with TV, Video, stereo and refrigerator into Jerusalem and checked into the star-studded Jerusalem Renaissance Hotel. In every city of Israel that we stayed for the two-week pilgrimage, we slept in star-studded hotels and were treated to the text book politeness of Israeli people and their array of food and fruits.

But pilgrimage is not a picnic. It requires some orientation in the Spartan lifestyle of the Port Harcourt Hajj Camp and Okada Air. It requires a certificate of endurance test and the courage of Paul of Tarsus to walk through the footsteps of Jesus. The buses could only take pilgrims to the nearest points of the Holy site and not the Holy site per se. The terrain is something like a dreamland. It is either you are ascending a mountain and descending into a valley. You are either walking on top of stone chips or a hot desert sand.

Sunshine is constant and rainfall is luxury. The volume of rainfall in Nigeria for one day is more than the volume of rainfall in Israel for one year. It is under these rigorous conditions that pilgrims go through.

And the signs were everywhere: back-pains, waist-pains, pain in the neck, pain in the joints, pains everywhere. Beginning from Day One, Dr. Valerie Obot and her nurse, Mrs. Regina Bassey were blessed with a sleepless night. Most mornings, you would see their eyes bulging and reddish as they hurry to grab their breakfast and meet up with other pilgrims. Why? Early morning "ward rounds."

Some nights, the number of patients and the nature of ailments would simply overpower the medical team and they would just dispatch an SOS for people to come and pray. "Bro Anietie, please come and help me pray for Prof," the lady's voice on the telephone said at about 12 midnight betraying some sense and sign of danger. I was beside my bed and on my knees praying with my room-mate Effiong Essien, when the phone call came. We flew into our 11th floor elevator and raced down to the eight floor of the Haifa Towers Hotel, where Professor Etim Udo was already in fits and half-conscious. His room-mate, Very Reverend Ekerendu of the Methodist Church along with Dr. (Mrs.) Obot and Mrs. Bassey (the nurse), stood beside his bed a bit unsure of what to do next.

But Dr. Obot knew of a world renowned physician by name JESUS. We put away stethoscopes, syringes and needles, and put in one hour of prayers, in Jesus Name. The answer was fast. The man was healed. Why not? After all we were in Jesus own country. And the next morning, even against doctors' advice, the Prof. stepped out kicking with other pilgrims on tour of Mount Tabor, the mount of transfiguration. Till we left Israel, the Professor never complained of any headache again. Instead he became stronger by the day. It was a miracle!

But a big headache surfaced just as we were winding up our pilgrimage in Bat Yam, near Tel Aviv. Okada Air would not show up on Sunday October 9, as scheduled. Our money had finished.

Sun Hotel had checked us out. And the Nigerian Embassy staff had deserted us. They were simply nowhere to the found. It was time to starve and sleep on chairs and floors again.

It was an anti-climax to an otherwise spiritually rewarding pilgrimage. The signs had been there that we might run into flight hitches. Some pilgrims from northern and western Nigeria had suffered the same fate, and the news had filtered to us. By the time we checked into Sun Hotel Friday, preceding our Sunday scheduled departure, tension and anxiety had quietly crept into our camp. Would Okada do to Eastern pilgrims what is did to northern and western pilgrims? Together we prayed to cancel flight hitches but that was to no avail. God did not answer that prayer, even in Israel. The trouble was not with God but with Nigeria.

Saturday was scheduled for shopping, but there was little left in our pockets for such luxury. We had bought enough holy oil and holy water from River Jordan, to drown our bank accounts even back home. Everybody was dead broke, down to his last shekel. Then our worst fears were confirmed. Okada Air would not make it because of "operational reasons." This news depressed pilgrims to no end. To worsen matters, the travel agent Philip Meyers insisted we must pay additional $50 each, in order to spend another night in the hotel. The flight cancellation was obviously not our fault, we pleaded with Mr. Meyers but the businessman would not budge an inch. Some Pentecostals began to pray in tongues. It didn't move Mr. Meyers one bit.

A task force led by Okon Nsabasi, the Akwa Ibom State Commissioner for Special Duties, was set up to handle the crisis and negotiate with Mr. Meyers. After three hours of negotiation, Mr. Meyers agreed to allow us stay one more night in Sun Hotel but on the conditions that we pay $30 each and forgo our launch on Sunday (of all days). The federal team and pilgrims from other Eastern Nigerian States could not strike any deal with the travel agency. The federal team, among whom were many Cross Riverians starved and slept outside the Hotel for two days before Okada Air finally came.

Akwa Ibom pilgrims fared better. We slept outside, many on the floor, others on chairs, for only one night. Throughout the night, Mr. Nsabasi, Rev. Fr. Eboh, Rev. Idara Ideh, this reporters, and other members of the task-force stayed awake, shuttling between the Airport and the Hotel and phoning everywhere possible to get starving pilgrims out of Israel.

Eventually a glimmer of hope appeared. A call to the Ben Gurioun Airport by Nsabasi and this reporter at about 1.30 am gave the arrival time of flight OKY 7772 from Lagos at 2.30 am. We were however, warned that the information is not from Israeli Air Port Authority but from Okada Air. By 5.30 am, we all headed to the Airport. Luckily Flight OKJ 7722 from Lagos, was displayed on the screens in the Airport along with 15 other aircrafts scheduled to land at the airport that morning. But of the 16 aircraft to touch down, Flight OKJ 7722 was flashing as the only flight rescheduled to touch down at 8.30 am. Said Mrs. Iniobong Ugot, a pilgrim on the federal team. "This pilgrimage has been very enjoyable until this flight problems."

Then again, the flight was rescheduled and displayed for 11.30 am to the agony of passengers. From 11.30 am. It was rescheduled for 12 noon. After 12 noon, the Israeli Airport Authority seemed to be fed up with the pranks of OKJ 7722 and simply refused to fiddle with the computer anymore. So, for two and half hours, the time for OKJ 7722 on the airport screens stood at 12 noon even when the time was about 3.00pm.

When the flight eventually came and it was time to board, the Israeli Airport Authorities did not even announce it. Two officials simply walked up to Gate 10 of the departure Hall, where we had been snoring away, (like Peter, James and John in the Garden of Gethsemane) and we scrambled forward the Nigerian way, struggling to beat each other to the gateway. Major Sonny Jackson of 6 Motorized Battalion, Nigerian Army, had a tough time controlling these anxious pilgrims. It was clear that home is now sweeter than Israel.

Then inside the aircraft, another waiting game ensued. We sat for one hour thirty five minutes inside the hot aircraft without any explanation to the delay by the captain or hostesses. Eventually the captain came on the P. A. system to apologize saying that the delay was due to a "technical hitch." At 5.00pm to the relief of pilgrims, Flight 7722 hit the skies, circled the Mediterranean Sea and headed southwards for a home-bound journey to home, sweet home.

Come to think of it. And sing it along with me. Adversities or not, nothing compares with the joy of being a pilgrim. Sing along with me. Nothing compares with the blessings of walking the footsteps of Jesus. Come to think of it. Nothing compares with the joy of having Jesus. Come rain or shine, I shall endeavour day and night to fly the flag of Jesus.

SOWING AND HARVESTING

Just as 1994 was winding up, my office witnessed a deluge of letters from readers, institutions and professional bodies. A streak of good news ran through the welter of letters, as each letter seemed to repeat the same message: "your team is doing a great job."

Bassey Udoidiong of No. 3 Military Street, Lagos, wrote to say "bravo for transforming *The Pioneer* into a full fledge national newspaper." He said Akwa Ibom indigenes in Lagos are very proud of the new look *Pioneer.* To curtail the "scrambling" for the newspaper, Udoidiong said we should increase our circulation figures in Lagos.

Killian Thompson of No. 15 Udo Street, Uyo, wrote also to say that our outing is "a feat which cannot be easily achieved." Dr. E. U. Uye, the Rector of Akwa Ibom Polytechnic wrote to express "deep appreciation" for our splendid features. Emman Asanga, who gave his address as No. 9 Itiam Lane, Uyo, described our efforts as "remarkable"; just as the Antiquity and Historical Research Association of Nigeria, wrote to classify our modest performance as "outstanding."

For the first time in the seven-year history of the company, honours and awards began to roll in. Altogether, seven awards came our way in 1994, among them the Rotary International Merit Award for our "outstanding publications in aid of humanity." And within a single week in December, I had the rare privilege of being a recipient of two personal awards. First, the Radio Television and Theatre Workers of Nigeria, RATTAWU, conferred on me the Excellence Award in Communications, and second, the Mboho Mkparawa Ibibio, MMI, an influential socio-cultural organization, gave me a Presidential Recognition for what they saw as my "immense contribution to the development of print journalism in Akwa Ibom State."

That night, history was made as I became the first member of MMI to be honoured by MMI. Standing on the same podium and being honoured the same night along with such titans as Chief Don Etiebet, the Petroleum Minister, Chief (Dr.) Clement Isong, the former governor of the Central Bank of Nigeria and first civilian governor of Cross River State, was one of the most humbling moments of my life.

A reporter walked up to me at Ibom Hall, just after the ceremony and asked: What's the secret of all these awards? The secret, I told him frankly, is a three-letter word: GOD. It's God that has made Obiota Ekanem, Ndueheidem Eshiet, Ekaette Ekpo, Sam Akpe, Ekikere Umoh, Patrick Essien; Victor Usimka, Boniface Okon, Lawrence Usoro, Mfon Ituen, and the entire 146 staff of Pioneer such a diligent bunch of staff. It's God that sent our publisher Yakubu Bako, a solider cum journalist to govern the state.

I'll like to say this and let the word go forth from here that, this newspaper would not have made the newsstands in 1994, except for one man: Yakubu Bako. It is not a mere coincidence that at a time that state government-owned newspapers are folding up or just printing a handful of dusty, token copies, *The Pioneer*, is adjudged the best state-owned newspaper in Nigeria. It is not a co-incidence that at a time that newsprint is hovering around N100,000 per ton, *The Pioneer* is expanding its coast. *The Pioneer* survived 1994, because God used Bako to back *The Pioneer*. Fully aware and conscious of the indispensable role an organization like our own plays for the government and the people, Bako simply threw all the weight he could muster behind us.

Today, one thing I can say about *The Pioneer* is that it has gained respect; it has won the confidence of its readers and it has made Akwa Ibom government and people proud. In a rather intricate and delicate balancing act, we have managed to protect and enhance the interest of our two sometimes antagonistic proprietors – the government and the governed. We have not betrayed the interest of government and we have not subjugated nor sacrificed the interest of the governed. And that is a miracle.

But 1994 was not a bed of roses – that is if there is any such bed anywhere in the world. We stumbled in our plans to complete our permanent site as we could only progress half-way. We failed painfully in the area of acquiring modern equipment to step up the quality and frequency of our newspaper. As I look around the News Room and the Production Department, I notice frustration and resignation on the faces of staff, who are literally producing this newspaper with their bare knuckles. For a newspaper house that is just as old as the State that owns it, its growth is anything but proportionate. For a newspaper house that has contributed so much over the years for the health and nourishment of the State, its health is a study in paradox.

But I see a light. I see a light in the uncharted tunnel of 1995. Over the years, *The Pioneer* has sown seeds, improved variety seeds, materially and spiritually. Every good sower expects a good harvest and I predict (you can call it a prophecy) that 1995 is the year of bountiful harvest for *The Pioneer.*

I see our operations computerized in the next couple of months. I see our permanent site gracing the skylines of our capital city. I see the newspaper building bridges across socio-political swamps and swatches. I see *The Pioneer* staying on top as one of the best state-owned newspapers in Nigeria. Stay with us.

THE CHARACTER OF VICTORY

When Sir Winston Churchill, war-time British prime minister was an old man, he was invited to give a speech to the students graduating from the University of Manchester. He arrived very late and after making his way to the platform learned that the certificates had already been given out and the occasion was about being rounded off.

Out of courtesy to the great men the organizers asked him if he would like to say a few concluding words. He rose to his feet, fixed the audience with his gaze and said: "Never give up. Never, never give up. Never, never, never give up." That was all. He sat down to a standing ovation.

Selywn Hughes, British gospel writer, who thrilled us last week with this tory had intended to drive home a message on perseverance. Coincidentally, that was the sharp message firmly stamped on the very souls of Nigerians after the sweet victory of Nigeria's football team at the just-concluded centennial Olympics Games.

Playing in front of 86,117 people at the great concrete bowl in Sandord Stadium, USA, and watched by estimated two billion television viewers round the world, the Kanu Nwankwo – led team rose from the ashes of defeat to pull off a thrilling and breath-taking 3-2 victory over Argentina. Nigeria went behind two times in that epic final but fought back each time to snatch the gold, only 90 seconds to full time.

Against Brazil, four times world champion, in the semi-final three days earlier, the Nigerian team was not really expected to win but bow out with, if possible, some respect. Trailing predictably with 1-3 margins, the Nigerian team equalized at 3 – 3 with only 20 seconds left in the clock and then punctured the myth of Brazilian soccer invincibility with a sudden death goal in the fourth minute of the extra time. With the emphatic defeat of Brazil and Argentina in a row, Nigeria became not just the first African nation to win the Olympic football tournament but arguably the most celebrated world soccer champion. The talk of the football world today right from Outer Mongolia to the jungle of Malaysia is Nigeria.

Nigeria's Olympic victory is a metaphor of perseverance and resilience. It is a token and symbol of our recovery and restoration on the dais of world leadership. I have forgotten the philosopher who said that "the gentleman who wakes up and finds himself a success hasn't been asleep." Nigeria hasn't been asleep. Nigeria may sometimes lapse into complacency but there is never mistaking our power of self-regeneration under God.

The final medal table last week showed that nearly a thousand medals were carted away by 76 countries. But all the medals of the centennial Olympics put together is wood compared to Nigeria's singular medal in soccer. Indeed, to some Nigerians, winning the soccer gold medal is the morale equivalence of landing in the moon.

Yet, one may know how to gain a victory, and know not how to use it. This is the challenge facing Nigeria now. We must be able to tap into the wind of this recovery and channel it into critical ramifications of our national life. Our economy, politics, not to mention our crises-prone educational system requires a fresh breath of this recovery wind. This is not in any way to detract from the important and impact of our victory. But it must be said that the Olympic victory is a function and product of merit, hardwork, teamwork, resilience, single-mindedness, loyalty of all Nigerians to the team and prayers. These are precisely the same recipe that are needed for the recovery of Nigeria's socio-economic and political life.

Take loyalty. To me loyalty is indivisible. The irreduceable minimum of loyalty is 100 percent. Any reduction or deduction from loyalty, no matter how infinitesimal, is no longer loyalty. It is disloyalty. That might sound a tall order. And you don't have to agree with me. But the point that is being made here is that every Nigerian team, be it in the concrete bowl of Sandford Stadium or in the concrete enclave of Aso Rock, will do well with loyalty.

Take prayers. I saw the leg of God in Emmanuel Amunike's decisive goal which went on record as the final goal of the final match in the centennial Olympics. A pastor friend of mine, told me the Brazilian – Nigeria semi-final match was an encounter between the god of Samba and the God of Miracle. A lot of Nigerian homes and churches gave up food, fasted and prayed for Nigeria's victory. And God heard and answered their prayers. It was Richard Nixon as American Vice President in 1954 who said at the gathering of the Full Gospel Businessmen Fellowship in California that: "America has become great because its great leaders have believed and put their trust in God." That's some food for thought.

Take resilience, I believe that the Olympic victory is a mirror, a true reflection of the country called Nigeria: the rare ability to rise like phoenix from the ashes of defeat to claim victory. And between Bonfrere Jo and his boys, there is this trait: they talk less and achieve a lot. This is certainly "not in our character." But this is the character of victory.

However, I was not happy that there was no "Calabar man" in the Dream Team. But who cares about tribe when a good job is done and seen to be done. Our first-eleven team in Atlanta gave us victory and fame around the world. Our first-eleven team in any sphere of national life will always achieve similar ovation for our country at any point in time. The trouble however with our march to socio-economic and political recovery is that, we often, out of sentiments, throw into the field of play our second-or even third eleven team at the very expense of our much-needed victory.

What the Atlanta miracle is saying to Nigerians, especially key players of the socio-economic and political ball game is: put your best leg forward and never, never, never give up.

AFRICA

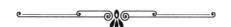

THE LAST DAYS OF A TYRANT

He looked dull and dismal as he walked into the posh sitting room to shake hands with his visitors. His grim visage showed he was in no mood for lengthy discussion. He had a cold and kept sneezing and blowing his nose in between each sentence. "Ya know, I've been down with bad fever for days now," Samuel Kanyon Doe, President of Liberia, said, his voice hoarse and barely audible. "Ya can be sure I'll grant ya an interview as soon as am better. No problem, my man," he said in his accented American English, blowing his nose once more as he took leave. He looked lonely and pensive as he walked away. There seemed to be very few civilian aides and allies left behind or visiting the president these days.

Outside, some 300 fierce looking soldiers armed with sophisticated weapons stood guard, encasing the executive mansion and shielding Doe against the reality of his war-torn country. Platoons of soldiers, couched like alligators behind huge sandbags, glared viciously at every visitor. Two armoured tanks, fitted with radar devices and stationed at the main gate completed the fortification of Doe's palatial official residence, located at the coast of the Atlantic Ocean.

His running nose aside, June 28, 1990, was not exactly a good day for Doe. News coming in from Freetown, capital of Sierra Leone, had finally confirmed his worst fears. The rebels of the National Patriotic Front of Liberia, NPFL, had, to his horror, turned down all entreaties by Liberian religious leaders and called off peace talks to end the seven-month civil war to oust him. To further compound his grief, virtually all his advisers and top government officials who went to Freetown to seek peace had dramatically turned their backs on him. With the rebels on the fringes of Monrovia, they could not risk a return to brief Doe.

Tambakai Jangaba, the "wise old man" and leader of Doe's delegation to the peace talks, who telephoned Doe to break the bad news, had himself arrived Freetown for the talks with his entire household, complete with his grandchildren and housekeepers. Boyish and randy information minister, Emmanuel Bowier, who had all along remained a vocal loyalist and spokesman of the embattled regime, had found the cosy serenity of the Three Star Mammy Yokko Hotel in Sierra Leone too absorbing to exchange for the all-night staccato gunshots in Monrovia. Dressed in a faded blue jeans and a gray T-shirt with the inscription "Bogle Boy: Commander of the Mountain Patrol," Bowier told *Newswatch:* "I came here to talk peace, man. Here I will stay to seek peace, rebels or no rebels." He had finally joined the long list of ministers fleeing Monrovia. One member of the peace talks delegation who went back to Monorovia was Moivabah Fofana, an assistant commissioner in the Bureau of Customs and representative of the Moslem community in the government delegation. "I am just going back to see whether I can get my family out in time," he told

Newswatch inside a car that took both of them from Kenema in Sierra Leone to Monrovia.

Monrovia, capital of "Sweet Liberia," stood last week at the edge of a precipice, surrounded by guns, deserted by men, gloomy: a shadow of its bustling past, a graphic sign that the days of Doe are numbered. Mass killings, abduction, destruction, confusion, tribal hatred, lack of food, water and light, anger and protest have conspired to make the last days of Doe a tale of woe. Wednesday, June 27, thousands of Liberians, for the third time in one week, poured unto the streets. Their message: "Doe must go," "Doe, please resign," "Sammy, come down today."

The past two demonstrations had been relatively peaceful. They were called "Peace March" and were mainly organized by Christian and moslem leaders who go by the name of Inter-Faith Committee. Today, the religious leaders had sought the backing of 20 professional and civic bodies, and they responded in sufficient number. They included the Press Union of Liberia, PUL; the Liberian Bar Association, LBA; the National Teachers Association, the Workers Union; and the Federation of Students Union. Traders, market women and shopkeepers closed their shops and joined the protest.

From an open field at Capital By-Pass in the centre of the city, the crowd defied a heavy rain and began their march, singing, chanting, waving placards; trailed all the way by pressmen. Destination: Executive Mansion, the residence and office of Doe. At a military barracks on a road called UN Drive, trouble struck. A company of soldiers, unable to stop the marchers, broke into the crowd, whipping the protesters with military belts. A free-for-all fight ensued between soldiers and the crowd. Soon, gunshots filled the air. Five men were down on the spot from gunshot wounds. Hundreds of others were injured in the stampede that followed. The crowd scattered and ran for safety. Even soldiers, who had mistakenly thought the shootings came from the rebels, were seen running for their lives. Any sympathy left for Doe had, from that moment, disappeared with the smoke from the gun shots.

The Unity Party (of Liberia), UP, the Liberian Action Party, LAP, and the Liberian Peoples Party, LPP, issued separate statements calling for Doe to quickly step down and make way for peace. In a press statement signed by Mambu David, secretary-general of the UP, the party said it had watched with dismay the tragic dilemma in which Liberia has been put by the government. "The gross human rights violation, the killings of innocent citizens, public harassment, the closure of schools, the collapse of the economy, as well as the inability of the government to deal with the insurgency by NPFL, which has resulted in thousands of deaths and refugees at home and abroad, are no longer acceptable," the UP said. In view of "this calamity," the Unity Party called on Doe to "resign immediately in order to save the nation from further bloodshed."

In its own statement, the LAP traced the rebellion, which began on December 24, to what it called "bad government." It was obvious that the regime had "crumbled," it said, and Doe had no choice but to "step aside." Said the party, "In a nutshell, the country is in disarray. The government has lost stamina and control. The credibility of the administration of Doe has been completely eroded at home and abroad. The image and future of Liberia under the regime is bleak. A state of anarchy now prevails which the people of this country cannot endure any longer. The Liberian Action Party is of the view that the continuous stay in office of President Doe one day longer does not augur well for the restoration of peace, stability, free and fiar democratic process in Liberia."

The LPP, pleading with Doe to quit, recalled a statement made by Doe May 25, 1990, when the youth wing of Doe's party, the National Democratic Party of Liberia, NDPL, visited the Executive Mansion. Doe had said then: "If the people of Liberia even say Mr. President, the only way the war will stop is for you to step aside and let us bring a new man to run the country, I will step aside." The LPP, therefore, said, in view of the massive calls made by a cross section of the society for him to step down, "we now call upon the president to honour his own promise and step aside because the party believes the resignation and departure of his government will create a fertile ground for peace and reconciliation." In the days that followed, virtually all newspapers in Monrovia wrote editorials explaining why Doe must resign.

Daily Observer, the leading tabloid in Liberia, for two consecutive days (June 26 and 27) devoted its editorials to Doe's resignation. In its June 26 editorial titled "Resign, Mr. President," the paper said Doe's resignation was the only way out of further bloodshed, destruction, hardship and misery. "We have reached the cross roads; the country as it is now is ungovernable; its resources are depleted; its people are distressed and confused. The people cannot take it anymore. There is now only one course left to save the nation, and that course must be taken as an act of mercy. The president must resign. Resign, Mr. President and secure yourself a place in history. Please, go away in peace," the paper said.

The next day, the paper adopted a harsher tone in its editorial titled "For the Love of God, Go." Doe was hardly referred to again as "Mr. President." The paper, just like the people, was beginning to run short of patience. Said the paper: "How long can Doe try the people's patience? How many more heads must be cut off? How many more must seek refuge in foreign countries before Doe realizes his resistance is in vain. We repeat, Mr. Doe, please resign. Do not wait any longer. Resign now before it is too late."

Said *the News,* owned partially by government June 27: "Since no government is indispensable and the fact that the taller a bamboo grows the lower it bends, the wishes of the people must prevail. We call for the immediate and unconditional resignation of President Doe?

As the demand for Doe's resignation mounted and the rebels tightened their choke-hold on the road to Monrovia, words leaked out from the Executive Mansion June 27 that Doe would broadcast to the nation later that night. Government watchers were confident the hour of reckoning had come and Doe was about to bow out. The public hooked on to the radio all night with subdued jubilation. But no dice. The former master-sergeant, who shot his way into power April 1980, had changed his mind to the discomfiture of Liberians thirsty for peace. Diplomatic sources attributed the cancellation of the "nationwide broadcast" to a last minute disagreement between Doe and the American government, who had promised Doe a safe passage to exile in the country of his choice. The Americans, diplomatic sources said, were ready to guarantee safe passage for Doe and 10 other people of his choice but Doe was said to insist on 150 people.

Instead of his expected resignation as demanded by the rebels and protesters, the information ministry put to circulation a six-page pamphlet on why Doe cannot resign. Titled "Resignation is no Solution," the document barely stopped short of saying Doe was indispensable. "Given the situation where no one is found suitable or acceptable, the question is: Must President Doe resign, leaving troubled Liberia without a leader? Absolutely No," the government document said. According to the document, "there is no precedence in the history of Liberia where the president of the republic had resigned contrary to constitutional provisions or where he was made to leave the office without the people first knowing the successor." The document cited the constitution of Liberia and said it makes no provision for the removal of the president either by force of arms or by compulsory resignation. As it put it: "For Dr. Doe, to quit in these times of national crisis would be setting a dangerous precedence for which present and future generations of Liberians will not forgive him. He would be leaving a vacuum which could create political disaster, national chaos and calamity." Instead of resigning, the document said Doe was willing to end his rule in October 1991, when his tenure will expire, without seeking a re-election.

In his efforts to buy time till 1991, Doe had, in addition, embarked on a series of fence-mending measures. He said he would facilitate and amend the constitution to permit rebel leaders and exiled opponents to contest the 1991 election. He was referring to the part of the constitution that requires aspirants to be resident in Liberia for at least 10 years. He said he would now allow opposition parties to have a say in the appointment of Electoral Commission, ECOM, officials and went ahead to dissolve the ECOM he had appointed a few years back. He announced an unconditional general amnesty to opponents who were either convicted, accused or suspected of committing offences against the State and lifted the ban on two banned political parties and the national students union. He even dropped charges of embezzlement against rebel leader Charles Taylor. The information ministry even dropped hints that he was prepared to meet with Taylor, a man Doe had earlier declared wanted.

Furthermore, he announced cuts in the prices of food, including rice, the staple food. He ordered that, beginning from June 21, a 100 pound bag of rice should be sold for $25, $10 short of the market price. Only last year, government had announced increase in the price of the same quantity of rice from $23 to $35. But in announcing the reversal of price, Doe said any dealer caught selling above approved price would be "arrested and banned from selling rice in Liberia."

In spite of his sudden generosity, there is no let up for Doe. Most angry Liberians who have rejected his "gestures" wonder what Doe is waiting for. Said George Drapper, a workers union official: "He is in a quandary. Maybe he thinks the presidency is a profession." But Henry Jallar, a student, thinks differently. "I think he want to leave power the same way he made Tolbert leave – in bits and pieces." Doe's predecessor, William Tolbert, was killed by troops led by Doe and reportedly dismembered, before 13 of his (Tolbert's) officials were strapped to wooden stakes on the beach and shot.

As the rebels gunning for Doe stepped into a part of Monrovia last week and cut off all communications with the city, there were no indications Doe had any significant defence outside roadblocks. There were no obvious trenches, bunkers or other positions being prepared around the city. Some of Doe's soldiers appeared even more scared of the rebels than stoic civilians. On June 27, when government soldiers fired warning shots to disperse anti-Doe demonstrators, many soldiers who thought the rebels had finally arrived were seen running in search of a hideout.

The army itself is ill-prepared and ill-equipped. Though Doe is said to have recently received plane-loads of arms from a friendly West African State, (which this reporter know but would not disclose), Liberia does not even have an air force that would have assisted its ground troops against the rebels. Doe's personal security, one African diplomat told *Newswatch*,is guaranteed by a handful of Israeli mercenaries. Obviously, because of the army's lack of firing power, Doe, in one moment of desperation, recently urged civilians to "take cutlasses, shotguns and bows and arrows to fight the NPFL." Hardly anybody heeded the call.

Army atrocities against helpless civilians may be part of the reason for apathy and disdain for Doe and his troops. The human rights group, *Africa Watch*, says the army responded to the initial rebel incursion by indiscriminate killing of unarmed civilians, raping women, burning villages and looting."*Newswatch* investigation and interviews last week in Liberia and Sierra Leone, where most Liberians have taken refuge, confirmed that Doe's last days are a sordid tale of atrocities. The army competes with the rebel troops in tribally-induced massacre.

Most victims killed by the rebels are the Krahns, Doe's ethnic group, as well as the Madingo tribesmen, considered as Doe's ally. Fofana, a Madingo and delegate to the futile Freetown peace talks, told *Newswatch* that more than 8,000 Madingo people have so far been killed by the rebels. Though that might be exaggerated, there is a reported case of 11 Madingo imams who were killed in Nimba County by rebels in one day. "The painful thing," said Fofana, "is that the international press had ignored our plight. We are now pleading with NPFL to spare the Madingo people because we are businessmen with minimal interest in politics."

But Doe's troops hold the ace in the Liberian pogrom. Last week, when the rebels stormed parts of Monrovia, there were still some court-marital cases pending on cases of kidnappings and killings by government soldiers. One of such cases was the case of abduction and killing of Vanjah Richards, professor and mayor of Clay Ashland by Andrew Gaye, a lieutenant of the Waterloo Checkpoint Command. When the murderous lieutenant appeared for trial June 20, he had told the court-marital board that his commander, Henry Johnson, a major, had ordered him to kill Richards. Similarly, David Toweh, a senator from Nimba Country, had his 17-year-old son abducted and killed in May. Hundreds of Gio and Mano people have similarly been abducted and killed in Monrovia. On the outskirts of Monrovia two weeks ago, 10 bullet-riddled and mutilated bodies strewed the sidewalk. There was blood all over. The victims were reportedly lined-up and shot in the early hours of the day by government troops. Government soldiers in the area were reported to say that the victims were "men targeted by the army as rebel sympathizers." They were identified later as Gio and Mano men from Nimba Country, where the rebel incursion began.

At a point, such killings were so appalling some top military officers felt compelled to take action. Henry Dubar, chief of army staff, said he had to personally spend several nights apprehending soldiers found at illegal beats. He arrested three enlisted soldiers. One of them, James Grear, a private with the brigade headquarters in Monrovia, had shot and killed one Edward Wellemongar for tribal reasons. Many believe most of the killings are hatched by a murder squad led by Harrison Pannue, a Khran and cousin of Doe, who once boasted that he personally murdered former President Tolbert.

Early in June, Khran soldiers stormed the United Nations, UN, compound in the capital city where several hundred Gio and Mano people had sought refuge. They abducted about 40 people at gunpoint and sprayed them with gunfire poles away from the UN premises. At least 30 of the refugees died on the spot. Doe later visited the UN compound along Tubman Boulevard to tell the panicky refugees that he would protect them. But the refugees did not believe him. They had received a similar pledge from a government minister a day before the killings. After that incident, Javier Peres de Cueller, secretary-general of the UN, ordered the withdrawal of all international UN staff and promised not to return until the war ends. The UN pull-out terrified thousands of refugees. They fled to the St. Peters Lutheran Church premises, where *Newswatch* found most of them last week. "We don't still feel safe at all, but most of us here are too poor to travel to the nearest border town," Fred Kporsor said.

In his last days, Doe had found out that the trouble with his army is not just lack of fire power but plenty of indiscipline. Most of the troops are drunk most of the time. It is normal in Monrovia to see a soldier on duty tottering with a bottle of gin in one hand and an automatic weapon in the other. In a bar opposite the information ministry, a few poles away from the Executive Mansion, even soldiers guarding the road leading to the president's residence are found drinking themselves to stupor. "Gi ma another bottle of criminally-cold beer, man," an already drunk sergeant armed with an AK 47 rifle, a grenade and bayonet, screamed at the top of his voice, sending shivers through the spines of foreign journalists who hurriedly emptied their glasses and disappeared.

In one of the checkpoints on the road to Kenema, the border town with Sierra Leone, a tipsy soldier demonstrating how he would deal with the rebels, two weeks ago, ended up spraying six of his colleagues with bullets. One died on the spot and five were rushed to a nearby hospital. Efforts to restore discipline, including missions by resident US military advisers to the war fronts, have failed to produce any tangible change. In the last three weeks, US military jeeps have simply restricted their job to patrolling around roadblocks in the city to rescue unfortunate victims harassed, ripped off their money and valuable items and still detained by trigger-happy troops. As a result of these endless harassments and suffering, anxiety has mounted and many in Monrovia are praying for Taylor to speed up the capture of Monrovia, if that will guarantee a return to normalcy. Said one hotel proprietor: "The only way out is for Charles Taylor to hurry up a bit."

The failure of the government to guarantee security, coupled with the not-so-good reputation of the advancing rebels, have contributed to the rapid desertion of Doe by top government officials. Ministers, security chiefs, top journalists and bankers, among others, have fled Monrovia. Said one minister who has taken residence in Kenema, Sierra Leone: "Nobody wants to be strapped to a stake and shot like a common criminal." As at last week, only two senior government officials, apart from Doe, were known to have remained in Monrovia. They were Harry Moniba, the respected vice-president who has succeeded in distancing himself from Doe without earning his wrath, and James Gongar, education minister. In the ministry of finance, none of the three ministers is in the country and this has created problems with workers' salaries. Emmanuel Shaw, the finance minister, fled to

London. His deputy, J. Harris, is in Freetown. The where-about of Jumita Neal, the assistant minister, is not known. A similar situation obtains in the Central Bank of Liberia where Thomas Hanson, the governor, has fled, just like his deputy Francis Hurton.

Other key officials who have abandoned Doe include Yudu Gray, minister of public works; Elijah Taylor, minister of planning; Martha Sendolo Belleh, minister of health; Rudolph Johnson, foreign affairs minister; Gblozuo Toweh, agriculture minister; Ansumannah Kromah, internal affairs minister; Yancy Peters Flah, presidential affairs minister; Emmanuel Gardner, the director of budget; as well as Patrick Kugmeh, the press secretary to Doe, who is now in Freetown. In the public corporations, the bosses of the Liberian electric corporations, LEC, the National Insurance corporation, the Housing Bank of Liberia, the Produce Marketing Corporation, the National Investment Commission, the Forestry Development Authority, among others, have all fled Liberia. In addition, the police director, Wilfred Clark, as well as the police chief of traffic, Deater Lincola, and the mayor of Monrovia, Kwia Johnson, are not in the country. Kenneth Best, one of the best known journalist in Liberia and boss of *Daily Observer*, is now in Accra, Ghana.

When the Liberian senate tried to hold a session two weeks ago in the midst of anti-Doe protests, only nine of the 36 senators were available and could not form a quorum. Moniba told reporters some senators were on sick leave, the common excuse given by run-away officials. Deluged by travellers, the foreign ministry said few weeks ago it had run short of fresh passports. An army transport plane for several weeks now has also been shuttling Khran people across rebel territory to their home country in Grand Gedeh, where Doe, according to diplomatic sources, had originally planned to return when Taylor takes over the Executive Mansion. As many as 2,000 soldiers are stationed there but cut-off by the rebels who invaded the country in such a way that they spilt the country into two and occupy the mineral-rich centre of the country facing Monrovia.

With all the key managers of the economy in exile and the NPFL controlling the major mines, timber and rubber plantations, the economy of Liberia in the last days of Doe is at a virtual standstill. Export earnings have nose-dived by more than 80 percent. Government coffers, as a result, are nearly empty. Salaries have become a luxury. Prices of food in Monrovia, when found at all, have gone through the roof. A 100-pound bag of rice, which Doe ordered to be sold for $25, now goes for $150. A tin of palm-oil which sold at $15, is now $45. A gallon of kerosene, sold a few months ago at five dollars, is now $15. In the interior areas such as Sinoe, prices are even higher. A bag of salt, sold at 75 cents, is now $8.50. The same quantity is sold at five dollars in Monrovia.

Fish can hardly be found in the market anymore due to lack of petrol (or gasoline, as the Liberians call it) for the Kru fishermen. Transportation has come to a near halt for the same reason and commercial life is in limbo. The Greenville general market, said to be one of the busiest, was empty when *Newswatch* visited. A bag of cassava, previously sold at $10, went for $75. Even then, women purchased it in a scuffle. In the rural parts of Greenville, acute shortage of kerosene has turned many homes into something like photographic darkrooms. Most families now make use of expensive palm-oil in place of kerosene. They place palm-oil in empty tins and insert pieces of cloth to form wicks.

Workers hardly go to work in Monrovia these days. When they do, they loiter outside for a while discussing the escapades of Charles Taylor. Schools are closed. All that was required to send the University of Liberian, UL, packing two weeks ago was telephone call from the rebels. Practically the only credible institution left in the country is religious. The religious institution is the one that initiated and spearheaded the Freetown peace talks. It is the same institution that started the internal anti-Doe protests. It has also taken the responsibility of hosting thousands of refugees from poor homes who are unable to leave the strife-torn country.

"When we lie down in our small homes and sleep peacefully, even when we eat nuts, we don't know how much we should be grateful to God," one woman heading for a refugee camp in far-away Sierra Leone with seven children said, tears welling up her eyes. The last days of Doe have succeeded in turning close to a quarter of the country's 2.5 million population into refugees. Some 150,000 are said to be in Ivory Coast. Another 100,000 are in Guinea. Sierra Leone refugee population is swelling up every day and hovers around 25,000 now. Friday, June 30, Martha Browne, a shop owner in Monrovia, broke down and sobbed as the taxi-driver parked to drop her and her two kids immediately after the Mano River bridge separating Liberia and Sierra Leone. "No, am not stopping here. I never been here, please, no, don't leave us here, we will die," she pleaded, crying. The taxi-driver and other passengers were in a dilemma. It was better she stopped like some other poor Liberian refugees around the Mano River villages, rather than continuing for another 80 miles to Zimmi or another 115 miles to Kenema, the driver argued.

Two women, their kids strapped to their backs and bundles of household wares balanced on their heads, walked past towards the direction of the village primary school. A group of children sat on the bare floor. Their mothers clamoured for a place in the queue for food. Then the queue collapsed and they began a battle with each other to get their plates filled. "Join them, they are Liberians," the driver told Browne, as he took off, leaving the woman transfixed on the roadside.

It was the cruel reality thousands of proud Liberians are finding hard to endure. Entire villages have been forced to flee their lands. Their homes have been shattered and scattered in different countries, cities and villages. Children, most of them hungry and sick, cry endlessly in the face of sudden hardship they cannot even comprehend. Those taking refuge inside Liberia numbering about 24,000, appear to be even worse off with lack of water and acute shortage of food and other basic commodities. Nigeria, the United Nations, the European Community, as well as the International Committee of Red Cross, ICRC, many aid and philanthropic organizations are rushing aid and relief to victims of the latest African war.

But what is needed most, according to diplomats in Monrovia, is the immediate political solution to the crisis itself. Barely a week ago, Joseph Momoh, president of Sierra Leone, who has watched the tragic events in Liberia from close quarters called on Nigeria, Togo and Guinnea, countries considered to be friendly with Doe, to "join efforts and prevail on (Doe) to resign." Many Liberians, both at home and abroad, seem to share Momoh's view as the only solution to the bloodshed. Many Liberians, who looked up to Nigeria in particular to help solve the problem, appear increasingly uncomfortable with what they call the "rather confusing signals from Nigeria." Said Amos Dukuly of the UL: "It does appear that Nigeria would prefer to rescue the political career of one man (Doe) than the lives of the people of Liberia." For

Fofona, delegate of the Freetown peace talks, "Nigeria is the only country in Africa that can help us out because Liberians have a lot of respect for Nigeria."

The role of the United States, too, appear somewhat passive, a kind of let-them-stew-in-their-own-juice policy. It refused Doe's request for arms. It ruled out any military intervention and tried half-heartedly to broker an end to the bloodshed, after it had ordered its citizens out. Taylor, who had initially said he wanted to get hold of Doe, "dead or alive," was persuaded by the US State Department to modify his position. He assured US he would allow Doe to leave Monrovia to avoid bloodbath and unnecessary destruction of property. It was left for Washington to persuade Doe to leave. Herman Cohen, assistant secretary of state for African affairs, shuttling between Taylor and Doe, two weeks ago, told the House of Representative sub-committee on Africa that "the current US policy towards Liberia was to seek to achieve a cease-fire and a freely held, internationally-monitored election." Taylor concluded America had been wasting his time. He sealed up the country and took the battle straight to Monrovia.

As it became apparent last week that Taylor meant business and seriously wants to kick Doe out in a battle for Monrovia, the US hurried back to the Executive Mansion to get Doe ready for a safe escape, possibly via one of its warships off the Liberian coast. It was almost certain at press time that the former master-sergeant would not last another week as the "beloved icon" of Liberia. Asked last week what Doe would possibly miss most if he quits, one Liberian Journalist said "the Mansion." There is a story in Monrovia that when Doe moved into the mansion in 1980 and had his first taste of the State House breakfast, he smiled at his wife and said: "Nancy, we never gonnna leave this place." Now he may have to hurry out.

THE FINAL HOURS OF SAMUEL DOE

When the end finally came for him, Samuel Kanyon Doe, the man who ruled Liberia with an iron fist for 10 years, was given the treatment that would have befitted only a common criminal. He was shot in both legs, dragged on the muddy grounds of the Monrovia seaport and hauled like a sack of potatoes into the back of a military jeep, then driven off for interrogation and trial.

Facing a mock trial for countless atrocities, Doe, like the executed Romanian dictator, Nicolae Ceausescu, would have railed at his captors: "I will answer only to the (Liberian) working class people." But Doe, according to Prince Yormie Johnson, the maverick break-away rebel leader who captured him, fainted a few hours after his arrest. He died later from "gunshot wounds." His "mutilated body" was put on display, outside Monrovia's Island Clinic owned by a Nigerian doctor. Doe, diplomats quickly concluded, was literally given a dose of his own medicine. It all seemed like story book justice for the tyrant, whose bloody regime tortured and murdered hundreds of opponents and publicly displayed their dismembered bodies as a "lesson" to other would-be opponents.

Doe's dramatic final hour was a comedy of errors. For almost three months, the self-styled "Commander-General" had not ventured out of his fortified presidential mansion. The last time he was seen in public was June 20, when he announced the reduction in the price of rice, after a surprise visit to the ministry of commerce. But this fateful Sunday afternoon, September 9, the beleaguered president wanted to prove that he was not a prisoner that he had unwittingly turned himself into. He took the short 10-minute drive from his mansion to the Monrovia seaport headquarters of The West African peace-keeping force, ECOMOG, without any incident. He had close to 100 Israeli-trained bodyguards with him. The body-guards waited somewhat leisurely downstairs, as Doe went upstairs for a chat with Arnold Quainoo, the Ghanaian general who is the commander of ECOMOG. Quainoo said the visit was "unscheduled and very surprising."

Their discussions over, Quainoo stood up to escort the august visitor downstairs, but another set of unexpected visitors stormed the premises. They were the crack rebel troops of Johnson, led by Johnson himself. An argument ensued. Then a burst of gunfire filled the air. Doe and Quainoo had to hurry back into Quainoo's first-floor office. At the end of the first salvo of gunfire, more than 60 bodies of soldiers, mainly Doe's body-guards, littered the ground. Several other soldiers, including ECOMOG troops, were wounded. Then the sharp-shooting Johnson troops forced their way into the ECOMOG secretariat, shooting from room to room and gunning down more men until they got to Quainoo's office, where Doe was hiding. Then Johnson ordered him shot in the legs and taken to his base camp in the centre of the city.

Doe had met his Waterloo. It was a Sunday when most of the half a million Liberian refugees would probably have been praying in various churches across West Africa for an end to the nine-month civil war. The casualty figure at press time had risen to 79 people. There was an unconfirmed report that seven of the victims were ECOMOG troops. Most of the wounded were still being rushed to military hospitals in Freetown and Lagos for treatment. *Newswatch* could not confirm that any of the victims was a Nigerian. The only Nigerian soldier known to have been killed so far is Lamidi Wasiu, a guardsman with the 123 Guards Battalion. He was killed by a sniper's bullet in ECOMOG's first clash with the main rebel troops led by Charles Taylor. During that incident, two other Nigerians soldiers D. Musa, a lieutenant of the 242 Recce Battalion, and Moses Ahmed of the 244 Recce battalion, were seriously wounded.

The death of the Liberian tin god and the circumstances of his death sent shock waves through The West African sub-region and even threatened to complicate the peace process in the war-torn country. There were many questions begging for answers. What was Doe's mission at ECOMOG headquarters? How did Johnson know Doe was with Quainoo at that material time? Was Doe set up and by who?

The first explanation of Doe's mission to ECOMOG's base was that he went to negotiate his flight from Monrovia. That seemed less likely for a stubborn man who had for months been offered safe passage, straight from his mansion, by the Americans to any country of his choice and even in company of his close family members and aides. Last week, amid the furore over Doe's death,

Abbas Bundu, Executive Secretary of Economic Community of West African States, ECOWAS, called a press conference in his Ikoyi, Lagos, office. In his written statement, he did not talk about the mission and circumstances of Doe's death until he was prodded by restive reporters. According to him, Doe went to protest to Quainoo that he would not accept the Amos Sawyer-led interim government backed by ECOWAS. Said Bundu: "I can assure you, and this I have been briefed by the commander (Quainoo) himself, that Doe's presence at ECOMOG headquarters was unannounced as, indeed, the subsequent presence of Johnson."

Reports quoting Liberian sources suggested that Johnson got to know of Doe's visit to Quainoo through a tip-off, either by America's Central intelligence Agency, CIA which has been very close to Johnson, or another foreign intelligence agency within ECOMOG. Doe's angry envoys in Lagos, who spoke to *Newswatch,* specifically pointed accusing fingers at Quainoo. "We knew from the beginning that the appointment of General Quainoo was a big mistake. It was no secret that President Jerry Rawlings and Doe were not the best of friends. So how can a general from Rawlings army be trusted in that circumstance?" The diplomat asked. Another Liberian, a refugee and close associate of Moses Duopou, Doe's former labour minister, said that even Sierra Leone could not be relied upon because President Joseph Momoh was the first ECOWAS leader to demand Doe's resignation.

There is no evidence yet to prove that either the Americans or ECOMOG had a hand in Doe's demise. If anything, Bundu said ECOMOG has demonstrated its neutrality conclusively by folding its arms and watching Johnson rain bullets on Doe and bundling him to his unmarked grave. As Bundu put it: "The incident that has taken place (Doe's death) surely confirms, at least, one point and that is ECOMOG was sent to keep peace. It is not a force that was instructed to take sides with any of the warring parties as Taylor says. If that were not the case, then ECOMOG surely would have been in a position to intervene on the part of President Doe and save him from being attacked by Johnson's forces."

It is assumed, at least for now, that Johnson, the dogged warlord himself, personally set the meticulous trap that finally got Doe out of the Executive Mansion and led him to die in shame. For six weeks Johnson, a Gio from Nimba county and a former Taylor commander, had courted the dethroned dictator. He suddenly declared war against Taylor, his former "commander-in-chief," and struck a truce with Doe. He literally served as cannon fodder between Taylor's forces and the presidential mansion. Doe loved the entire episode. And when, on the eve of ECOMOG's arrival in Monrovia, Taylor mounted an all-out battle to force Johnson's troops out of the port area and prevent ECOMOG from landing, Johnson asked Doe for support. Doe sent some 300 soldiers and tons of ammunition which helped Johnson repel Taylor. Doe kept congratulating Johnson by telephone and Johnson pledged he had no problem with him.

For instance, when Doe and his guards ran short of food, Johnson, on September 3, sent 1,000 bags of rice and other food items to the Executive mansion. He promised Doe "absolute security" whenever he wanted to step into the city and urged him to "try and go to the port and say hello" to ECOMOG officials. When Doe refused, he taunted him publicly in an interview with Nigerian reporters covering ECOMOG. Said Johnson: "You see, Doe is too afraid. ECOMOG is here and he cannot even come and say hello." Beneath this veiled love tango, it appeared Johnson had always relished the idea of personally gunning down the elusive despot at sight and was desperate to lure him out. For one, many believe Johnson had not forgiven Doe for the way Thomas Quiwonkpa, Doe's former deputy and Johnson's childhood friend, was killed and his dismembered body put on display.

The day Johnson was sure he would meet Doe face-to-face was September 6, when he and Doe were scheduled to formally sign "an agreement to join forces' against Taylor. The ceremony was billed to take place at ECOMOG's office. Johnson arrive that afternoon to discover that Doe had only sent a six-man team led by Wisseh Maclain, a minister of presidential affairs, and one Hezekiah Bowen, a brigadier-general of the presidential guards. Doe had signed the prepared agreement back in the Executive Mansion before he despatched Maclain and Bowen to the meeting. Johnson was furious. "Why is he (Doe) scared? The man should not be scared. He only knows how to deploy missiles and rockets from the mansion,"*The Guardian* correspondent, Kayode komolafe, who was on the spot, quoted Johnson as saying. Johnson, however, signed the agreement and sent a message back to Doe through Maclain, to "please find time and meet with ECO-MOG." Doe's defences might possibly have crumbled because of these endless baits.

Immediately he finally got Doe last week, a jubilant Johnson declared himself the president. He said, however, he was willing to step down after a general election at an unspecified date. He promised to continue his co-operation with ECOMOG but warned the remnants of Doe's guards to quit the Executive Mansion or face his fire-power. He said he attacked Doe because he came into the part of Monrovia under his control without due permission, adding that any of the warring parties that strays into his territory would face the same penalty. Inside the barricaded Executive

Mansion, the jolted elite presidential guards declared their commander, David Nimley, a brigadier-general, as the new president to succeed Doe. With Amos Sawyer, the ECOWAS-backed interim head of state named two weeks ago, and Taylor, the main rebel leader, also claiming the presidency on July 27, the tiny West African country had the unenviable honour of being saddled with four separate heads of state at one go.

Though the sad end of the young Liberian tyrant was regarded in diplomatic circles as "good riddance," it instantly created a huge credibility problem for ECOMOG and sent the confused ECOWAS thinking just what next to do. An emergency summit of the sub-region's heads of state was supposed to hold last week but by Friday, no clear indication had been given as to where the meeting might hold and how ECOWAS would now tackle the problem with Doe out of the way. Dauda Jawara, president of The Gambia and incumbent chairman of ECOWAS, who was on tour of Zimbabwe when Doe was toppled and killed, sent directives to the ECOMOG peace-keepers to "do everything possible to ensure that members of Doe's family and close associates are protected." He said although the sub-regional grouping had called on Doe to step down, nobody wished him dead.

President Ibrahim Babangida of Nigeria described Doe's death as an occupational hazard. "What happened (Doe's death) is one of the hazards of a developing nation," Babangida said with philosophical calmness. He sent a message to Johnson and Taylor: "Spare your country the agony of further destruction and unnecessary killing." Ghana was worse hit by the news of Doe's death, especially because Quainoo, a Ghanaian and leader of ECOMOG, was playing host to Doe at the time he was captured and killed. Mohammed Ibn Chambas, Ghana's deputy foreign minister told reporters in Accra that it's government might even pull out of ECOMOG as a result of Doe's death. He described the circumstances of Doe's death as "very embarrassing," adding that the incident "has exposed the difficult and complex posture of ECOMOG forces."

America's reaction to the escalating bloodbath in a country it describes as its "closest ally in Africa" was, at best, passive and, at worse, hypocritical and confusing. A state department spokes-person merely said it had confirmed Doe's death from "various sources, including representatives of the rebels." It said it would not recognize any of the four Liberian so-called leaders, including ECOWAS-backed Sawyer, which it had earlier endorsed. The next day, the state department took another step and said it was suspending fresh pacts with Liberia. "We're going to avoid signing new agreements for the time being then we will review the situation and may resume full-scale diplomatic relations with Mr. Doe's successor," the state department official said.

A professor at the Nigerian Institute of International Affairs, NIIA, suggested last week that the US state department "appears not to have given any serious attention to the Liberian crisis, as all its foreign policy machinery is focused on Iraq."

As the international community remained in a quandary over the Liberian crisis, the bloody fight to take control of the Executive mansion was intensified last week. Taylor's National Patriotic Front of Liberia, NPFL, which had earlier sounded conciliatory to Johnson soon after Doe was captured, later declared a "total and final onslaught" on Johnson, just as Johnson's forces battled to uproot the remnants of Doe's troops at the mansion. By press time, the entire elite presidential guard was in disarray and hundreds were said to have dropped their arms, changed into mufti and fled to safety.

Amidst the bombardments, Johnson and Nimley permitted ECOMOG to enter the presidential mansion where the peace-keepers on September 13 successfully evacuated 1,000 associates and family members of Doe to the ECOMOG base of the port. Nimley and a few other top aides, a BBC report said, were not really in a mood to continue the fight but were "too scared to come out because of the fighting and what the two rebel forces might do to them." Nimley is believed to be more scared of Johnson's troops due to the torture Johnson once underwent in Nimley's hands after the 1985 Quiwonkpa coup. Johnson was prominent in that coup. He was caught and, according to his (Johnson's) account to Nigerian journalists, "Nimley singled me out for torture and detained me inside a tank for days; but I managed to escape."

When Doe, a mere master-sergeant, terminated the 133-year-old rule of the America-Liberians in 1980, he, as Willie Givens, his speech writer, said, probably confirmed Napoleon's adage that "every ordinary soldier carries a marshal's baton in his rucksack." Despite the carnage that heralded his assumption of power, Doe came with some hope of "making Liberia a better place for every Liberian." But that hope was soon to be dashed by his ruthless style. Apart from William Tolbert, his predecessor, whom he boasted to have personally killed, Doe quickly ordered the public execution of 43 top government officials. But before they were tied to the stakes and killed, the top officials, including the 72-year-old speaker of the House of Representatives, Richard Hens Henries, were paraded naked in the streets, beaten and showered with insults.

Doe, Quiwonkpa and Weh Syen were the triumvirate that

headed 15 other Non-Commissioned Officers, NCOs, who took over power and formed what was called the "People's Revolutionary Council, PRC. Soon, Doe took on the PRC and began to dish out the kind of rough justice that he had given to Tolbert and his key officials. Of the 17 NCOs who formed the original PRC, 16 were either killed, detained or retired under one pretext or another. Syen, his first deputy, called the vice-head of state, was taken care of quite early in 1981, when he was arrested, summarily tried and executed for plotting a coup. Nicholas Podier, the vice-head of state who succeeded Syen, was also to go the same way three years later. Nelson Toe, the youngest member of the PRC, was executed to same day with Syen. Even before their deaths, Fallah Varney, also a PRC member, was killed in a mysterious motor accident.

Quiwonkpa, the popular head of the army, who was more respected than Doe, was redeployed to an inferior post. When he rejected the post, he was dismissed from the army, an action that annoyed his kinsmen in Nimba county. Quiwonkpa went into exile in America and returned in November 1985 to stage a coup. In his radio broadcast, Quiwonkpa called the coup "the ultimate gamble in the task of national liberation." It surely was for the charismatic Gio man. When the coup failed, Doe exacted his retribution with ultimate ruthlessness. Quiwonkpa was not only executed. He was castrated by Doe's guards and his mutilated body put on display. The brutality that accompanied Quiwonkpa's death and the subsequent victimization of officers from the Gio and Mano tribes marked the turning point in the geo-political relations in the country. Whole villages were razed in a macabre man-hunt for opponents. At least 500 Gio people were killed in the wave of repression that followed Quiwonkpa's coup. Recalled on Liberian refugee in Sierra Leone three weeks ago: "It was an atmosphere of total terror, with countless mass graves."

With time, Doe steadily lost his best advisers and began to suffer gradual erosion of well-trained technocrats in government. In his last days, some of his ministers could pass for clerks in other neighbouring countries. He developed a style of government that bypassed normal governmental and judicial processes. More and more people from the Grand Gedeh county, his ethnic county, were given jobs for which they had little or no qualification. Said a Liberian refugee in Nigeria: "Opposition was soon to manifest in every form: From the legitimate (formation of political parties) to the illegitimate (series of coup plots), as well as bloody students and workers' riots."

In 1984, Doe, then a field-marshal, said he wanted to become a civilian president. He set up his party and named it National Democratic Party of Liberia, NDPL. Sawyer, who also set up a party, was bundled into detention with key members of his Liberian People's Party, LPP. The detention brought the University of Liberia students onto the street. Doe responded by sending his palace guards after the students. At the end of that day more than 50 students lay dead in the streets, while another 200 were injured. This was seen as an attempt to frighten Doe's opponents out of the elections. And it worked to some extent.

After delaying the election result for one week, Doe said he won with 51 percent vote. He lost only in Nimba county. America praised the elections as "genuine." Doe, many argued, could after-all have proclaimed a one-party state like Ethiopia's Mengistu Haile Mariam or simply refused to hold elections like Idi Amin and claim mandate from God. Besides all that, Doe scored himself only 51 percent, when other tyrants like Zaire's Mobutu Sese

Seko and Togo's Gnassingbe Eyadema would have scored themselves a landslide 99 percent vote.

Doe, to his credit, tried to mend fences after the elections, except that there were no more fences left in Liberia to mend. He had virtually destroyed everything. The economy was in shambles, even with $500 million aid from America. It was not long before Doe ordered an across-the-board 25 percent reduction in the salaries of all workers and pensioners receiving up to 200 Liberian dollars. It was an ironic twist for a man whose first actions as head of state in 1980 was to double the salaries of soldiers and civil servants. That single act had upped the annual wage bill by $34 million.

Doe is dead. But the bloodshed, and many other odious legacies of his 10-year misrule, will persist. Liberia is entering a perilous new phase with several would-be successors still at each others throat. West African nations, too, have been torn into factions and the much sought after economic integration appears, for now a much longer journey than envisaged, all because of Doe. When the Liberian leader died last week, it was as if Johnson had exorcised the ultimate demon from the country's tormented soul.

But was Doe the only problem? Can Taylor and Johnson and other parties in the conflict that has claimed thousands of lives lay down their arms and negotiate their country's future? As one diplomat said last week: "If Taylor, Johnson, Nimley and Sawyer do not sit down fast and talk peace instead of war, they will soon find that there may be nobody left in Liberia to rule."

BY FORCE AND FURY

A Nigerian solider was the first casualty of the West African peace-keeping force, ECOMOG, as the regional troops battled with the Charles Taylor-led rebels for much of last week to establish a stronghold and impose a cease-fire in the eight-month-old Liberia civil war. The soldier, a guardsman in the 123 Guards Battalion, was according to military sources here in Freetown, shot to death by "a single sniper bullet" in the port area in Monrovia, as ECOMOG tried to install emergency defenses in empty warehouses within the dockyard. The body of the slain soldiers, along with six other wounded soldiers, were quickly ferried by a small boat to the *NNS Damisa,* a Nigerian fast attack craft, FAC, mid-sea, for preservation and treatment. Three of the wounded soldiers, including an officer, were riding in an armoured car that was blasted by a rocket-propelled grenade fired by the rebels. Nigeria has a 1,358-man contingent in the ECOMOG.

ECOMOG arrived the Liberian port August 25 amid artillery fire exchange between the two rival rebel forces of Taylor and Prince Yormi Johnson. Taylor was desperate to drive the Johnson-led troops away from the port area and prevent ECOMOG from anchoring its warships in Monrovia. But after a 13-hour battle, the Johnson troops successfully repelled the attack by Taylor's forces; and the peace-keeping troops, ferried by a Ghanaian naval vessel, *Tano River,* eventually docked without immediate opposition. Then Johnson, dressed in combat fatigue, walked down to the dockside to meet ECOMOG officers, as his troops fired welcoming shots in the air.

From that point, it was over to ECOMOG. Some soldiers quickly set about securing strategic positions around the port. Others worked on the habour cranes, in preparation for other heavy-duty ships, particularly *NNS Ambe,* the Nigerian landing ship, to dock. *NNS Ambe* was loaded with the bulk of the tanks, armoured cars and other equipment needed by ECOMOG. Two other Nigerian warships, *NNS Ekpe* and *NNS Damisa,* had surveillance duties, while the entire naval convoy was closely escorted by another Nigerian ship, *MV Northern Naavigator*, an oil tanker. While some soldiers quickly unloaded the tanks, vehicles, ammunition and other supplies, other troops set up offices and field kitchens in the port buildings. Several hundred more stood wet and bedraggled on the quayside, under a steady downpour, as more than 200 trucks, tanks and armoured cars were hoisted off sophisticated Nigerian warships by cranes. The wharf was littered with spent cartridges from recent fighting and reporters inside the warships saw bodies in civilian clothes floating nearby.

Despite the immediate casualty, ECOMOG troops were in high spirits. They quickly consolidated their hold on the port area, securing strategic positions, including two bridges over the Mesurado River leading to the centre of Monrovia. On August 27, two days after the peace-keepers landed, Taylor suffered his first major setback when his naval boat, named *NPFL Navy,* was apprehended and seized by *NNS Damisa,* along with 27 rebels. The *NPFL Navy,* fitted with radar and automatic weapons, was believed to be on a sabotage mission when *NNS Damisa,* commanded by Gani Adekeye, a lieutenant-commander, caught sight of the rebel gunboat some 15 nautical miles from the Monrovia seaport. A dialogue then ensued:

NNS Damisa: what are you doing there?
NPFL Navy: This is a Liberian Navy patrolling Liberian waters.
     We are not patrolling Nigerian or Ghanaian waters.
NNS Damisa: Stop or I blast you
NPFL Navy: Okay, I will comply.

The arrest of the rebel gunboat, it was believed last week, partially crippled the rebel navy, said to consist of only two vessels. By press time, ECOMOG operation, code-named "Liberty," was still trying to inch its way out of the port area, but it had successfully liberated some 50,000 refugees.

Yet, "Operation Liberty" last week appeared to be in danger as West African countries seemed sharply divided over its mission. At least five members of the Economic Community of West African States, ECOWAS, by press time, had raised objection to ECOMOG. They included Cote d'Ivoire, Burkina Faso, Senegal, Togo and Mali. The objections by the French-speaking countries, apart from strengthening Taylor's hands, also threatened to develop into something of a diplomatic row between

English-speaking (which make up 80 percent of ECOMOG) and French-speaking ECOWAS countries.

Senegal, the latest country to be at odds with ECOMOG, said it was disgusted because members of the ECOWAS mediation committee which set up ECOMOG did not even care to inform other ECOWAS member-states of their decision to deploy troops to Liberia. Togo, which had all along egged on Nigeria to intervene in the Liberian crisis and had pledged to contribute troops to ECOMOG, suddenly backed out. It said it would no longer join ECOMOG unless the warring parties first agree to a cease-fire. Last week, Tom Woewiyu, Taylor's defence minister, said he even met with Gnassingbe Eyadema, president of Togo, who assured him Togo would have nothing to do with ECOMOG unless there is a total cease-fire. Some African diplomats in Freetown last week argued that Togo's about-turn may have something to do with its aversion to Ghana, whose army general, Arnold Quainoo, takes charge as the commander of ECOMOG.

Burkina Faso, one of the first countries to raise strong objections against ECOMOG, went one step further last week and sent troops and weapons to Taylor, further complicating the crisis. A Libyan plane, according to report reaching Freetown, touched down last week at the burnt-out Robertsfield International Airport, carrying "highly-trained" Burkinabe troops as well as military hardware, including grenade launchers and automatic rifles. Tons of weapons from Libya were also reported to have passed through Burkina Faso and Cote d'Ivoire by land into rebel hands. Blaise Compaore, president of Burkina Faso, who is the son-in-law of the Ivorian leader, Felix Houphouet-Boigny, is considered to be spearheading the drive for support for Taylor, with active backing of Abidjan. Abidjan, though opposed to ECOMOG, has, however, denied facilitating weapons delivery to Taylor through its border with Liberia.

Amid the risk of an escalation of the Liberian crisis, ECOW-

AS mediation committee went ahead last week to convene the scheduled Liberian all-party conference in Banjul, Gambia. But the principal parties to the conflict Taylor and Samuel Doe refused to take part in the conference which was expected to come up with an interim government for Liberia. Woewiyu reiterated the stance of the NPFL last week, saying it cannot participate in the Banjul conference "unless ECOWAS is able to properly address the critical issues of the conflict." But the surprise was Doe, who had all along appeared to fully support ECOWAS' plans for Liberia. Doe showed clearly last week that he supports ECOWAS only to the extent that it would imposed a cease-fire, drive his enemies out of the way, while leaving him behind to continue as president.

Selly Thomson, Doe's spokesman, speaking late last week on the Banjul conference, said the question of telling Doe to step down for an interim government was completely unacceptable. "President Doe's position remains that the most pressing problem in Liberia was that of the imposition of the cease-fire and not an interim government. How can they (ECOWAS) be talking of an interim government, when there are bullets flying all over the place,?" Thomson said angrily in a BBC telephone interview. According to him, Doe feels it is "an offence" to talk about an interim government. As he put it, "Doe is the elected president of Liberia. He will call of a national conference of Liberia to decide the future. If, after such a conference, the people of Liberia want Doe to step down, he will do so. Why should he (Doe) send a representative to the conference in Banjul while he remains the elected president of the people? (Dauda) Jawara (president of Gambia) should rethink the entire ECOWAS strategy."

Jawara, ECOWAS chairman, opening the Liberian all-party

conference last week, reiterated the goals and objectives of ECO-MOG. Said Jawara: "The deployment of the ECOWAS peace-keeping force in Liberia is aimed at creating conditions necessary for Liberians to discuss freely the political future of their country." Present at the conference were Liberian church leaders and former politicians such as Amos Sawyer, Ellen Sirleaf Johnson, Baccus Mathews, John Potto Tambakai Jangaba and George Washington. One of them was expected to be named to head the interim government. The choice at press time appeared to have been narrowed down to Sawyer, Washington and Jangaba. Sawyer, 46, an academic, was at a time head of the Liberian Constitution Commission. Jangaba was the speaker of the Liberian senate until the civil war, while Washington is the head of a Liberian exile group in America. A strong point in Washington's favour, some Liberians argued last week, is his ethnic background. He is a member of Kru tribe, which has remained neutral in the ethnic war. But many delegates at the conference were believed to be opposed to his status as a former military officer, indicating that a concensus was more likely to form around Sawyer.

Whatever comes out of the Banjul conference, there is only a slim chance that it would be implemented, as the crisis appears increasingly out of control. Last week, as Johnson capitulated to ECOMOG and took a back seat in the crisis, Taylor did not only win sympathizers but reportedly went ahead to round up thousands of West African nationals, mostly from Nigeria, Ghana and Guinea, as hostages. One diplomatic source in Freetown said Taylor was evacuating his captives from Monrovia to Buenanau his stronghold, and plans to shoot them in retaliation if his troops are seized or killed by ECOMOG troops.

But Woewiyu debunked the claim that the hostages, including two Nigerian journalist, would be shot. He said speculations about killing the hostages were propaganda peddled by Nigeria, Ghana and America to smear the reputation of the NPFL. Said Woewiyu in a BBC telephone interview: "We are not threatening to shoot anybody. We have no reason to shoot our fellow Africans who have been in our country. We will never think of anything like that." However, the rebel defence minister said there is a great risk of ECOMOG killing the hostages because of the heavy equipment used by the regional troops to bombard rebel positions. "They (ECOMOG) are the ones doing the shooting. They are the ones using all the heavy weapons in Liberia. They are still at the port area but they are using their heavy weapons to shell all the neighbourhood. Now I hear they have sent for more troops in Sierra Leone. There is a danger that they might be killing their own people too with their weapons," Woewiyu said.

Possibly, the biggest danger ECOMOG faced last week was the prospects of failure as some member-states of ECOWAS and Liberians themselves seemed to have no faith in the ability of the regional forces to solve the seemingly intractable fracticidal conflict. Last week, even as the Banjul conference was in progress, Kwia Johnson, the mayor of Monrovia, pleaded with the United Nations, UN, and America to "hurry now" and intervene in the crisis, as they hold the only wherewithal to end the bloodbath. Johnson, who is currently the president of the 1,500-member World Council of Mayors, questioned the refusal of America to force Doe out and send a peace-keeping force to the troubled country. Said Johnson: "The United States and the UN have a moral obligation to save Liberia from self-destruction. God will not forgive us while we sit idly and allow defenceless people to be so massacred."

Many Liberian refugees in Sierra Leone last week believed ECOMOG was quite capable of solving the Liberian crisis. Said Fredrick Stemn, a Liberian refugee: "Let Doe go. Let Taylor lay down his arms. Let ECOWAS speak with one voice. Let them all stop playing politics with our lives and give the peace-keeping force a chance to restore normalcy to our country,"

FROM PEACE KEEPERS TO PEACE TAKERS

The war appeared to have reached the zenith. Bombs were dropped everywhere even by the peace-keepers. Scores of bodies littered the city. Houses went up in flames. Monrovia, once the beautiful capital city of Liberia, stood charred, a ghost town. Then at the end of what might have probably passed as the bloodiest week in the nine-month civil war, a desperate diplomatic offensive brought the battle closer to the end, more than ever before, as all the warring parties indicated their willingness to negotiate a peaceful settlement to the bloodbath.

The tonic for the last-ditch battle was the capture and execution of Samuel Doe, the stubborn Liberian despot, September 10, by Yormie Johnson, leader of the breakaway rebel forces. In the scramble for Doe's prized Executive Mansion that followed, even the West African Peace-Keeping Force, ECOMOG, could not avoid being brought into a bloody face-off with the two rebel troops led by Charles Taylor and Johnson. First, Johnson wanted ECOMOG to assist him bomb out the remnants of Doe's loyalists left in the mansion. Then Taylor declared a "total war" against ECOMOG, in an effort to neutralize the peace-keeping force, which he regarded as the obstacle between him and the Executive Mansion. One of Taylor's artillery shells landed at the ECOMOG seaport headquarters, damaging the building and killing three Nigerian nurses. Another artillery shelling from rapidly advancing Taylor's troops landed inside ECOMOG's headquarters. Three Ghanaian soldiers were killed while 18 others were wounded.

From that point on, ECOMOG knew it was fishing in troubled waters and had to adopt what it called the "military alternative" in keeping peace in the small West African country. Three small Ghanaian jet bombers, stationed for weeks at Freetown, Sierra Leone airport, were ordered to rescue ECOMOG from the fast-advancing rebel forces. When the Ghanaian jet fighter went into action September 16, the rebels found nowhere to hide. They had to beat a fast retreat. The arrival of roaring Nigeria's Jaguar, MIG and Alfa jets in the Monrovian skies the next day completely turned the tide against the Taylor-led troops as the sophisticated air fighters raided and bombarded rebels' strongholds, crippling further rebel advances at least within Monrovia.

At the same time, Nigeria ordered an additional 1,400 troops from its Airborne Brigade in Makurdi to join the first Nigerian contingent of 1,358 soldiers. For most of last week, trailer-loads of arms and ammunition including tanks, armoured personnel carriers, etc., were being shipped to Monrovia. Ghana, which had almost pulled out its troops from ECOMOG, changed its stance following the visit of Nigeria's foreign affairs minister, Ike Nwachukwu, and announced it was similarly sending an additional 1,000 troops to Liberia to help fight back the rebel forces. ECOMOG said by increasing its troops it had effectively ceased to be a peace-keeper but a peace enforcer. When later in the week Arnold Quainoo, Lieutenant-General and Commander of ECOMOG, visited Nigeria to brief government on the crisis, he gave indications that the problem had become so complicated that ECOMOG would have to pull all the stops to rout the rebels. Said Quainoo, who has been severely criticized for the death of Doe: "We have got a new mandate now to carry out enforcement action to ensure that all the aims and objectives of ECOWAS authorities are carried out. What we are trying to do now is to enhance our effectiveness by reorganizing the whole force structure and sending more reinforcement."

Soon after Quainno left Nigeria, a government spokesman announced that the Ghanaian general was being dropped as ECOMOG commander. He was quickly replaced by Joshua Dogonyaro, a Nigerian major-general, who is currently the director of training and operations at the army headquarters, Lagos. Quainoo has been on the firing line since Doe was captured in his office and subsequently slaughtered.

Just at about the same time Quainoo was speaking in Lagos, Harman Cohen, American assistant secretary of state for African affairs, was meeting with Taylor at the Liberian-Ivory Coast border. Cohen, who had only two days earlier met with Johnson inside the American embassy in Monrovia, later broke the good news that both Taylor and Johnson are "very concerned" about the escalating bloodbath and were now willing to embark on a negotiated settlement. It was not certain at press time when the negotiation proper would begin, but the intervention of the American government was seen as weighty and capable of reconciling the rebels with ECOWAS intention of Liberia. Cohen's diplomatic shuttle, which also took him to many ECOWAS countries, was seen as America's readiness to expand its role in the

Liberian crisis. Amos Sawyer, the ECOWAS-backed interim head of state of Liberia, also spent most of last week shuttling across West Africa in search of goodwill for the interim government. In Burkina Faso, he asked President Blaise Campaore, leading supporter of Taylor, to persuade the main rebel leader to agree on a negotiated settlement.

Though prospects of a negotiated settlement looked bright last week, Taylor's National Patriotic Front of Liberia, NPFL, which controls more than 90 percent of Liberia, vowed to retaliate ECOMOG's attack against its positions. "Whatever pains they are inflicting on us, we will reverse all of that on them too." Tom Woewiyu, Taylor's defence minister, said in a BBC interview. Woewiyu said the air raid and other "aggression" mounted against the NPFL has only served to strengthen the resolve of the rebels to drive ECOMOG out of Liberia. "We have done nothing to Nigeria, Ghana or any of the (ECOMOG) countries to provoke the type of aggression that they have mounted against us. And they have to pay dearly for this naked aggression," Woewiyu said.

According to Woewiyu, some of the bombs dropped by ECOMOG "landed on a girls' school housing refugees, in which several hundreds of them were killed." He said that it was futile for ECOMOG to bomb rebel-held territory in the hope of displacing rebel troops because "we do not have a specific location and our fighting force is not concentrated on any spot where anybody can throw a bomb." He warned that plans by ECOMOG to parachute into rebel territory "is like committing suicide because every living Liberian on our territory is a soldier." He also told some ECOMOG countries to "start to think and realize that we will strike back against them by any means possible." And in response to this threat, security along Nigerian border routes and ports were reported last week to be tightened, to forestall a suspected attack by Charles Taylor's allies.

But, perhaps, the greatest scare in Lagos last week, at least in media circles, was the possible harm to two Nigerian journalists taken hostage by Taylor's men two months ago. The scare was heightened by a report in the British Sunday observers that Nigerian refugees in Taylor's territory "were executed in front of reporters." The report said "the two Nigerian journalists (Krees Imodible of *The Guardian* and Tayo Awotusin of *The champion)* have disappeared and rebel sources have hinted that they too have been shot as spies."

AU REVOIR KEREKOU!

"The Knock-out Blow That Saves The Nation." That was the banner headline of a Cotonou newspaper last week, announcing the defeat of Mathieu Kerekou by Nicephore Soglo at the March 24 presidential election. The newspaper called *24 Heures* (Twenty-four Hours), had an accompanying cartoon to dramatize the story. Victorious Soglo stood at the centre of the ring, his hands raised by Isidore Souza, Bishop of Cotonou and Chairman of the interim parliament called the High Council of the Republic. A dazed Kerekou, seeing stars, lay on the canvas muttering some words to himself: *"Le type la! Ii est trop furt quoi,"* meaning *"I have never been hit by this type of blow."* Apt. Kerekou had, in his 17 years of iron-fisted rule, won the presidential election three times as the sole candidate, perhaps god, of his party and country. But faced with a multi-party election last week, he was floored by lesser known Soglo, who won a 67.6 percent of the vote leaving Kerekou with just 32.3 percent.

As the defeated president kissed the political canvas, the president-elect was himself bed-ridden, knocked down for two weeks running by what Beninoise citizens called a "sudden and mysterious disease." Soglo's campaign aides told *Newswatch* that since the second week of March when Soglo was stoned and violently chased out of Natitingou, Kerekou's home base in the northern region, he has not been able to step out again to campaign. On Election Day, Soglo appeared in public for the first time in two weeks, to cast his vote at the Cocotier Primary School near his residence. He looked pale and emaciated. His hands and legs were tremling. He could not walk on his own and had to throw his two hands over the shoulders of two relatives, who virtually lifted him into a classroom where he voted. He seemed stricken from waist down. Attempts by *Newswatch* to interview him was futile as his voice too was shaking and his words slurred. Honore Odoulami, Soglo's personal physician, told *Newswatch* the president-elect is very sick. He said that from his examination, what he has "found out for now is typhoid fever." Odoulami, who is also Soglo's brother-in-law, talked about "complications" arising from acute pains in his spinal cord and waist. By press time, a team of Beninoise doctors had recommended that Soglo be flown to France for treatment.

But for thousands of Soglo's supporters, the ill-health of the president-elect is not a matter for "whiteman medicine but the hand work of *juju* men and voodooists." And their accusing fingers are pointed in one direction: Kerekou's.

With the illness of the president-elect, which puts in serious jeopardy his April inauguration, and the grumbling of the defeated Kerekou, which threw the country last week into a bloody post-election inter-tribal violence, a thick cloud of uncertainty hung over the political horizon of this tiny West African State. Last week, as violence spread in Kerekou's home base in

The North and southerners working in the troubled areas fled in droves back home, there were strong speculations about the possibility of a *coup d'etat.* Souza had to go on the air March 27 to plead for calm. In his nation-wide broadcast, first aired at 7.00am, he called on Kerekou to "take a trip to the two northern provinces" of Atacora and Borgou and effect an end to violent attacks against southern citizens. With thousands of workers fleeing The North, Souza said, social services and public utilities such as water, electricity, telephone and postal services were on the verge of being crippled.

The election had appeared smooth nationwide until about 3.00pm March 24, when the national radio first announced an outbreak of trouble in Parakou, Borgou province. The cause of the violence was traced to a press release issued by Kerekou earlier in the day, in which he said his supporters in Zou province, Soglo's home base, were molested. The allegation by Kerekou was later found to be false as the national radio correspondent reporting live from Zou said the election in the area had been "very peaceful without any ugly incident." But before then, two people, a man and woman, had been killed in a revenge attack on Soglo's supporters. Churches and houses were set ablaze and hundreds of people were admitted in hospitals around Borgou province. Later in the day, Kerekou had to go on air to appeal for calm. But the harm had been done. From that point, it was difficult to stop the exodus of the southerners.

The Parakou violence was a rather odd exception in an otherwise smooth and well-conducted election. In Cotonou, voters streamed out of their homes as early as seven in the morning and completed their task even before they headed for the Sunday services. In Zougo, a swarming suburb in the capital city, *News-*

watch found out that voting in two polling stations set up under a tent close to a new mosque, was so orderly that soldiers posted to the station turned their attention to draughtboard games and East African *Makossa* music coming from their transistor radio. In virtually all polling stations, ballot-counting centres and the national tabulation centre at the interior ministry, reporters and international observers were struck by efficiency and diligence of electoral officers.

Said Carl Noble, an American observer: "We found (except in Parakou) a high level of conscientiousness, diligence and competence at the polling places, the enthusiasm of both election officials and the voters, was testimony to the widespread support for free and fair election in Benin.

Yet, there were clear indications during the last week of the campaign that trouble was lurking somewhere along the road. In most of his last minute campaign stops, Kerekou was treated with very little courtesy. Kerekou's aides said last week that "angry mobs and stone-throwing Soglo's men" did not give Kerekou the "chance and confidence to deliver his message fearlessly and persuasively." In the Cotonou suburbs of Sainte Cecile, Zogbo, Zougo, Dantokpa and Akpakpa, the "Chameleon" as Kerekou nicknamed himself, did manage to speak before boos from the crowd drowned his speech. But Cove, Zou province, he was much less successful as the crowd kept throwing stones and shouting hostile slogans. In Mono and Oueme provinces, his campaign, just like in Zou, was a flop and ended with stones raining down his platform.

Most politicians attributed the reception accorded Kerekou in the southern provinces, to the maltreatment earlier given Soglo in Kerekou's home province. By the time Kerekou was rounding off his campaign, he had almost replaced his message of "change in continuity" with threats of not minding to "fight and die with my gun in hand." With his earlier threats that there may be no president on April 1, most of his opponents realized it was time nobody fooled with the "Chameleon."

But the threats did not in anyway douse the anti-Kerekou sentiments. A large section of the country's press held the fort for bed-ridden Soglo. They accused Kerekou of a wide range of misdeeds ranging from his "two decades of incompetence" to "large-scale fraud." One newspaper, *La Gazette da Golfe*, even said the former dictator got $2.5 million in 1988 from a foreign company, Sesco Gibraltar Ltd., in exchange for the dumping of toxic waste in Benin. Another newspaper said: Kerekou's campaign was bank-rolled by "other unwanted dictators in Ivory Coast and Togo." Yet again, he was accused of buying voters cards in large quantity in the southern provinces, in an effort to undercut Soglo's support base.

On the other hand, Soglo was praised for putting the country back on the path of recovery during his one year as interim prime minister. At the same time, workers who were owed backlog of five months salaries by Kerekou, rooted for Soglo, who paid up the salary arrears and made it possible for them now to collect their salaries regularly. Said Michel Soumanou, a teacher: "This election was a choice between the economic uncertainties of the past and the economic hopes of the future. It was a choice between delays in payment of salaries and regular payment of salaries." Soglo, to many therefore, represented the high hopes of the future.

But perhaps, the biggest factor in Soglo's favour was geo-politics. He hails from the southern part of the country which, apart from being more populated, has four of the country's six provinces. He won convincingly in the four southern provinces, polling 93.2 percent in Atlantique, 91 percent in Oueme, 90.7 percent in Zou, his home province, and 81.5 percent in Mono. Kerekou on the other hand won 96.4 percent and 93.6 percent in the two northern provinces of Borgou and Atacora respectively. But there were some analysts who insisted last week that the regional factor was only "coincidental." Said Jean-Claude Soehou, a trade unionist: "The big factor was the anti Kerekou sentiment. Everybody was fed up with him. And in fact, any other candidate beside Soglo would still have defeated him."

Last week, as the "Chameleon" sulked over his defeat, the immediate concern of the interim administration was how to finally ease Kerekou out of power without making him feel humiliated. "That is the key strategy now because he can risk everything and try something bloody," one member of the High Council told *Newswatch*. According to the High Council member: "We have instructed prominent friends and supporters of Soglo to keep their heads down. Everything has to be done to make sure he (Kerekou) is guaranteed a graceful retreat. The issue is so important that everyone has to be on guard to avoid a last-minute mistake." This strategy was very apparent when Soglo issued what was regarded as his victory statement. In the carefully worded one paragraph statement Soglo thanked the "masses" for giving him the mandate and urged everyone to be "law abiding and calm."

Soglo, his supporters hope, should be able, before long, to overcome both his illness and the man called chameleon. But Soglo, an economist and former World Bank director, will certainly find the task of governing the poverty-ridden country by far a tougher venture. Saddled with an external debt of $7.2 million, 70,000 workers whose productivity level the World Bank describes as one of the lowest in the world, the Benin economy is practically at a standstill. There is scarcity and high prices of virtually every essential commodity. A bottle of 29cl coke in most hotels go for the equivalent of N10. And with the harsh backlash of the Structural Adjustment Programme, SAP, underway, observers are certain it would not be long before the public begins to cry aloud.

Still, Soglo's backers, including five presidential candidates who dropped off in the first round of the election, believe the most important task was to get Kerekou out of the way, and everything else would just fall into place. As Moses Adjile, a political scientist at the Benin University, said last week: "The people have jointly given Kerekou a slap on the face. They will have to join hands in fighting the decline of the last two decades."

THE FALL OF ADDIS ABABA

The battle for the capital city itself was brief. After a three-hour bombardment, the defenses of loyal government troops collapsed. The rebel troops rolled in more tanks. And the fabled city of New Flowers bowed to superior fire-power. That was the fall of Addis Ababa, capital of Ethiopia, Africa's oldest independent country. It was the climax of 31 years of what has gone into history books as Africa's longest running civil war.

The rebel units of the Ethiopian People's Revolutionary Democratic Front, EPRDF, entered the city in a disciplined fashion, urged by top American officials. At 10 o'clock in the night, flashes of red and orange lit the skyline. It was the first indication of artillery exchange. Soon, intense sounds of heavy gunfire followed. The rattle of light machine-gun fire was interspersed with the crack of heavier caliber weapons, and then complemented with occasional outburst to shelling and huge explosions.

The rebels were attacking the city from several directions, capturing first, the ministry of information, before turning attention to the presidential palace, home of Mengistu Haile Mariam, the iron-fisted ruler, who fled into exile a week earlier. A direct hit at the presidential palace immediately blew up an ammunition dump, releasing huge balls of flames and deafening explosions. In another hour or so, the palace, sandwiched by mountains, south-west of the city, had changed hands. An Ethiopian journalist who saw the tank column entering the city described the scene to foreign newsmen: "They drove slowly, with very proud movement. They drove like they were not at war. It was like they were driving into Rome."

By dawn, however, bodies littered the streets. The Red Cross, quoted by the British Broadcasting Corporation, BBC, reported that some 200 people were killed. More than 800 were wounded. Inhabitants of the city packed into the premises of churches for protection and prayers. For much of last week, Addis Ababa, the cradle of the Organization of African Unity, OAU, and home of the United Nations Economic Commission for Africa, ECA, was a city holding its breath, waiting to see whether the transition from government to rebels control would be accompanied by general disorder and revenge executions or not. That was yet to happen by press time, as diplomats and millions of restless Ethiopians awaited the return of the rebel leader from the aborted London peace talks, to begin the day-to-day administration of the country.

Maile Salawi, the 36-year-old leader of the EPRDF and now head of the interim government, said in London that his immediate concern would be to establish a lasting peace and prepare for democracy. "The priorities of the interim Ethiopia's administration will be to improve law and order situation, facilitate the distribution of relief aid, maintain essential services, create a lasting peace and prepare for democracy," Salawi told reporters.

The new interim administration, Salawi said, has scheduled an all-party conference for July 1, during which a broad-based government would be established.

However, another major rebel group, the Eritrean People Liberation Front, EPLF, which has complete control of Northern Ethiopia, said they will not be part of the transition government. Ande Michael Kassai, a spokesman of the EPLF, said the group, one of the three rebel groups which participated in the London talks, had not been fighting to have ministerial posts in future Ethiopian government, but a separate country. There were indications that the SPRDF would probably not stand on the way of the Eritreans, who started their "liberation" war in 1960.

As anxiety and concern about possible anarchy mounted, thousands of Ethiopians, both military and civilians, continued to flee the embattled country in search of sanctuary in neighbouring countries. Last week, the government of Djibouti, Ethiopia's small north-western neighbour, appealed to the international community for food, medical supplies and blankets to help comfort the more than 30,000 refugees, just arriving from Ethiopia. Six hundred French troops, on their way home from the Gulf war, had to be diverted to Djibouti to help settle the refugees. Diplomats in Djibouti estimated that 70 percent of the refugees were government soldiers.

With the flight of Mengistu a week earlier, most people connected with his regime, especially top military officials were just grabbing the next available means of transportation out of the country. Two air force pilots simply laid hands on their MIGs-23 and flew it to Djibouti. Another two pilots from the air force training school arrived in a training aircraft. Similarly, a group of 2,000 soldiers arrived in five transport aircraft, one of them flying a general who commanded Asmara, the second largest city, before it fell to the EPLF. In addition, two Ethiopian air force pilots hijacked a commercial aircraft with 53 people on board and flew it straight to Djibouti. By the last count, 14 Ethiopian military aircraft, 12 helicopters and 11 civilian airliners landed in Djibouti just before the rebels took over Addis Ababa.

In Kenya, Ethiopia's southern neighbour, 60 fleeing military top shots arrived May 28, in three air force planes. Airport officials at the Nairobi's Jomo Kenyatta International Airport said a total of 14 Ethiopian planes, including two Soviet-built military cargo planes, had so far landed, with unspecified number of military and civilian officials. In Yemen, north-east of Ethiopia, officials also announced last week that the whole of Ethiopian navy escaped across the Red Sea to the country. Twelve Ethiopian naval vessels, carrying 3,000 people, were seen anchoring at the southern, Yemen port city of Mocha. "We believe it is the entire navy," one official said. Sudan, Ethiopia's neighbor to The West, recorded probably the largest influx of military and civilian refugees. As at Wednesday, May 29, Sudanese authorities said more than 150,000 refugees had arrived at their border, within the first 24 hours of the fall of Addis Ababa. Another 200,000 were estimated to be on their way.

Just before the rebels took over Addis Ababa, Israeli jets flew all night to pluck 16,000 black Ethiopian Jews, called Falashas, to safety in Israel. It was a remarkable operation, even by Israeli usually dramatic standards. Four Israeli air force Hercules and every plane in the El Al fleet, shuttled between the two countries, in an airlift prepared secretly in both countries and code-named Operation Solomon. Seats were stripped from aircraft and replaced with foam mattresses, on which the Falashas were crammed in their flight to "the promised land." One Boeing 747 was crammed with 1,087 passengers, the largest number in aviation history ever carried by a single aircraft. Yitzhak Shamir, the Israeli prime minister, was at the airport to welcome the first plane-load of the black Jews, who joined some 200,000 other black Jews to swell the population of the tiny Jewish state.

Though the EPRDF took over the government last week, trouble looms yet. Barely 24 hours after the fall of Addis Ababa, Ethiopians at home and abroad protested the role of America in the final capitulation of their government, as well as in the setting up of the interim government and the plan by the EPLF to secede. Several hundreds of Ethiopians took to the streets in Addis Ababa in a demonstration that resulted in the death of at least two people. In Washington, USA, a group of Ethiopians rallied at a park across the street from the White House and later marched to the state department to protest the US decision to invite the EPRDF to take over the Ethiopian capital. Protest demonstrations were also held in Los Angeles, San Francisco, Seattle, Toronto and Ottawa. "We are outraged, baffled and at a loss to explain the US position," said Abera Yemane, a member of the executive committee of the Coalition of Ethiopian Democratic Force, COEDF. "Ethiopia is not for sale, America, be warned," a banner carried by the protesters said.

The US had, in the past few weeks, attempted to broker peace talks between the Tigrean-dominated EPRDF, EPLF and a third guerrilla group, the Oromo Liberation Front, OLF, of southern Ethiopia. But in a sudden change of strategy, the US urged the EPRDF to take over Addis Ababa, making the peace talks irrelevant and possibly complicating the Ethiopian crisis. Margaret Tutwiller, state department's spokeswoman, was hard put last week to explain America's role and interest in the crisis. She said Washington instructed the rebels to move into Addis Ababa after the Ethiopian acting president, Tesfaye Dinka, told US *charge d' Affaires* in Addis Ababa, that they were no longer in control of basic law and order situation in the city.

But African affairs experts in the state department told *New York Times* last week that the US wants to regain some influence in the region with the collapse of the leftist regime of Mengistu. "Because of the ending of Soviet interest in Ethiopia, Washington wants to fill the vacuum," the paper quoted officials as saying. Another reason for America's support of the take-over by EPRDF, some officials also said last week, was that the administration was haunted by memories of the horrors in Monrovia, Liberia and Mogadishu, Somalia, after rebel forces rampaged through the fallen capitals. "If we had the kind of situation in Mogadishu reoccur in Addis, it would have been a disaster on a far larger scale for years to come," a senior administration official told the *New York Times.*

But said another official: "Let's hope the Ethiopian disaster is not only being escalated."

FROM HUGE JOKE TO BIG JOLT

In the beginning, it looked like a huge joke. No one took Uganda's guerrilla leader Yoweri Museveni seriously when he declared a guerrilla war against the government of Milton Obote, in protest against widely rigged elections which returned Obote to power in 1980. Museveni was dismissed as inconsequential. Whenever Obote wanted to ridicule his opponents, he would sarcastically advise them to "join Museveni in the bush."

Unknown to Obote was the caliber of the Ugandans who joined Museveni in the bush. They were university graduates, doctors, architects, engineers, surveyors, nurses, men and women trained in commerce and business. Soon, the military activities of the Museveni guerrillas began to bother even the Ugandan soldiers. Museveni became an enigma. And even before he came out from the bush, Obote has lost his job to his army commanders, led by Tito Okello. Obote fled. Museveni peeped from the bush. He realized that what was left of Obote's army was too feeble to resist a chase. He chased them. They fled. And Museveni triumped.

On January 26, exactly six months after Obote was toppled

for the second time in 14 years, Museveni's National Resistant Army stormed Kampala on a chilly evening, took over the Government House and installed Museveni as the fifth Ugandan head of state since independence. Only last July, Museveni has boasted to reporters that "even now I can kick Obote out of Kampala but I would invite problems. I need more preparation so that when I kick Obote out of Kampala, I am able to control the disorder in the whole country." Despite his preparation, riotous orgy followed the capture of Kampala. Stores and homes were looted by retreating Ugandan soldiers.

The battle for Kampala had raged for two days and reached a climax at daybreak, Sunday. Hundreds of bodies littered the streets. The loyal troops of run-away head of state Tito Okello, holed up in parliament buildings and government offices, using anti-aircraft guns in defence of the capital. The staccato rhythm of bazooka and artillery guns filled the air. First, the NRA guerrillas quietly took the radio station and the main post office, then shot their way down the main streets, of Kampala in a house-to-house combat, avoiding embassies and churches, where most civilians had taken refuge for days. Their troops were orderly and disciplined. They surrounded the parliament building, the secretariat, the banks, fired a chorus of artillery shells, sending government troops scurrying for safety. AK-47 bullets slammed and smashed hundreds of windows and glass panels.

As run-away government soldiers rained bullets on the city from hilltops on their way to the eastern suburb of Jinja, the NRA back-up relief officials announced messages to civilians from loud speakers mounted atop jeeps: "Lock your doors, draw your curtain and take cover." Hours later, Museveni speaking on Radio Uganda which came back on the air after two days of silence, announced that NRA had taken over Kampala and the ruling military council of Okello had been dissolved and replaced by National Resistance Council. Jubilant civilians poured on the streets in thousands to celebrate the NRA take-over. Amid jubilation in Kampala, Museveni said he would soon set up a broad-based government after adequate consultations with all parties and interest groups. Museveni is believed to include heads of state of countries bordering Uganda, especially Kenya and Tanzania in the list of those he wants to consult before setting up a government.

Museveni also said he was ready to talk to Okello "as a person" at any venue of his own choice. Dressed in combat fatigue but looking relaxed, Museveni said "Uganda's problem is not as insoluble as they may look from outside," adding that what Uganda lacked was leadership, organization and planning. He urged the international community to assist Uganda saying he could encourage a mixed economy. The next day, the US became the first western nation to recognize Museveni's government. State department spokesman Benard Kalb said, "The United States expects to have friendly and amicable relations with the new Ugandan government.

Meanwhile, the ousted troops of the military council were continuing their rapid retreat; looting and killing civilians on their way after having abandoned their important industrial town of Jinja, 80 km east of the capital, where they had regrouped after the fall of Kampala. Jinja was reported to be quiet and firmly in the hands of the NRA advancing troops. So far, more than 6,000 loyal troops have surrendered to the NRA in various parts of the country. However, the ousted Ugandan military leader Tito Okello reportedly said he would fight to the bitter end to regain power in Uganda. A Kenyan weekly, the *Sunday Nation* reported

January 26, that Okello, accompanied by seven fleeing officials, told a group of Kenyans and Ugandans at the border town of Busia that, "I am going back to fight and regain power." Basilio Okello, the army commander and cousin of the deposed augandan leader, was reportedly shot and killed by his unwilling troops, who would not do anything but run.

Observers see the fall of Kampala and the emergence of Museveni as the new Ugandan leader, as a logical culmination of five years of dedicated, disciplined, popular and purposeful guerrilla warfare against an imposed leadership and government. Museveni took to the bush after Obote's Ugandan Peoples Congress, UPC, party was declared the winner of the still disputed 1980 elections. Museveni believed that the Democratic Party, DP, led by the mild-mannered Paulo Ssemogerere won the election and that the UPC victory was in fact, a fraud. More than half the country agreed with him.

At the start of the guerrilla war, many people predicted defeat for the rebels. But they were wrong. Obote's tactics for winning the war were inhuman. His soldiers led by Tito and Basilio Okello massacred so many innocent civilians including women and children that Obote's western backers started to grumble. In April 1985, Amnesty International and American human rights groups said between 1981-84, Obote's soldiers had massacred 20,000 innocent civilians purported to be supporters of NRA. The United Nations High Commission for Refugees said more than 300,000 people had fled Uganda within that same period in fear of Obote soldiers. The figure was more than the 250,000 who fled Uganda during the eight years of Idi Amin's reign of terror. Five years earlier, it would have been inconceivable that any other Ugandan leader could have had a worse image than Idi Amin. But

Obote did. As one Ugandan once made the comparison: "Amin killed men, many men, but at least he left widows and orphans. But Obote soldiers killed even the women and children left by Amin, indiscriminately." The NRA was therefore, seen as a savior that deserved support.

Where Museveni got the money and weapon to wage the war is as puzzling as Museveni himself. All that is very well known is that he started by raiding banks and government army barracks for money and ammunition. After every bank raid, the guerrillas would leave a note behind promising to pay back the money "as soon as we come to power." Museveni is nevertheless known to be a close friend of Prime Minister Robert Mugabe of Zimbabwe and President Samora Machel of Mozambique, whom he helped to fight the Portuguese colonialists in Mozambique. Some months ago, it was speculated that Libya might have been assisting the NRA, but the speculation was dismissed as a ploy to woo American support to the side of the Ugandan government.

Despite NRA's victory, the end to the Uganda's two decades of political turmoil is still not in sight. Underlying such pessimism is the statement by fleeing Ugandan External Affairs Minister Olara Otunnu, who said only a few months ago that, "if Museveni comes out of the bush and takes over Kampala, those of us who are in Kampala now will go into the bush." Crucial is the tribal factor and the fundamental disagreement over how each warring factions wants the country to be governed. For Okello and his group, the overthrow of Obote was the logical solution to Uganda's problems. In Okello's thinking, "everybody who had opposed Obote should back the government which overthrew him and the country should carry on more or less as normal." Not so, according to Museveni. The NRA had been waging a guerrilla war, not only against Obote but the whole system which Obote created, including his army. For the NRA, therefore, concrete and down to earth reforms and in some cases, a complete break with the past is of a necessity.

For three months, Okello and Museveni argued in Kenya under the watchful eyes of Kenyan President Daniel Arap Moi, on how these differing views could be converged to make way for peace in Uganda. After countless adjournments and consultations, the text of a peace agreement was placed before the warring faction on December 27, 1985. Museveni was a wary signatory. And so warily he implemented it. It was reasoned then in diplomatic circles that the NRA leader just signed the papers because Arap Moi (who had provided sanctuary for the NRA political office) had invested so much personal and national prestige in search of peace, to be ditched. Actually, he hated everything about Obote soldiers, especially their alliance with discredited Idi Amin. He said so and insisted he cannot work with them. "They are murderers of our people; there will be no compromise with criminals," he said.

In the aftermath of the peace agreement, when it appeared Okello could not control his soldiers and make Kampala safe for the implementation of the Nairobi agreement, Museveni insisted on a scrupulous respect for human rights, as a precondition for his alliance with Okello. Restless, he left for Dares Salaam and Nairobi and told Presidents Ali Hassan Nwinyi and Arap Moi that: "I have notified the Okello government in writing that if they fail to maintain peace in Kampala and cause death to the people, we will assist them in maintaining security." Few days later, Museveni kept his words. Backed by his 8,000 strong guerrillas, he took over Kampala and has been maintaining security. A man to be taken seriously, you may say.

THE TRIAL OF A TIN GOD

Jean Bedel Bokassa, 65, one-time self-proclaimed emperor of Central African Republic, CAR, went on trial November 27 for mass murder, theft and cannibalism. The trial contrasted starkly with the pomp of his coronation in 1977 for which the country's coffers were emptied to pay for an intricately fashioned crown and imperial robes embroidered by 25 Parisian seamstresses.

But Bokassa, though in shackles, was still his old imperial self, at least from the way he spoke. He roared like a lion and continuously attracted cheers from a large crowd that massed outside the courtroom. In CAR, where rumour runs faster than the Ubangi River, there were speculations that the old fox could turn the table and use the trial as a platform to launch himself back to power.

Moments before the trial started, President Andre Koling-ba, who five years ago succeeded David Dacko, (the man who stepped into Bokassa's shoes after the French overthrew him,) suddenly developed cold feet. For some undisclosed reasons, he ordered a change of venue for the trial from a specially prepared

3,000-seat sports stadium, where Bokassa had once lowered a glittering diamond-studded crown on his head, to a colonial courtroom called the "Palace of Justice."

While some 2,000 Bangui residents jostled that morning at the entrance of the stadium to catch a glimpse of their ex-emperor, some 100 journalists, 20 witnesses and hand-picked members of the public squeezed into the old, dusty courtroom. Bokassa, dressed in a sky-blue three-piece suit with a tie to match, and looking cheerful, told the court in his very first sentence "I returned to face my judges." Switching from the charges against him, Bokassa made it clear that he was going to dwell on the embarrassing subject of his gifts of diamonds to former French President Valery Giscard d'Estaing. Bokassa blamed him for his overthrow in what he described as a *"coup d'etat* which violated the sovereignty of my country." He launched a tirade against the French for their interference in CAR, and his attack struck a sympathetic chord among a section of his countrymen that had been demanding the withdrawal of French troops from CAR.

The speech, which was transmitted live from the court by radio, was stirring in its patriotic appeal. Said one French journalist: "Bokassa has many enemies, but as loud cheers outside the court showed, he still has some fans too." After a four-hour hearing, the trial was adjourned until December 15. And Bokassa's conviction, which had initially looked like a foregone conclusion, is now far from certain.

Kolingba, who had widely publicized the trial of Bokassa in the hope of making some political gains, is believed to be finding his home-coming a little bit difficult to handle. Jean Claud Mansion, a French army colonel, who is the chief military adviser to Kolingba, has put his 450-man presidential guard and the 3,000

French troops in CAR on full alert to prevent any disturbances that may be caused by remnants of Bokassa's supporters. It was Mansion who bundled Bokassa unceremoniously into a blue Peugeot car at the Bangui airport when Bokassa arrived from Paris a few weeks ago.

Why Bokassa decided to return home has remained a mystery. He is believed to have been tricked into taking the decision by a woman who convinced him that an agreement had been struck between the French and the CAR government to ensure a reprieve. Bokassa left Paris apparently hoping for a hero's welcome with his gold embroidered uniform packed. But when he found himself in a cell in the hilltop fortress of Camp Duroux, he knew that he was in trouble. He refused food and drinks for two days for fear of being poisoned. A day later, he was told he would be facing trial for murder, theft and cannibalism, which he allegedly committed during his tenure.

During his 15-year reign, Bokassa's personal brutality was legendary. At his Berengo palace, he meted out his own brand of justice, seated on a marble throne under a mahogany canopy, interrogating prisoners who lay on slab of rough concrete opposite him. Most prisoners had no chance in Bokassa's court. It was either they were murderedor mutilated and left to die.

In 1981, Bokassa was convicted in absentia. He and six other people were found guilty of participating in the torture and murder of school children in Bangui in 1979. The six, including his son-in-law, were executed in 1981, following the trial. Bokassa had ordered school children to wear expensive uniforms that he had designed. Students who protested were imprisoned and beaten and 59 of them died in the cell.

The incident led the French to force Bokassa into exile

through a *coup d'etat.* He fled to the Ivory Coast and later moved to Paris, where he barely survived with a pension of £600. His water, electricity and telephone were periodically cut off because he was unable to pay the bills. The ill-treatment is believed to be part of the reasons Bokassa decided to return home.

HELLO, IS MOBUTU STILL THERE?

Ten, nine, eight, seven, six, going--- going --- going. Is Mobutu Sese Seko Kuku Ngbendu Wa Za Banga still there? I mean the supreme guide, and life-president of Zaire. Is he still there?

Forget about the "shinning spear" for a while. Now, who can help me talk sense to a drunken friend who's in grave danger. If there is anyone out there, please take the next available flight to Kinshasha and ask for a man called Mobutu Sese Seko Kaka Mgbendu Waza Banga (the man who killed lions with his bare hands). Otherwise the "lion killer" himself and six million residents of Kinshasa may be dispatched to thy kingdom come by the Laurent Kabila troops, who are demanding for keys to the State House that Mobutu has occupied for 32 years.

Which is why I have lost patience with frenzied diplomats who think they can lure Mobutu into premature exile. They have missed the point of the whole matter and have grossly misunderstood the condition of my friend. The fact is that a power drunk is worse in perception, judgment and discernment than a man soaked in a barrel of Spanish rum.

Like any drunk, a power drunk cannot see well, hear well, reason much or understand much. He is completely stripped of every sense of danger and can even attempt to stop a moving train with his chest. This was the trouble with Samuel Doe. This is the trouble with Mobutu. And this is why we need more than diplomats to guide the "supreme guide" out of grave danger.

Kyungu Wa-Kumnwanza is a Zairean cardiologist based in Kinshasha. Two weeks ago he fled to safety in neighbouring Zambia with his head on his neck. Musangu Muhendi is another Zairean doctor who escaped Kinshasha to Lubumbashi just last week as Kabila closed in on Kinshasha. Kadima Katengwa is an engineer, who fled with his three children to Ndola. He said he sensed bloodbath in the battle for Kinshasha, the only city of substance left under Mobutu's control. But Mobutu has not sensed any danger and has vowed to retain and defend his palatial home till the end.

The Americans, French, Belgians and Canadians are begging Mobutu just as they begged Samuel Doe to jump into their luxury yatch at the shores of Zairean river for safety, all to no avail. Zimbabwe's ruling party (ZAMU-PF) of President Robert Mugabe on Monday congratulated Kabila over his victory so far and requested Mobutu to accept exile while it is not too late. But the comical Field Marshal replied by saying Mugabe had better donated his head for dinner than take him out of his fortified lodge.

The real nemesis of Mobutu however is not Mugabe but "the Museveni boy's spearheaded by the burly warlord called Kabila. Yoweri Museveni, the Ugandan professor of economics, who emerged from the bush to overthrow Milton Obote in 1986, is actually the secret of Kabila's adventure. Kabila has acted beautifully the script written by his good friend Museveni.

Six months ago, Mobutu never really thought Kabila could pose any threat to his dreaded regime. Convalescing on the French Riviera while his country was burning, Mobutu displayed a "Nero-like aplomb," turning a deaf ear entirely to Kabila until the Patrice Lumumba's disciple became unstoppable.

If Mobutu cannot stop Kabila again as it seems, the sick man can at least bank on his legacy. For years his style of rule had combined "charisma with a flair for draconian repression." He dealt brutally with all forms of political agitation and sacked as many prime ministers as his number of years in power.

In an effort to strip Zaire of its European tendencies, he banned bow ties, public kissing and Christmas. And to quote Kevin Fedaro, one of Mobutu's journalist-friends, he successfully marketed his country to The West as a bulwark against Soviet expansion in Africa, until the collapse of the Soviet Union robbed him of his usefulness.

While clinging tenaciously to power, Zaire's plunderer-in-chief has stockpiled much of the country's wealth for himself. He is reported to be worth $30 billion, while his country is steep in debt and poverty. An extravagant man, Mobutu used to fly in barber from New York every two weeks to cut his hair at the cost of $5,000 per cut. Mobutu according to various reports defended his actions by saying he was afraid African barbers could use his hair for charms and witchcraft. Similarly, he has always defended his wealth by insisting that in African tradition, the king owns everything in the kingdom.

The 65-year-old thief surrounded himself with witch doctors from Benin and Uganda, who told him he would live forever if only he lives drinking water alone. For a man whose favorite meal is fufu, the witch doctors' panacea for long life was next to suicide.

But his veritable road to suicide is following the footsteps of Samuel Doe. This is certainly the last days of Mobutu's regime. The countdown to his exit is in the last few digits: five, four, three. I wish the longest serving head of state in Black Africa can spare the world the horror of Samuel Doe.

WHO'S RUNNING THIS COUNTRY?

Pieter Botha, the frail and stubborn president of apartheid South Africa, tottered when he appeared on television last week, soon after returning to work, in defiance of the sack notice served on him by his party, the ruling National Party, NP. His right hand groped unsteadily, missing the target, as he tried to offer a handshake to some waiting State House aides. The black bowler hat in his left hand shook all the way, as he shuffled through the small crowd of loyal aides, into his office.

For his growing band of political opponents in the ruling NP, who had unanimously endorsed Fredrick De Klerk, the party's new leader, to succeed Botha, it was clear that this grand old patron of apartheid was yet to recover from what was officially called a "mild stroke." But Botha, 73, a man reputed to have the "constitution of a bull," proved last week that there was still some fire left in him. He told off his party in an unprecedented political tug-of-war and balked at the decision of the party to forcefully shove him out office. "I have informed them that I have resumed my task as the state president today," Botha told a handful of loyal ministers at his first, formal meeting with them in two months.

The return of Botha to office, after his party had voted to strip him of leadership of the party and named De Klerk as successor, led last week to a complex political deadlock and precipitated a fierce power struggle described as the worst constitutional crisis in South Africa since 1948. Asked *The Beeld,* an Affrickaans language daily, on the stalemate; "Just who, exactly, is running this country?"

The ruling NP had attempted to find an answer to that question the previous day, when it summoned an emergency meeting in Cape Town. After hours of closed-door deliberation during which the party clearly expressed anger at Botha's refusal to step down "honourably," the party's 29-members Supreme Federal Board (an advisory body which consists mostly of the cabinet members and party chietains) and the 133-member party caucus (which is made up of all the party's legislators) voted unanimously to withdraw Botha's mandate to rule. De Klerk, 52, the education minister, who was elected the leader of the party after Botha was struck by stroke, was mandated to replace the ailing Botha. "The national caucus had told Botha to pack his bags," Con Botha, the spokesman of the party announced. According to the party spokesman, "the decision in principle was that the leader of the National Party should be the state president." Indicating that the party was aware of Botha's stubborn determination to hold on to the presidency, the party spokesman warned Botha to "avoid confrontation" and ensure a smooth handover to De Klerk. "This decision leaves the door open for Botha to retire. It is now expected to be merely a matter of time and procedure to arrange for his (Botha's) departure from Tuynhuys (the State House) and public life. There is a strong feeling by the caucus that confrontation should be avoided if at all possible," the party spokesman added.

De Klerk, the president-elect, who was also given a vote of confidence by the party for the way he handled the party's "toughest leadership crisis," added weight to the party's call on Botha to "quietly retire." Said De Klerk after the emergency meeting: "I am in principle the leader-in-chief of the National Party, and the decision was in principle, that the leader-in-chief of the National Party should be the state president."

But as at press time, Botha had continued to ignore De Klerk. In a television interview, he merely described De Klerk as "one of my good advisers" who, he said, was only being "misused by some people" in the party. He stunned party members when he said he would not even call for an early election this year but until the end of his tenure in March next year. In a separate interview earlier in the month while still recuperating in his private residence, in a place called Wilderness, Botha had indicated that he might seek re-election after his five-year term expires.

When Botha put pen to paper to resign the party's topmost post on February 2, two weeks after he suffered a stroke, he had made it clear that he would not compromise his job as president of the apartheid enclave. "In my opinion," wrote Botha in his notice of resignation as party leader, "the role of state president and the role of chief leader of the National Party should now be separated so as to put me in a position to continue just with the role of the president. The time has come when the two offices should be separated so that the president could assume the role of a unified force, free from party politics."

"No way," said an opinion poll, "the time has only come for you to quit and give the party leader the traditional opportunity to double as the head of government." Results of the poll, commissioned by the *Johannesburg Star,* the country's biggest daily newspaper just as the crisis deepened, showed that 47 percent of the people in six major urban areas, believed that it was time for Botha to bow out, while 33 percent wanted him to stay put and 20 percent were undecided. Those who want, and are urging, Botha to stay, are the "beneficiaries of his 10 years of imperial presidency," especially the powerful men in the president's palace, thousands of members of the armed forces, the police and the intelligence service, who staff the pervasive National Security Management System, NSMS. "Those toadies," complained *The Beeld,* "are worse than enemies."

Political pundits and newspaper commentators throughout South Africa last week predicted a prolonged power show-down between Botha and the party-backed De Klerk. "Botha is impregnable," said *The Citizen*, pro-government Johannesburg newspaper, in an editorial March 15. Though the Star said Botha had lost the vital party support, the paper contended that "if Botha chooses to delay elections and stay in office until early next year, he is capable of weathering the storm."

Pik Botha, the country's foreign minister, who also vied for the party leadership when Botha took ill, also foresaw a prolonged battle and suggested last week in London that a "dignified solution" be found to the debacle. The minster, who talked to reporters after a meeting with Prime Minister Margaret Thatcher, said if Botha wants to step down, "he should be allowed to do so with dignity, having served the country creditably well."

As Botha cut short his sick-leave by two weeks and hurried back to work last week, what became more frustrating for the ruling party was that it lacked the legal and constitutional power to force the president out of office before his term of office expires. In addition, says the constitution, it is the president, not the party, who sets the date of a general election. And for that reason, many believe it is only a pacified and gracefully treated Botha who holds the key to solving the crisis. Even if Botha were to change his mind and call for elections right away, analysts believe the damaging public fight would certainly hurt the party and give an edge to its main rival, and Andries Treurnicht's far-right Conservative Party, CP.

As the cracks in the racist ruling party widened into a gulf last week, watchers of the racist enclave were beginning to weigh the implication of the power struggle against the back-drop of The South Africa situation. If De Klerk takes over, will that mean a significant shift, a change of heart or a perpetuation and reinforcement of the apartheid *Status quo,* to the detriment of the black majority? Or, are Botha and his close aides better disposed to speed up the "reforms" – a case of the enemy you know being better than the one you don't know?

In his decade as the country's leader, Botha, stung by international outrage, legalized mixed marriages and scrapped laws that reserved many jobs for whites and prevented blacks from moving into the so-called white cities. Coloured (mixed race) and Asian South Africans were given their own chambers in parliament. But blacks were kept out, and they rejected subsequent attempts to offer them anything less than full voting rights in a colour-blind democracy.

Though clumsy and often adamant, Botha sometimes appeared, at least, to his Western mentors, as the man who realizes the limits of the apartheid system: that apartheid has no place in today's world. Botha, it seems sometimes, also recognizes the limit of South African power: that South Africa cannot sustain forever terrorism against neighbouring Frontline States or afford to go on losing soldiers in Angola or pay for the occupation of Namibia. That much is known about Botha.

But who is De Klerk? What does he stand for? Is he likely to invigorate Botha's cripple reforms? "De Klerk," say the *Economist,* the conservative British magazine, "is unlikely to be in a hurry to (continue) with the reforms." As a leader of the party's Transvaal branch, the bastion of the right-wing racial onslaught, he resented the so-called "wide-ranging reforms" that Botha embarked upon. As education minister, he tried unsuccessfully to cut down the number of blacks enrolling in white universities and to stop political activities there. In his first major address after his election as party leader February 8, De Klerk told the white parliament that the government needed to develop a constitution that protected the rights of both whites and blacks in South Africa. "I want to state unequivocally that the National Party is against domination of any one group by others. White domination, in so far as it still exists, must go," De Klerk said. But he seems to be a master of double-speak as he also said that the government remained committed to segregated neighbourhoods, schools, and other facilities under the principle of "group rights." "A strong emphasis on group rights, alongside individual rights, is based on the reality of South Africa and not on an ideological obsession or racial prejudice," he said. That statement led watchers of The South Africa apartheid government to quickly cast De Klerk in the mould of the grumpy and "blood-thirsty" John Vorster, Botha's predecessor, who was chased out of office by a huge scandal in 1978.

The party crisis is a good enough cause for "small celebration" for the oppressed blacks and coloured peoples of the country, who have often been portrayed by the racist government as people who cannot live together in peace. Said a black South Africa miner in Carltonvile, a Transvaal mining town: "For now, we are not gladiators but glad spectators." At the same time, the power struggle has robbed the gloss off the ruling white party by factionalizing and weakening it, not only against the rival Conservative Party, but the anti-apartheid campaigns.

To worsen the racists' problems, the feud came just at the time the Afrikaners' Dutch Reformed Church (the largest and the white minority's most influential church) made a historic declaration that apartheid is a sin, and expressed guilt for its role in providing spiritual sustenance for the racist ideology. Said the church is a communiqué issued after a week-long meeting: "We confess with humility and sorrow the participation of our church in the introduction and legitimization of the ideology of apartheid and subsequent suffering of people." According to the church statement, "apartheid cannot be accepted on Christian ethical grounds, because it contravenes the very essence of reconciliation, neighbourly love and righteousness." The statement by the more than one million-member church was the most explicit condemnation made by such a large white body, to which Botha and virtually all his cabinet ministers and senior officials of the party belong. For a church that provided the spiritual foundation for apartheid and actually codified racial segregation, its repentance, observers said, is a big blow to apartheid.

The disarray in the apartheid territory was further stirred last week when the government-appointed Law Commission published its report that called for an end to all apartheid laws and the creation of voting rights for the black majority. The

Commission which was appointed by Kobbie Coestsee, the justice minister in 1986 and which included officials of the justice ministry as well as some of the country's top-ranking judges and legal scholars, said all attempts at race reforms were unlikely to succeed unless the government allows the country's 28 million blacks to participate fully in national elections. "A bill of rights will not be accepted as legitimate if the black peoples in South Africa are not given the vote," the Commission said, adding. "The right to vote is one of the fundamental human rights that must be enshrined in any constitution." To this effect, the Commission recommended that as a first step to the new constitution that is being prepared, the present statute books should be purged of all discriminatory legislations.

The embattled government, still virtually incapacitated by Botha's confrontation with his party, is yet to comment on the report. But the church's stance and the Commission's total rejection of the murderous racist ideology is certainly the beginning of the inexorable end of apartheid.

THE KING OF AFRICA

Hero. Legend. Healer. Unifier. Superstar. True Prince of Africa. Citizen of the World. Extraordinary Human Being. Just a few of the names the man has been called. Words, writers have discovered, are not adequate to describe the international impact of this gracious old man. One thing is, however, certain: Nelson Rolihlahla Mandela, 72, anti-apartheid crusader and deputy president of the African National Congress, ANC, emerged in 1990, as one of the most important and admired figures in the world, whose courage, dignity and integrity, and whose humanity and willingness to sacrifice personal gratification for the good of all, captured the imagination of the world.

"Mandela represents the kind of moral leadership we need throughout the world," Zaria Griffin, an American entrepreneur, said in July as Mandela charmed America during his historic trip: "He is something tangible, not just someone in the history book." Another admirer said: "He is among the two or three undisappointing figures in the world." Amanda McMurray, a New York teacher, said in a *Time* magazine interview. "He is unique among heroes. His magnetism is palpable. In this era of cynicism, such legendary figures have all but disappeared,"*Time* magazine itself said. Said Thelma Cagatno, a Guatemalan woman: "I want to see this man."

Jailed and cut off from the world for nearly three decades, his honesty of purpose, steadfastness, tolerance in the face of all odds and political savvy before and after his release February 11, 1990, put Mandela in the distinct domain of legendary political giants such as Mahatma Gandhi, Martin Luther King Jr.; Marcus Garvey and John F. Kennedy. The great difference is that Mandela is a living legend. Everywhere he has set his foot in the world since he regained freedom, a red carpet has been rolled out for him. In Africa, America, Europe, Asia, he got reception worthy of a visiting head of state. In New York, US, more than 750,000 people lined the streets as Mandela waved from a bullet-proof glass vehicle called Mandelamobile. As Mandela delivered his address in July to the packed chamber of the US House of Representatives, his appearance before the American Congress marked the third time in US history that a private foreign citizen had addressed the combined House of Representatives, the Senate, the president's cabinet and the diplomatic corps.

Everywhere Mandela went, he cut the image of a man for all seasons:

The great leader: "When a leader starts thinking of himself as a hero or messiah, then he becomes a problem to his people. He might even become a disaster," he said while visiting Nigeria in May.

The humble public servant: "Whatever honours we receive must be understood to be honours given to the organization to which a man belongs and to the people he represents. It would be in this spirit that I will receive whatever gifts and honours meant for me and my wife," he said also in Lagos last May.

The conciliator: "We don't mean to dominate anybody," he said during his British trip.

The man of peace: "Let not a single head, nor a window be broken when you leave this place," he said in Soweto, February 13, at the end of a rally to welcome him back from 27 years of captivity.

But this is one exhortation the blacks in South Africa have failed to heed, to the dismay of Mandela and the world. Black-against-black violence escalated to an unprecedented record in 1990, claiming more than 1,000 lives since last August. But Mandela has continued to push for peace and normalcy not only between blacks but with the racist government of President Frederick de Klerk. And if there is any glimmer in the horizon that apartheid would be crushed, that hope has been kindled in 1990 and kept aglow by one man: Mandela.

AMERICA

NO TO REAGAN, NO TO APARTHEID

The showdown was imminent. The determination of the American congressmen to impose sanctions on South Africa was as steely as the will of President Ronald Reagan to veto the congress bill on sanctions.

Since he came to office some six years ago, Reagan has successfully used his veto power 44 times. But the latest veto on September 24, to stop the sanction bill against South Africa proved to be one veto too many. The American House of Representatives on September 28, defied personal appeals by Reagan and voted overwhelmingly (313-84) to override the presidential veto.

The legislation prohibits new American investments in South Africa; private or public loans, extensions of credit and the importation of South African uranium, coal, textile, iron and steel, arms, ammunition, military vehicles, agricultural products and gold coins. The legislation also bans the export to South Africa of crude oil, petroleum products, munitions, nuclear energy equipment and computers. And it cuts off direct air link between the two countries.

In the weeks leading up to the veto, the White House was searching frantically for ways of winning enough Republican votes to sustain a presidential veto. Reagan quickly proposed 500 million dollars in new economic aid to the nations of southern Africa called Frontline States. An African trip by the Secretary of State, George Shultz was proposed. An executive order imposing limited new sanctions against South Africa, like the ones announced last year, was to be issued. And just as the House of Representatives was preparing to override the veto, the belated appointment of Edward Perkins, a black career diplomat as the American ambassador to South Africa was announced, all to soften the heart of congressmen. But the gambit did not pay off.

It was too late for Reagan. Americans spoke their hatred for apartheid through their congressmen. No more doubt, the honeymoon between America and apartheid has petered out. A wild wind of confusion and panic blew across South Africa as the long awaited American economic sanctions swung into gear. For The South African government, the eleventh hour attempt to avert the sanctions by threatening American senators not to vote in favour of them turned out to be a fruitless exercise. The threat boomeranged as angry senators overwhelmingly voted 78-21, to join the House of Representatives in overriding President Ronald Reagan's veto of the congressional decision. The American Congress decision dealt a fatal blow to the dwindling support and fortunes of the racist government.

Defeated and desperate, The South African government quickly announced, in retaliation, a ban on the importation of farm goods from the United States. Last year alone, South Africa imported farm goods worth $108 million from the United

States. There are indications also that the racist government may prevent American grains from reaching other southern African countries as South Africa's Foreign Minister Pik Botha hinted in his threat to American senators.

But Reagan, one of the biggest losers in the fight with congress over sanctions, has taken the defeat gamely. Reacting to the congress decision, Reagan said the vote for sanctions portrayed the strength of anti-apartheid feeling in the United States. He expressed his new determination to press Pretoria for change. "The Congress vote should not be seen as the final chapter in America's effort to address the plight of the people of South Africa. Instead, it underscores that America – and that means all of us – opposes apartheid, a malevolent and archaic system totally alien to our ideas," Reagan said. He called on South Africa's government to "act with courage and good sense to avert a crisis and ensure that moderate black leaders who are committed to democracy are not kept waiting."

In the wave of American resentment against South Africa that followed the sanctions, the directors of Harvard University decided to sell $160 million worth of shares that the institution held in companies in South Africa.

The euphoria of the congress' victory immediately spread outside the United States. Officials in some European and African capitals welcomed the American decision as a very bold step towards achieving peace in southern Africa. In Brussels, European Economic Community's diplomats said that the action of the Congress was likely to revive pressure for tougher European Economic Community measures against Pretoria. Members of the EEC who favour sanctions are expected to push hard when the community's foreign ministers meet in Luxembourg, October 27, to consider measures to match those imposed by the United States. It was believed last week that Japan would feel strong pressures to follow suit if the EEC decided to approve tougher sanctions.

In London, Shridath Ramphal, the secretary-general of the Commonwealth, welcomed the Congress vote as "an historic contribution to the ending of apartheid." He said that the sanctions bill demonstrated that the concerted international efforts urged by Commonwealth leaders during a meeting in August were now on.

Robert Mugabe, the prime minister of Zimbabwe and chairman of the Non-aligned Movement, congratulated the American congress for the passage of the sanctions bill. Mugabe dismissed arguments that the sanctions would hurt Zimbabwe more than South Africa. He warned that if Pretoria imposed sanctions against his country, "we will block the payments of dividends and, if necessary, nationalize." While South Africa has investments in Zimbabwean corporations, Zimbabwe has no investments in South Africa.

The British government, in its typical hypocritical attitude to apartheid, said it had no plans to toughen its sanctions against South Africa. But political opponents of Prime Minister Margaret Thatcher said that the American Congress vote had isolated the British leader in her refusal to adopt punitive economic measures to end apartheid. And in Bonn, a West German government spokesman said that the country planned no new sanctions against South Africa. Friedhelm Ost, the spokesman, said the government still doubted the effectiveness of economic sanctions.

West Germany and Britain are the strongest West European op-ponents of measures against South Africa, although the EEC, of which they are key members, had agreed to limited sanctions.

Many African countries hailed the congressional vote but Nigeria was "cautiously optimistic" about the outcome of the legis-lation. Archbishop Desmond Tutu, of 1984 Nobel Peace laureate, who last year called for international sanctions, said the Ameri-can Congress decision was "not anti-South Africa, it is anti-apart-heid and anti-injustice."

South Africa is expected to devise various means of circum-venting the impact of the sanctions. But others say the sanctions will have a far reaching effect on South Africa's Foreign Trade Organization: "The sanctions package will certainly hit hard but it may not be devastating."

The United States was South Africa's most active trading partner in 1985 with exports to South Africa totaling $1.3 billion and imports totaling $1.37 billion. Computer headed the list of American sales to South Africa last year accounting for $87 mil-lion. In addition, South Africa sells more than $40 million worth of agricultural goods and buys more than $108 million worth of agricultural goods every year from the United States.

Economic analysts in Washington calculate that the ban on all new American public and private investments in South Afri-ca would be "certain to slow industrial growth," although they said it was too early to estimate the loss. American investments in South Africa totaled about $30 billion as at last year.

The American ban on landing rights for South African airlin-ers will affect an estimated 95,000 passengers. But South African Airways said last week, that beginning from October 12, it would provide additional flights to London, Frankfurt, Zurich and Lisbon so that passengers could make connections.

But the sanctions can still be overruled if the racist government makes major concessions on apartheid. Said Tutu last week: "The sanctions are conditional. The onus is on The South African government. If it takes the actions we have been advocating then there will be no sanctions."

THE TRAVAILS OF RONALD REAGAN

His first experience was frightening. For five hours, William Casey, 67, the director of the American Central Intelligence Agency, CIA, sat confused, exhausted and short of words as angry Congressmen, December 11, grilled him for his part in the illegal arms shipment to Iran.

He spoke with a deep halting voice. His facts, Congressmen said, were incoherent. His answers to questions too, were mostly evasive. The Congressmen said Casey still had much more to say to help them get to the bottom of the matter. On December 15, barely 24 hours before Casey was to make another appearance before the Congressional committee, the man collapsed in his office and was rushed to a Washington hospital. Doctors diagnosed his sickness as "cerebral seizure," a mild form of heart attack. But this did not end the scandal.

As Casey was convalescing in the hospital last week, the scandal deepened with startling revelations that some $5 million from the arms sales was also diverted apparently through the CIA to a conservative political group in Washington. The money, according to *New York Times,* was used to undermine Congressional opposition to the Reagan administration's support for the Nicaraguan rebels. The allegation sent shock waves through Washington, and presidential spokesman Larry Speakes reacted with a statement that the White House had no evidence to support the allegation. "If the money was used in political campaign," Speakes said, "It would be morally and politically wrong. The White House condemns it and those responsible should be brought to book at the earliest possible date."

The Congressional committee said it was digging further to find out everything that the profits from the arms sales were used for. The emerging details of Casey's role in the whole deal have angered members of the two intelligence committees probing the scandal. Casey, according to committee sources, actually encouraged the White House initiative towards Iran by "providing his own intelligence evaluation."

Contrary to statements made by Casey, the congressional committees discovered last week that the CIA director, together with dozens of arms merchants and foreign middlemen, knew and supervised the 18-month arms sales to Iran. At the same time, the CIA also proposed the idea of keeping the Iran arms sales secret from Congress and President Ronald Reagan later ordered Casey, in January this year, not to notify the Congress about the deal. During his appearance, December 11, before the Congressional Committee, Casey admitted under pressure for the first time since the crisis began, that he knew much about the arms sales and the subsequent diversion of funds to the Nicaraguan rebels through the CIA bank accounts in Switzerland.

As investigations into the scandal gained momentum last week, John Kelly, the American ambassador to Lebanon, further undermined the Reagan administration's claim that it sold arms to Iran mainly to improve links with Iranian "moderates," rather than to obtain the release of American hostages. Kelly was summoned to Washington two weeks ago to explain his role in the affair. He told investigators that John Poindexter, the national security adviser, who lost his job because of the scandal, instructed him to co-operate with another dismissed National Security Council aide, Oliver North in securing the release of the hostages after the arms deal had been struck. According to Kelly, Poindexter stressed that the order was from the president and must be kept secret. Thereafter, Kelly said, all communications with Poindexter on the deal came through a "back channel" using CIA communication facilities.

With the noose tightening around the neck of Reagan and some of his top officials, there were growing pressures last week that the White House chief of staff Donald Regan, secretary of state George Shultz and possibly Reagan himself be compelled to appear before investigators. The White House issued a statement, December 15, to the effect that Reagan had urged all his officials to co-operate with the investigators, and that the president himself would not hesitate to testify, if asked to do so. Reagan's close friend, Senator Paul Laxalb said last week that the embattled president might make a dramatic appearance before the Congressional investigating committee.

But there was a feeling among investigators that the White House was reluctant to co-operate fully with the congressional investigators. Senator David Durenberger, the Republican chairman of the Senate intelligence Committee, reacted angrily after a third administration witness, Robert Earl, a National Security Council official, refused to testify before the committee. Earl said he had not had enough time to prepare his testimony. A fourth witness, Howard Teicher, the senior director of the NSC for political military affairs, also requested additional time to find private counsel hours before Casey was admitted in the hospital. Said Durenberger: "The attitude to dodge investigators smacks a great deal of suspicion. Nobody will escape justice."

There was more bad news for the White House in the shape of an opinion poll conducted jointly by the *Economist* and the *Los Angeles Times* which found that 82 percent of Americans believe that Reagan knew something, if not everything of the diversion of money of the Nicaraguan rebels. The poll also found that 86 percent of West Germans and 87 percent of Britons felt the same way.

Meanwhile, the Democratic leaders who met in Williamsburg, Virginia, to shape the party's agenda for the 1988 presidential campaign, found themselves overwhelmed with a sudden surge of hope that the Iranian scandal would deliver them the White House without much of a fight. Though the Democrats are less eager to capitalize on the scandal, they could not resist the surge to joke about the Iranian affair. Said Charles Robb, the chairman of the Democratic leadership council: "What did the president know about the Iranian affair and when did he forget it?"

NO RESPITE FOR RAMBO

He is tough, stubborn and controversial. President Ronald Reagan calls him a "national hero" but others condemn him as a "common criminal." Last week, amidst growing indications that his troubles would not end yet, Oliver North, 47, the marine lieutenant-colonel at the centre of the illegal arms shipment to Iran, took his travails to God. "I refer you to Psalm 7, verse 1," he said defiantly to reporters keeping vigil at his Washington' suburban home. Reporters who had not read the Bible for years, rushed to their office libraries to discover that the passage reads thus: "O Lord, my God, in thee do I put my trust. Save me from all them that persecute me."

But it seems God may not answer North's prayers, at least for now. As North remained adamant and refused to testify before investigators probing the arms sales scandal, the United States Justice Department announced just before Christmas that it found a secret memo in files of the former National Security Council aide, outlining his plans to divert Iran arms profits to rebel forces in Nicaragua. Attorney-General Edwin Meese informed congressional investigators last week, that the discovery of the secret memo in North's office next to the White House suggests that top Reagan's aides may have broken the law in the Iran affair. Meese who himself is currently under investigations by his own department for his "partial" handling of the early stages of the arms scandal, told investigators that the memo was undated and suggested North had contacted customs officials to try to undermine possible investigations.

Following these grave allegations, frustrated congressmen, who have been unable to get the key figures in the arms scandal to testify, terminated their hearing abruptly, thus paving the way for an independent prosecution (similar to the Watergate prosecution) of the scandal. The Congressional Committee said it was "very disappointed" that there were more questions raised than answers. "The major fact we don't possess', said Senator David Durenberger, chairman of the Senate Committee on intelligence, "is how much money was diverted and who had the overall responsibility for this policy." He repeated one of the key questions in the whole scandal: "Did President Reagan authorize the arms shipment?" Answers to that question are many and conflicting. Robert McFarlane, the former National Security Adviser, said the president gave a verbal approval. Donald Regan, White House chief of staff, said Reagan was opposed to any sales and condoned it only after he discovered it had happened, while Meese, said Reagan approved the first shipment, but "may have been under sedation" when he approved it because the approval was given when the president was recovering from surgery last year.

The second issue still unresolved is who authorized the transfer of the profits from the arms sales to the Nicaraguan rebels at a time when it was illegal for the US to help them because of a Congressional ban on military aid to the *Contras.* Yet another riddle is how much money was involved in the whole deal. Meese said some weeks ago that between $10 million and $30 million was diverted to the rebels. But the rebel leaders have denied getting any of that money. There have been accusations that middlemen misappropriated most of the money. Another issue still to be clarified is whether North acted on his own.

Lawrence Walsh, 74, a former judge and prominent diplomat named two weeks ago as the independent prosecutor, has been saddled with the task of unraveling the puzzle of the arms scandal. Like the special Watergate prosecutor, Archibald Cox and Leon Jaworski, Walsh has been granted full powers of prosecution. He can make criminal indictments if he finds any laws were broken in the secret sales of arms to Iran and the alleged diversion of the profits to the *Contras* and some political groups in America. He is also to "investigate the provision or coordination of support for persons or entities engaged as military insurgents in armed conflict with the government of Nicaragua since 1964." Said the three-man court that appointed him: "Judge Walsh is one of the outstanding lawyers of the nation and brings to this very broad investigation, the judgment and ability acquired through years of experience as a prosecutor, federal judge, government official, trial lawyer and as a recognized leader of the bar of the nation."

In a development that appeared ominously similar to the Watergate Scandal, the *Washington Post* revealed last week that meetings related to the arms deal may have been taped. The White House according to the paper, has a sophisticated communication system that records some telephone calls and meetings and preserves messages and documents written on the NSC computer terminals. The communication system includes an inter-office network used by members of the NSC, including North, who is said to have used the computer system extensively.

While the Reagan administration simmers in the stew of the scandal, one of the president's top advisers and director of the Central Intelligence Agency, CIA, William Casey, who was rushed to the hospital on the day he was to appear before the Congressional Committee, has been recuperating in the Georgetown University hospital where he had a cancerous tumour removed from his brain. Casey may not return to his position as the nation's highest-ranking intelligence officer. His 43-year-old deputy Robert Gates, who has been performing Casey's duty since he took ill, has been tipped to replace him.

The issue of dismissing some of his key advisers, including Casey and Regan, has been a source of serious friction between Reagan and his wife, Nancy, over the past few weeks. Nancy has adopted opposing views to her husband's on some of the key issues and has consistently and publicly asked the increasingly embattled president to weed out most of his top advisers who misled him in the Iranian arms sale. Nancy said last week that Reagan could recover from the current "valley" in his presidency if the two dismissed aides, North and John Poindexter, would publicly reveal their roles in the secret arms deal. "These men should tell the public what they know because they are obviously the ones who know what went on."

THE CONFESSION OF RONALD REAGAN

At last, the man admitted it 'all'. But investigators say all doesn't appear to be all. They want to know all President Ronald Reagan knew and know about the Iran arms scandal that has practically brought the tough talking president on his knees.

For ten weeks, President Ronald Reagan was virtually in confinement. When seen in public, it was only for very brief moments when he waved from the White House lawn or when delivering his carefully rehearsed addresses on television. American newspapers reported that he could only work for 90 minutes a day and needed even longer naps than usual. When he woke up, one reporter said, "it took him hours to focus his thoughts again, his mind wanders and he tells silly, pointless anecdotes."

But on January 28, Reagan, 75, the oldest president in American history, appeared before the American Congress and live on national television for 45 minutes to deliver the annual State of the Union address. While Congressmen were all ears for what Reagan had to say, being his first full-length public speech since the breakout of the Iran's arm sales scandal; millions of Americans were looking out for signs of ill-health. Would he last the 45 minutes? Would he falter or would he sound secure and confident as usual?

Reagan lasted the full 45 minutes. He did not quite miss his lines. But he was no more the cocky and confident Reagan Americans have come to adore for the past six years. The return of the charming, folksy image which White House had hoped for and worked hard to achieve failed to click, even when Kenneth Khachigian, one or Reagan's favorite inspirational speech writers, was brought back from his retirement to add flavor to the speech.

Reagan's speech underscored his determination to keep America strong as well as the desire to reach arms control agreement with the Soviet Union. He, as expected, also reaffirmed his commitment to Strategic Defence Initiative, SDI, popularly known as Star Wars, a subject that has thrown spanners in the works at the recent arms control negotiations with Soviet Union. And on the Iran arms sales scandal, which has grounded his highflying presidency, Reagan said his administration's policy to establish contacts with moderate Iranian leaders was not wrong, neither was it wrong to secure the release of kidnapped Americans in the process.

But he was soon to go on his knees, metaphorically speaking. He accepted "full responsibility for the serious mistakes" made in the arms transaction and the subsequent unauthorized diversion of funds to the rebels in Nicaragua. He confessed and admitted for the first time, that the scandal had become his "one major regret." He promised to cooperate with investigators and do everything possible "to get to the bottom of the matter." He got a rather subdued applause from the congressmen but outside Congress, very few Americans cheered.

The latest polls show that 68 percent of Americans still disapprove of Reagan's handling of the Iran arms deal and a clear majority – 56 percent – thinks he is lying. On January 27, barely 24 hours before he delivered his State of the Union address, Reagan was for the first time grilled in his Oval Office by investigators probing the arms sales scandal. After a one-hour tense session with the president, the investigators, led by former Senator John Towers, left with a promise to keep another date with Reagan.

Reagan was reported to have told the Tower's committee that he did not recall authorizing Israel to sell American arms to Iran. The investigators had for weeks had problems of getting an audience with the president. They had asked "five or six times" for an interview with the president. Repeatedly, they were told it would have to wait until after the State of the Union speech. The investigators rejected the excuse and insisted on having an interview "soonest" since their scheduled deadline for submitting the report was originally set for January 28. In the end, the investigators got their way and Reagan faced them a day before his State of the Union speech.

Since the investigators insisted on "getting more facts to finish their report, White house sources said last week that, Reagan needed to be coached and drilled on how to face the investigators the second time. "The president needs to be drilled on what he knew and when he knew it. This doesn't necessarily mean that he is being taught to fib" a White House sources said.

Earlier on January 21, the first signal of how the new Congress intends to relate with the White House, was indicated. The

Democratic-controlled senate voted to uphold a $20 billion water-cleaning bill which Reagan had vetoed last year. The margin was 93 to six, a majority which implied that the president's view had become irrelevant.

Meanwhile, it is becoming impossible to know who is actually running American foreign policy. George Shultz, the secretary of state, is doing all he can to distance himself from the administration which has encouraged die-hard Reaganites to ignore his opinion. He had been denying that he intends to resign, though few people believe him. Frank Carlucci, the new head of National Security Council, NSC, is said to be "too busy" re-organizing the council to have time for foreign policy matter. Donald Regan, now firmly back in control as White House chief of staff, is believed to know "almost nothing about foreign affairs." Even the special adviser appointed by Reagan some weeks ago to manage the arm sales scandal, former NATO ambassador David Abshire, is said to be scrambling to keep himself informed about the details. What is more worrying, said a report in *London Observer,* is Reagan's air of disengagement and the loss of his old spirit. "The feeling in Washington is that Reagan doesn't really care much anymore."

HOW NOT TO COMMIT SUICIDE

The man has been under severe strain since the Iran arms scandal blew open November, 1986. He was grilled by stern-faced investigators both from the Central Intelligence Agency, CIA, and the Federal Bureau of Investigations, FBI. He testified before several congressional committees as a prime witness in the ensuing investigations. And he dared the White House and accused President Ronald Reagan and several White House officials of telling "total lies" about the secret arms sales to Iran.

But last week, "Robert McFarlane, 49 the former National Security Adviser to Reagan and a key player in the Iran arms scandal had wanted to end it all. He took an overdose of valium tranquilizers in a bid to kill himself but he failed. Doctors at the Bethesda Naval Hospital, where Reagan underwent a prostate surgery a few weeks ago, drained his blood of the deadly drug and put him back to life.

The suicide attempt was not a perfect birthday gift for Reagan who turned 76, February 6. Instead it tightened the noose around the neck of his administration, more so, as congressional investigators were just beginning their second round of probe into the scandal. Already, investigators have given indications that they would brook no-nonsense in their attempt to get to the root of the scandal. In a dramatic and unexpected move, they demanded to see Reagan's personal and private diary. The American president, investigators believe, keeps a confidential diary of handwritten notes for his memoirs, which contain some crucial materials on the "Irangate" scandal.

The first reaction by the White House was to reject the demand for the president's diary which it said contained "private records within the bounds of confidentiality." But as the pressure mounted, the new White House spokesman, Martin Fitzwater announced that Reagan was "willing to make available relevant excerpts from his personal notes." This according to Fitzwater, "is consistent with Reagan's commitment to co-operate fully with investigators. He wants to get to the bottom of the matter and fix what went wrong."

What exactly went wrong and who were responsible for the wrong doing have proved elusive after several months of inquiries by several congressional committees. Investigators say they are still facing three unanswered questions, namely: Was the Reagan administration's Iran policy justifiable? How was the policy made? Were crimes committed as the policy was carried out? The Senate Intelligence Committee's report, the most authoritative account of the affairs to date, which was made public three weeks ago, dealt to some extent with some of the unanswered questions. But the chairman of the committee, David Boren, emphasized last week that their investigation was "preliminary" and did not answer the "principal questions." Said Boren: "We must try to discover whether laws have been broken: who violated the law? Were the violations serious enough to warrant removal from office? Did Reagan violate the law in a manner that will be an impeachable offence?" The Boren committee also listed 14 major "unresolved issues" ranging from "curious activities" in the White House to "intricate financial transactions."

The White House said it would surrender "relevant excerpts" from the private diary, and last Wednesday, it kept the promise thus avoiding a long legal fight similar to the battle over the Nixon's tapes which were handed over only when the Supreme Court decided the president must submit relevant evidence in a criminal investigation.

While Reagan battles with nosey investigators, there were fresh reports last week that a major crisis was brewing inside his cabinet. At the centre of the crisis is Donald Regan, the White House chief of staff. The *Washington Post* reported some republican big wigs as saying that unless the president sacks Regan, the secretary of state, George Shultz would resign and a powerful group of other cabinet officials would follow him.

According to the report, long-term republican faithfuls such as James Baker, the treasury secretary, Malcolm Baldridge, the commerce secretary and Bill Brock, the labour secretary, were determined not to let "Don Regan drag their party to ruin." Amid the looming crisis, Michele Daniels, the White House political director, and the chief political adviser to Reagan, who was in the forefront in demanding for Regan's resignation over his handling of the "Irangate" scandal, resigned in protest. Daniels said he was leaving to pursue "economic opportunities." His resignation coincided with the "retirement" of William Casey, the director of the Central Intelligence Agency, CIA, who had a sudden heart attack two months ago, on the day he was to appear before the congressional committee probing the "Irangate" scandal. In the last two weeks, Reagan has also lost his director of communication, Patrick Buchanan, who was regarded as one of the last "right wing zealots" to desert Reagan.

Similarly, James Miller, the director of the office of management and budget, has already given notice of his resignation. Yet another top official likely to quit soon is Richard Perle, the deputy defence secretary. The spate of resignations has caused serious concern among the Republican law makers. Said Robert Michell, a Republican congressman; "The time is coming when the White House is going to contain just two persons – Reagan and Regan."

THE MAJESTY OF DEMOCRACY

In his moment of glory, George Bush, 64, the president-elect of the United States, was short of words. "Our hearts all full. We love you all. We love this country. God bless America," Bush said as he stepped out of his Houston, Texas home, to meet his supporters soon after he won a massive victory into the most powerful office in the world. "I have just received the most gracious telephone call from the Democratic Presidential Candidate, Massachusetts' Governor Michael Dukakis," he continued smiling nervously, his voice drowned by the deafening cheers of his jubilant supporters. "He has congratulated me and I must tell you, he was very sincere."

It was a historic moment for a man who had just been declared the 41st president of America and became the first American incumbent vice-president in 152 years to capture the White House. Bush won in 40 of the 50 states, polling in all 54 percent of the popular vote. In the process, he amassed 426 electoral votes, 116 more than the 270 required to win the presidency. What was left for Dukakis was only 112 electoral votes which he won in

10 states. This represented 46 percent of the popular vote. For Dukakis, the last minute surge in the polls proved too little, too late. By the time results in 32 states had been flashed on the ABC television and Bush had already swept 26 states and 271 electoral votes, Dukakis knew Bush's next stop would be No. 1160 Pennsylvania Avenue (the White House).

He telephoned Bush and congratulated him. Then, he jumped into his navy-blue suit and went down from his top-floor Boston headquarters to meet thousands of his loyal supporters still waiting to see him. "The man has won," he told the crowd in his concession speech. "He will be our president. We will work with him. Kate (his wife) and I talked to the vice president a few minutes ago and congratulated him."

Dukakis was not the only one who sent a congratulatory message to Bush. World leaders joined Americans in rejoicing with the triumphant Republican candidate. Yasuhiro Takeshita, the prime minister of Japan, while congratulating Bush, said he looked forward to co-operating with his administration in "solving trade problems" between the two countries. Margaret Thatcher, the British prime minister, in her message offered Bush her "warmest congratulations." Said Thatcher: "we offer our staunch support to this leadership of the western world. We are a staunch ally of the US. It was particularly easy during President Reagan's time because I knew him before he was president and he knew me before I was prime minister. We have each other and we had similar views and similar policies. That too is true of George Bush. He has been part of the American success under Reagan."

In China, senior leader Deng Xiao Ping, who described Bush (a former US envoy in China) as an "old friend," expressed the hope that Sino-American relations would continue to "develop in friendship and stability." President Ibrahim Babangida in his message hoped that the existing cordial relations between Nigeria and the US would be further strengthened during the Bush administration. However, diplomatic circles in Africa expressed subdued concern that the US policy towards Africa under Bush may not change for the better, especially with regard to southern Africa's problems. Said Joseph Garba, Nigeria's permanent representative to the UN and the chairman of the United Nations Committee Against Apartheid: "The election of the Republican Party's George Bush will translate to business as usual between United States and South Africa."

As at press time, there was no official comment from Soviet Union on the outcome of the elections, but Radio Moscow said Soviet Union hopes to continue its disarmament dialogue with the president-elect but expressed regret that Bush endorses Ronald Reagan's "Star Wars" and based his foreign policy on "the principle of strength." Similarly, in European financial and stock market circles, reaction to the Bush victory was somewhat cold as a result of what stockbrokers saw as "the vagueness of Bush's economic programme."

Though Dukakis lost to Bush, the Republicans failed to gain control of the American Congress. In the senate and House of Representatives elections conducted also on November 8, the Democrats tightened their hold on the Congress, capturing additional four and two seats in the senate and House of Representatives respectively. One of the re-elected Democratic senators was Llyod Bentsen, Dukakis' running mate, who retained his senate seat, with a landslide victory in Texas. Ironically, Texas voted for Bush the same day, in the presidential race.

The ominous sign of what lay in stock for Dukakis emerged

early morning on Election Day. Dixville Notch, a tiny hamlet in the north-eastern state of New Hampshire, which has a tradition as the first community to cast ballots in US elections, completed their enviable task within a few hours. The result was: Bush, 34 votes; Dukakis three votes. This voting pattern was to haunt the embattled Democratic candidate for the rest of the day, in spite of his frantic last-minute efforts to change to tide. That morning, even while elections were under way and Bush had returned to his palatial Houston home to rest and await the result "the Duke" was still hopping around television stations in Boston doing interviews and urging voters to go out and give the country a November surprise." At a point, he telephoned Jesse Jackson, the black civil rights leader, and urged him to "go out and campaign." Jackson obeyed. But that was medicine after death.

"The Duke" was facing an electorate that had already made up its mind and appeared to be satisfied with the way the country had been faring under President Ronald Reagan. To complicate his mission, Dukakis had allowed the Bush campaign to successfully label him as a "liberal" who is "right out of the mainstream of American political values." His campaign managers had disregarded and miscalculated the effect of the negative campaign mounted by Bush against him. So much distortion had been done to his records and image, the smear had stuck. He had tumbled from a double-digit lead in the opinion polls to a double-digit deficit, in a bitter and "sound bite" campaign that was noted more for "idiotic political insults" than sensible political issues. By the time the Dukakis campaign shed their gentleman galland and poised for a fight the fight was over. The battle had been won and lost, and the polls said so.

Despite his gloomy prospects, Dukakis ignored the polls and

put in a final sprint, worthy of any of his predecessors including the obsessive "marathon man," Jimmy Carter. Sleeping only in his campaign plane, he criss-crossed America in a frenzy of last-minute "tactical switches." In the last two days, he flew to Washington, Cleveland, St. Louis and then back west to San Francisco, before he headed home to Boston via Los Angeles, Iowa, New Jersey and Ohio. He shed his stiff, technocratic style. He sharpened his message. His popularity surged and sent jitters to the Bush camp. "They are slipping and sliding, we are rocking and rolling," Dukakis told a cheering crowd at Ohio. Pollsters, for once started talking about an "upset."

Dukakis, "the broccoli of American politics," as he is sometimes called had hoped to confound opinion polls and repeat the feat of President Harry Truman, who was written off by pundits in 1948, but who turned the tables in the last minute to floor Republican challenger Thomas Dewey who was billed to win by landslide. "Do a Truman," thousands of supporters shouted at his last rally in Cleveland on the eve of the election. "They talk a lot about October surprise. Tomorrow, we're going to give them a November surprise," Dukakis said, rolling up the sleeve of his shirt and punching the air. The new Dukakis forced the Bush campaign to return to the television to mount a last-minute million-dollar attack on Dukakis, with a fierce five-minute advertisement criticizing the Democratic candidate for his approach to issues ranging from crime to the environment.

Bush, who had almost ended his campaign, swung back in a hectic bid to bolster his narrowing lead over Dukakis. He mocked Dukakis as a "desperado" and promised to continue with the prosperity of the Reagan years. Reagan, "the grandest cowboy of them all," whose "coat-tail" Bush hung on to success, headed back to California, the state with the largest electoral votes of 47. He pilloried the "Doomo-crat," urging them to vote for Bush. "I feel a little like I'm on the ballot myself this year," Reagan said in his velvet baritone voice. His audience broke into a prolonged cheer. "Reagan for Pope," they shouted. Reagan's aides joined in the final onslaught too. "He really likes George Bush," Marlin Fitzwater, the White house spokesman, said. "And he's truly angry at Dukakis for misleading people about his liberal beliefs and about the Reagan record."

As part of the last-minutes strategy by the Republicans, Dan Quayle, the vice-president-elect, whose nomination as Bush's running mate nearly cost the Republicans the White House, was consigned to campaign mainly in remote hamlets, where he would be very far away from the television cameramen and would not be heard by reporters. But whether in a remote hamlet or in New Hampshire, Quayle remained a major final-hour campaign topic hoisted by the Democrats to raise doubts about Bush's ability to make good decisions. Said Dukakis in his last stop at San Francisco: "This Quayle is a crisis who has to be managed."

But last week, the president-elect sought to blunt the criticism and taunting that accompanied the choice of Quayle, when he named James Baker, his campaign manager and former treasury secretary, as his secretary of state. The appointment, the first by the president-elect, was widely applauded. Said George Shultz, the out-going secretary of state: "Baker is a wise choice and Bush has taken a good step in the right direction." As Bush made a triumphant return to Washington November 10, he was full of poise and grace as he spoke to thousands of supporters led by Reagan, who turned up at the airport to welcome the new president. "We can now speak the most majestic words that democracy has to offer: "The people have spoken," he said.

WORLD

FROM IRON LADY TO WOODPECKER

Some call it the worst political crisis of her 11-year grip on power. Others described the crisis as her veritable political graveyard. One way or another, Margaret Thatcher, 65, British prime minister and one of the best known world leaders, is in deep trouble. The Iron Lady, as she is popularly called around the world, stands a good chance of losing the leadership of the Conservative Party, this week, when the faithfuls meet to decide whether or not she could continue to lead them.

Amid a fierce and devastating attack by Geoffrey Howe, her deputy, who resigned in protest two weeks ago, another party stalwart, Michael Heseltine, stepped forward last week to seriously challenge Thatcher for her top jobs as prime minister and Conservative Party leader, in an epic election that is scheduled for Tuesday, November 20. If conservative members of parliament, MPs, give their overwhelming votes to Heseltine, Thatcher would be automatically overthrown and Heseltine named prime minister on the spot.

The resignation of Howe and his damaging indictment of

Thatcher's government strongly reinforced Heseltine's political platform last week and could help to deal a mortal blow on Thatcher's enviable political career. Heseltine, the 56-year-old flamboyant politician, popularly called Tarzan, looked quite ready to snatch the job, when he told his supporters: "See me on Tuesday at No.10" (Prime minister's official residence on Downing Street).

But Thatcher, the longest serving British prime minister this century, did not seem to be in a hurry last week to quit No. 10, as she reduced the tough political battle to metaphor of cricket game, Heseltine's well-known favourite sport. The Iron Lady promised she will "knock" Heseltine and his supporters "for six." As she put it: "I am still at the crease though the bowling has been pretty hostile of late. And in case anyone doubted it, I can assure you there will be no ducking the bouncers, no stone-walling, no playing for time. The bowling's going to get his all-round the ground. That's my style."

Come Tuesday, Thatcher said she will send Heseltine's hopes crashing because as prime minister, she has broken the "post war mould of bureaucracy and decline." Flaunting her record, Thatcher said her government has set standards of sound finance not seen since the World War II. "Most striking of all," she said, "for the last eight years, we have maintained our share of world trade ending the progressive decline that dates back to 19870." Thatcher got a rousing ovation at the Lord Mayor's banquet where she fired the salvos.

But most of the conservative MPs who will decide her tenancy at Downing Street Tuesday, are not applauding so loudly. By press time, the Heseltine camp had reported about 100 "hard pledges with more to come." Thatcher needs a simple majority of 214 of the 372 MPs to win outright. But Heseltine could force a second ballot if he polls up to 159 votes, which is just one vote short of the simple majority Thatcher requires. After Howe's scathing attack on Thatcher, pundits said Heseltine's sure votes had risen to about 140 and he may snatch a dozen more uncommitted votes before "Super Tuesday." In case of a second ballot (that is if Heseltine gets up to 159 votes), other candidates army join the race. Douglas Hurd, the foreign secretary and John Mayor, Chancellor of the Exchequer are already tipped as strong contenders to be called upon by the Thatcher camp to do the "Stop Heseltine Job." Political tacticians, even in Thatcher's camp, said last week that if Heseltine gets just more than 120 votes, Thatcher would be "so seriously damaged," she will become a lame-duck Prime Minister.

Conservative MPs are sharply divided between the two candidates and precisely along the lines of those who favour Thatcher's style of leadership and cautious approach to a federal Europe on one hand and those who are averse to one or both issues on the other hand. Said Teddy Taylor, MP and one of Heseltine's most outspoken critics: "If the Conservative Party is stupid enough to be led into unseating Thatcher, I think the savage backlash from the constituencies will be unbelievable. MPs won't know what hit them. You will find large scale resignations." Thatcher's supporters are also drumming up the Gulf crisis, saying it is not the best time to sack Thatcher Said William Whitelaw: "I believe profoundly that at this time, our country badly needs her courageous, determined leadership as prime minister." But for Howe: "I fear the prime minister is increasingly leading herself and others astray." Norman Tebbit, the former party chairman, described the crisis in the party as a "civil war."

The opposition Labour Party is enjoying every bit of the "civil war." Neil Kinnock, Labour leader, capitalized on the Conservative Party's disarray and said what is actually needed was not the conservative change of leadership but a general election because "the Tories are now incapable of governing." The Labour Party, which is currently enjoying a 14-point lead in public opinion polls, however, prefers Thatcher's victory over Heseltine. Said one Labour MP: "Heseltine is our worst fear. He is the only one who has stood up to her openly and if he has stood up to her, he might be seen as a strong leader. Besides, he will not be haunted by the poll tax issue. He is much closer to us (Labour on Europe) and he is popular, good-looking, well-known, and full of energy. He'd make Kinnock look old. He could be tailor-make for the job." The Labour, therefore, prefers a "bitterly contested election," which should even go to a second ballot, in which Thatcher nominal charge of a sharply divided party.

However, Thatcher is a known survivalist, whose "obituaries" as one commentator said, "have a habit of proving premature." But whatever the outcome of the epic political clash, Thatcher, her Conservative Party and probably British politics, which she has dominated for the past decade, may never be the same again.

END OF THATCHER'S ERA

It was a stormy end to an era. After dominating British politics and the global stage like a colossus for more than a decade, Margaret Thatcher, 65, the longest serving British leader this century, threw in the towel last week, sending shock waves around the world. Under intense pressure from her party members in the last two weeks, Thatcher, known the world over as Iron Lady, was bended, smelted and then became a plastic lady. By 7.am, November 22, when she summoned an emergency meeting of her cabinet to break the news of her resignation which was helped along by Geoffrey Howe's resignation, the deputy prime minister, two weeks ago, she looked like any other leader in deep trouble, emotional and melancholic: "It's a funny old world. Here I am with all the majority and yet I have to go," Thatcher said, trying to force a smile.

It was not a smiling matter for her faithful cabinet members, most of whom could not immediately imagine a Conservative Party without Thatcher's resolute leadership. Thatcher had spent a sleepless night alone struggling to decide whether to go on a full scale political war with Michael Heseltine, her arch-rival, who had fought her to a standstill, or bow out honourably and save the party from a bitter "civil war." Now, with pains in her heart, she told her cabinet, she had decided to quit "in the interest of the party." She pleaded with members of the cabinet to unite behind one of the cabinet members who would be vying for her job against Heseltine. Kenneth Clarke, Education Secretary and Thatcher's loyalist told reporters, "it was a very, very emotional and sad cabinet meeting."

By 12.45pm, last Thursday, Thatcher, dressed in a blue skirt-suit, emerged from 10, Downing Street, her home for almost 12 years, slid into her black Rover car and headed straight for Buckingham Palace to tender her resignation letter to Queen Elizabeth II, the British monarch. As British political ritual and protocol demand, Thatcher asked the Queen to name a new prime minister. But the Queen would not do that until Tuesday this week, November 27, after the Conservative Party leadership election.

Soon after Thatcher's resignation hit the airwaves, Douglas Hurd, the foreign secretary and John Major, the Chancellor of the Exchequer (treasury chief), two Thatcherites, announced they were in the race with Heseltine, for the posts of party leader and prime minister. For Thatcher, the decision to step down was a sharp turning point of a brilliant political career that spanned more than three decades. Only the previous day, she had boasted on her return from Paris: "I will fight on. I fight to win."

In Britain, Europe and the rest of the world, the news was received with mixed feelings, shock and consternation. "This is a very sad day for all of us," Cecil Parkinson, British transport secretary said. Neil Kinnock, Labour Party leader said he was "delighted" by Thatcher's departure but praised her courage to step down and called for immediate general elections. "I will frankly say that I respect the manner of her departure. No doubt about it I have respect for her courage and resilience but she has left behind an infamous chapter in the political history of Britain," Kinnock said.

Other Labour Party leaders trying to score political points accused the Conservative Party "war lords" of viciously "forcing" Thatcher out of office. Said Gerald Copman, Labour Member of Parliament, MP: "I am pretty disgusted by the way she has been forced out, not by a general election, in which she is defeated by the votes of the people, but by some selfish, backroom, Conservative Party war lords." Heseltine, who sounded a bit uncoordinated in his reaction, said Thatcher's departure "opens the way for the election of a new leader."

In the Soviet Union, where Thatcher is held in high esteem, people interviewed on the streets expressed sadness and sympathy about her exit. Guedy Grasmoy, Soviet foreign ministry spokesman praised Thatcher's "immense stature" in the world and said no matter who emerged as the new British prime minister, "good relationship between the two countries will continue uninterrupted." George Bush, American president, who was in Saudi Arabia with the American troops said Thatcher was "an outstanding prime minister and staunch ally of the United States." Ronald Reagan, former American president said that during his tenure he "always counted on her (Thatcher's) loyal and wise counsel as well as strong leadership." One analyst on American Cable network News, CNN said, "When Reagan was president, it was a very special relationship between Thatcher and Reagan, and when Bush came in, it became a very special relationship between America and Britain." Saddaam Hussein, Iraqi president said: "I had no personal quarrel (over the Gulf crisis) with Thatcher but I am not displeased by her resignation." There was no negative reaction in the financial market. The *Financial Times* share index in London was up by 10 points, while the pound sterling gained about one cent against the US dollar.

Three hours after submitting her resignation letter to the Queen, Thatcher arrived at Parliament to deliver her valedictory speech and defend her record of all most 12 years of uninterrupted rule. Sounding confident throughout the session, Thatcher enumerated her achievements in a superbly delivered speech. Said the fallen prime minister: "Britain stands tall today in the councils of Europe and the world. We have given power to the people on an unprecedented scale. We have given back control to the people over their own lives and their livelihood by curbing the monopoly power of trade unions to control and even victimize the individual worker, we have enabled families to own their homes, we have enable parents have a say on which school is right for their children, which course is best for the school leaver, which doctor to choose to look after their health and which hospitals they want for their treatments." Thatcher criticized the Labour Party for seeking power to limit these freedom and choices.

According to Thatcher, II million people in Britain now own shares, while 7.5 million people have now indicated their interest on buying electricity shares alone. In addition, she said two million more jobs have been created and though she admitted that inflation has risen to 10.9 percent during her tenure, she said it is a lot less than 26.9 percent that was recorded during the last Labour government. Said Thatcher: "Mr. Speaker, there is a reward for hardwork. Four of the industries we have privatized are now in the top ten British businesses. At the very bottom of the list of one thousand British businesses lie the nationalized industries. There have been 400,000 new businesses since 1979. It is our companies that now lead the world in pharmaceuticals, in telecommunications and in aerospace. These are rewards for hardwork." She was still her fighting self all the way.

However, Labour MPs who questioned Thatcher for her records accused her of "succeeding only in widening the gap between the rich and the poor." Said one Labour MP: "She (Thatcher) says she has given power back to the people. Those people, over two million of them are jobless. Is that giving power back to the people?" The house erupted with "No -o-o." At press time, a confidence debate tabled by Kinnock against Thatcher, was still being debated. Political punters, however, said it was not likely to go against Thatcher since her party still controls an overwhelming majority.

As Thatcher defended her Downing Street years, world attention was already shifting quickly to the battle for the next occupant of 10, Downing Street. Who wins on Tuesday? Heseltine, Hurd or Major? Political pundits in Britain agree that with the exit of Thatcher, the battle is much more confused now and would be "very bloody." In the first ballot last week, Heseltine won 152 of the 372 Conservative votes, while Thatcher won 204, just two votes short of victory. Sixteen MPs abstained from voting. Some analysts said last week that Heseltine had already established a "commanding lead and momentum" to see him through this week. Opinion polls two weeks ago showed Heseltine was better placed than any other Conservative Party candidate to win a general election. He is ready to scrap the controversial poll tax, a flat tax on every man and woman, irrespective of his or her income, which made Thatcher very unpopular. The "caring capitalist" as Heseltine is called, is also a "great European," ready to go along with other European countries on the concept of federal Europe.

But Heseltine is not likely to get the crucial support of Thatcher's faithfuls. Said John Macgregor, an analyst on British ITN television: "Thatcher's supporters are very angry about the way Thatcher has been treated and they will take a revenge on Heseltine and unite either behind Hurd or Major." Steel, the former Liberal leader predicted that Hurd is likely to emerge as prime minister "because he is very respected by party members." But probably the man to watch is Major, 47, the youngest of the contestants who is said to have the secret support of Thatcher. Said Michael Stern, conservative Party MP: "(John) Major represents the new generation of Conservatives. He has stature, he has the fire. He is one candidate who can actually unite the party." However, Major is regarded by some party faithfuls as "very new in the scene and the man who will carry the can for the fat deficit and other unpopular economic legacies of Thatcherism.

Given the good credentials of the three candidates, Hugh Dyke, a Conservative backbencher, described the election as "an agony of choice," Said Dyke: "All three will make excellent prime ministers." Gerald Copman, a Labour MP, however, saw the three in a different light. "Heseltine is a very shallow man. The other contenders are all rag bags who have put Britain in its present economic predicament. They don't make any great difference to us," Copman said. Labour MPs say they are poised to wreck any "honeymoon," the Conservatives hope to enjoy, with the departure of Thatcher. However, Hurd, the foreign secretary is considered by many Labour leaders as the strongest choice the Conservatives could make. He is judged to have had a "good Gulf crisis," impressive under pressure, and a man who walks the world stage like a statesman and who would be a unifying force for a party which had torn itself apart.

A BULLY ON THE RUN

B attle weary and broke, the Soviet Union is desperate to quit Afghanistan, the small neighboring state it invaded on Christmas Day 1979. Soviet leader Mikhail Gorbachev, in a dramatic turn of events, February 8, said the estimated 115,000 Soviet troops in the tiny wild country will pack its deadly load ready to go home within three months. In just 10 months, he promised, no Soviet boot will be found anywhere in Afganistan. This is a time span surprisingly close to the eight months persistently demanded by America and its allies, which the Soviets hitherto blatantly rejected.

Gorbachev, whose novel approach to the management of Soviet affairs is gradually dismantling the foreign policy legacy of his predecessors, said the pull-out would be implemented regardless of whether the warring Afghan people themselves are ready to live in peace or not. The Soviet leader also indicated that his government had no interest anymore in who rules Afghanistan. Whether the incumbent Soviet backed government in Afghanistan remains in power after the withdrawal, according to him, is "purely an internal Afghan issue."

The only important conditions given by Gorbachev are that Afghanistan and its neighbor, Pakistan, the principal supporter of the rebels, sign an agreement on mutual non-interference, as well as an international guarantee (already agreed to by America and its allies) on non-interference in Afghan internal affairs. To meet the deadline for the withdrawal of its troops, the Soviet Union is even seeking the assistance of the American government to help iron out some frictions threatening to delay the withdrawal. "There are considerable chances," said Gorbachev, "that the next round of UN sponsored peace talks on Afghanistan (billed for March 15 in Geneva) will become the final one."

The announcement by Gorbachev was the clearest indication yet that he was seeking to rapidly extricate his country from a conflict that he described in his speech as a "bleeding wound" for his country. Reactions to the announcement were mixed. The Reagan administration made a positive assessment of the Gorbachev plan. Marlin Fitzwater, White House spokesman, said Gorbachev "does seem to take a very good step in the right direction" while the State Department termed it "a positive signal of serious Soviet intent to withdraw from Afghanistan." In New York, Diego Cordovez, the United Nations mediator in the Afghan peace talks, said Gorbachev "has closed the gap (of conflict) to a point where I think a specific agreement at Geneva is foreseeable."

However, in Pakistan, the government of Mohammed Zia ul-Haq expressed misgivings about the Soviet withdrawal timetable. Top government officials insisted the Soviets could not "runaway" unless it helps to set up an interim coalition government in Kabul, capital of Afghanistan. Said Zain Noorani, Pakistan's minister of state for foreign affairs: "Pakistan will sign the Geneva agreement with the legitimate government of Afghanistan as and when the time for signing same comes."

The statement infuriated Soviet officials, who accused Pakistan (which is representing the rebels at the UN talks) of sabotaging moves to end the civil war. But far more threatening to the Soviet plan is the disarray among the various guerrilla groups fighting to overthrow the soviet-backed regime; they remained bitterly divided, especially on the proposal for an interim government. Said Younis Khalis, head of three moderate guerrilla groups: "I cannot accept any coalition with the present Kabul regime." With some of the guerrilla groups determined to fight their way to "total victory," some observers said last week that the Soviets may be forced to prolong their stay to prevent a military defeat or the kind of disorganized, humiliating withdrawal the Americans suffered in Vietnam in 1974. But in spite of the looming specter of an escalation of the war, the Soviets appeared bent on leaving Afghanistan, "reconciliation or no reconciliation."

The scenario reflects, for the Soviets, a deep frustration with the misadventure in Afghanistan. After eight years of bloody efforts to stabilize Afghanistan, which have resulted in the death of more than 18,000 Soviet soldiers and airmen, the Soviets have found that they are no way near their objective. Though an estimated 80,000 Afghan rebels have been killed, the resistance by the guerrillas continues to be formidable as more than three quarters of the country's villages are controlled by them. By one conservative estimate, the Soviets, last year alone, lost 270 military aircrafts worth about $2.2 billion.

In a recent poll by the Soviet Academy of Sciences and the French Poll Organization, IPSOS, 53 percent of the respondents in Soviet Union favoured total disengagement. They voiced unusually acute awareness of the terrible toll the war is exerting on the country's military as extensively reported on Soviet television. In letters only recently published in some Soviet newspapers, men who have served in the war complained that Soviet reporters had, over the years, given false impression of the fighting. Soviet citizens at home, they said, were denied the knowledge that thousands of Soviet troops were being killed continuously. A television documentary aired early in January was more daring. It informed its viewers that "cease-fire, reconciliation and peace are on the lips of every Afghan," suggesting that the Soviets are the war mongers. Said a *Pravda* commentator last month: "Everybody is starting to know the truth of the situation and there is grumbling everywhere... the sort of thing that broke American policy in Vietnam."

Even worse, the Soviet-backed Afghan leader, Bullah Najib, has failed to gain significant support despite the Soviet sponsored campaign for national reconciliation. More than a third of Afghanistan's pre-war population have fled abroad, while the rebels say the reconciliation campaign is a "puppet show." Even Najib's own brother, Khali defected to the guerrillas last November, a blow which the Afghan leader tried to brush aside as a sign of "democratic spirit now flourishing in Afghanistan." In the face of these setbacks and the increasing cost of the war, Gorbachev seems to be very eager to stop the "bleeding wound" in order to concentrate on his *perestroika* (economic reconstruction) at home.

Apart from halting the drain on the economy, ending the intervention in Afghanistan will yield diplomatic benefits for the Soviet Union. For one, an agreement to end foreign involvement in Afghanistan looks like the only possible substantial platform for the Gorbachev-Reagan summit, which is due to take place in Moscow in June. A "successful summit" is needed by both sides – by Reagan to boost the Republican Party's chances in the US presidential elections in November, and by Gorbachev to enhance his standing at the important Soviet Communist Party convention, also in June. A bigger pay-off for Gorbachev may come in improved relations with China.

But then, doubts still persist even in the Soviet Union whether Moscow really means to withdraw from Afghanistan and abandon its Afghan allies. "You can't just pack and go," says a Soviet official quoted by the Voice of America. "People will ask, "why did my son die?" The problem is why did we fight for eight years? What is the result? We have to say something – that Afghanistan is stable or something. You have to explain somehow." Many observers believe the Soviets have tried to weave Afghanistan into a net of relations with Moscow that will remain after the withdrawal. "To think that you can remove all Soviet influence is unrealistic," Slieg Harrison, a US expert on Afghanistan, said last week.

Even if the Soviet Union wants to keep its promise, diplomats in Kabul say its plans for an orderly pull-out will be thwarted by "the blood-thirsty chaos that is part of Afghanistan culture." The Afghan rebels, who are mainly sustained by US financial support, believe they can obliterate Najib and his supporters. On the other hand, Najib and his supporters believe it will be impossible for the rebels to remove them from office. Whether the Soviets quit or tarry awhile, the ethnically divided Afghan warring factions are still expected to be hostile to one another. Said a UN diplomat: "There will always be fighting in Afghanistan – Afghan versus Afghan."

REBELS ON THE MOVE

Along the narrow streets of Jali, a small hilly town in the Paktia province of Afghanistan, little Afghan boys dressed in dirty native tunics played on top of a shot-down Soviet helicopter. They fingered and fiddled with every part of the intimidating wreckage, marveling at its size and screaming happily in their native *Urdu* tongue. Some reached for empty shells strewn on the ground. Other dashed away and jumped on top of destroyed tanks. Down the street, another group of boys made an effigy of a Russian soldier and dressed it in dark green woolly rags. Armed with sticks, they sang, as they thrashed the effigy into pieces.

For these kids, the war between their parents, called Mujahideen, and the Afghan soldiers seems to be terrific fun. But for their American-backed parents, who are fighting to oust the Soviet-backed government in Kabul, capital of Afghanistan, the bloody war is no child's play. The guerrilla tactics they have adopted since 1979 are giving way to a conventional warfare. Missiles, rockets, bombs and tanks of the computer age, are finding their way to the war fronts. Death toll on both sides, in the last three weeks, has risen steeply. The Geneva Accord of April 14, which set in motion the withdrawal of Soviet troops from Afghanistan and a possible end to the conflict, has been severely threatened. The Russians are slowing down their withdrawal as the rebels unleashed a relentless attack on their convoys. Said Shyid Hussain, an Afghan engineer and guerrilla officer: "It's as if this war has only just begun."

Behind the escalation of the conflict is the calculation by the Mujahideen, (defenders of the faith), that they can easily depose Muhammed Najibullah's regime and take over the State House in Kabul, as soon as the Soviets complete their withdrawal. Boosted by the additional arrival of tonnes of sophisticated weapons from America, they have now taken over three provinces abandoned by the Soviets. The provinces include Paktia, Nangarlar and Logar, where the last column of Soviet troops departed on June 15. At the moment, the Mujahedeens claim they are just 30 kilometres away from Kabul, although there is no independent confirmation of this claim. Kabul Radio, however, admitted for the first time last week that rocket attacks by the rebels on June 13, destroyed a section of Kabul's air field, killing a number of guards on duty. Another airport, at Sindad in Farah province, was similarly destroyed by a ground-to-ground missile. About 80 Soviet troops were reported killed during the missile attack, while several Soviet helicopters at the airport were destroyed.

Casualty has not been limited to the Soviet-Afghan side. The Resistance, as the Mujahideen is also known, has suffered great losses in men in two weeks of fierce fighting to capture Kandahar and Jalalabad, two key cities which lead to the strategic Torkam-Khost-Kabul road. Though the rebels played down their losses, claiming that they had killed about 217 government troops, injured 300 and captured 200, they recorded more casualty than their enemies. One rebel commander, who described the casualty figure as "extremely high," said 10,000 Mujahideens from all seven rebel groupings were involved in the Kandahar offensive which began on May 31. As at June 17, when *Newswatch* visited one of the Mujahideen military camps in Pershawa, more troops were being recruited and trained for the Kandahar and Jalalabad fronts. The fighting, according to one of the rebel officers, is particularly heavy inside Spin Buldak town, where rebels "reinforcement is urgently needed."

Though the Afghan government troops June 14, lost Air Force Major-General Aziz Sarwari in the battle in Kandahar, they still maintained superiority in the air, often striking deep into Pakistan, where the rebels are headquartered. The Soviet-backed government troops are known to be well-equipped and very effective on the ground. Their on-going retreat and surprise abandonment of about 10 major garrisons, some without any visible threat, is seen as a trap, which rebels should try to avoid. Said Naim Mahjrooh, Mujahideen strategists and editor, at the Afghan Information Centre, AIC: "By abandoning outposts and strengthening the cities, the (Kabul) regime may be intending to lure the Mujahideen into the cities and, therefore, into large set-piece battles. We are not suited to this kind of warfare, neither do we have the equipment, nor the organization necessary." The rebels, Mahjrooh said, are at their best and most effective in waging guerrilla warfare. "If we are tempted to concentrate our forces, the consequences could be disastrous," Mahjrooh told *Newswatch.*

Not many Mujahideen commanders are ready to accept Mahjrooh analysis. They believe the Soviet-backed troops had to run away because of Mujahideen's superiority in the battle field.

They say that the morale of the Kabul troops is low because of the decision of the Soviets to withdraw their backing. "They have been abandoned, besieged and defeated. What they do now is just to waste ammunition, shoot guns at random to scare us as they retreat," one fierce-looking rebel officer told *Newswatch* in a military camp in Pershawa.

In Kabul, thousands of troops arriving from the abandoned regions and garrisons have been deployed to replace the Russian soldiers in cities and other strategic locations. Indications are that Kabul actually needs the troops to ensure the security of the home-bound Russians between Kabul and Kairatan Port. However, the Najibullah administration said it was withdrawing troops from the Pakistani border provinces and garrisons, in order to create a demilitarized zone for the return of the 2.7 million Afghan refugees, resident in Pakistan, in accordance with the Geneva agreement.

This claim may be true to some extent but not in the case of Zazi, a small garrison town near Pakistan. In Zazi, the Afghan soldiers were forced out. Before they departed, they mined the city and set booby-traps. The mines, rebels soldiers argue, could not have been aimed at refugees. Abkar Jan Darwikai, a commander with Mahaz, one of the rebel factions, told reporters that while the Afghan soldiers were laying the mines, the rebels surrounded and ambushed the Afghan garrison for eight days. On June 15, the rebels stormed the garrison from different directions. The garrison of 700 Russian-backed troops made a last minute bid to escape by helicopters. The Mujahideens launched a close range attack with their shoulder carried anti-aircraft missiles, mortars and recoilless rifles. The bodies of 30 soldiers including six Russians were alter picked up in the wreckage. Among the war booty captured at Zazi were 33,000 artillery guns, 20 military trucks, two tanks, 200 boxes of helmets, etc. As the Mujahideens celebrated their victory from one end of the town to another, they stepped on booby-traps and mines. More than 100 rebels were killed while some 230 arrived hospitals in Pershawa without legs, hands or both.

The morale of the rebels, however, still remains very high. Determination bordering on religious fanaticism is the propelling force. "We are fighting against a power that is called superpower but we believe there is no superpower except Allah," Shaharuk Kran, a medical doctor and chief of army staff of one of the rebel groups said. "This is a war between the Warsaw Pact and the Afghan people," Ghulam Kurshan, 64, a senior editor with Afghan Media Resources Centre said. "We have killed and captured soldiers from Cuba, Yugoslavia, Poland, etc. *InSha Allah* (By the grace of God) we are at the verge of disgracing Warsaw Pact." Inside the captured Afghan territories as well as in Pershawa, the border town between Pakistan and Afghanistan where the rebels are based, they pray and dream of the day Kabul would be in their hands and peace would return to Afghanistan. For now, the rebels claim that 80 percent of the countryside is under their control. "In this hilly countryside," said Mahjrooh, "there is no way the Russians or any other power can defeat us... Fighting is normal for us here. The (Russians) don't know where to find us, or what to do and this makes things very difficult for them."

Things seem to be getting even more complicated for the Russians especially with the difficulty in implementing the Geneva Accord. The accord had envisaged the withdrawal of Russian troops within nine months. After the occupation of Afghanistan for nine years, which they found difficult to justify even at home, the Russians had hoped to withdraw peacefully with some respect and prestige. But with arms from America and Pakistan, the Afghan rebels have harassed, molested and humiliated the Russians in their retreat. Last week, the accord appeared doomed. On Thursday, June 16, the Soviet Union became so furious; it summoned Pakistani ambassador in Moscow, Bhahid Amin, to the ministry of foreign affairs for tongue-lashing. "Your country is committing a gross violation of the Geneva Accord and there may be no counting on us if this kind of situation continues any longer," Eduard Shevardnadze, Soviet foreign minister warned Amin. Amin sent the message home. Two days later, Shah Nawaz, Pakistani UN delegate, sent a reply to Moscow, "Pakistan," he said, "rejects as baseless Kabul-Soviet charges that Pakistan was violating the United Nations mediated agreement." Nawaz, who was addressing the UN General Assembly on behalf of President Zia Ul Haq, said "the difficulty, if any, which may be experienced in the implementation of the Geneva Accord, will be directly attributable to the absence of a transitional government, acceptable to the people of Afghanistan," an earlier unsuccessful position which Pakistan had canvassed to replace the Najibullah administration in Kabul.

As the Soviet bicker with the American sponsored Pakistani government, the Mujahideens themselves are quarrelling with the composition of the future government. They disagree on everything from who should become the leader of the Resistance to whether a rebel government should be formed either in exile or in part of the territory that they control. Last week, when one of the Mujahideen groups announced a government in exile, it was roundly condemned by other groups. In an interview with *Newswatch* June 16, Sayd Mahjrooh, editor of the Afghan monthly bulletin admitted that "the question of rebel or exile government is a bigproblem, it won't be accepted, it won't be recognized. We are not united. Solution depends on a broad-based decision taken by all the tribal leaders, religious leaders, war commanders and all the groups in Afghanistan." Afghan numerous groups, despite the seeming unifying influence of Islam, have always found it convenient to antagonize one another. The joke now on the rebels is "united we fall."

This poses a serious threat to peace even if they defeat the Soviet-backed regime. Last February, Professor Sayd B. Mahjrooh, one of the most respected Afghan intellectuals and a notable voice against the Soviets was shot dead outside his home in Pershawa, by extremist Mujahideens, when he suggested that the former leader of the country King Mohammed Shah be made the interim head of state of a future coalition government in Afghanistan. Right now, rebels are torn between fundamentalists and moderates. They have a shaky arrangement whereby one of their bearded leaders is chosen as acting chairman of the rebel alliance for a tenure of three months. The current alliance chairman is Gulbudin Hekmatyer, leader of the Islamic Party of Afghanistan. "They call us moderates," said Shararuk Kran, chief of staff of the National Islamic Front, "but we see ourselves as fundamentalists. The fundamentals of Islam call for moderation in politics." Kran is convinced that none of the present Mujahideen leaders would be acceptable to all the seven factions to lead a future government. "Conflict among leaders will lead to making a third-party president of liberated Afghanistan," he said.

Pakistan, which together with international relief agencies, has generously provided food, shelter and employment to the Afghan refugees, may find it difficult to exert any influence on the future direction of any Afghan government. So also will America, which has bankrolled the rebellion. Afghan rebel leaders say they have been resisting all forms of domination since Alexander The Great and they are ready to resist not just the Russians but any other invader. As Kurshan of the AMRC puts it: "When this war is over, we shall thank all those who came to our aid. But we will make it very clear to them that the defeat of the Soviets was not as a result of their aid but the blood and determination of the Afghan people." Kran put the point more directly: "We hope America would not come and dictate to us at the end. If they come, they will get the same treatment, given to the Russians."

THE FALL AND RISE OF GORBACHEV

The end was as dramatic, shocking and audacious as the beginning. The dreaded men who plotted the coup had lost their nerves at the most crucial point. Mikhail Gorbachev, 60, the Soviet president and probably the most admired living political actor on earth, was back to power, rising incredibly like the proverbial phoenix from the ashes of defeat. The surprise putsch that toppled him August 19 had crumbled 72 hours later. Then the world, as it is wont to treat Gorbachev, rose like one to hail the super *tsar*. It all looked like a megahit movie straight from Hollywood. It was the most memorable 72 hours in modern history, when the predicament of one single man touched the heart-strings of millions of people around the world.

"This is a major victory for *perestroika*. What we have been doing since 1985 has borne fruits. (Soviet Union) has changed and that has proved to be the major obstacle on the way of the adventurers," Gorbachev said in his first statement just after alighting from the blue and white executive aircraft that brought him from Crimea, where he was kept under house arrest for three days. The usually robust Gorbachev looked tired and a bit worn out as he spent five minutes with reporters at the foot of the aircraft that returned him to power. He wore a light grey shirt without a tie and a grey V-neck sweater atop a casual jacket.

He looked calm at the beginning of his chat with reporters but could not bottle his anger for long. He launched an attack on the coup plotters and described them as "reckless gamblers." Said Gorbachev: "Their objective was to crush me morally. They wanted to push the people on the road to catastrophe. They have failed. The law of the land is going to deal with them. There is no question about that." The visibly shaken president heaped praises on his savior: Boris Yeltsin, the maverick president of the Russian Republic, as well as workers and thousands of protesters who barricaded roads and defied the emergency laws of the coup-makers. "I am grateful to the Soviet people, I am grateful to the President of the Russian Republic, Boris Yeltsin, I am grateful to the Russian people and the workers who stood up to the challenge of the reckless gamblers," Gorbachev said.

Just before he got into his waiting car, he promised to tell the world the whole story of his three-day ordeal. "the whole world must know what they wanted to do with me. I will talk more about it later at a world press conference," he said as he zoomed off to his Moscow residence. Tens of thousands of people jubilated and waved from the road. Millions of others round the world sat glued to satellite television, watching the unfolding of an historic event that bore no parallel in Soviet history.

World leaders and friends of Gorbachev reacted with joy and hailed his miraculous return to power. "It is a good day. It's a very good day. It's a fine day for US-Soviet relations. Democracy and freedom will go on," an elated US President George Bush said August 22, soon after speaking to Gorbachev on phone. To a question by reporters on what he would be discussing with Gorbachev later, Bush said: "I would say, stay with your principles, stay with your reforms, stay with your commitment to democratic process." Bush praised Yeltsin for his heroic opposition against the coup. "He has shown tremendous courage. I think he will have a well-earned stature around the world," Bush said.

John Major, British prime minister, who kept close contacts with Yeltsin throughout the showdown, welcomed the second coming of Gorbachev and said he was delighted the coup had failed. Douglas Hurd, British foreign secretary, speaking on a radio interview in Brussels, where an emergency meeting of The NorthAtlantic Treaty Organization, NATO, was going on, said the collapse of the coup was a "huge relief." "The main victory," said Margaret Thatcher, former British prime minister, "is that of Soviet people under the leadership of Yeltsin." Peres De Cuellar, secretary of the United Nations, said he was "encouraged" by the turn of events.

Later that afternoon, Gorbachev addressed a world press conference and threw more light at the crisis which he described as "the most difficult trial" in the history of his regime. He said Gennady Yanayev, his vice-president, and other key coup plotters were his very close friends, whom he trusted a great deal. When some of them went visiting his holiday resort at Crimea, Gorbachev said his chief of guards, knowing his very close, personal relationship with them, readily allowed them to see him. Instead of the usual friendly chat, the team, led by Vladimir Kryuchkov, the KGB chief, told Gorbachev to resign and hand over authority to Yanayev. Said Gorbachev: "I said who sent you. He said the State Emergency Committee sent us. I said who appointed such a committee? He said you have to hand over your authority to the vice-president and resign. I said I will not resign convey that to those who sent you. Tell them categorically that I said you are definitely going to meet with defeat."

Gorbachev was locked up in his holiday home, protected, however, by his loyal bodyguards, as the coup went ahead as planning. But the political tide receded very fast against the coup plotters, culminating in the collapse of their bid. By press time, all but two of the eight members of the junta had been arrested. Boris Pugo, the interior minister and a leading member of the gang of conspirators, was reported to have committed suicide before he could be arrested. The report said Pugo's wife and Prime Minister Valentine Pavlov, who also attempted suicide on hearing of the failure of the coup, had been hospitalized. Agency reports quoted Konstantin Kobets, Yeltsin's defence minister, as saying the coup plotters should face a firing squad. "I will be perfectly calm when I personally command the firing squad that will shoot those junta bastards," Kobets said.

The news of the coup itself, first broken by the Soviet news agency, TASS, caught world leaders off-guard, sending shockwaves round the world. Just before Gorbachev's planned return from a vacation in Crimea and before most Russians had risen from their beds that morning, eight men had seized power with military backing. A stern-looking Yanayev, surrounded by other coup-makers, told the world he was taking over as acting president and head of an eight-man State Emergency Committee. He said Gorbachev was incapacitated by ill-health, a lie cooked up to justify Article 127, Section 7, of the Soviet constitution, which says a president can only be replaced as a result of severe ill-health.

Yanayev quickly decreed a six-month state of emergency 'with a view to protecting the vital interests of the people." Under the state of emergency, the newfound press freedom in the country was terminated, with a ban on all but nine pro-communist newspapers. Then Yanayev pointed to Gorbachev's policy of *perestroika* as being responsible for the "woes" of the country. Said the colourless hardliner in a nation-wide address: "Fellow countrymen, citizens of the Soviet Union, a mortal danger hangs over our great homeland. The policy of reforms initiated by Mikhail Gorbachev, conceived as a means to ensure the dynamic development of the country and the democratization of the life of the people, has come to a dead end."

Yanayev went further to say that Gorbachev's rule had created an atmosphere of psychological and political terror, as well as a sharp decline in the standard of living. "Crime is growing quickly, becoming organized and politicized. The country is sinking into a abyss of violence and lawlessness. Propaganda of sex and violence (has) reached a scope never known in our history threatening the life and health of future generations. Such is the bitter reality. And we intend to restore without delay legality, law and order and declare a merciless war on the criminal world, to root out shameless manifestations which discredit our society," Yanayev threatened. Although the coup leader said the policy of reforms will continue and all Soviet international obligations honoured, the substance of his speech sent cold shivers down the spines of the Soviets and the world.

Most Soviet quickly interpreted the threats as a "return to the reign of terror." Yeltsin, the quirky, boisterous populist who is well-known for fighting Gorbachev's "snail-speed to reforms," summoned courage to stand up against the dreaded hardliners.

By the end of the first 24 hours of the coup, the maverick volleyball enthusiast had become the rallying point of opposition against the coup plotters. A decree was quickly issued for his arrest. But part of some 100 tanks heading for the Russian parliament to rout Yeltsin and his supporters switched loyalties on the way and took sides with Yeltsin.

Standing on top of one of the tanks, Yeltsin spoke to a large crowd of soldiers and civilians that had gathered around his office. "Soldiers, officers, generals and countrymen, the clouds of terror and dictatorship are gathering over the whole country. They must not be allowed to bring eternal night," Yeltsin said, to the deafening cheer of the crowd. "Soldiers," Yeltsin, a gifted orator, continued, "I believe in this tragic hour, you can make the right choice. The honour and glory of Russian men shall not be stained with the blood of the people. Do not allow yourselves to be ensnared in the net of lies. Do not allow yourselves to be ensnared by promises and demagogic calls to "military duty." Think of your loved ones, think of your friends, your people. Raise not a finger against them." Yeltsin urged the security agencies to regard the coup plotters as criminals. "It is only criminals who steal power by placing themselves outside the law. This pack of criminals and opportunists have betrayed the Soviet people. Don't deal with them," he said.

The message won the hearts of the soldiers. "I am not going to order my troops to shoot," one of the commanders of the tank column told Yeltsin. "How can you even take part in a military coup," one woman, quoted by agency reports, shouted at a soldier. "We won't fire," the soldier replied. From then on, clusters of protesters huddled with some confidence under freezing temperature, analyzing the coup. "Gorbachev is an idiot, he should never have gone on a holiday," one man, quoted by *The Independent,* a British newspaper, said. "Let's worry how to get him back first," another man replied.

Soon the Yeltsin campaign paid off. And official order to storm his headquarters was rescinded unilaterally by one of the KGB chiefs. The battle line was being gradually redrawn. A showdown became imminent. Cracks quickly appeared on the walls of the hardliners. With the split of the KGB and the sudden dropping of the Prime Minister, Pavlov, from the junta leadership, there were clear signals that Yanayev and his men were having problems asserting their authority. For two days running, the world reacted with rage, condemnation and fear.

Industrial nations, led by the United States, demanded the reinstatement of Gorbachev and announced the suspension of economic aid to the country. Eastern European countries were uneasy that Moscow's new rulers could threaten their fledgling democracies. Most developing countries were cautious in their reaction, while the totalitarian ones among them hailed the overthrow of Gorbachev. Bush, who kept constant telephone contacts with Yeltsin throughout the ordeal, described the crisis as a "straightforward, old-fashioned garden coup" that was quite "a disturbing development." Helmut Kohl, regarded as Gorbachev's closest friend in The West, broke off his Australian vacation and returned to Bonn, with a warning that Western powers have "a very clear responsibility to assure stability in Soviet Union."

Nigeria expressed "disquiet" over the coup and praised Gorbachev Lavishly for his policies and achievements, "especially his contribution to the wave of democratization sweeping across the world and the settlement of intractable regional problems, including some in Africa." India described the coup as "hogwash."

The Vatican expressed concern over the crisis and prayed for peace. But Iraq, Cuba, Libya and the Palestinian Liberation Organization, PLO, jubilated over the coup and welcomed the Yanayev regime.

Iraq claimed responsibility for Gorbachev's downfall and said his departure from power "deals a decisive blow" on the US and The West. "Iraq is one of the main reasons for the fall of Gorbachev. This refreshing development will restore the correct international balance," the defence ministry newspaper, *Al Qadissiya,* said in a front page report. In Tunisia, the PLO found themselves on the wrong side again (reference Gulf war). "We hope the fall of Gorbachev will help to solve the tragic internal problems facing the Soviet Union, especially Jewish immigration, which affects the search for a just solution in the Middle East." And in Libya, Muarnmat Gaddafi congratulated Yenayev and said the move was a "magnificent act" that would restore Soviet prestige. "It is our pleasure to congratulate you for carrying out this historic and brave act," Gaddafi said.

In every corner of the world, in news-rooms, classrooms sympathizers, who had back led under for years, resurrected and found a new impetus for heated pontification. Alexander Bourdakin, the Soviet envoy in Nigeria, August 20, condemned Gorbachev and gave justification for the coup. Said Bourdakin: "There were very many reasons for changes in the Soviet leadership. The state of the national economy is really on the verge of collapse. Reforms were introduced in a hasty way. There was a sort of vacuum in the national economic system. Nothing worked, nothing is working."

Edwin Madunagu, former university teacher and a well-known Nigerian Marxist, told *Newswatch* on the first day of the coup that "the putsch was long overdue." He, however, praised *perestroika* but said what Gorbachev implemented was not the real *perestroika*. Said Madunagu: "What was actually happening under Gorbachev was a conflict between *perestroika* and oppositions; thesis and anti-thesis and the synthesis is the communist offensive (coup)."

The coup plot was for months an open secret, a well-rehearsed affair, but the warning signals, it seems, fell largely on deaf ears, Eduard Shevardnadze resigned last December as foreign minister, in protest, warning of an increasing threat of right-wing dictatorship. Boris Fyodorou, the Russian Republic finance minister, also left in frustration. Besides, forces of the KGB, army and the interior ministry had, according to reports, practiced their coup roles at least three times in recent months. There were "certain movements" of the armed forces in the Baltic Republics and other parts of the country, beginning from February, which, for the trained eyes, were just more than mere military exercises. Around Leningrad and Moldavia, the military had also conducted exercises on working together and sharing responses in meeting unrest and terrorism. In Moscow itself, arrays of forces had several times in the last few months been unnecessarily called out for exercises. One such exercise was on February 25, which was publicly interpreted as preparation for coup. But defence minister, Dmitri Yazov, said at that time that "thousands of soldiers seen around Moscow are helping with harvest."

It seems now that speculations about a coup against Gorbachev had become so monotonous that observers and Western intelligence agencies alike relaxed their vigilance and the coup plotters used that to their advantage. So while the coup was not a "strategic surprise," it certainly achieved what military planners like to call "tactical surprise." That was, of course, a sufficient source of embarrassment to Western intelligence, particularly the American Central Intelligence Agency, CIA. Said one commentator last week: "How could Western intelligence be taken by surprise again the August in Soviet Union as it was last year in Kuwait?"

With the collapse of the coup, kremlin watchers went back to the drawing board last week, searching not just for the cause of the coup but why the coup failed. Beginning from the early 1990, Gorbachev, to many, seemed to have fallen from grace, not only at home but even with his loyal friends abroad. Aurel Braun and Richard Day, two respected political scientists at the University of Toronto's Centre for Russian and East European Studies, described Gorbachev in *Time magazine* of March last6 year as a loser who has been "mishandling reforms and desperately trying to cling to power."

The view gained wide currency and, in spite of the Gorbachev hosannas sung by Western governments, it became clear that he may end up a rebel overtaken by his cause. American *Newsweek* magazine June last year described him as a brilliant failure, who "lacks the understanding and the vision needed for his main goal." Though he has shouldered an enormous task, his inability to make significant progress out of *perestroika* has always been attributed to his personal shortcomings. He lacks economic expertise. His vision of the future is regarded as narrow and vague. His triumph in diplomacy hardly translates into domestic success. And he remains more popular abroad than at home.

Most of his policies, analysts say, produced unintended results, partly through miscalculations. Wanting to promote like-minded reformers in Eastern Europe, Gorbachev instead provoked the collapse of communism across the world. In the process, he realized a primal Russian fear: the rise of a powerful united Germany. Then, his political indecisiveness and efforts to steer a middle course between the conservative hardliners and liberals propelled Yeltsin to political prominence as the forefront reformer and made him the President of Russian Republic, the largest Soviet republic with 148 million of the country's 289 million people.

It became clear that Gorbachev merely wanted to give the face of communism a little make-up and not to change it. Then he became a sitting target for both pro and anti-reformers, two irreconcilable forces he helped to create but could not control. In the case of the anti-reform hardliners, Gorbachev personally appointed them and tolerated them even when they brazenly challenged his policies.

But the spark that kindled last week's take-over was, by all indications, Gorbachev's acceptance of the new union treaty that promised the final demise of the old Soviet order and a massive surrender of power to elected leaders in the republics. According to opponents of the pact, the pact which was scheduled to be signed last Tuesday with Yeltsin and other republic leaders "poses an imminent threat to the power of the military, the KGB, the communist Party and the state bureaucrats, the overlords of the state economic." Said Bourdakin, the Soviet envoy in Nigeria, last week: "The treaty had so many shortcomings, so many weakpoints. If we had signed that treaty, there would have been so much problems in the relations between the republics and the centre."

But if things were so bad as some analysts and anti-reformers say, why did the coup fail? Lack of cohesive support for the coup plotters has been identified as one reason. "There was tremendous confusion about who was in charge and what was going on," said Henry Dodds, editor of Britain's authoritative *Jane's Intelligence Review.* "It was as if the system was almost paralysed. They didn't know who they should be following," Dodd said.

Another analyst at Britain's Soviet Studies Centre blamed the failure of the coup on ideological split among army officer corps. Top-ranking generals were said to be mostly conservative right-wingers but many of the officers in the middle and junior ranks were reformists. Yet the failure of the coup has been traced to the fact that the army is orientated to be an army of the people. "To turn against the people and fellow soldiers would be tremendously traumatic and they simply refused," he said.

Then there was a tribal factor, Eugene Kogan, a researcher at the German defence ministry, said ethnic divisions and rivalry among troops created tension and made any attack on Russian parliament and Yeltsin a tricky affair.

But above all, the coup failed because of *perestroika.* "What defeated the coup was the commitment of the ordinary Soviet citizen to being a free person, living in a free society. And that is what *perestroika* is all about," Bolaji Akinyemi, former Nigerian external affairs minister, said in a television interview late last week. Perhaps it is the same point Gorbachev made last week in his first interview with reporters after the coup failed, when he said: "This is a major victory for *perestroika.* What were have been doing since 1985 has borne fruits."

Perestroika may have rescued its god father from the jaws of the Soviet bears last week, remained somehow in a state of suspended animation, uncertain about the future. The political mood of the world continued last week to oscillate like a pendulum, sometimes turning 360 degrees. From the early hours of the coup, when a dazed world began to contemplate life without Gorbachev, the mood swung later in the week to a world that began to contemplate how to live with a resurrected Gorbachev.

Still, the future somehow remains somewhere near uncertainty. What was pretty certain last week were the rising profile of Yeltsin and the fact that the men who wanted to turn the hand of reforms back had invariably accelerated the momentum of reforms.

A TYRANT BITES THE DUST

The man died violently. His body was mangled, battered and difficult to identify from a heap of smouldering rubble. As desperate rescue workers braved the ravaging flames and picked 30 completely burnt bodies, they stood aside drained but certain that the 11 years of draconian rule in Pakistan by Muhammed Zia-ul-Haq, had ended.

Zia, 64, had left Islamabad, capital of Pakistan, August 17, at the head of a high-powered military delegation to inspect newly-constructed military depots at Bahawalpur, west of Pakistan. The brief reception for the delegation at Bahawalpur airfield was impressive. Zia himself, bubbling in confidence appeared very impressed with the sophisticated and strategic depots constructed with the help of the United States. But as his C-130 military transport aircraft, carrying 17 of officials and 13 crewmen, took off amidst tight security on its way back to Islamabad, it exploded in a deafening sound and crashed in flames, a few kilometres outside the airport.

Killed with Zia were Arnold Raphel, the amiable American

ambassador in Pakistan and Mike Wassom, American brigadier of the American Central Command in the Indian sub-continent. The crash, however, took a more fatal toll on the Pakistani army. It killed a generation of army top brass including six generals, five brigadiers, a colonel, a captain and four senior air force officers among them, Rahat Saddiqi, Squadron leader and aide de-camp to Zia. The generals killed were Akhtar Abdul Rehman, Chairman Joint Chiefs of Staff; Mian Muhammed Afzaal, Chief of General Staff; Abdus Sani, Vice Chief of General Staff; Muhammed Sherif Nasir, Director of Military Intelligence; Muhammed Hussani Awan, General Officer Commanding 23 Division and Najeeb Ahmed, Military Secretary.

Shortly after the disaster was announced on Pakistani radio, Ghulam Ishaq Khan, a retired civil servant and chairman of the senate, said he had taken over as president in accordance with the constitution. In a nation-wide television and radio broadcast, Khan, who was hand-picked by Zia in 1985 to head the senate, said the crash was a "great national tragedy." He declared a state of emergency, 10 days of national mourning and fixed August 20 for the burial of Zia. Khan, who said "sabotage cannot be ruled out as a cause of the crash," added that investigations were being carried out to track Zia's killers. He praised the former Pakistani strongman for building a strong Pakistan and making "an unforgettable contribution towards its stability and security."

In what was regarded as a shrewd political move, he formed what he called emergency caretaker cabinet and named three new armed forces chiefs into the cabinet. That, according to Pakistan watchers, served to lessen the immediate possibility of a military take-over. The new president also announced that elections would be held on November 6 as scheduled and said the country would "continue to march along the path of democracy." Pakistani foreign policy, bilateral and international treaties, he said remain unchanged. He called on Pakistani citizens to co-operate with the caretaker government. "We have to keep our eyes on our enemies and be vigilant," he pleaded.

The news of the tragedy was received in Pakistan with surprise and mixed feelings. There were no placard-carrying protesters on the streets. There was no pointing of fingers at any country or group of terrorists. Though Pakistani radio speculated that the ill-fated *Charlie*, as the aircraft is called in military circles, "may have been hit by a ground-to-air missile." Many Pakistani were clearly nonplussed and barely restrained themselves from jubilating over the demise of the dictator. Said Benazir Bhutto, leader of the Pakistan People Party, PPP, and daughter of former Prime Minister Ali Bhutto: "During the long years of his rule, we never knew when we would be raided, when trumped up changes would be made against us. Suddenly, it just seems so unbelievable that the entire shadow of death and threat that we have lived under is actually gone. It's really unbelievable."

The United States, a principal ally of Pakistan, said it was shocked at the death of Zia. President Ronald Reagan, who was told of the tragedy by his security adviser, Collin Powell, said the tragedy was a "great loss." Secretary of State George Shultz said Zia was a "great man and a fighter for freedom." British Prime Minister Margaret Thatcher said Zia had won "the admiration of the world" for his support for Afghan people.

Tributes to Zia also came from Indian Prime Minister Rajiv Gandhi and his Bangladeshi counterpart Mohammed Erashad, who spoke of an "ardent friend who had contributed to the cause of Islam." The general assembly of the United Nations observed a minute silence in Zia's memory and UN Secretary-General Perez de Cuellar said Zia was a "far-sighted and widely respected leader." In Nigeria, President Ibrahim Babangida expressed sympathy for the late Pakistani leader and praised his contribution to the Non-Aligned Movement.

Zia seized power in a bloodless coup in July, 1977. Just a year before the coup, Ali Bhutto had promoted him to the rank of a full general and named him army chief of staff. As soon as he took over power, he imprisoned Bhutto and later hanged him after being convicted of complicity in the murder of a political opponent. The hanging of the widely-respected former prime minister, despite worldwide appeal for clemency, marked Zia out as a brutal leader.

After 10 months of domestic turmoil and external threats, Zia changed his mind and cancelled his promise to hold elections in 90 days and return the country to democracy. Instead, he perpetuated a ruthless rule under the cover of marital law. Thousands were sent to jail and many simply disappeared. The list included more than 2,000 journalists who dared to report the true events in the country. Some journalists, who were jailed, were publicly flogged or dismissed from their jobs.

The reign of terror thawed a bit under international pressure in 1985 and Zia eventually held elections but on his own terms: no parties, no campaigns or "other political activities." The opposition led by Benazir Bhutto did the next best thing: they boycotted the elections. Zia went ahead and formed a party called the Moslem League and got their members elected into the national and regional assemblies. One of the "elected" assemblymen, Mohammed Junego, was made prime minister. But in one fell swoop last May, Zia sacked the entire federal and provincial assemblies and cabinets. Some of the governors and the ministers sacked were barely two weeks in office. One of them, Ali Kazi of the Sind region was just in the process of forming his cabinet when he was sacked.

The accusation against Junego was that he was getting "too big for his shoes." His other sins were that he had a passion for foreign trips and was not just content with this title and "extravagant perks" but "wants some power to go with that all." The sin of the national assembly which led to the punishment of all the regional assemblies as well, was that it "insisted on scrutinizing defence expenditure." Zia, who was usually addressed by some Pakistani newspapers as the "giver of the constitution," promised another election in 90 days. Because of Bhutto, who was likely to be elected prime minister in a free and fair election, he got it enshrined in the constitution that no woman can be prime minister. The sacking of the national and provincial assemblies was followed a few days later with the imposition of sharia, the Muslim law.

The entire drama, described by some Pakistani newspapers as "constitutional arm-twisting," infuriated the entire nation who greeted Zia with a loud protest. Said the *Mag Weekly:* "What is obvious is that the political system created by General Zia has failed dismally. It is more apt to say that it had been failed by him and his military colleagues who back him." Other newspapers, such as *The Dawn*, accused him of "betraying even the constitution he created" and trying to "perpetuate a strange system that will see him not only as the apex but the dominant centre-piece." The protest angered Zia and he shifted the date of the "party-less election," to November 6.

Now that Zia is dead, the political uncertainties in Pakistan, according to observers, "have multiplied many times." David Taylor of the London School of Oriental Studies, told the BBC last week that with Zia gone, the opposition that united to fight him will run short of a common enemy and may resort to "street fighting." He, however, predicted that Bhutto will become the next prime minister of the country in a free and fair election. Oliver Foster, former British high commissioner in Pakistan, made a different kind of prediction: "There will be within the army a very strong lobby which will say, "We cannot hand over power to the civilians at this point in time."

While Zia's death had caused tremendous uncertainties on the domestic scene, it also left so many question marks in the international arena. Strategically placed next to Afghanistan, Soviet Union and Iran, Pakistan has been the focus of American policy of confronting Soviet occupation of Afghanistan and the Islamic radicalism of Khomeini's Iran. Zia, for one, made Pakistan serve as the conduit for US weapons to Afghan rebels, a situation which cannot be guaranteed by Zia's successors. Secondly, Pakistan's traditional tense relations with India are left up in the air. Indian leaders, despite many points of conflict with Zia, are far from reassured by the prospect of Pakistan with him. The new Pakistani government, India fears, may try to play the anti-India card as a strategy to hold the country together. All these combine to usher in a period of uncertainty in the Indian subcontinent. Perhaps, the only consolation is that the wiping away of the Zia's era may have closed the chapter of agony and political despair in Pakistan.

UNITED STATES OF DEBTORS

Debtor countries are angry. Creditor nations are jittery. The saying that a beggar has no choice may not be entirely true after all. The burden of heavy debt repayment is becoming unbearable for Third world countries and they have come together to say no to their creditors.

Africa alone alone owes $170 billion to The West. Latin American countries indebtedness to the same Western nations stands at a staggering $360 billion. Can the third world ever repay debts owed Western creditors? Indications are negative. Dissent voices against repayment are mounting. There is an increasing unity in poverty. Finance and foreign ministers of eleven Latin American debtor countries recently met quietly in Cartegena, Colombia, to define "the most appropriate initiative and means of action for dealing with creditors." They told creditors firmly to their face that there was a limit to the deprivation that could be imposed on their people.

The final communiqué represented a detailed reply to the conclusions of the London Economic Summit, where the rich countries proved unwilling to accept joint responsibility for debt problems. The communiqué reminded creditors that debt service payments had grown twice as fast as exports. It urged greater flexibility in the IMF policies and a rapid elimination of tariff barriers by industrialized countries. The communiqué also called for immediate and drastic reduction of interest rates and referred optimistically to a "mechanism for regional consultation and follow-up." Since then the crescendo of protest against Shylock creditor countries has risen higher.

Presidents of Argentina, Brazil, Colombia and Mexico met before the ministers and blamed indiscriminate and successive increase in interest rates, the prospects of new increases and the intensity of protectionism by IMF and other creditors, for causing "untold hardship" for their countries. They declared: "We cannot indefinitely accept these risks."

Said an Argentine foreign ministry official, Jorge Oscar Romero: "Unless there is a big change in financial conditions, there will be a debtors club."

In Africa too, IMF is about to feel the heat. The growing momentum for a united approach to debt problems owes much to Tanzanian President Julius Nyerere. In a speech to the Royal Commonwealth Society in London, earlier in the year, Nyerere called on Third World countries to wield the power of their debts and force the rich nations into a new economic dialogue. He said: "If the Third World stands together in seeking better terms, there could be real threat to financial stability and discussions would be held." Delving more into the issue before the British audience, Nyerere said: "Africa debt burden is intolerable. We cannot pay. You know it and all our other creditors know it too."

Two weeks ago, echoes of another dissent voice was heard

from Cuba. Fidel Castro, addressing an international conference on foreign debts in Havana, said, the third world countries' debts to The West should be cancelled "forthwith as unpayable and un-collectable." He added: "What we propose is that, we simply put our hands in our pockets and don't give anything. If we don't do that, they are not going to talk."

Combating debt, Castro said, amounted to a "struggle of na-tional liberation and a decisive battle for independence," adding, "it is actually the "West who are owing us for all our wealth they have exploited."

Observers believe creditors, especially IMF, appear to be guilty of false economic analysis and projections; guilty of mis-leading poor debtor countries; guilty of exploitation and destroy-ing the economies of Third World countries; guilty of precipitat-ing riots and political instability and guilty of causing hunger, starvation and death.

Said Francis Nkhoma, general manager of Zambia's Barclays Bank: "If a black man has a fever, the IMF says give him a polio injection regardless of whether it is malaria he is suffering from." Even voices inside IMF admit that "IMF endeavours in Africa in the 80s have been a total blunder." A paper examining the IMF's recent record in Africa by Justin Zulu, a former director of IMF, and Saleh Nsouli, its divisional chief, showed that only a fifth tar-geted level of economic growth. Less than a half achieved their inflation goals and only about a third, their targets for the current account of the balance of payment.

Nyerere recently challenged "whoever knows it, to give an example of a country which has prospered as a result of an agree-ment signed with IMF." Replied Tunde Idiagbon, Nigeria's No.2 strongman: "The IMF has never cured any economically sick country."

In Zambia, government is walking on an increasingly precarious tightrope. "It is getting to a point where we seem to be borrowing just so that we can pay our debt," said a Zambian State House official. Zambia owes IMF $700 million and has suffered one of the world's steepest and most sudden economic downturns.

Sudan owes $11 billion in foreign debts. It has one of the biggest outstanding commitments to the IMF in Africa. As many as 11.5 million Sudanese face starvation in the next few months. In Ghana, (the testing ground of the tough policies advocated for Africa by Western financial institutions), progress looks good only on paper. At present, industries have seen average income per capita fall by 10 percent and in some cases as much as 25 percent.

The point is, debtors use a greater part of their export earnings to pay interests on already accumulated debts. Bolivia spends 57 percent of its export earnings to service debts; Argentina, 52 percent; Chile, 45.5 percent; Nigeria, 44 percent; Mexico, 36.5 percent, Peru, 35.5 percent; and Brazil 36.5 percent. The implication is that it is impossible for any country to develop under such debt servicing burden.

The snares of debt trap extend beyond developing countries. Western financial institutions are also taking the backlash. Several of the US bank have already lent the equivalent of 100 – 200 percent of their primary capital to a handful of countries in Latin America and rumours are rife that the banks are in trouble. Experts say a major debt default in the third world countries, coupled with one or two big company bankruptcies, can trigger classic collapse of the lending agencies.

During the Cartegena Summit of eleven debtor countries, US banks lobbied Brazil to torpedo the accord. They succeeded partially as Brazil rejected most of the radical views expressed by the Latin American debtors.

The pressures on IMF can be gauged by the number of countries in arrears with repayments. Until recently no Third World country defaulted on IMF loan. But "declaration of ineligibility" has now been made against Vietnam and Guyana, under a process that leads to expulsion from the IMF. The IMF never allows the money it is owed to be rescheduled. Even a country's vital imports of food must wait for IMF repayment. Zambia, Sudan and Liberia are behind with their repayments and complaints have been made against them before the IMF board. According to an estimate earlier this year, Sudan could be as much as $250 million in arrears by the end of this year. The new regime in Sudan seems to care less for the debts incurred by the ousted government of Nimeiri.

With the present campaign against IMF and other creditors, chances are that the number of defaulters will increase because in most cases the interest charges alone have exceeded the initial loan. Thus, they cannot afford to pay their debts and ignore the needs of their people, without incurring serious political wrath.

Said a high-ranking Zambian bank official: "They (IMF) cannot get money out of a country that has not got. You don't give what you don't have. Do you?." Richard Erb, deputy managing director of IMF, warned African central bankers in Nairobi, last May, that "any failure to repay IMF loan undermines the institution's unique role to help Africans. This mild threat was a clear indication that IMF is quite troubled by the new trend towards default.

Analysts believe this might well be the beginning of a troublesome era for IMF and other creditors, if the demands of the debtors are ignored.

To avoid a block default which can be catastrophic for creditors, experts say Third World countries will need a big increase in aid and a generous rescheduling over several decades. Further delay, as President Belsisario Bentancor of Colombia said, may bring about "a legally binding framework of cooperation between debtors" that will complicate the situation.

INTERVIEWS

THE OJUKWU INTERVIEW

"We Are a People without Backbone"

"Having mandated me to proclaim on your behalf and in your name, that Eastern Nigeria be a sovereign Independent Republic, now therefore, I Lieutenant Colonel Chukwuemeka Odumegwu-Ojukwu, Military Governor of Eastern Nigeria, by virtue of the authority, and pursuant to the principles recited above, do hereby solemnly proclaim that the territory and region known as and called EAST-ERN Nigeria, together with her continental shelf and territorial waters shall henceforth be an independent sovereign state, of the name and title Republic of Biafra." These were the historic words of a 33 year old, Oxford trained Nigerian Army officer, which threw Nigeria into a bloody civil war that claimed an estimated three million lives. Since this monumental and cataclysmic event, his life has never been the same again. Enigmatic, aristocratic and unmistakably mystifying, his aura and carriage command and compel deep respect and awe. It is sometimes easier to secure an interview with a serving head of State than with the self-acclaimed 'most misunderstood Nigerian'. As The West Africa Regional Editor of the London-based Africa Today magazine, I tracked him for six months and eventually cornered him one-on-one, for two hours plus, in his modest Enugu residence, his beautiful wife, Bianca hovering and

eavesdropping to make sure he stays out of controversy. Literally venerated by his people, I met a man that some Nigerians love to hate, others hate to love and everybody long to meet.

Anietie: So good to sit down with a legendary, iconic and fabled figure like you (handshake and smiles). I think I want us to talk politics first and I want to begin with the just concluded registration of political parties in Nigeria. Out of 29 political associations that applied for registration as political parties, nine were registered and your association, the People's Democratic Congress, was curiously not registered. Your supporters are outraged. Many are surprised. How do you interpret all this?

Ojukwu: I thank you. And may I take this unique opportunity to send my humble greetings to the very many readers of *Africa Today* across the continent of Africa and indeed beyond. I choose to start this way because actually I am one of those old Africans who believes still very much in pan-Africanism, and I feel that, that the moving away of the substance of pan-Africanism from our politics has left us all soft and mushy and we are like an invertebrate animal today. We haven't got a backbone; neither do we know where we are going. I think that the pan-Africanist element of our politics is what is really, sadly, lacking.

Having said that let me turn my attention to your question. Yes I was very, very surprised that the PDC was not registered. Looking at the various requirements they demanded for the registration of parties, I am absolutely confident that we fulfilled the various requirements for the registration of

PDC as a party. We applied to be registered. We obtained the forms; we returned the forms duly completed. I set up offices of the PDC in 34 of 36 States, including Abuja, the federal capital. I gave addresses of all our offices and we had staff in all the offices. We had more than the five required staff in all the offices. We presented the list of PDC executives in every state.

I make no bones about this: After the war, it is true that the Igbos of Nigeria have always had this bond of marriage with me. So you find that in Nigeria, wherever there is an Igbo community, particularly an Igbo community outside Igboland, there is a feeling that they are in the battle front and they have a greater need for Emaka Odumeguwu Ojukwu. Generally they are part of my constituency and incidentally there is no part of Nigeria where Igbos alone will not constitute the 10 percent required by the INEC (Independent National Electoral Commission), so there are two possible reasons I see for refusal to register the PDC. One, you can bear in mind the Nigeria factor, which boils down to corruption. I know that it could be in the interest of one or two people to pay some money to some quarters to ensure that my party does not appear in the list. But more importantly I feel that within the army there are nonentities, whose only claim to pre-eminence in Nigeria is that they conducted and took part in a destructive civil war against me, leading the Biafrans. There are men who refuse to accept the free unconditional and total pardon granted me by President Shehu Shagari. They queried it when the thought was mooted. Ever since my return, they have been waging a rear guard action to nullify the effect of my return to Nigeria. To these people of course,

I continue to say without the slightest doubt that they are going to fail. I am already back; I am a Nigerian; I will remain a Nigerian and I will do everything a Nigerian is expected to do.

Anietie: Do you feel intimidated?

Ojukwu: I will not be intimidated. I just laugh at them because I am made of much sterner stuff. I don't think they can even outlast me. You saw the crowd of politicians here this afternoon. They could not even find a space inside and outside the premises.

Anietie: Does this mean you are joining hands with other political parties?

Ojukwu: Well, other political parties are seeking to join hands with me. In fact, I am laughing and enjoying myself. I said to them (delegation of political parties) at one stage that I wake up in the morning and I have my bath, comb my hair, and apply the various lotions and powder because I enjoy being the beautiful bride. So basically I believe that whoever tried to disenfranchise members of my party by refusing to register our party will be disappointed. His intention will fail because I will come out in another party. I will take my supporters into another party. We will take part in the transition programme and have an effect on the outcome of the transition programme.

Anietie: One very interesting topic of political discourse today is a power shift to Southern Nigeria, since power has resided in The Northfor 34 of the 38 years of Nigeria's independence. But it seems that when Nigerians talk about a power shift to the South, the assumption is south-west, not south-east where you hail from or south-south, where I come from. Is this your understanding?

Ojukwu: I feel that Nigeria being a federation, we should always talk about Nigeria in that federated frame of mind. You see, in actual fact there is no such thing as south in Nigeria. In the context of a federated unit we have east, west and north. There has never, politically, been a south in Nigeria. I think the introduction of south at this time is purely to confuse and a lot of people have bitten on the bait. What is the south? I know the east. I know The West. But I have to think hard to find out who The South really is. I don't say that you cannot design a south. Of course you can. But you see, for me, you have to build The South first before you use it politically. So when somebody in a federation where there were clear three federating units (which we have now modified and made six) say to me that power shift is between north and south, my reaction is that there is no such thing. There are either three or six areas as far as power shift is concerned.

Now, I am by nature, by philosophy, indeed by education and training a democrat. I believe in democratic practice. Now you say, do you believe in power shift? My answer is that I believe in any shift occasioned by democracy. If that power shift is democratic, I go for it. Put it this way, should suddenly something happen, an army officer from the south-south zone with some of his colleagues take over power in Nigeria tomorrow, I wouldn't support it, even though power shifted. So what I am after is a democratic shift. When we went to the constitutional conference in 1995, we discussed for a long time the whole question of power. There are two things wrong with power in Nigeria. People think power should be exercised. Of course that is right. The emphasis should be on power-sharing, not exercise or shift. Then you find that, unfortunately for us, it appears that all forces at the command of The North have been concentrated at securing power. To the extent to which the election that took them to power is free and fair, I have no objection. But each time they have taken power by force of arms, I oppose it. Now there has been this unholy alliance between the military and The North, which seems to have a stranglehold on Nigeria. And this has made it possible for The North to be ruling Nigeria, practically all the time.

It is because of the difficulty of easing the military out that as a national compromise we worked out the formula for a shift of power. I have to go to this length to explain it because everybody just looks at it as the right formula or philosophy. No. it is a philosophy which arose out of the painful necessity of looking for any way to find a sense of belonging in Nigeria. So we opted at the constitutional conference (of which I was a member) for power shift. And it then became a popular topic. It's still mere talk because nobody is sure what the constitution would say.

Now the question of whether it is the turn of The South-West, south-east or south-south is a media problem (hype). The media in Nigeria being in the hands of The South-West interprets everything to the advantage of The South-West. The South-South can't say much, The South-East can't say much because they have no voice in the media. We have been crowded out of the media. So whenever anybody says power shift, you tend to hear only The South-West laying claim to it. Their reason is that they have been wronged, that they were wronged by this June 12 business. I say to The South-West, the sooner they drop that argument the better for them. They should find what all of us in The South actually can subscribe to and let us join hands and face this question of concentration of political power in the north. Each time they want to get it as an advantage. Why should The South-East or the south-south accept? Because this idea of looking for an advantage where no advantage is called for is one of the failures of The South-West political struggle in Nigeria. There are gestures you should make for the solidarity of the entirety of the south.

Anietie: Sure, you were at the constitutional conference that decided on this issue of rotating the presidency of Nigeria around the six new regions. Is a rotating presidency really the ideal solution to Nigeria's political problems?

Ojukwu: The important thing to bear in mind is that no political solution is perfect. Now there are countries that actually run on a rotational presidency. The one that come to mind immediately is Switzerland. But my point is that all politics in a federation is an interaction between the federating units, each wanting to protect its own rights. A federating unit is that unit in a federation that actually acceded to the federal agreement. That means a tacit acceptance that power belongs to you but you have given some to the federal centre. So when you talk about the rotation of the presidency of Nigeria, I say again this is the major compromise actually made because when you are a Nigerian and you are faced with 38 years and find clearly for so many reasons that the route to the presidency is blocked, you are looking for a way around it. And if you can't get there because you are quite willing to falsify the census figures and maintain that you are bigger than everybody and if you have no qualms about rigging elections, if you have no qualms about riding into the presidential palace any time you want on the back of army tanks; so let's write it into the constitution, that this power must rotate. The idea was to nullify a lot of the Nigerian aberrations. That's why we went in for rotation. I support rotation and it is a support which I look upon as a Nigerian consensus in 1995. And I said instead of going back each time, let us base our future on the 1995 consensus and let's move from there forward.

Anietie: So where do we start the rotation from?

Ojukwu: Let's start it from me (general laughter). So what I've said actually is that everybody wants it to start from the area most advantageous to himself. It is in fact in an effort to ensure which area it would start that the question of power shift has begun to take currency. I believe that since it is now being offered to the south, that the choice should be democratically made within the south.

*Anietie:*There seems to be a lot of political schism in the geographical south. The much expected handshake across the Niger doesn't appear to be forthcoming. Can the Igbos of The South-East and Yorubas of The South-West ever cooperate politically to form a strong southern bloc along with the minority tribes of the south-south?

Ojukwu: I don't see why not. In fact if we are true politicians, the beginning of wisdom is an understanding between The East and The West, since we are being confronted face to face with the bloc called the north. When I was at school, I know it's many years ago but I am sure they are still teaching the same thing, the opposite of The Northis the south, it's never been east and west. So we must create a south that will become the opposite of north. And how do we do it? I say, even today that the PDC and the Alliance for Democracy (AD), which is essentially a south-west party, were the only two ideological parties in Nigeria before INEC. For inexplicable reasons INEC refused to register the PDC. These two could have worked together whether you like it or not. In a situation that finds the AD struggling and the PDC struggling, then you can be sure all Igbos, all Yorubas, all Ibibio, Efiks, Ijaws, will find a need to coalesce and come together to win this battle. And actually there are so many things in Nigeria that The Eastand The West can look into and decide who, where and what goes where. If the presidency has to go to The West, that can never be my problem. My problem is, when that happens, what goes to the east. Now if you are prepared to then satisfy me, then we have a basis for discussion. But if you refuse constantly to discuss that other side, particularly after this age-long suspicions, then you are in trouble for ever. We can sit round a table. And I will put this bluntly to you: if you want to be president, Mr. Akin Oluwole, with my support, do you agree that Mr. Ibechukwu Onuara should be the next governor of Lagos? Then we balance it out. Look at Lagos, for example, there should be many non-Yoruba judges in the court. Why shouldn't there be non-Yoruba permanent secretaries in Lagos. I agree that you Akin should be president but to balance it out, I want ministry of defence, etc. that's how brother share their patrimony.

Anietie: At the moment, are you, I mean east and west talking with regard to this power shift?

Ojukwu: We are sending messages to each other instead of talking. Again I am saying to my friends, my brothers and sisters of The South-West, let us start the dialogue now, no matter what it cost us. The future lies in the east. East and west making a success of an enterprise rather than constantly having their heads twisted backwards, looking at their failures of the past. If you are looking on failure, you are fixated on failure but if you move on from this point and say let us cooperate and collaborate, I can assure you, we can achieve a lot and after that everybody would be swearing by the efficiency of the east-west collaboration.

Anietie: I was speaking to someone here in Enugu this morning and he churned out what he called a "history of betrayal" of The East by The West. He said The West deceived The East into the civil war and this among other things has made it difficult for The East to trust The West. Would you subscribe to that as the basic problem plaguing east-west relations?

Ojukwu: If I say, which I always say, that The West betrayed the east, I am sufficiently democratic to accept the possibility that a westerner would say that The East betrayed The West. But the only way to reconcile this is through dialogue. But I have gone beyond dialogue because waiting for this has cost us three decades. And it is for this reason that I say let us drop it all. Nobody should apologise to anybody again. Forget it. Those who are dead will not come to life because of apologies. Let us just get together, discuss our present predicament, plan our strategy for overcoming it together and go in for victory together. That way, things of the past would just fade from our memory.

Anietie: One of the 'things of the past' was the civil war. You were the Biafran leader and commander-in-chief. Did you personally feel let down or betrayed because The West did not secede as their leaders promised after you declared Biafra?

Ojukwu: Naturally. Every suffering I have had derives from that word betrayal. And when I say betrayal, I put it in inverted comas, because they might have a different interpretation and I believe that every family in The Eastthat lost a loved one during the period certainly still feels the pain. But you see, nobody should carry pain as a badge of honour on his chest. Pain is private. Keep it private. Suffer it. The only thing that can wipe out pain is something pleasurable. So let us get together and seek pleasure instead of dwelling in pain. We cannot create a nation of masochists. No. What we want is people who look forward. When I came back from exile I said this and I still maintain it. God is so powerful that if he wished He could have put our eyes, either two in front or two behind so that we can be looking in both directions at the same time but in His infinite wisdom He put the two eyes in front. What God is saying to us is "look forward to the future." That's where we should be looking.

Anietie: With the benefit of hindsight, without necessarily looking backwards (laughter), do you think that the geographical area now called Nigeria would have been a better place, if The West and north had gone their different way to form their own country at the time you led The Eastto secession?

Ojukwu: I generally refuse to answer "If" questions. But I believe that a credible threat of east and west pulling out at that time would have brought The Northto its senses. (And please let my brothers and sisters in The Northforgive me when I say the north, it's just for ease of communications because there was a northern military and civilian, etc.) That is what actually went wrong. I would have expected from The West up to a point to make that threat. And I would have expected it even after the declaration of the state of Biafra, rather than find my philosophical partner becoming the minister of finance and the anointed crown prince, etc. But the most painful was our brothers and sisters in The West turning their weaponry against us and actually shooting at us.

Anietie: From media reports, some respected names in The West and pro-democracy groups are still insisting on a sovereign national conference. We have also seen banners and heard talks about the Oduduwa Republic, meaning that Nigerians are still far from satisfied with the political structure of the country. If The West seceded, would The Eastfollow suit?

Ojukwu: My name is Ojukwu (general laughter). My name is not Obafemi Awolowo. The problem today, first of all, is that 1967 bears very little resemblance to 1998. A great deal has happened. Nigeria cannot go back to the truth of 1967. We have to face the realities of 1998. Having said that, the problem which The West sees and, believe you me, I have every sympathy for them, cannot be solved by pulling out unilaterally. And then I find it even more painful that in this period, this threat does nothing but produce confusion. But I know that The West will not do it. They cannot take that type of initiative. So let us stop raising the temperature and heating the polity. Let us sit round the table to discuss.

I have said that there are two ways of ending military rule. If you want, you can take your stone or whatever and stone the military out of power. It can be done. Some countries have done it. But if you are not prepared to do this and you are always afraid of the bullets, then be reasonable. Sovereign national conference? (pause). You really think that the military will say one day, come and hold the sovereign national conference? What sovereign national conference means is that the conference will be for that period the sovereign of Nigeria, the government of Nigeria. And whatever it decides goes. What it then means is that the military has abdicated power. And can you see the Nigerian military abdicating power just by your screaming on the pages of newspaper? Ask anytime for a national conference, you will be right. In fact, I see the (last) constitutional conference as a national conference and I know the limitations we had from the military on that conference. I say therefore, let us accept the compromise of the 1995 constitutional conference and insist that succeeding civilian governments should immediately set the stage for a sovereign national conference, where in greater freedom, we can repair a number of things we did not dare to touch under the military. This is my attitude. But when you say sovereign national conference now, you are bringing confusion and very often, a number of the proposals from The West, with all due respect, tend logically to anarchy. And that is the weakness of their posture. My God, I love The West. I was brought up in The West. I spoke the Yoruba language even before I ever spoke Igbo. I went to school there. But they make this mistake of going at everything with blinkers on. They don't see side-wards. They don't even understand the need of taking The Eastalong with them. When you are weak, and you have problems, you go out and seek friends. You don't sit in your house expecting friends to come to you. But precisely that appears to be their policy.

Anietie: Recently, the Nobel Prize winner Wole Soyinka returned to Nigeria briefly and he was so concerned about the situation in Nigeria that he said another Biafra could happen.

What do you say to this?

Ojukwu: I congratulate him in his use of English words, but I don't think there is much sense in it.

Anietie: Your people, the Igbos, have been talking of late about marginalization. Some would have thought marginalization is a subject for smaller and minority Nigerian tribes and not one of the big three. How are the Igbos marginalized?

Ojukwu: We are marginalized in every way. (Angry, with his voice rising and his eyes bulging). Again, you might call this semantics but this concept of the big three I find very odd. In actual fact, it is only now that Igbos realize that we are the biggest minority tribe in Nigeria. And this is how we should be looking at ourselves. I don't know where you have been since you crossed the Niger to come to this house but look at our roads, you will see clearly the evidence of marginalization. If you can, compare the Enugu you knew in 1959, if you were born, with the Kaduna you knew in 1959, you will see clear evidence of marginalization. I am talking of The Eastin general and not only Ndigbo.

We started at independence with Nigeria accepting that the national income would be distributed on a 50-50 basis, based on where the produce emanates from. I find Nigeria today giving only 11-12 percent instead of the agreed 50 percent at independence to the area where the produce emanates from. There is marginalization there. In the constitutional conference, I fought very much and brought it up to 13 percent but even then it hasn't been done. That is marginalization. I find marginalization in education. Policies of quota, catchment areas, etc, have marginalized people from the east. (More angry) Whenever it becomes necessary to get a job by denying your own origin, that is marginalization. People join the armed forces by faking their origin, that is marginalization. There is certainly marginalization in the high echelons of the armed forces and indeed all the security services. The catalogue of marginalization is so much. You see marginalization in political appointments. You see certain departments of government where people from The East are never allowed to have access to such offices. Nothing will make me accept that all the drug-pushers in Nigeria come from the east. It is not true. Nothing will make me accept that all the smugglers come from the east. I don't agree. Nothing will make me believe that all those that have defrauded banks are easterners. I don't agree. These are all efforts to marginalize the east. In this country you are not permitted to be honest. In my own way, I, Emeka Odumegwu Ojukwu sitting before you, Anietie Usen of *Africa Today* magazine in my house here in Enugu, am marginalized in politics. They simply ensure that my party is not registered. Why? I should be a citizen. But I am one person not permitted to be a Nigerian, not to talk of being a good Nigerian. Nobody wants to hear of it. That's marginalization.

Anietie: (Paused briefly to allow Ojukwu's temper to thaw) Who is marginalizing you? Who is marginalizing the Igbos?

Ojukwu:(*Still angry*) That question has very often been thrown at me as a challenge. But I will give you the answer bluntly. The person marginalizing me is the person who thinks he has something to gain by maintaining the war situation without the fighting. They are the ones marginalizing me. They don't allow you to fight but they want to keep the war situation alive. It is so easy to seize my father's property by calling me a rebel. By the year 2000, they will still hold my property and because they had called me a rebel they justify their banditry. That's marginalization.

Anietie: Are you saying that Nigeria's politics and polices today are a continuation of the civil war by another name?

Ojukwu: To a large extent (and because you ask the question), yes. But to make it more correct, let's put it this way: Nigerian policies appear to the easterners as though they are still a continuation of the civil war by another means.

Anietie: But what do the Igbos really want as a people, that they are not getting?

Ojukwu: I would answer with modesty because I am not the entirety of the Igbo people. But having said that, we want to be free to live anywhere. We want to be equally Nigerians as any other Nigerian anywhere. We want to develop without hindrance provided we do not cause an upset to other people's development. We want to ascend to any position in the land just like any other Nigerian. We Igbo-Nigerians have so much that we can give to Nigeria. In fact our greatest disappointment and frustration derive from the fact that we can proudly say that given the chance we are very capable of moving Nigeria to the 21st century and competing favourably with any other people on earth. We have the means, the knowledge, the men and the women. Can you imagine how frustrating it is that we have so much to offer but are now being consigned to the backyard as carriers of water and hewers of wood? What can be more painful than the people of The Eastsitting on the wealth of Nigeria and having no say whatsoever in the sharing of that wealth? I want to take this opportunity to say to the Jesse people of Delta State, that I am very sympathetic to their plight. I offer my self for any job that can be done to alleviate that sorrow. Any country that loses in one single event nearly 1,000 citizens deserves to be declared a disaster area. And I want to take this opportunity to plead with the federal government not just to pay medical bills but to take it up to rehabilitate our brothers and sisters who have survived that catastrophe.

Anietie: The Niger Delta problem, running from Isaac Boro to Ken Saro Wiwa and now the Ijaws and the Jesse tragedy, along with the clamour for independence or self-determination in most parts of Nigeria, seems to suggest that things you had foreseen way back in the 60s and asked for, which resulted in the civil war are what most parts of the country are agitating for today. Some people believe you are vindicated.

Ojukwu: There is no doubt about that. I believe that I am vindicated. But rather than wallow in self-praise, there is a need to bring about a greater understanding in Nigeria. I have said to you already that power should be…decentralized. I said and I maintain it that people should feel part of government rather than make it exclusive to a few. These oil-producing people are perhaps the most exploited people in Nigeria. Actually they are not seeking to move away as a separate entity. They don't want to. But it is their frustrations that make them now question their manhood. This is what has brought about their reaction. This is the problem.

Anietie: Some minutes ago I asked you what the Igbo people really want. Now let me ask you: what does Ojukwu want for himself:

Ojukwu: at 65, I want to die in peace. At 65, I want to have the opportunity of becoming the best Nigerian of my time. I want to leave a mark on Nigeria, that forever people will remember that Emeka Odumegwu Ojukwu was a Nigerian. I would like to be loved by Nigerians, all of them.

Anietie: Would you also like to be in Aso Rock as the President of the Federal Republic of Nigeria and Commander-in-Chief of the Armed Forces?

Ojukwu: You see, people always ask me that question. It isn't the object of my living. It can never be a do or die affair. I have been head of state of the Republic of Biafra and I am very proud of that fact. So I know the limitations of the head-ship of state. But what I am telling you is this: my religion has taught me that the presidency is something given by God. At the same time that religion has taught me also that it is my duty at all stages to preserve and polish up myself so as to be a suitable vessel for carrying God's responsibility wherever He chooses to bestow it. So God gives the presidency but it is my duty to prepare and polish myself just in case he says, Emeka, take it" (Prolonged laughter).

Anietie: (Still laughing) Ikemba sir, there is an Igbo son, whose political profile, with regard to the presidency, appears to be on the rise right now. I am talking about former vice president Alex Ekwueme. Are you rivals?

Ojukwu: (Long pause) He is shorter than me; I am taller than him. He is lighter than me; I am darker than him. I call him my brother, he calls me the same. Rivals? I don't think so. Alex and I were at king's college, Lagos, together. He was my very good friend at school. During the war we maintained a certain friendship and so on. Rivals? Rivals for what?

Anietie: For the presidency and Igbo leadership.

Ojukwu: For the presidency? I have never declared my wanting that job. If he gets it I will be happy and I will be proud to serve not just under him but him. We are certainly not rivals. What I have he cannot have and the vice versa.

Anietie: Another friend and contemporary of yours, I believe, is General Olusegun Obasanjo. What advice would you give him with regard to reports that he is being pushed by the military to contest the presidency?

Ojukwu: No, no,no, no. In this business nobody pushes you. Let's get that very straight. The thing I would like him to bear in minds is this: let him make sure that whatever decision he takes is his own decision. Very often we find ourselves trying to impress but whenever you do that and you don't actually make up your mind, you tend to run into difficulties. I must say this because Segun and I actually met and served together in the fifth battalion of the Nigerian army. That was at Kano in 1965. And ever since then we've known each other. Now if at this stage, what he wants is a repeat performance, then I hope that in going into it, he would remember that Nigerians are brothers. He should remember also that the only validity he has since is what the Yorubas think of him. Therefore, start from home being pretty before you present yourself to the world.

Anietie: Some analysts have said that he is more highly respected overseas than in Nigeria and more acceptable in Nigeria than in his home base in The South-West.

Ojukwu: That is the problem. It should be the other way round. He is a man who seems to be running upside down, from front to back. God did not make a mistake when he created him a Yoruba man.

Anietie: What is your perception of the on-going political transition programme. Is the optimism of Nigerians and the international community justified or misplaced?

Ojukwu: The military is still very firmly in control of Nigeria. I do not see too much of a difference between the Abacha regime and the Abubakar regime, other than in the realms of public relations. But that notwithstanding, Nigerians are so anxious to ease the military out of power that Nigerians would take anything to achieve that purpose. We are just looking for a way out of the predicament of having to suffer military governance. And I am one of those who have to be optimistic about the transition programme. But there are many shortcomings. The very first one is the registration of parties. I have already spoken on the registration of parties. How come voters' cards were scarce in some parts of the Nigeria and not in other parts? Indeed I would like to see the international observers for the elections arrive here in Nigeria long before the elections so that they can get to know about the Nigerian before we vote. You cannot assess elections just by arriving hours before the elections and being taken on a tourist ride around the polling stations by government.

Anietie: Do you think that the sudden deaths of General Abacha and Chief MKO Abiola have paved the way for Nigeria to make a fresh attempt at democracy? **Ojukwu:** The deaths of these two gentlemen certainly leave a lot to be regretted. Pave the way? No. But we can use their deaths to pave the way to a new Nigeria. When we look at them we see the ephemeral nature of life, position and we become wiser in knowing that in life death is always present and that we as human beings can plan anything but the Almighty will have His way.

Anietie: How close were you to Abacha and Abiola? How would you assess them now?

Ojukwu: You know in Nigeria everybody want to be friends with great people. So it is possible that I can now boast that Abacha was my friend. He wasn't. I respected him, I must say. And he respected me a great deal. Of all the military men in power I met on my return from exile, he was the one who gave me the greatest respect. No doubt about it. I certainly acknowledged that fact and reciprocated it. But having said that, friends? I don't think so. I was already a lieutenant colonel when he joined the army, so how can we be friends. I don't think I even trained those who trained him.

Anietie: But during the early part of his administration, you were one of those he sent to Europe to polish his image.

Ojukwu: I must say that I am old-fashioned in my concept of patriotism. I will never wish ill on Nigeria. I felt that I had enough contacts abroad, particularly when some people were insisting on economic sanctions against Nigeria. So I said no, let me go forward and show them that there are two sides to the Nigerian economy. There are those who think the answer is violence and confrontation and there are those like myself, who perhaps because of my age, believe in constructive engagement. I also believed that the points that were arrived at the constitutional conference are landmarks in our constitutional development. But for Abacha we would never have gotten this in our books.

Anietie: On Abiola.

Ojukwu: Yes, Abiola was also a friend. We were in SDP together. When I found him on the path of presidency, we had a lot of discussion. My subject was always: what do you have in store for your brothers and sisters from the east? Even though we couldn't agree on specific things, we were certainly close. In fact, the last time I saw him he ate in my house. We had lunch together in my house in Lagos.

Anietie: What's your dream for Nigeria?

Ojukwu: Ever since I was a child, the motivating factor has been the racial issue. I have always wanted Nigeria to be a beacon of hope for all black people on earth. I have always felt that if Nigeria does not fulfill that function for the Black man on earth, then we have not begun. Therefore, my dream for Nigeria is that Nigeria should become a safe haven for all black people on earth. We should not just be takers but givers to the development of God's earth. That in a nut shell is my dream for Nigeria.

THE EKWUEME INTERVIEW

"We Must Make a Nation of this Country"

All eyes are on him, so to speak. Dr. Alex Ekwueme, wealthy architect, respected lawyer and former vice-president of Nigeria, is hopefully one of the leading contenders for the presidency his beleaguered country in the up coming, given the leadership role he played and is playing in the campaign to return Nigeria to a democratically elected government. He sat down with AfricaToday, Editor in charge of West Africa, Anietie Usen, for this exclusive interview. It is vintage Ekwueme.

Anietie: You have just come in from another overseas tour. You have spent the better part of the last five weeks in the US and Europe. What have you been up to?

Ekwueme: First of all, allow me to note with appreciation the wonderful job Africa Today is doing in reporting Africa to Africans and Africa to the rest of the world. Most of us look forward to each edition of your colourful magazine to learn what is going on in the continent. You must keep this good work going. Now to your question: I was in the US initially to participate in the Nigerian Investment Summit and to help urge the international community to renew their interest in Nigeria. During the summit, many Nigerians in the US came to see me and ask questions about what is really happening back home. They said they have got bits of information on the internet and would really like to know first hand the situation from someone like me. They persuaded me and I agreed to return to have a session with them. It was organised by the Nigeria People's Forum in the US. It was a very pleasant visit and they are very excited about what is happening now in Nigeria.

Anietie: But some people thought that you were intimidated by the international stature of General Olusegun Obasanjo, your main opponent in the PDP, and you were trying to run around a bit to add some international gloss to your credentials.

Ekwueme: No that's not correct. Don't forget that I was the vice president of Nigeria for more than four years. And I conducted several bilateral talks for Nigeria and was closely involved in running Nigeria's international relations. I had bilateral talks with then vice president George Bush in US, who also came to Nigeria for talks with me. Before then my American counterpart was Walter Mondale who, like Bush, had several bilateral talks with me. I enjoyed very good relationships with these men. So in my position as vice president, I had wide international contacts. In any case, the truth of the matter is that the decision as to who will be the presidential candidate of our party and who will be Nigerians' president rests more on Nigerians, so I do not need to go all over the world to canvass for support. Well, naturally, while I was there, I had a lot of American friends who had discussions with me, trying to find out and know more about the true situation in Nigeria; and I was able to convince them about the wind of change that is blowing.

Anietie: Many people were struck by the enthusiastic reception you were given on your arrival at the airport. It was as if you had been away for years. Were you expecting anything like that?

Ekwueme: In fact, I was very surprised and happy. You know, before I travelled I had indicated my interest in the presidency and maybe that announcement which I made just before I travelled made people turn out in large number to welcome me, when they heard I was returning. Recall that the PDP was facilitated by the Group of 34, a group of respected Nigerians who had taken risks and made a strong case against Abacha's self-succession, and I was chairman of G34. Ever since I said that I would be contesting the presidency, so many people have shown tremendous excitement and good will. In fact, I was quite surprised at the airport reception. I couldn't even get out of the place. My first attempt to step out and greet the people and say hello to the press was so tumultuous, my staff had to pull me back to the VIP lounge for a while. It was an ambush but I decided to advance (general laughter: this was a veiled reference to General Obasanjo's remark that he was ambushed by people who want him to contest the presidency).

Anietie: Talking about ambush and advance: General Obasanjo coincidentally that afternoon formally declared his candidacy at a big rally near Lagos. It seems your supporters were trying to retaliate and send a strong message to General Obasanjo.

Ekwueme: I don't know what really happened because the impression I got before I travelled and the news I was getting on the internet was that he was going to make his declaration on Thursday not Tuesday. So I decided to come back on Tuesday, two days ahead, to see what will happen. But when I got to Nigeria, I was informed that he had just declared his candidacy that afternoon. So I don't know whether his announcement motivated the PDP people to come for me in the airport, but I rather doubt it.

Anietie: There has been a sustained campaign in the media against the candidacy of General Obasanjo, especially in his home base in the south-west. I was just reading a comment in the papers today by Ola Vincent, the former governor of the Central Bank of Nigeria, who said the candidacy of General Obasanjo is a recipe for chaos. Would you agree with this view?

Ekwueme: No, I wouldn't really want to discuss anybody's candidacy in that terms. As 1 said at the airport that night:, every Nigerian has the constitutional right to aspire to any office in the land provided he is qualified according to the laws of the land. That General Obasanjo chose the PDP as a vehicle to pursue his ambition is a credit to the PDP and members of G34, who with other credible Nigerians gave birth to our party. It is a confirmation that PDP is a great party. Now, it is left to the electorate to determine the fate of every candidate who is interested in public office. Not just General Obasanjo and myself. We have at least five other presidential aspirants as at today. And I am sure the number of candidates to choose from will increase before close of nominations. This is what democracy is all about.

Anietie: You are trying to sound more like a statesman than a politician. But do you really and honestly think that it is right for a retired general, a former military head of state for that matter, to come forward and campaign for the presidency, especially now that Nigerians are yearning for a clean break from three decades of military rule to which he was party?

Ekwueme: You have said that Nigerians are yearning for a clean break from military rule. If that is the case, let Nigerians themselves say so at the polls. But I want to believe that 100 per cent of Nigerians cannot say that retired military men like General Obasanjo should not contest elections. After all, we are made to understand that a group of PDP members invited him to contest.

Anietie: This group of PDP men who invited him to contest have been described as the "military wing" of the PDP (general laughter). Are you worried? Are you intimidated?

Ekwueme: How can I be intimidated? No. I am not.

Anietie: Notice sir, that the PDP supporters of General Obasanjo belong to the late General Yar Adua's group. Speculation in the local media has also linked General Ibrahim Babangida, among other generals, to the candidacy of General Obasanjo. This must worry you.

Ekwueme: It does not. Now I am not in the race for fun or personal reasons. I have a great dream and vision of what and where this country ought to be. I have worthy ideas that can make a positive difference, a world of difference between where we are now and where we are supposed to be. I am totally committed to these ideas. And for that reason I don't get easily discouraged. We have a mission and we have a duty to justify the potentials which God has endowed this country with. I have offered myself to help this home of more than 100 million black people move forward, yet I keep saying this that it is left to the electorate to decide who they want to do business with, to lead this country beyond this point. You may be the best candidate without having the support of the electorate or vice versa.

Anietie: Who are those supporting you? At least we have read about those supporting General Obasanjo. Who are those behind you?

Ekwueme: I expect support for nomination from every member of the PDP, every member without exception. As I said before, the PDP is a child of G34. And when we started G34, I was not thinking of running for the presidency at all. That was not my concern. My concern and the concern of these eminent Nigerians in G34 was the terrible direction Nigeria as a nation was heading under General Abacha's transition programme and we stepped forward to say this cannot lead Nigeria to a good future. Our mission was a commitment to integrity, accountability and transparency in governance that will lead to alleviation of poverty and improvement in education, health, utility and the general well-being of Nigerians. Now, I believe that these ideas have motivated the bulk of the PDP members to have confidence in me. So I am not backed by any particular bloc or wing of the party. I simply happen to have a lot of friends in the party.

Anietie: Who founded G34?

Ekwueme: The G34 actually originated from what we called the

Institute of Civil Society (ICS). After the All Politicians Summit of December 14, 1995 under my chairmanship —remember, Nigerian politicians of every ideological view, from every part of the country gathered together at Eko Hotel, Lagos, to assess the broadcast which General Ahacha made regarding transition to civil rule. The summit was disrupted by security agents —we set up a 21-man committee, under my chairmanship, to discuss in a friendly manner with Abacha the future of the country, what we think is good for Nigeria and present it to government. We were not confrontational or controversial in any way. The next thing we heard was from some of his ministers who said: who are these people after all that want to talk to the head of state. They are people whose mandates have expired, former vice-president, former governors, former ministers, former senators; so they have no mandate. We were a group of people who felt the transition programme of General Abacha was not well-intentioned and was lacking in transparency and cannot lead Nigeria to the Promised Land. Very soon, it was clear to all that we were not shouting wolf. Soon political associations which appeared to the public to be credible were not registered as parties. Instead some that were not heard of and were formed overnight were registered. So we thought that if a few of us should get together and form a small caucus to address the issues in our own way without being adversarial, it could help. So we set up the ICS and nine of us formed the board of governors.

Anietie: Do you remember the nine members of the board?

Ekwueme: I was chairman of the group. Others were Chief Solomon Lar, Chief Bola Ige, Chief Olu Falae, Alhaji Adamu Ciroma, Alhaji Abubakar Rimi, Senator Francis Ellah, Professor Jerry

Gana, and Sule Lamido. So we got together, had it properly registered as a non-governmental organisation. Our mission was to try and educate civil society as to its responsibilities, role and functions in sustaining democracy and combating dictatorship.

Within a few months of our registration, government picked up Olu Falae, accused him of something and locked him up (general laughter). You know how Nigeria was in those days. So our number was reduced. But we went on. When we saw the way things were going with regard to total violation of societal norms, some of our members from the north said the impression was being given that all northerners supported what General Abacha was doing, and that it was important to disabuse the minds of Nigerians. They said they were going to call a meeting specifically of northern elders with like minds, to say that they do not endorse Abacha's self-succession. So 18 of them met on February 25 this year at Kaduna under the name of G18 and a statement was issued which said what Abacha was doing was wrong and not conducive to Nigeria's unity. That same day, they picked up Abubakar Rimi and Sule Lamido and locked them up. So our number kept going down. We [ICS] had scheduled a meeting for April 27 to discuss the whole problem of Nigeria created by Abacha's transition programme. But 10 days before that, all the five political parties in Abacha's government convened an abnormal convention. All of them incredibly nominated Abacha as the sole candidate for the presidential election. So when we met on April 27, we decided that we should forget all the other problems we were going to address and focus on Abacha's self-succession. We prepared a well thought-out statement under the aegis of G34 and gave nine good reasons why Abacha should not accept that abnormal nomination by the five parties. I signed the letter as chairman and forwarded it to all media organisations. At that time people thought we were crazy. Some people even ask me to confirm that I have written my will. You know three or four days after we issued the statement, on May 2, Bola Ige was picked up. In fact the next meeting we had one week after, we were asking ourselves: whose turn next?

Anietie: Were you not concerned that you could be picked up too by Abacha's security agents?

Ekwueme: Certainly, there was no doubt that I could be picked up at any time. But the rightness of our action and the conviction that things were really going out of hand, was stronger than the fear of Abacha or detention. To further strengthen us, the general public supported the steps we took. It was like a dam had been opened. Many people came on board. Chief Gani Fawehinmi made a statement immediately that our argument was incontrovertible and unassailable. Chief Rotimi Williams, eminent Nigerian jurist, who normally does not get involved in matters like this, came out and said there is no way General Abacha can succeed himself under the law. University teachers got involved and even former heads of state started making statement directly and indirectly to caution General Abacha. So the G34 became a very respected and weighty voice against General Abacha and dictatorship. And within six weeks, unfortunately, General Abacha himself died unexpectedly from heart attack.

Anietie: But the sad point now is the breaking away of the Bola Ige-led People's Consultative Forum to form the Alliance for

Democracy (AD) which is now a strong party in the south-west. What happened?

Ekwueme: It is a great pity that it happened. The intention of our group was to really have a broad-based national movement, that will involve Nigerians from every part of the country so that the type of experience we had in 1959 (First Republic) and 1979 (Second Republic) will not be repeated again. Fortunately G34 had eminent people from all parts of Nigeria, which was unusual. Now, after the broadcast of the head of state General Abubakar on July 20, in which he outlined the on-going transition programme, the G34 met two days later on July 22. We were under a lot of public pressure to transform into a political party because they felt that we had a certain amount of credibility. We decided at that meeting that we did not set out ab initio to form a political party but to form a group that will sensitise the people to their rights, obligations, duties and responsibilities. So we ruled against turning into a political party. But then we decided that we should facilitate the formation of a broad-based national political party that will be anchored on accountability, integrity, transparency and that would give good governance to Nigerians. The motion as to how this will come about was in fact moved by Chief Bola Ige. He moved that we should invite the political associations which General Abacha refused to register, to which many of our members belong, to come together to form the nucleus of the party. So we did that. We met a few days after that on July 28 at Abuja, passed a resolution that these groups have joined together and we were going to invite others. So it is not as if the Afenifere [PCF] was at the periphery of things. They were central to everything.

After that we met again on August 4, briefly and on August 13, where we passed a resolution. It was the first time in Nigeria, a political party said it was committed to power shift; true federalism; transparency, accountability and integrity in governance. I was the chairman of that meeting, but the three persons who were asked to draft the constitution was Alhaji Adamu Ciroma, Chief Bola Ige and Chief Ayo Adebanjo. So again, this shows that the PCF was central to decisions. The next meeting we had was on August 18 in Abuja. We met from 4pm to 12 midnight because we were going to present the party to the public the next day on August 19. So we took time to discuss the resolutions, which we all signed, setting out the vision we have for Nigeria. The same day, we looked at the decree setting up the Independent National Electoral Commission (INEC). Overnight we prepared a memorandum setting out our views on the decree because the next day, August 19, INEC had called a first meeting with all the political associations at 11 o'clock. So we [the PDP to he] went there as six groups: ANC, SPP, PDM. PNF, PCF and SSG. The memorandum which we prepared for the meeting with INEC was presented by Chief Bola Ige on our behalf. It was very beautifully presented. You know, he is a very good orator. He was sitting next to Chief Abraham Adesanya, the leader of the PCF. In fact, our memorandum presented by Ige became the reference point for the rest of the associations. After his presentation he received a big ovation and he walked across to where I sat and we embraced each other warmly. Now, that afternoon at 4 o'clock at Sheraton Hotel, we presented the 11)1) to Nigerians in a most memorable occasion. You couldn't even find a space to stand. We set up various com-

mittees and each of the committees was headed by a representative from each of the associations. And Chief Bola Ige,
representing the PCF, was chairman of the constitution committee. A week later at Lagos during the steering committee
meeting, I got a handwritten note from Chief Bola Ige saying that because of certain developments at Abuja last week
during the launching of the party, he was sorry that the PCF
members will not be able to come to the steering committee
meeting. This took all of us by surprise. Immediately we set
up a committee under Alhaji Bamanga Tukur to go and discuss with them and find out what the problem was. But within five days we discovered that they had gone to join the APP,
which was a great surprise to us because the whole basis for
forming the PDP was joint interest in a political norm which
we canvassed for during Abacha's regime and the new party
they were going to was formed by those who were very active in the Abacha transition programme. We really couldn't
understand what their grievances was. Quite frankly, up till
now, I can't fully understand it.

Anietie: Are there things the PDT' or you are doing to resolve
your differences?

Ekwueme: Well, we don't know what the differences are. But we
have set up a committee headed by Alhaji Bamanga Tukur to
resolve whatever differences may exist. The committee has
met with them several times, the last meeting being last week,
Monday, October 26. This time we are now talking about a
merger because they have formed another party. We need to
have this party as a truly national party with everybody that
is important in Nigerian politics on board. My mission was
that we would not duplicate the situation we had in 1959 and

1979, which generated instability in the country and brought us to the present situation we are finding ourselves in. So the matter is still open. They are our friends and natural ally.

Anietie: But is it right to say, as some of your opponents have said, that the PDP is a military party? There appear to be so many retired generals in the PDP: General Obasanjo, friends of General Yar 'Adua, General David Mark, etc.

Ekwueme: (laughs) Well, that is a funny presumption to make. I have already traced the history and birth of the PDP for you and this is public knowledge. But I must say that our party is an inclusionary party. We cannot exclude any good citizen of Nigeria from our party. In fact, we are not allowed to do so by law. You cannot convert a political party into a cult or club. That they are coming to join this party is evidence of the respect the party enjoys as a truly national movement. So they are all welcome. So far, none of them is an officer or on the national executive committee of the party. I am the chairman of the board of trustees of the party and no retired general is on the board of trustees yet. So it is a mistake for anybody to label us a military party.

Anietie: But you must be facing some threats.

Ekwueme: What threats?

Anietie: The threat of incursion and influence of these retired generals in the party. Are the retired generals not capable of eroding the influence and vision of the civilian leaders that founded the party?

Ekwueme: I don't know how that can be. I don't know how an increase in membership, quality membership, should be a problem or a threat. The party is formed, our mission and vision are clear and things are moving well.

Anietie: Let me put this question in another way. Is General Obasanjo a threat to the PDP?

Ekwueme: Why should he be? How can he be a threat to a party that he is a member of?

Anietie: What about General Babangida?

Ekwueme: General Babangida is not a member of the party as at today. They are no threat whatsoever. In fact, when Chief Bola Ige was unable to take up the chair of the constitution committee, it was General David jemibewon, who is also a very good lawyer, who did the job. I don't think they constitute a particular club within the PDP. In other parties you have retired officers.

Anietie: Is it right to say that your wing of the PDP is now anxious to bring back the AD into the fold, probably as your own "military" wing?

Ekwueme: (prolonged laughter) First and foremost, let me tell you that there is no wing to talk about in the PDP. We took a decision on August 26, that as at that date, all the political associations which came together to form the PDP (at the last count we were 105 associations) ceased to exist. So we are not an amalgamation of parties. We are a party. It is true, perhaps, that the PDM elements still maintain some identity within the party, but that identity is on a transformation process. It will fade out over time.

Anietie: Some Nigerians don't seem to know the difference between all these parties. You hear some people saying they are one and the same thing. So what is really the difference between say the PDP and the APP?

Ekwueme: It is not easy to draw a fine line because there has been a lot of movement of people. But basically it is safe to say that the PDP is essentially peopled by those who did not take part in General Abacha's transition programme. On the other hand the APP was founded basically by people who participated in General. Abacha's transition programme. Simply put, PDP is pro-democracy while APP is pro-military.

Anietie: So much has been said about power shift and rotational presidency between north and south. But the impression is that power shift for now means rotation of the presidency to the south-west. Is that your understanding?

Ekwueme: You see power shift is a funny terminology. And we must situate it within the historical framework. In 1994, when General Abacha decided to have constitutional conference, various parts, segments and groups in the country presented memoranda. Nigerians of every shade thought it was an opportunity to discuss Nigerian's problems as a modus vivendi to reduce tension and promote unity and stability. Those of us who felt that such an opportunity should not be lost availed ourselves of the opportunity. It was at that conference, based on a minority report, which I presented, that the six geopolitical zones we are now using were set out. You will not find it anywhere else in the document of the constitutional conference except in the minority report submitted by me. And...

Anietie: (cuts in) So the six political zones in the country now were your idea?

Ekwueme: Yes and were embodied in the minority report which I submitted in the conference: the report from the committee on structure and framework of the constitution. Based on that and the issues that arose from it, we decided to have a consensus committee. Of the more than 1,000 memoranda we got, not one of them said we should not have one Nigeria. Everybody wanted Nigeria, but they wanted a Nigeria in which everybody will have a sense of belonging, a true country everybody can owe allegiance to. Now, a consensus committee was constituted to look into this problem. We spent time discussing it. And on a motion moved by a delegate from the northern part of the country, it was agreed that the presidency of the country should rotate between the northern and southern parts of the country. This was embodied in section 229 of the constitution as rotation of the presidency. Now that was in 1994/95. Those who were not contributory to that decision and who in fact were abusing us, saying that we were wasting time at the conference; they are the same people who have now christened the rotational presidency clause as power shift; as if it is something they have just originated. Now, that clause is clear that rotation will be between the southern bloc and the northern bloc. My minority report created three zones in the northern bloc (north-east, north-west, north-central) and three zones in the southern bloc (south-east, south-west, southern minority — which we now call south-south). Therefore if the president is going to come from the south, it means it will come from any of the southern zones and if from the north, any of the northern zones. And again this is not new. In September 1978, when General Obasanjo, as head of state, lifted the ban on politics, the National Party of Nigeria (NPN) was formed and the leaders got together and said, look, let us sit down and work out how we are going to apportion positions, so that we don't quarrel over it and so that we can carry Nigerians along. They said, to start with, the 10 northern states should produce the president. After they complete two terms, the nine southern states should take their turn. On the basis of that agreement, nobody from the south presented himself for nomination. We have six candidates from the north: Alhaji Shehu Shagari from Sokoto state; my friend Maitama Sule from Kano; Oluso-la Saraki from Kwara; Joseph Tarka from Benue, Adamu Ciro-ma from Potiskum, then Bornu state; Professor Iya Abubakar from Mubi, in then Gongola state. You can see the spread. Every part of the north (Tiv, Yoruba, Hausa, Fulani etc) was offered the opportunity. And when we fixed our convention on December 9 at Casino Cinema Hall, Lagos, Shehu Shagari was nominated. If the military had allowed us, the south would have since taken its turn. So it's not as if we are doing it for the first time.

Anietie: Obviously, you played quite a prominent and principled role at the constitutional conference. Would you say that you left the conference a hero?

Ekwueme: I wouldn't say so. Quite frankly, there were some people who didn't like the role I played at the conference. But I said and did everything I said and did at the conference because I love Nigeria. I didn't want us to create a situation that will lead to problems for our children and children's children; when we are no more here. And therefore if it is possible for us to arrest friction and cleavages among our children, we should do so. That was my purpose at the conference. Some people like it, some don't; and that's natural in public service. It is .true that The Vanguard [a leading Nigerian newspaper] did a survey of all the journalists who covered the conference and asked them to pick an outstanding contributor and performer at the conference, and unanimously they picked me. But that was the view of journalists and not mine.

Anietie: Somehow, there is still a clamour for a sovereign national conference, especially by some politician in the south-west of Nigeria. What do you make of this?

Ekwueme: I have no quarrel with a national conference. Legally and constitutionally, the quarrel I have is with the word "sovereign". Now my understanding of it is that a sovereign national conference has all the attributes of sovereignty. Such a conference becomes the government of Nigeria. In a situation where you have a government in place already, a sovereign national conference is therefore a recipe for chaos. So I think that at any time Nigerians ought to he able to sit down and discuss the problems of the country in a peaceful atmosphere and solve them. During our colonial days, our founding fathers, starting with the Ibadan conference in 1950, discussed the best form of government ;Ind arrived at a federal form of government, which Was embodied in the independence constitution. So, at any time we want, we should be able to have a conference because we ought to be able to sit down and discuss amicably among ourselves. But to insist on a sovereign national conference when there is a government in place is a recipe for disorder.

Anietie: Let us turn attention to the issue of marginalisation. How come the Igbos of the south-east, from where you hail, who are the third largest ethnic group in Nigeria, are saying they are marginalised? We used to think that the issue of marginalisation is the exclusive subject of the minority ethnic groups.

Ekwueme: In fact, all Nigerians are marginalised. It depends on what aspect of our existence you are talking about. Now, there are Nigerians who are marginalised politically. They are kept out of the position of authority in government. There are Nigerians who are marginalised economically. They are kept out of the commanding heights of the economy by those who control it, kept out of the banking institutions, industries, etc. There are Nigerians who are kept at the margin of the bureaucracy. Of a large number of federal permanent secretaries, they can only find one or two from their part of the country. So they feel that the bureaucracy, which is really the effective executive arm of government, does not include them. There are those who feel they are left out of the armed forces: so many generals, admirals, air vice marshals, and they are not there. And I tell you, there are those who are marginalised educationally, which many Nigerians don't react to. Some Nigerians are blessed with crude oil in their soil and waters, from where the wealth of Nigeria for decades has come from, but they don't even have roads to their villages or clean water to drink. They are highly marginalised. So every Nigerian suffers from one form of marginalisation or the other. My mission as president, if I become one, is to ensure that all these areas are properly addressed. So far, some of them have been swept under the carpet but we must do something about it. We are fortunate that the constitution allows the president to create ministries or departments, depending on the country's needs and I will create the ministry for national integration, which will specifically address ethnic cleavages; the type of problems we have in Delta and Ondo states. All these things complicate our relationship and we should look into ways of making everybody have a feeling of belonging instead of a sense marginalisation?

Anietie: In which areas are the Igbos marginalised?

Ekwueme: No, no, no. it's not fair to draw me into specifics. This is a national issue.

Anietie: Okay, sir. But someone once said that Aso Rock is not for an Igbo man.

Ekwueme: Who said that?

Anietie: I read it in the papers.

Ekwueme: If anybody said that he should leave Nigeria. Aso Rock is for any Nigerian whom Nigerians elect to serve them as president. The whole purpose of democracy is for the people to exercise their right to choose. They can choose an Igbo man, a Hausa man, a Yoruba man, a Fulani man, Ibibio man, Ijaw man, Efik man, Jukun man or Kutep or Angas. Whoever they choose, Aso Rock belongs to him for the duration of his tenure. It is not a personal property or the birth right or inheritance of any body.

Anietie: There is a suggestion also in the press that if the next president of Nigeria emerges from the south-east, the vocal agitation for a president from the south-west could escalate and split the country.

Ekwueme: It is an extremely dangerous position to take. I don't think any responsible Yoruba person can say that.

Anietie: Now, how soon can we expect a handshake across the Niger: political unity between the south-east and the south-west. I was speaking with one of the political leaders in the north recently and he said to me that they have agreed to power shift to the south, but that the "fight" between the south-west and south-east can cost southerners the job.

Ekwueme: Whoever said that power shift to the south will depend on the unity of the south does not understand the political parameters under which it will work. For example, if we have three political parties at the end of the day and one of those parties have a presidential candidate from the south-west and the other party nominates a candidate from the south-south, while the other chooses its candidate from the south-east, it will be the responsibility of all Nigerians to vote for those three candidates. To expect that the south should come together and present one candidate to the rest of Nigeria is a ridiculous proposition. A party should be free to take its presidential candidates from any of the southern zones and it is for Nigerians to decide which of those candidates they will elect as president. The effort we are making at PDP is to have all Nigerians from the six zones in our fold; and notwithstanding the little hitch with the AD we have largely succeeded.

Anietie: Do you really trust the north when it comes to this issue of power shift?

Ekwueme: It is not a matter of trusting the i north. First, it is a function of the provisions of the constitution. Apart from the constitution, my reading of the situation within our own party is that we have said categorically that on August 13 and on September 8, we will nominate our presidential candidate from the south, which is why I resigned my position as chairman of the steering committee. I understand that APP after a lot of dilly-dallying has also made a statement that they will nominate their presidential candidate from the south. The AD, I understand, has also made that known. There may be more. So I trust them. I trust that these parties will implement their decisions.

Anietie: Most Nigerians believe that you can emerge as the next president but they also worry that you will be a lame duck president because the army and other security agencies are in short supply of senior officers from your part of the country. Do you consider this a handicap?

Ekwueme: The implication of your question is that the Nigerian army is tribalised and each person there is out to defend his ethnic group. I don't think that is fair on the Nigerian army. I expect that the military will be loyal to any president, no matter where he comes from.

Anietie: Military coups appear to be at the root of Nigeria's many problems. Are there constitutional ways to outlaw coups?

Ekwueme: Yes, there are. The surest way to stop coups is to have such a government that will be glaringly good and will make a difference between the type of government that we are used to and the type of government that will be in place. For me, it means running the best government possible, so that if anybody brings his gun to seize power, Nigerians themselves will rise up to say: no, you can't do that.

Anietie: So the solution to coups is good government?

Ekwueme: That is one solution to coups. It is not the only solution. There are other solutions.

Anietie: What are the other solutions?

Ekwueme: Well. It is a long story. We discussed this at length at the constitutional conference. We made recommendations, for instance, to the effect that anybody who attempts to destroy constitutional order should be guilty of a crime punishable at all times under the general law. There were other suggestions. But certainly a good government that make a positive difference from the past and in the lives of Nigerians will go a long way to discourage coups.

Anietie: For some people, Nigeria's problem is not so much the soldier as the politician. The Nigerian politician appear to be a special breed. For many they are very unreliable, unprincipled, unable to accept defeat and maybe a cash-and-carry individual. What is really the matter?

Ekwueme: Nigerian politicians are not different from politicians anywhere else. Given the opportunity to govern, make mistake and correct it, he would be one of the best you can find. How much of politics and civil rule have we really experienced in Nigeria. The army has been there for three of nearly four decades. How many?

Anietie: But we have politicians who abandoned M K 0 Abiola and instead helped General Abacha extensively in his pet project to remain indefinitely in power.

Ekwueme: Are they politicians?

Anietie: I would call them politicians.

Ekwueme: I won't call them politicians (general laughter).

Anietie: One of the things that bothers Nigerians about their politicians is corruption. And the Shagari administration that you served as vice-president left a legacy of corruption. What...

Ekwueme: (interrupts)I will contest that. I will never stand up to defend corruption but I will contest that statement. First, go and look at some of the ministers who served in that administration. Go to their homes. Go and see the cars they ride. Some of them are still living in bungalows they built before coming to government. There are some of them when you see them and they tell you they were ministers at a time that people say was seething with corruption, you can't believe it. Naturally, we had a few bad eggs. I will be the first to admit it. During our second term, on my insistence we tried to prevent that. First, we insisted that anybody who was appointed a minister must sign a letter of resignation ahead of time, so that if we have the slightest inkling that so and so was engaging in corrupt practice and we verify it, your resignation was already in our hands, and all you have to do is to say to us: "I am the minister of X and for personal reasons I have tendered my resignation". And we will say: "We have accepted, farewell". Now, if you do that to ministers, the chairmen of boards, heads of parastatals, etc will receive a strong signal. And the effect will be felt down the line. Then of course the code of conduct bureau was there. But within three months the military took over. Now, let me tell you about myself and not other people. Immediately the coup was announced on the December 31, 1983, I was one of the first persons to be picked up by the military. They had free access to my house and my office. They took every paper that was there. They set up a judicial tribunal headed by the high court judge, Justice Uwaifor, with two military and two police members, both lawyers. They went through all the records. And they unanimously made a pronouncement that I came into government and left it much poorer than when I came in. They also made a pronouncement that my conduct was such that if I were to be charged, I would set a standard too high even for saints. Go and check it.

Anietie: You came into the government a very rich man. You were already a multi-millionaire in the 1970s. How...

Ekwueme: (laughing) I don't know about that. I am telling you what the tribunal said.

Anietie: It is public knowledge that you were very rich. How rich were you when you came in as vice-president and how poor where you when you left or vice versa?

Ekwueme: My assets were declared and you can have access to them. All assets of all politicians should be available for everybody to scrutinise, so that anybody who notices anything funny can raise it with the code of conduct bureau.

Anietie: Can you say the same of President Shehu Shagari, your boss?

Ekwueme: Yes, of course. He was acquitted by the tribunal as well. And, as I said, he noticed problems, and the important thing is that he took steps to correct these problems. Then we were thrown out by the military.

Anietie: Now, what is really the agenda of the PDP? What are you out to do for Nigerians?

Ekwueme: The immediate agenda of the PDP is giving Nigeria a good government that can raise the country from this present level of poverty to a point where an average Nigerian can at least be comfortable. I don't know where you live, but I live in a village, and we have reached a point where an average Nigerian is not talking about three square meals but what students call 001 or 010. The worst part of it is that we are degenerating to a 000 situation. You may not believe it. But this is unacceptable. More so because this country is rich enough and so endowed by God that a good and efficient management of our resources can cater for not just Nigerians but our neighbours. So, the alleviation of poverty is PDP's number one goal. Then we must look at the future. Take education, for instance. We were going to a campaign yesterday and we saw hundreds of children littering the streets, hawking oranges when they should be at school. This is unacceptable, because it is not the best way to plan for our future. And we Nigerians have become so insensitive that we don't even notice it. We just take it for granted, without remembering that these are the people we are living for. So we must have a regime of free and compulsory education. We must invest in our children because that means we are investing in our future. For the PDP, that is a very wise investment to make. So many things have to be done as a priority. Take our refineries, for instance. How do you explain a situation whereby all our refineries are down and the sixth largest oil producer in the world cannot provide petrol for its citizens? Somebody told me yesterday that he bought a litre of petrol for N50 instead of N11. Government may have to divest a fraction of its shares and sell them to Nigerians and others. Run them efficiently and the money you derive from divesting, you put it in productive areas such as agriculture, etc, We must build a nation out of this country called Nigeria, Look at the oil producing areas, Look at the very sad incident at Jesse town, where nearly a thousand poor villagers were set ablaze in a flash of fire. On one stretch of road between Port Harcourt and s ALA Abosi, we have a petrochemical plant, two refineries, a fertiliser complex and the aluminium smelting plant. That road is impassable, in spite of billions of dollars invested in these projects. To even evacuate fertilisers out of that road is a big problem. That road had been slated for dualisation since 1986 but nothing has happened till today. We must get our priorities right. This country is a great country by any standard if we know what to do. And the calibre of men and women we have in the PDP know what to do and how to get this country back on its feet.

Anietie: ECOMOG is almost synonymous with your country. Nigeria has committed enormous resources and men into the regional force. As president, will you continue on the path of the present administration or you will chart a fresh path in foreign policy objectives?

Ekwueme: By providence Nigeria has the largest concentration of black people in the world. This confers on us responsibilities not just in our sub-region but beyond. We are very proud of the record of our soldiers in Liberia, Sierra Leone and even in UN peace missions. It is not going to be possible for any country to treat our might lightly in the continent and we will not allow that to happen. At the same time we are not going to make ourselves the policeman of the sub-region or the continent but must act in concert with other members of Ecowas and OAU in order to promote stability. Similarly, we have to draw a balance between spending our resources externally and ensuring that our citizens are adequately provided for. I believe too that Nigeria has done enough in international arena to be accorded a permanent seat in the Security Council of the UN.

Anietie: By the way sir, what is former President Shehu Shagari, your former boss, saying about your presidential ambitions?

Ekwueme: He has made it clear that he is no longer going to be involved in partisan politics. He explained that recently at Kaduna. And I think it is a good position to adopt really, because in a developing country and even in the developed world like the US, once you are made the head of state, it would be useful for you to stay away from partisan politics, so that if things go in the wrong direction, you can objectively intervene as an elder statesman and in a way that will not be regarded as partisan political views. I expect that from all our former heads of state. This is the position Shehu Shagari has taken and I commend him for that. I don't expect him to descend to the point of moving from place to place campaigning for me. Naturally if he does that, I will be very delighted because it will help my candidacy, but I respect his decision to remain an elder statesman.

Anietie: Now you have finally taken a shot at General Obasanjo.

Ekwueme: (laughing) No, no, no. I am talking about former President Shehu Shagari, who after all has said and conducted himself as a statesman not a politician.

OUR SOLDIERS, OUR PROBLEM

ADAMU Ciroma, scion of Northern Nigerian political elites,
and former minister of several portfolios, in both civilian and
military administrations, spoke with Africa Today's Editor (West
Africa), Anietie Usen, in his Kaduna residence, on several issues
affecting Nigerian politics.

Anietie: Most parts of your country are agitating right now for
power to shift from the north to south. The North of which
you are a leader has held on to power for 34 of 38 years of
Nigeria's independence. Why are the northerners reluctant
to cede power to the south?

Ciroma: It is not true that we don't want southerners to rule Nigeria. We do want southerners to rule Nigeria and that was
proved and demonstrated conclusively and beyond doubt in
the June 12, 1993 presidential elections in which northerners
voted massively for Chief M.K.O. Abiola, a southerner. Recall
that Abiola won in virtually all the northern states and in fact
most states in the north voted for him more than some states

in the south. Even in Kano state, where his opponent Alhaii Tofa hails from, the people in the heart of the north voted for Abiola and showed their preference for a southerner rather than their own son. So this issue of a power shift to the south is what indigenes of the north without any pressure had already made up their minds to do, as a demonstration of their sense of fairness and faith in one united Nigeria where every section of the country has a sense of belonging. But we have to be careful to make a distinction between the military and civil rule in Nigeria. I am a known antagonist of military rule in Nigeria because the military are without doubt blameworthy for stifling and complicating the steady political maturity of Nigeria. Now if you take away the military men who seize government illegally by force and do as they like, you will notice that the issue of northern domination does not exist under democratic dispensation.

For instance in 1960, Nigerians opted for Dr Nnamdi Azikwe, a southerner, and Abubakar Tafawa Balewa, a northerner as governor-general and prime minister respectively. When Nigerians had another opportunity to vote in 1979, they voted for Shehu Shagari, a northerner, as president, and Dr Alex Ekwueme, a southerner, as vice president respectively. And the third time, Nigerians were allowed by the military to choose their leader on June 12, 1993, Nigerians massively chose Abiola, a southerner and Babagana Kingibe, a northerner, respectively as their leaders. So if you look at our democratic experience and experiment so far, you will agree completely that northerners have not dominated the southerners. Our problem and misfortune are our soldiers.

Anietie: But has it not been said often that key civilian elites in the north are usually the unseen hands who encourage their sons in the military to seize and remain in power at the expense of the south which is not strategically positioned in the military?

Ciroma: How can that be true? To begin with, the first coup in this country was carried out by southern officers. Did northern elites sponsor Generals Buhari, Idiagbon, Babangida and Abacha to overthrow President Shagari, who was also a northerner? As recently as a few months ago, is it not the Emmanuel Inwuanyanwus, the Arthur Nzeribes, the Jim Nwobodos, the Sam Mbakwes, the Ebenezer Babatopes; Olajumokes, Farumbis, Adedibus (all southerners) who publicly sponsored and campaigned for General Abacha, a northerner, to turn himself into a life president? Our brothers in the south are not fair enough to those of us in the north. Let us not forget so soon that if General Abacha encountered any serious opposition in his plans to remain in power, that opposition came from the north. We northerners formed a group of 18 elders and wrote to him and publicly advised him against self-succession. The group of 18 later led to G-34, which included some respected southern leaders.

Anietie: Collectively northerners (both soldiers and civilians) have ruled Nigerians for 34 of the 38 years of independence. Should power now shift to the south?

Ciroma: I have already answered that question. This issue is already settled in the minds of northerners as demonstrated in the June 12, 1993 election of Chief Abiola. These soldiers who plan coups and rob civilians of their legitimate and constitutional duties are not doing so because they are northerners; they are doing so because they have guns and are power-hungry. In the process they have created problems for the north itself... As far back as 1979, we politicians in the NPN [National Party of Nigeria], which was regarded as a northern-oriented party, were the first to come out with a formula of zoning and rotating power between the north and the south, because we realised that political inequality or any semblance of dominance of each other was a sure prescription for political instability, which could cost Nigeria its important place in the comity of nations. Now in the draft 1995 constitution, now before government, that idea — which was just a political formula — has been elevated to a constitutional issue and I have no objection whatsoever to it.

Anietie: Would you say that the north has used the opportunity of its 34 years, in power to better the lot of its people in terms of economic, educational, infrastructure and industrial advancement?

Ciroma: Unfortunately, the answer is no. Frankly, and I am sure most northern leaders will agree with me, the north benefited more when General Obasanjo [a southerner] was the head of state between 1976 and 1979, than any other administration in this country.

Anietie: At this juncture what in your opinion is the way forward for Nigeria? Do you subscribe to the suggestion that a big step forward would be the proper operation of a federal constitution, which Nigeria opted for at independence?

Ciroma: Definitely, definitely. I feel that it is vital to go back to operate a federal system. The founding fathers [of Nigeria] knew what they did when they founded this country on the basis of a federal constitution. It was intended to allow unity in diversity; to allow [our] various people to do things in

the way they know how. But because of the military's uni-
tary command [structure], we have now reached a ridiculous
situation where everything is literally in uniform all over
the country; where a local government on the shore of Lake
Chad or on the verge of the desert must act in the same way
as Brass local government on the shores of the Atlantic. The
uniformity is too excessive and in fact stifling. There is need
for us to return to a federal system. [Already], this week, the
Yorubas in their meeting have made certain demands. They
want a return to the federal system, the restructuring of the
federation, they want the commissioners of police to be people of their own states. They don't want internal colonialism; I have no quarrel with any of those [demands]. Even the
controversial ones, including their request for a sovereign
national conference to discuss the basis of our relationship,
should be discussed. We should be open with ourselves and
discuss these matters. Definitely, we must go back to a federal system.

"OBASANJO IS MISCHIEVOUS"

Duro Onabule, Chief Press Secretary to President Ibrahim Baban-gida, in an interview with Newswatch Dodan Barracks correspon-dent, Anietie Usen, December 1, 1987, reacted to General Oluse-gun Obasanjo's criticism of the President Babangida's policies. Below are excerpts:-

Anietie: What is President Babangida's reaction to the criticism of some of his policies by former Head of State, Gen. Olusegun Obasanjo?

Onabule: The president has been very disappointed about the behaviour of an otherwise respected officer like Obasanjo. He is quite disappointed.

Anietie: What is the view of Dodan Barracks on Obasanjo's call for the release of Buhari and Idiagbon?

Onabule: Obasanjo's record in office proves that if he were at the helm of affairs, he would have submitted Buhari and Id-iagbon to a harsher treatment. It is quite disappointing if as a retired general, Obasanjo does not know the difference between restriction and detention. The two former officers in question are being restricted and not detained. If they were detained, you (*Newswatch)* would not have reported that they were free to jog, play games, receive visitors and other liberties denied every other detained person. It is ordinary restriction. So, Obasanjo was only being mischievous. Quote me, he is mischievous.

Anietie: Isn't it possible that Obasanjo's statement concerning Buhari and Idiagbon will put serious pressure on the government to release them?

Onabule: Any decision at all to release them will not be as a result of Obasanjo's recent utterances. The minister of defence and chairman, Joint Chiefs of Staff, General Domkat Bali, is on record as saying that no charges will be brought against them. Bali has also said that both men will be released at the appropriate time. So, that's position of the government as at today.

Anietie: What about Obasanjo's statement on the political programme of the administration?

Onabule: Obasanjo was a party to Gowon's decision to extend the handover to civilians beyond 1976. He was. Yet, didn't he use the same excuse of Gowon not handing over in 1986 as one of the reasons to overthrow him?

Anietie: Now, how does Dodan Barracks view Obasanjo's statement on the economy, particularly SAP?

Onabule: I challenge Obasanjo to suggest an alternative to SAP. It is not enough to criticize. Admittedly, SAP is biting. But everybody in this country agreed all along that Nigeria's economic problems required a surgical operation. Tell me anywhere in the world where such operations are performed without some pains. Britain, for instance, has had its economic problems since 1964 when Harold Wilson became prime minister. What were the symptoms? Were they not huge deficits, high rate of unemployment, inflation, etc.? Only in the last couple of years has Britain gone out of the woods. Ours is only two years and people are expecting miracles. It is not possible. Nigerians tend to forget so soon the kind of economic problems this administration inherited.

Anietie: Do you mean that what Obasanjo said were uncalled for?

Onabule: Tell me a single aspect of Obasanjo's speech which is original. It's just a rehash of what other people have been saying. It's not original. He has just jumped into the bandwagon. Take his views on religion, for example. Is it different from what the president said in Kuru during the graduation ceremony at National Institute for Policy and Strategic Studies and in Abuja during the meeting with traditional rulers? Obasanjo is either ignorant of what the president said at those two places or he did not understand the speech or both.

Anietie: Some people are saying that Obasanjo may not have had access to the president to personally tell him his piece of mind.

Onabule: The man has a direct and unlimited access to the president but he never makes use of it.

Anietie: Are there chances that the government may apprehend Obasanjo if his statements are found to be inciting?

Onabule: Although his statements are quite distasteful, the best thing to do is to ignore him. As a former head of state, he is entitled to some respect. The reaction of the public is enough rebuke for him.

SPORTS

TEXTBOOK FOOTBALL COMES TO TOWN

They are all university students. They boast and lay exclusive claim to "textbook football based on research." At least, they have the prestigious Cross River State Challenge Cup trophy to show for it. That trophy is sitting prominently right now in the office of their vice chancellor back in University of Calabar, waiting for more trophies to come.

Top Division One Rovers FC of Calabar was beaten to their free-flowing game, when the all students' team defeated them in a thrilling Challenge Cup final and captured the imagination of football fans nationwide. At the end of the 90-minute duel Rovers' nine-year monopoly of the State championship was terminated with a 1-0 shocker.

Said Bassey Okon, 25, a Rovers FC fan,: "It was like Big League Soccer in England, when a students' team would defeat league champions Liverpool. It was unthinkable…" But boasted Wellington Johnson, Calabar university (UNICAL) Geography student and team manager of Acada United: "We are better than Rovers in all departments of soccer."

How did Acada United FC evolve?

The story is a short one. On December 23, 1984, at No. 121 Fosbery Road, Calabar, three young University of Calabar Students, Abang Ating, Udosen Inwang and Akpaka Inwang, were discussing arrangements for their Christmas party over some bottles of drinks. Suddenly, the discussion veered into football since the three friends were good footballers.

As the discussion heated up, the three felt unhappy that Rovers FC is the only team in the State participating in the national league. They thought there were no other avenues for younger talents to exploit. "Can't we raise a team ourselves? asked Abang Ating. "Sure we can raise a team that can beat Rovers," Udosen Inwang charged. "Jokingly, we decided to start something, even at the expense of our lectures," Ating narrated to *Newswatch.*

Throughout the Christmas holiday, the idea dominated the minds of the three friends. Back to school, they sold the idea to their senior colleague, Umoh Bassey. Bassey who had played "big-time football" with Flying Eagles, Rovers FC, etc, loved the idea. He talked to other footballers on the campus and the initial team came into existence as a backyard side at "Malabo" – Unical's new site.

The backyard side and their fans decided to sponsor Bassey for the students union post of Director of Sports. "We had neither money for facility, so we wanted to operate under the umbrella of the students union," Bassey explained. He won the elections and got the union to own up the Acada United embreyo.

Meanwhile some campus footballers who went to register for the Central Bank FC in Calabar were each offered a miserable purse of N300 a month. Furious, the boys returned to campus and teamed up with their colleagues at no fee. Then, the boys decided to register for the State Challenge Cup.

But time was running out and they needed more players. Bassey, now the teams' co-ordinator, rushed to nearby Calabar Polytechnic, hoping to recruit Aniefiok Ekarika (Uwem's brother) but Rovers had registered him. Bassey took the next fast-moving taxi to University of Cross River State (Unicross) Uyo, about 100km away, where he convinced dare-devil striker Tony Essien to join the club. Tony laid hands on some other good footballers at his campus.

It was the last day of registration for the State Challenge Cup. A bigger problem soon emerged. Money. The Students Union had only pledged kits and moral support. Determined, the Acada boys decided to contribute N10 each and about N200 were realized on the spot.

It was not enough. Desperate, Udosen Inwang, a UNICAL Geography student and one of the brains behind the team decided to let go N200 out of his pocket money. A good Samaritan photographer quickly snapped the required passport photographs at the cost of N160, as loan.

Time had almost run out when Bassey and some colleagues stepped into the office of the State FA to register Acada FC for the Challenge Cup.

When they started preparing for their first match, the boys had no coach. However, one of them, Celestine Nsekwe alias Tino, was chosen as a coach. "We decided to obey whatever instructions he gave because we needed a coach," one of the players said later. Nsekwe turned out to be a good coach and it is evident. So far, Acada United have not lost a match. They have played eight matches, wining all, scoring 18 goals and conceding only 2. "We don't know what it means to lose a match," Ating said, but before he could complete his statement, team manager Willington Johnson cut in "we are not playing football with our legs, brainwork matters. That's why we are a bit too much for some Nigerian clubsides," he said confidently.

The team list itself looks like a small national team: Celestine Nsekwe (Sociology) ex-Bendel academicals, Sylvanus Udobong (Medicine) ex-Cross River academicals; Ejike Ekwueme (History) ex-vice-captain of 1982 YSFON, which captured the world cup; Umoh Bassey (Management Studies) ex-Flying Eagles, ex-Rovers etc.; Tony Essien (Education) ex-Jetimo FC; Abang Ating (Geography) ex-Cross River academicals, Okon Akpabio (Education) ex-Rovers; Gerald Etuk (Physics) ex-Jetimo FC and Udosen Inwang (Geography) and others.

Said Paul Oluwa who works with the NEPA at Calabar "The boys are just too good. They made Rovers look like a village team. They sky is their limit."

But problems abound. A major one is the regular clash of academic time-table with scheduled football matches.

Acada United is complete with all the trappings of a school boys' team: nicknames, die-hard and loquacious fans, little or no kits, high team spirit and offcourse, "Acada girls."

Meanwhile Acada United are billed to play the Challenge cup preliminaries at Bauchi against such crack Division One team like Rangers FC of Enugu, Spartans FC of Owerri and Sharks FC of Port Harcourt.

Acada United may require more than textbooks to cross the first hurdle.

THE FAMOUS KNOCKOUT

There was a pervading wind of confidence bellowing through the indoor sports hall of the National Stadium as Billy Famous, 25, Commonwealth and African light welterweight champion took a seat at the ringside to watch two of the three supporting bouts, preceding his title defence fight with Langton "Schoolboy" Tinago of Zimbabwe. "This is the most important fight of my life and I am going to do it right and quick," Billy Famous said to *Newswatch*.

Two hours later, he discovered he needed every ounce of his 61.5kg and all his newly-acquired American ring craft to keep the sticky jabs of his lanky Zimbabwean challenger from bursting his head. The fight lasted 32.2 minute of the scheduled 36 minutes and the memory of its explosive tail end will linger.

In the weeks leading up to the fight, Famous fumed as many sports analysts gave him a narrow chance of beating his more exposed opponent, who had won many hearts during his previous ring appearances in Nigeria. Famous' pride was sorely stung and a deep burning anger wrote his battle plan.

The strategy was simple, one that would have been designed by Joe Frazier: "keep the sword swinging until there are no more heads to roll. There will be only one direction – forward." It was a gamble, for Famous would be exposing his young 25-year-old body to the cannon that had subdued 80 out of the 95 men that his 35-year-old challenger had faced.

As the challenger, Tinago came in first, lean and strikingly lanky at 62.1kg, wearing a purple robe with yellow trimmings. He jumped up and down to limber up his leg muscles, his two bandaged hands held preciously up to acknowledge cheers from the capacity crowd.

A large singing crowd accompanied by talking drums heralded the appearance of a dancing Famous, clad in a white shinning robe over trunks of the same colour. The crowd went wild with tumultuous ovation. Billy jumped into the square ring, fixed Tinago a scowl across the ring, shadow-boxing. A beautiful Zimbabwean lady stood up behind K.D. Dhiliwayo, Zimbabwean High commissioner to Nigeria, and spread a large Zimbabwean flag, beckoning on Tinago to see. Tinago got the message and sparked into flashy blasting of the thin air.

When the bell rang, war broke out instantly, with Famous firing the first shot which bounced off Tinago's guards. A good part of the first round was spent psyching and sizing each other. At the end of the round, only 20 blows were exchanged: 10 each way. None made impact.

"I think Billy will come all out to satisfy his anxious fans, so you'll just stick and move," Taylor, the challenger's manager said, wiping the trickling sweat on Tinago's face. "Then Billy will be tired after seven or eight. And we'll go for a late knockout," the manager added.

By the third and fourth rounds, Tinago's stinging jabs had started hitting targets with such precision and accuracy that visibly disturbed Famous' fans. Shouted Jimoh Aremu, the champion's manger: "Go for his head, go for his body, go, go, take him out..." Famous moved in and during the violent toe-to-toe exchanges that ensued, both fighters rocked themselves with thunderous blows that could have left lesser boxers flat on their backs. Midway in the sixth, Famous started developing a running nose, which seriously disturbed his concentration. A fierce roundhouse landed openly on Famous' left eye making him look very ordinary.

Worried, Famous stepped up his offensive in the seventh and eighth rounds, connecting telling punches to the ribs and body of Tinago. Twice, during the eighth round, the challenger was dazed by Famous' staccato rhythm of left-right-left-right hooks. Tinago's guards started dropping dangerously. An abrasion had developed under his left eye.

Returning to his corner, Tinago sat down for the first time, wearing a drained expression that signaled trouble. "What are you doing?" Taylor screamed, "You've got to stick and move. Jab! Don't fight him." In the champion's corner confidence has started building up. "Don't change" Aremu advised Famous. "Just keep your hands up a little higher. Keep charging and keep the pressure up."

"O.K., ok" said Famous. And he came out ready to bulldoze whatever was in his path. But Tinago had introduced spring into his feet. He was jabbing and moving. A powerful right flew like a missile over Tinago's ducking head and sent the champion off balance. Tinago closed in and rattled Famous with a quick succession of heavy shots to the head and jaw, but it was clear the jabs lacked the effectiveness of the earlier rounds.

It was also clear, Tinago was staging his last act of bravado. The champion knew that too. "How is the situation?" Famous asked his manager, and without waiting for a reply, he said, "Don't worry. Don't worry," spitting a mouthful of water and blood into a bucket, "I've taken his best shots, now I'm going to give him mine."

Two minutes, twenty seconds into the fateful eleventh round, Famous waded through the challenger's jabs, first firing a shot left and then a smashing right on Tinago's head. Dazed, the challenger staggered backwards and dropped on the canvass, siting and trying to get up. But his legs failed him.

As referee Howard Jones moved in to do the counting, Tinago managed to his feet, floundering across the ring. The pursing champion unloaded left and right barrages that thundered again on Tinago's head. On instinct, Tinago tried to clinch but Famous pushed him away, charging. "Throw in the towel. Throw in the towel," shouted fight promoter Peter Erutayo. Tinago's manager wasted no time in throwing in a yellow towel.

Said Taylor, Tinago's manager, "Billy is good, no doubt about it." Tinago agreed, saying: "Billy deserves it." The fight has improved Famous' reputation, who is billed to fight the WBC world champion, Billy Castello later in the year for the crown. At present, Famous is ranked 9th in the world.

NIMBLE SKILLS MADE IN HEAVEN

Every superlative that sports writers could contrive has already been deployed to describe him: golden boy, football genius, soccer wizard, phenomenal schemer, predatory finisher, king of goals. Yet words always seem to fail sport writers and fans bewitched by the immense talent and courage of Nwankwo Kanu, Nigeria's imperious 23-year-old striker, who last month joined the London football giants, Arsenal.

Joining the Gunners, as Arsenal is also known, after months of speculations was a dramatic new twist in the Kanu's tale, especially after an open-heart surgery had threatened to terminate his career. His miraculous comeback from hell, as it were, yet with skills made in heaven, represents, for many, the ultimate triumph of human spirit. For heart surgeons around the world, the thrill is a different kind of triumph: the triumph of medical science and technology.

The faulty valve in his heart was corrected and Kanu returned as Kanu: the same player to watch, "so lofty, so lanky, running with his head high, scenting opportunities and going for it with startling deftness; scoring, dribbling and could still fob off markers with his beguiling skills. He can with the ball between his feet shoot, without giving away any hint of which foot he would strike with." So says Christo David, a Lagos fan. "His deceptive on-field machination is used to disarm markers and serve as a decoy," he added.

Though it is in continental Europe and playing for the Super Eagle – the Nigerian national team – that Kanu has plied his trade and displayed his soccer artistry, playing for Arsenal in England, in the Premiership, will expose him to some of the most passionate football fans in the world. They will want to waste no time to unravel the Kanu puzzle. One so slender does not look like a typical predator. But that is precisely what he is at any position and angle on the field. Roy Hodgson, former coach of English premier league club Blackburn Rovers and formerly coach of Kanu's Italian club, Inter Milan, has warned defenders that: "Kanu is more dangerous with his back on the goal post." To borrow Roberto Baggio's apt metaphor, he plies his trade with a certain confidence of a rendezvous and a rare knack for doing the unimaginable. Says M Amadi, a Lagos lawyer and football fan: "His 360-degree vision on field, his camouflage tactics and split-second run-ins mark him out as a virtuoso of the game."

August 1996. With swaying hips and swinging dance steps, the Super Eagles of Nigeria do their lap of honour round the Georgia Bulldogs stadium in Atlanta. It is the action-packed final of the Olympic Games and Nigeria has just beaten Argentina 3-2. Around the world, most football analysts and fans feel that the Nigerian deserved this victory after beating the favourites, Brazil, a few days earlier in a sparkling semi-final. It was Kanu, said football experts, who kept Nigeria in that competition with "a peerless performance." A metre from the goal-line, with his back to the goal, he conjured with the ball and then managed to flick it past the bewildered Brazilian goalkeeper on the dot of 90 minutes. It was 3-3. Five minutes into extra time it was Kanu again. He collected a loose ball outside the 18-yard box and feigned a pull-out but kept the ball to himself. Waltzing sideways, he executed a body movement that sent his markers off the way and released a left footer that curved its way into the right corner of the Brazilian net.

But millions of football fans around the world were still savouring the dazzling performance and prospects of the football whiz kid when tragedy struck. A routine medical check-up in Italy, where Kanu had just signed a multi-million-dollar contract to play for Inter Milan, revealed a serious heart defect known as valvular insufficiency of the aorta. Cardiologists who diagnosed the ailment said the condition could lead to heart failure and he would never play serious football again. Said Bruno Caru, a heart specialist and consultant for Inter Milan: "It means an operation to remove the valve. It is serious enough to prevent him from playing. It is regrettable when it concerns an athlete of world standing, especially one that is very young, but the man is more important than the footballer."

Of about 350 Africans earning their living as professional footballers in the European League, Kanu, at just 20, was one of the best known and most promising. But how to save his life, not his career, became more urgent to his admirers around the world. "It is unfortunate to have to be so pitiless towards a player of world class," Piero Volpi, team doctor of Inter Milan announced. "But the cardiac specialists are categorical. We have to think of the man before we think of the player." Said Kanu in desperation:

"I knew nothing. Nobody told me. What am I going to do now?"

In Nigeria, the news was devastating. Virtually all churches declared weeks of fasting and prayers for a miraculous cure. "Don't let it happen, God,"*Newswatch,* a leading Nigerian news magazine, implored in a bold headline. "God has not finished with me ye," Kanu Said, in a display of courage.

Caused, according to specialist, by previous rheumatic illness, the damaged aorta valve allowed blood to seep back into his heart. Neither doctors nor insurers gave him any hope of performing to professional levels again. But by the time he was booked into the Cleveland Clinic in Ohio for open-heart surgery, Kanu was defiant, declaring that he would play again and that he intended to be available for the 1998 World Cup. As he was wheeled into the theatre for the surgery he gave a V for Victory sign to his friend Bello Osagie. "Mr. Bello," he called, "I will be back." For four and half hours, doctors tinkered with his heart, successfully repairing the weakened valve instead of, as had earlier been expected, replacing it with an artificial one.

Once out of intensive care and given the go-ahead to return to light training, he pushed his programme to the limit. "I have never seen somebody who went through that kind of rehabilitation in my life," Osagie says. "Five times a day, wake 6 o'clock in the morning, come back again, train in the evening. He was training five times a day throughout the rehabilitation until the very first day he played his makeshift match and scored three goals."

Osagie was there to watch that first match after surgery. "His first goal came in from a corner kick. He chested the ball down and as two defenders were coming on him, he sent the two of them in wrong directions with a stylish body movement, then hit a shot into the net." It was a game between a Spanish selected

side and the American UCLE team. His performance was celebrated in medical circles as a rare feat. Says Osagie: "I was very
happy."

The final test to ascertain his fitness was to take place in the
Cleveland Clinic. He had to undergo what experts call the "echo
test." It is a very stressful test on a troche mill. World-class marathon runners can only survive for 20-25 minutes on a troche
mill. Kanu worked the troche mill for 21 minutes. Doctors were
so excited with his recovery that Dr. Bruce Lytle, the head of the
Cleveland Clinic, told Kanu, "if you were my younger brother, I
would say, play in your club tomorrow." That was five months
after the surgery.

The clean bill of health sent Kanu and football fans in Nigeria into wild jubilation. Said Kanu: "With God, doctors have been
able to mend not just my football career but my ability to live
a normal life." In his first professional match after surgery, he
played for 22 minutes for Inter Milan, showing no trace of being
someone who had undergone surgery.

He play his first full 90 minute game for the world class club
side in February 1997 and scored his first goal since his recovery. "This shows that people should not give up hope even when
they are down," Kanu said after the match. "I never allowed some
negative comments made about me after the surgery to deter me
from proving that I am still the person I was before the surgery."
By January 1998, he was firmly back on the bench of Inter Milan.
Despite the frustration of having to wait for the likes of Ronaldo,
the Brazilian wonder reckoned to be the best footballer in the
world today, and Ivan Zamorano, who dominated Inter Milan's
forward line, he broke into the team in April and was in the squad
that won the 1998 UEFA cup in May. "I am lucky to have been

blessed with a natural distinctive talent. Whatever happens to me in life, that would not go away."

It was in Conakry, Guinea, that Kanu stepped onto the pitch for Nigeria for the first time since the surgery, during the 1998 World Cup qualifying series. While recuperating in hospital, he had been voted African Footballer of the Year by the Confederation of African Football (CAF) and ranked sixth in the world by FIFA. So his arrival and performance in Guinea became a befitting celebration of African ruggedness. He was mobbed like a pop star, borne along on people's shoulders and showered with gifts.

In the 1-0 defeat of Nigeria by Germany in Cologne weeks before the World Cup Finals in France, Kanu completed his first full match for Nigeria. For most football analysts, this was his true comeback. "Nigeria lost narrowly but Kanu came through stronger and stronger," Ian Hawkey of the *Sunday Times* of London said. "He showed many things he can do, an excellent disposition and discipline. I am so happy with the way he plays," said the Nigeria coach Bora Milutinovic.

In his young life, he has won the FIFA JVU Junior World Cup for Nigeria, a European Champions Club cup medal for Ajax of Amsterdam, a runners-up medal in the same competition and a World Clubs Champions medal also for Ajax; and a European Cup-winners' Cup medal for Inter-Milan; he has capped all this by winning for his country the Olympic Gold medal in soccer. All of these enviable accolades before his 23rd birthday, something that would normally take even the best of football players a career lifetime to achieve.

With his heart literally in the hands of God, Kanu has undoubtedly done enough to remain the focus of the football world for years to come. "The only thing that you can talk to me now that will interest me is not the surgery but the future," he told some Nigerian journalists. Clearly, the future for Kanu now lies with the London club Arsenal. The club's French manager, Arsene Wenger, said: "In terms of strikers, Kanu is probably the most important player we wanted. If I wanted to gamble I would go to the casino. But I've calculated the risk with Kanu and, for a player of his talent and potential; he is not a huge gamble in my evaluation. He has convinced all the doctors, including our own heart specialist, that there is no problem."

"I'm relieved that the move is finally over," said Kanu.

INDEX

Printed in Great Britain
by Amazon

82020871R10410